EPILEPSY AND OTHER NEUROLOGICAL DISORDERS IN COELIAC DISEASE

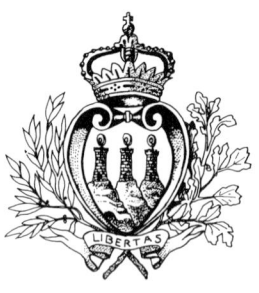

Republic of San Marino
Department of Health and Social Security

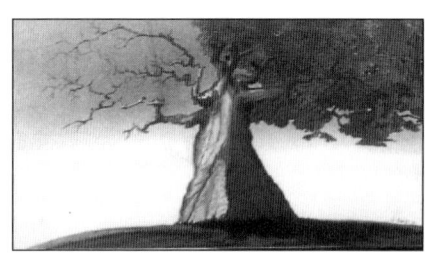

Fa.Ce.
Associazione Famiglie Cerebrolesi

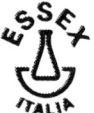 Essex Italia S.p.A.

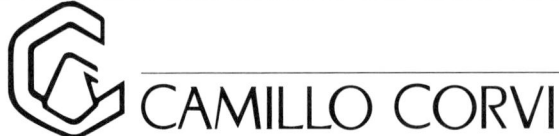 CAMILLO CORVI

Eurospital®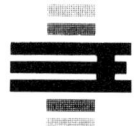

Acknowledgements

The editors wish to thank the Republic of San Marino Department of Health and Social Security, Fa. Ce. Associazione, Essex Italia S.p.A., Camillo Corvi S.p.A. and Eurospital S.p.A., for their generous financial support.

EPILEPSY AND OTHER NEUROLOGICAL DISORDERS IN COELIAC DISEASE

Edited by

Giuseppe Gobbi
Frederick Andermann
Salvatore Naccarato
and
Giacomo Banchini

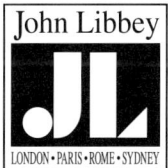

John Libbey
JL
LONDON · PARIS · ROME · SYDNEY

British Library Cataloguing in Publication Data

Epilepsy and other neurological disorders in coeliac disease
   1. Coeliac disease 2. Neurological manifestations of general diseases
   I. Gobbi, G.
   616.3'4

ISBN: 0 86196 537 X

Published by

John Libbey & Company Ltd, 13 Smiths Yard, Summerley Street, London, SW18 4HR, England
Telephone: 0181–947 2777 Fax: 0181–947 2664
John Libbey & Company Pty Ltd, Level 10, 15/17 Young Street, Sydney, NSW, 2000, Australia
John Libbey Eurotext Ltd, 127 Avenue de la République, 92120 Montrouge, France

Printed in Great Britain by WBC Bookbinders Ltd, Unit 5, Waterton Industrial Estate, Bridgend,
Mid Glamorgan, CF13 3YN, U.K.

C O N T E N T S

Foreword

Iwas enthusiastic when Giuseppe Gobbi asked for my opinion about the organization of a meeting in San Marino concerning the neurological features of coeliac disease, and about the publication of a book on this topic.

There are many correlations between the central and peripheral nervous system and the small bowel. It is sufficient to consider the relationship that links these two systems by means of neuro-endocrine mechanisms which allow them to control each other, and how such feedback can be greatly altered in both functional and organic pathology. Highly significant clinical relationships are thus created, some of which, however, are still not fully recognized.

While some of the stimulating signals produced by the nervous system and numerous mediators released locally can lead to significant alterations in both the quality and quantity of the secretory and peristaltic activities of the small intestine, there are also numerous amines and hormones that are released into the digestive system and which may cross the blood–brain barrier and affect the control mechanisms of the brain, either directly or though receptor alterations. Irregular secretions can lead to intestinal dysfunction. A more serious result may be found in neurological diseases, with alterations in the behaviour of the organism, caused by the secretions released by a severely diseased organ no longer capable of processing the numerous substances that should be absorbed, as occurs in the small intestine in coeliac disease.

The clinical features dependent on the malabsorption present in the 'classic' form of coeliac disease were known 60 years ago, when this disease was known as idiopathic sprue. Many studies have been carried out in the last 40 years on the psychological reactions to gluten-free diet, the relatively recent identification of the 'mono-symptomatic' and 'latent' forms of the disease. This has made it possible to recognize many other typical signs and symptoms which may represent the only clinical expression of coeliac disease.

On the neuro-psychiatric side, only a few research groups have provided interesting information to date: the English group, which described a correlation between schizophrenia and coeliac disease; the group which reported the association between coeliac disease and Down's syndrome and, more recently, the Italian group which described the association between coeliac disease, epilepsy and cerebral calcifications.

The complex physio-pathological mechanisms must now be clarified and the etiopathogenetic causes which can link the two systems must be investigated: are they immunological and/or vascular, genetic and/or receptorial diseases, or is direct biochemical damage involved?

Due to the high prevalence (1:200) of coeliac disease and since non-invasive means now exist for its diagnosis, including the 'silent', 'latent' and perhaps even 'potential' forms, epidemiological screening, especially if carried out in 'high risk groups', will provide new data on the actual number of associations between the small intestine and neuro-psychiatric diseases and will also make it possible to understand why these associations occur.

This volume brings together many of the results and opinions of the world's leading researchers in the fields of neurology, psychiatry, internal medicine, gastroenterology, immunology, genetics and imaging.

Giovanni Gasbarrini
Professor of Internal Medicine
Università Cattolica
Rome

Epilepsy and other neurological disorders in coeliac disease, edited by G. Gobbi *et al.*
© 1997 John Libbey & Company Ltd, pp. 1–4.

Introduction

Overview and historical background

J.A. Walker-Smith* and J.K. Visakorpi**

*University Department of Paediatric Gastroenterology, 3rd Floor, Royal Free Hospital NHS Trust, Pond St, London NW3 2QG, UK, and **University of Tampere, Tampere, Finland*

Coeliac disease is classically described as a gastrointestinal disorder which affects both children and adults. The first modern description of this disorder was made in 1888 by Dr Samuel Jones Gee at St Bartholomew's Hospital, London. He described chiefly a disorder of children presenting most often between the first and fifth birthday. Later the concept of adult coeliac disease arose and it came to be appreciated that it was a life-time disorder which could in fact present at any age of life although its clinical expression varied a good deal at different ages.

Dr W.K. Dicke in Leiden in 1950 recognized for the first time that this disorder responded to a gluten-free diet and the notion of gluten intolerance arose. It later came to be accepted that this state of gluten intolerance was permanent, although its clinical expression could vary with age.

In 1957 Margot Shiner performed the first small intestinal biopsy on a child with coeliac disease and demonstrated the typical flat mucosa (Sakula & Shiner, 1957). This abnormality was then shown to be reversible by a gluten-free diet (Anderson, 1960).

Diagnostic criteria

In 1979 the Interlaken or ESPGAN diagnostic criteria were proposed whereby the key diagnostic criterion was the presence of small intestinal mucosal damage, i.e. enteropathy which responded to gluten elimination. The mucosa healed on a gluten-free diet only to relapse again after gluten challenge albeit at variable time intervals, although usually less than 2 years (Meeuwisse, 1970).

Implicit in this complicated diagnostic approach including at least three intestinal biopsies was the conception that another syndrome of gluten intolerance existed which was transient or temporary. Thus the diagnostic category of transient gluten intolerance arose (Walker-Smith, 1987).

More recently ESPGAN revised the diagnostic criteria, basically no longer recommending such a complete procedure of gluten elimination and challenge in every case but only: (1) in those who presented under two years of age, the age group when transient gluten intolerance occurred; (2) in those children who wanted to depart from a gluten-free diet; (3) in those cases where there was no previous biopsy or the diagnosis was uncertain (Walker-Smith *et al.*, 1990). This move came largely from the collaborative Italian study (Guandalini *et al.*, 1989).

1

In recent times various antibody tests of high diagnostic specificity and sensitivity for coeliac disease have been developed. The best of these diagnostically are IgA anti-endomyseal antibody (EMA) and IgA anti-gliadin antibody (AGA). Whilst these are of great assistance diagnostically most authorities have continued to insist that small intestinal biopsy remains the gold standard for diagnosis of coeliac disease. The use of antibodies however has enabled cases of coeliac disease to be recognized that have not been readily diagnosed before, the so-called atypical forms of the disease.

Examples of such atypical presentations of coeliac disease include extraintestinal manifestations such as short stature, delayed puberty and iron or folic acid deficiency anaemia as well as non-specific and often rather mild gastrointestinal symptoms such as recurrent abdominal pain.

A recent multi-centre study (Greco et al., 1992) demonstrated that there is an overall increase in the age at diagnosis in children with coeliac disease in Europe. When the symptoms and signs at the time of presentation were studied by dividing children into two groups, those with typical symptoms and those with atypical, it was found that geographical areas with a high mean age at diagnosis reported high frequencies of atypical symptoms and vice versa. At one extreme of children diagnosed as atypical 'coeliac disease' are those without symptoms. This concept of 'coeliac disease' in a completely asymptomatic form arose first from studies investigating the relapse of patients treated first with a gluten-free diet and then provoked by gluten challenge, according to the ESPGAN diagnostic procedure. In the majority of cases, small intestinal mucosal relapse occurred without clinical manifestations. The second way asymptomatic patients were recognized was when first-degree relatives of known patients were biopsied and shown to have an abnormal mucosa. Today we can say that this asymptomatic state is not exceptional. Instead of the term asymptomatic, it has been suggested that the term 'silent' be used for these children (Visakorpi, 1992). These patients may have some minor symptoms but these are noted only after diagnosis has been made and treatment started. Then the patients may feel generally better after a gluten-free diet than they did before treatment.

The diagnosis of coeliac disease has become even more complex with the proposal that intolerance to gluten in patients may not be life-long and may be variable during life.

Therefore we now have to consider so-called latent (or potential) coeliac disease. The first observation was made two decades ago by Weinstein (1974). Many recent observations support this concept. Latency in coeliac disease means that the disease exists but is not currently manifest. This term should be applied only to patients who fulfill the following conditions: (1) a normal small intestinal mucosa on biopsy when on a normal diet and (2) at some other time, before or since, the biopsy finding of a flat small intestine mucosa which recovers on a gluten-free diet (Ferguson *et al.*, 1992).

Clinical associations

For some years it has been known that coeliac disease is often associated with other well known disorders. The best example perhaps is dermatitis herpetiformis (DH), where the rash as well as the coeliac-like small intestine mucosal damage respond to gluten elimination. Thus DH is a manifestation of coeliac disease which expresses itself outside the gastrointestinal tract and is not just an associated disease. Another manifestation is dental enamel hypoplasia (Aine, 1990).

The most clearly verified disease association of coeliac disease is juvenile diabetes mellitus (Maki *et al.*, 1984). Several screening studies show the prevalence of coeliac disease among diabetic children to be 2–6 per cent. Other associations have been found especially with autoimmune diseases such as thyroiditis, Addison's disease, vasculitis and chronic liver diseases.

In 1966, Cooke and Smith reported 'unexplained unconsciousness' in five adult coeliac patients. Then in 1978 Chapman and colleagues reported an increase of epilepsy in coeliac disease. Various psychic disturbances and even schizophrenia as well as chronic, progressive neurological disorders have been described in association with coeliac disease (Hallert & Derefeldt, 1982).

Sammaritano *et al.* proposed in 1988 a specific syndrome associating coeliac disease with intracranial calcifications and folic acid deficiency. In the same year Malten *et al.* (1988) also described the association of coeliac disease, epilepsy and intracranial calcification. Since then there have been many Italian studies concerning this issue. The Italian Working Group on Coeliac Disease and Epilepsy (Gobbi *et al.*, 1992) has been particularly active with a very large study: 77 per cent of patients with epilepsy and intracranial calcification on computer tomographic (CT) scanning had the characteristic small intestine lesion of coeliac disease.

Of particular importance for paediatrics is the observation by Bardella *et al.* (1994) that epilepsy may be preventable in children with coeliac disease who adhere strictly to a gluten-free diet. They found that not one of 81 patients who adhered to a strict gluten-free diet, compared to four of 47 patients on an unrestricted diet, had epilepsy and calcifications.

These observation suggest that epileptic patients should be screened by EMA testing and if positive should have a small intestine biopsy to diagnose coeliac disease.

What is now clear from these and other observations is the concept that coeliac disease may not only be associated with skin disorders, bone disorders and malignancy as well as the classical gastroenterological manifestations, but also with significant neurological disease.

Thus whilst the small intestine appears to be central for pathogenesis the concept arises that coeliac disease is a multi-system disorder. It must now be considered in the differential diagnosis of patients with neurological disease of unknown origin especially unexplained epilepsy. Certainly in adult life it would seem that coeliac disease may be far commoner (at least in Italy) than generally realized. This may be true for children too. Catassi *et al.* (1994) in their important study of 3351 school children (aged 11–15 years) found a high incidence of 3.87 for 1000 subjects (1 in 320). Clearly there is still much to be learned about the clinical importance of coeliac disease, in a wide variety of clinical situations.

References

Aine, L., Maki. M., Collin, P. & Keyrilainen, O. (1990): Dental enamel defects in celiac disease. *J. Oral Pathol. Med.* **19,** 241–245.

Anderson, C.M. (1960): Histological changes in the duodenal mucosa in coeliac disease. *Arch. Dis. Child.* **35,** 419–423.

Bardella, M.T., Molteni, N., Prampolini, L. *et al.* (1994): Need for follow-up in coeliac disease. *Arch. Dis. Child.* **70,** 211–213.

Catassi, C., Raetsch, I.M., Fabiani, M., Rossini, M., Bordicchia, F. & Candela, F. (1994): Coeliac disease in the year 2000: exploring the iceberg. *Lancet* **343,** 8891: 200–203.

Chapman, R.W.G., Laidlow, J.M., Colin-Jones, D., Eade, O.E. & Smith, C.L. (1978): Increased prevalence of epilepsy in coeliac disease. *BMJ* **ii,** 250–51.

Cook, W.T. & Smith, W.T. (1966): Neurological disorders associated with adult coeliac disease. *Brain* **89,** 683–722.

Dicke, W.K. (1950): Coeliakie: een onderzoek naar de nadelige invloed van sommige graansoort op de lijder aan coeliakie. MD Thesis, Utrecht.

Ferguson, A., Arranz, E. & O'Mahoney, S. (1992): Definitions and diagnostic criteria of latent and potential coeliac disease. In *Common food intolerances 1: Epidemiology of coeliac disease,* eds. S. Auricchio & J.K. Visakorpi, pp. 199–127. Basel: Karger.

Gee, S.J. (1888): On the coeliac affliction. St Bartholomew's Hospital Reports, 24, 17.

Gobbi, G., Bouquet, F., Greco, L. *et al.* (1992): Coeliac disease, epilepsy, and cerebral calcifications. *Lancet* **340,** 439–443.

Greco, L., Maki, M., DiDonato, F. & Visakorpi, J.K. (1992): Epidemiology of coeliac disease in Europe and the Mediterranean area. In *Common food intolerance 1: Epidemiology of coeliac disease,* eds. S. Auricchio & J.K. Visakorpi, pp 25–44. Basel: Karger.

Guandalini, S. Ventura, A., Ansaldi, N. *et al.* (1989): Diagnosis of coeliac disease: a time for change? *Arch. Dis. Child.* **64,** 1320–1324.

Hallert, C. & Derefeldt, T. (1982): Psychic disturbances in adult coeliac disease. 1. Clinical observations. *Scand. J. Gastroent.* **17,** 17–19.

Maki, M., Hallstrom, O., Huupponen, T. & Vesikari, T. (1984): Increased prevalence of coeliac disease in diabetes. *Arch. Dis. Child* **59,** 739–742.

Meeuwisse, G.W. (1970): Diagnostic criteria in coeliac disease. *Acta Paediatr. Scand.* **59,** 461.

Molteni, N., Bardella, M.T., Baldassarri, A.R. & Bianchi, P.A. (1988): Coeliac disease associated with epilepsy and intracranial calcifications: report of two patients. *Am. J. Gastroenterol.* **83,** 992–994.

Sakula, J. & Shiner, M. (1957): Coeliac disease with atrophy of the small intestinal mucosa. *Lancet* **ii,** 876.

Sammaritano, M., Andermann, F., Melanson, D., Guberman, A., Tinuper, P. & Gastaut, H. (1988): The syndrome of intractable epilepsy, bilateral occipital calcification and folic acid deficiency. *Neurology* **38** (supp. 1), 239.

Visakorpi, J.K., (1992): Silent coeliac disease: the risk groups to be screened. In *Common food intolerance 1: Epidemiology of coeliac disease,* eds. S. Auricchio & J.K. Visakorpi, pp. 84–92. Basel: Karger.

Walker-Smith, J.A. (1987): Transient gluten intolerance: does it exist? *Netherlands J. Med.* **93,** 1356–1362.

Walker-Smith, J.A., Guandalini, S., Schmitz, J., Shmerling, D.H. & Visakorpi, J.K. (1990): Revised criteria for diagnosis of coeliac disease. *Arch. Dis. Child.* **77,** 891–894.

Weinstein, W.M. (1974): Latent celiac sprue. *Gastroenterology* **66,** 489–493.

Part I
Gluten intolerance

Epilepsy and other neurological disorders in coeliac disease, edited by G. Gobbi *et al.*
© 1997 John Libbey & Company Ltd, pp. 7–11.

Chapter 1

Clinical and biological characteristics of gluten intolerance

Gino Roberto Corazza, Federico Biagi, Maria Laura Andreani and
Giovanni Gasbarrini

*Dipartimento di Medicina Interna dell'Università, dell'Aquila, Patologia Medica dell'Università di Bologna,
Clinica Medica dell'Università, Cattolica di Roma, Italy*

Coeliac disease (CD) can be defined as a chronic disease in which there is a characteristic mucosal lesion of the small intestine, which impairs nutrient absorption by the bowel and which improves on withdrawal of gluten from the diet (Trier, 1991). In this context gluten collectively refers to prolamins of wheat, rye, barley and oats.

In recent years evidence has accumulated in favour of an increasingly broad spectrum of gluten-sensitive conditions and Fig. 1 shows the range of all the possible forms of gluten intolerance. As well as the frank form, defined as active by some authors, the potential form and the latent form, which, respectively, may develop or do in fact develop into a frank form, there is also evidence of extraintestinal and gastrointestinal gluten intolerance other than CD. The existence of naturally occurring CD in animals currently represents a clinical-pathological curiosity, but from a biological standpoint it can constitute a useful model in understanding the mechanisms of gluten toxicity.

Frank CD

Frank CD is the form normally encountered. From a pathological point of view, it is characterized by villous atrophy, hypertrophy of the crypts and abundant infiltration of the small bowel mucosa by inflammatory cells. Clinically speaking, it is represented by an extremely varied range of clinical signs (Corazza & Gasbarrini, 1995). Within the limits of frank CD, the distinction between the classic variety, characterized by the presence of malabsorption symptoms (diarrhoea, steatorrhoea, weight loss), the subclinical form, characterized by minor, transitory and extraintestinal symptoms, and the silent variety, characterized by a complete absence of symptoms and recognizable only through the screening of an at-risk population, thus undoubtedly represents an oversimplification. This is, however, useful on clinical grounds. It was first realized in adults and then in children that patients with the subclinical or silent forms constitute the majority (Corazza *et al.*, 1993; Logan *et al.*, 1983). The biological reasons for this clinical variability are not immediately obvious, although

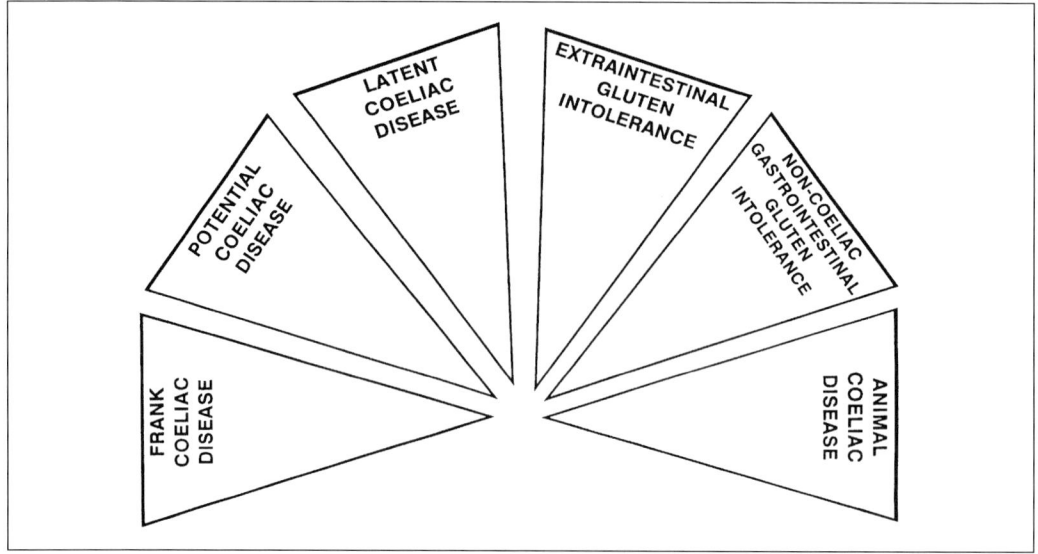

Fig. 1. The spectrum of possible forms of gluten intolerance.

earlier reports suggested that this may be due to a greater or lesser extent of the lesions along the small intestine (MacDonald *et al.*, 1964).

From a clinical point of view, the diagnosis of patients with subclinical or silent forms has been greatly aided in recent years by the availability of non-invasive serological tests (Corrao *et al.*, 1994), such as antigliadin, antireticulin, antiendomysial and antijejunal antibodies. These tests have made it possible to diagnose patients who were otherwise unsuspected in a series of at-risk populations, such as first-degree relatives (Corazza *et al.*, 1992), patients with insulin-dependent diabetes (Mäki *et al.*, 1984), Down's syndrome (Zubillaga *et al.*, 1993), epilepsy with cerebral calcification (Gobbi *et al.*, 1992), iron-deficiency anaemia (Corazza *et al.*, 1995a), alopecia areata (Corazza *et al.*, 1995b), autoimmune thyroiditis and Sjögren's syndrome (Collin *et al.*, 1994) and even in the general population (Catassi *et al.*, 1994). The importance of screening for silent or subclinical CD in patients with conditions which, like those mentioned above, are frequently associated with this disease is two-fold. It is in fact clear that the only clinical signs of silent CD may be those of the second disease and, on the other hand, the treatment of CD may favour a remission of the associated disease (Corazza & Gasbarrini, 1995).

Latent and potential CD

The term latent CD was coined by Weinstein (1974) to indicate patients with dermatitis herpetiformis and normal jejunal biopsies in whom flat lesions developed after their normal diets were supplemented by extra doses of gluten. Currently, in agreement with Ferguson *et al.* (1993), the definition of latent CD should be applied only to patients who had a normal jejunal biopsy while following a normal diet and who subsequently developed a flat jejunal biopsy which recovers on a gluten-free diet. In agreement with this definition, the diagnosis of latent CD is retrospective, occasional and sporadic. To date, only a few cases have been described, mostly in coeliac relatives (Mäki *et al.*, 1990) or in patients with normal mucosa but positive antigliadin and/or antiendomysial antibodies (Collin *et al.*, 1993). We have observed three adult cases and, among the various serological markers, only the antijejunal antibodies were constantly positive (Fig. 2) when the intestinal mucosa was still normal (Corazza *et al.*, 1996).

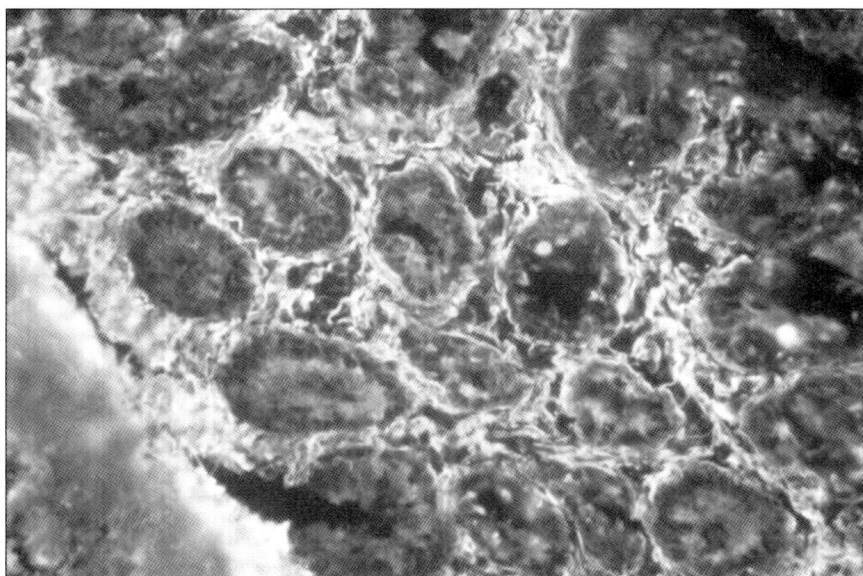

Fig. 2. Antijejunal antibody positive pattern in a patient with coeliac disease.

From a biological standpoint, latent CD could be very useful in understanding the pathogenetic mechanisms of CD when reliable indicators are available for predicting the transition from normal mucosa to flat mucosa. The increase in the γ/Δ intraepithelial lymphocytes (Mäki *et al.*, 1991) and the increased secretion of IgM and IgA in the intestinal juice (Arranz & Ferguson, 1993), proposed as markers of latent CD, are not specific to this condition. With regard to the factors that can, in susceptible individuals, predispose to a transition towards a frank form, many authors indicate an absolute or relative excess of gluten in the diet. Doherty & Barry (1981) showed that the administration of an extra dose of 40 g of gluten per day for 6 weeks induces villous atrophy in healthy relatives of coeliac patients. This demonstrates the possibility of triggering a latent form of CD, transforming it into a frank form through the administration of high doses of gluten.

Unlike the latent form, the diagnosis of potential CD is prospective and identifies those patients with normal mucosa that might develop a frank form of CD (Ferguson *et al.*, 1993). This includes healthy individuals, such as first-degree relatives of coeliac patients, subjects with 'false' positive antibodies, increased γ/Δ lymphocytes, increased IgA and IgM in the intestinal juice, all considered to be conditions which indicate an increased risk for CD. From a clinical standpoint, these individuals should be carefully monitored in order to detect promptly their potential transition towards a frank form of CD.

Extraintestinal gluten intolerance

The close association between CD and dermatitis herpetiformis is well known (Fry, 1995). Nevertheless, even in those cases in which dermatitis herpetiformis is not accompanied by a frank enteropathy, the cutaneous lesions are controlled by a gluten-free diet (Reunala *et al.*, 1977). Even in the absence of a frank form of CD, significant clinical improvement after gluten withdrawal from the diet has also been described in recurrent aphthous stomatitis (O'Farrelly *et al.*, 1991) and in IgA nephropathy (Coppo *et al.*, 1986).

In biological terms, this confirms that the spectrum of sensitivity to gluten is truly wide: it always originates in the intestine, but the consequent pathological lesions may appear elsewhere.

Non-coeliac gastrointestinal gluten intolerance

There is evidence, mostly in the form of anecdotes, of the existence of gluten intolerance in syndromes and diseases of the gastroenteric tract other than coeliac disease. As far as functional disorders are concerned, nine patients were described with symptoms that were completely identical to those of irritable bowel syndrome and negative biopsy for CD. Pain, abdominal distension, diarrhoea and general malaise improved after gluten-free diet and worsened again after a single dose of 30 g of gluten, administered in a double blind study (Cooper *et al.*, 1980). It is known that there can be physiological malabsorption of the starch contained in bread and pasta (Anderson *et al.*, 1981). It is possible that in some healthy individuals this physiological defect becomes more pronounced and induces this syndrome.

A positive response to gluten-free diet has been reported in HIV intestinal diseases (Quiñones-Galvan & Lifshitz-Guinzberg, 1990), in Crohn's disease (Rudman *et al.*, 1971), in tropical sprue (Bayless & Swanson, 1964) and in chronic dyspepsia (Pock-Steen, 1973). The results of these studies should be confirmed with stricter methods, and with the aim of identifying the mechanisms that regulate the sensitivity to gluten in these conditions.

Animal CD

It appears that the spectrum of intolerance to gluten is so broad that it even includes several animal species. In the Irish setter dog a naturally occurring rather than experimentally induced intestinal disease is present, which is manifested first by increased intestinal permeability (Hall & Batt, 1991), whereas there is no evidence of an alteration in the immunological response to gluten (Hall *et al.*, 1992). These results confirm the possible occurrence in nature of mechanisms other than immunological ones in determining gluten intolerance.

Conclusions

Coeliac disease is a heterogeneous condition, probably mediated by various mechanisms. There is still much to be clarified regarding the relationships between the various clinical forms of frank CD and between the latter and latent/potential CD. It is possible that a study of the minor forms of gluten intolerance (extraintestinal, gastrointestinal and animal) may contribute to a better understanding of these relationships.

Acknowledgement

Supported in part by a grant from the 'Associazione Ricerca in Medicina'.

References

Anderson, I.H., Levine, A.S. & Levitt, M.D. (1981): Incomplete absorption of the carbohydrate in all-purpose wheat flour. *N. Engl. J. Med.* **304**, 891–892.

Arranz, E. & Ferguson, A. (1993): Intestinal antibody pattern of celiac disease: occurence in patients with normal jejunal biopsy histology. *Gastroenterology* **104**, 1263–1272.

Bayless, T.M. & Swanson, V.L. (1964): Comparison of tropical sprue and adult celiac disease (nontropical sprue). *Gastroenterology* **46**, 731.

Catassi, C., Rätsch, I.M., Fabiani, E. *et al.* (1994): Coeliac disease in the year 2000: exploring the iceberg. *Lancet* **343**, 200–203.

Collin, P., Helin, H., Mäki, M. *et al.* (1993): Follow-up of patients positive in reticulin and gliadin antibody tests with normal small-bowel biopsy findings. *Scand. J. Gastroenterol* **28**, 595–598.

Collin, P., Reunala, T., Pukkala, E. *et al.* (1994): Coeliac disease-associated disorders and survival. *Gut* **35**, 1215–1218.

Cooper, B.T., Holmes, G.K.T., Ferguson, R. *et al.* (1980): Gluten- sensitive diarrhea without evidence of celiac disease. *Gastroenterology* **79**, 801–806.

Coppo, R., Basolo, B., Rollino, C. *et al.* (1986): Dietary gluten and primary IgA nephropathy. *N. Engl. J. Med.* **315,** 1167–1168.

Corazza, G.R., Valentini, R.A., Frisoni, M. *et al.* (1992): Gliadin immune reactivity is associated with overt and latent enteropathy in relatives of celiac patients. *Gastroenterology* **103,** 1517–1522.

Corazza, G.R., Frisoni, M., Treggiari, E.A. *et al.* (1993): Subclinical celiac sprue: increasing occurence and clues to its diagnosis. *J. Clin. Gastroenterol.* **16,** 16–21.

Corazza, G.R. & Gasbarrini, G. (1995): Coeliac disease in adults. *Baillières Clin. Gastroenterol.* **9,** 329–350.

Corazza, G.R., Valentini, R.A., Andreani, M.L. *et al.* (1995a): Subclinical coeliac disease is a frequent cause of iron-deficiency anaemia. *Scand. J. Gastroenterol.* **30,** 153–156.

Corazza, G.R., Andreani, M.L., Venturo, N. et al. (1995b): Celiac disease and alopecia areata: report of a new association. *Gastroenterology* **109,** 1333-1337.

Corrao, G., Corazza, G.R., Andreani, M.L. *et al.* (1994): Serological screening of coeliac disease: choosing the optimal procedure according to various prevalence levels. *Gut* **35,** 771–775.

Doherty, M. & Barry, R.E. (1981): Gluten-induced mucosal changes in subjects without overt small-bowel disease. *Lancet i,* 517–520.

Ferguson, A. Arranz, E. & O'Mahony, S. (1993): Clinical and pathological spectrum of coeliac disease-active, silent, latent, potential. *Gut* **34,** 150–151.

Fry, L. (1995): Dermatitis herpetiformis. *Baillières Clin. Gastroenterol.* **9,** 371–393.

Gobbi, G., Bouquet, F., Greco, L. *et al.* (1992): Coeliac disease, epilepsy, and cerebral calcifications. *Lancet* **340,** 439–443.

Hall, E.J. & Batt, R.M. (1991): Abnormal permeability precedes the development of a gluten-sensitive enteropathy in the Irish setter dog. *Gut* **32,** 749–753.

Hall, E.J., Carter, S.D., Barnes, A. & Batt, R.M. (1992): Immune responses to dietary antigens in gluten-sensitive enteropathy of Irish setters. *Res. Vet. Sci.* **53,** 293–299.

Logan, R.F.A., Tucker, G., Rifkind, E.A. *et al.* (1983): Changes in clinical features of coeliac disease in adults in Edinburgh and the Lothians 1960-79. *BMJ* **286,** 95–97.

MacDonald, W.C., Brandborg, L.L., Flick, A.L. *et al.* (1964): Studies of celiac sprue. IV. The response of the whole lenght of the small bowel to a gluten-free diet. *Gastroenterology* **47,** 573–589.

Mäki, M., Hällström, O., Huupponen, T., Vesikari, T. & Visakorpi, J.K. (1984): Increased prevalence of coeliac disease in diabetes. *Arch. Dis. Child* **59,** 739–742.

Mäki, M., Holm, K., Koskimies, S. *et al.* (1990): Normal small bowel biopsy followed by coeliac disease. *Arch. Dis. Chlld.* **65,** 1137–1141.

Mäki, M., Holm, K., Collin, P. & Savilathi, E. (1991): Increased in gamma/delta T cell receptor bearing lymphocytes in normal small bowel mucosa in latent coeliac disease. *Gut* **32,** 1412–1414.

O'Farrelly, C., O'Mahony, C., Graeme-Cook, F. *et al.* (1991): Gliadin antibodies identify gluten-sensitive oral ulceration in the absence of villous atrophy. *J. Oral. Pathol. Med.* **20,** 476–478.

Pock-Steen, O.C.H. (1973): The role of gluten, milk, and other dietary proteins in chronic or intermittent dyspepsia. *Clin. Allergy* **3,** 373–383.

Quiñones-Galvan, A. & Lifshitz-Guinzberg, A. (1990): Gluten-free diet for AIDS-associated enteropathy. *Ann. Intern. Med.* **113,** 806–807.

Reunala, T., Blomqvist, K., Tarpila, S., Halme, H. & Kangas, K. (1977): Gluten-free diet in dermatitis herpetiformis. I. Clinical response of skin lesions in 81 patients. *Br. J. Dermatol.* **97,** 473–480.

Rudman, D., Galambos, J.T., Wenger, J. & Achord, J. (1971): Adverse effects of dietary gluten in four patients with regional enteritis. *Am. J. Clin. Nutr.* **24,** 1068–1073.

Trier, J.S. (1991): Celiac sprue. *N. Engl. J. Med.* **325,** 1709–1719.

Weinstein, W.M. (1974): Latent celiac sprue. *Gastroenterology* **66,** 489–493.

Zubillaga, P., Vitoria, J.C., Arrieta, A. *et al.* (1993): Down's syndrome and coeliac disease. *J. Pediatr. Gastroenterol. Nutr.* **16,** 168–171.

Chapter 2

Non-gastrointestinal manifestations of coeliac disease

Pekka Collin and Markku Mäki

Departments of Medicine and Paediatrics, Tampere University Hospital; Medical School and Institute of Medical Technology, University of Tampere, Tampere, Finland

Introduction

Dicke (1953) was the first to show that ingesting wheat is harmful to patients with coeliac disease (CD). Today it is well known that in susceptible individuals, dietary cereals will result in small intestinal mucosal atrophy together with crypt hyperplasia. Dietary gluten or gliadin peptides are the toxic fragments in cereals.

In recent years the clinical picture of CD has changed dramatically. The disease can be clinically silent and even totally asymptomatic, the patient still having the gluten-sensitive jejunal flat lesion. Moreover, CD develops gradually from normal mucosa to villous atrophy typical for CD (Ferguson *et al.*, 1993). Some individuals having a normal villous architecture, and eating normal amounts of gluten, can later develop a mucosal lesion compatible with CD. It is today possible to detect patients who presumably have such a latent form of CD. They do have intestinal markers of latent CD such as an increased density of intraepithelial lymphocytes, and especially T-lymphocytes bearing the gamma delta receptors (Mäki *et al.*, 1991b).

The susceptibility to CD is strongly genetically determined. CD is associated with chromosome 6 HLA B8 and DR3 haplotype. An even stronger association has been shown with the HLA DQ2 α, β heterodimer, encoded by the DQA1*0501 and DQB1*0201 alleles (Sollid *et al.*, 1989).

Immunological factors are most likely involved in the pathogenetic mechanisms seen in CD. In genetically susceptible individuals, dietary gluten or gliadin causes inflammation, activated T-cell response and increased DR expression in the gut mucosa. The precise mechanisms are not known so far.

Provided that CD is an autoimmune disease triggered by gliadin, one could expect some manifestations even outside the gastrointestinal tract. It is well known that CD patients have an increased risk to develop several associated conditions, especially autoimmune diseases. Circulating immune complexes originating from the atrophic mucosa may deposit in and damage other organs as well (Scott & Losowsky, 1975). Subjects with HLA DR3 haplotype have an increased risk of autoim-

13

mune diseases in general, which may explain the concomitant occurrence of these diseases with CD. On the other hand, the prevalence of CD is higher than previously anticipated. Therefore, many associations may be fortuitous.

For a true extraintestinal manifestation of CD, certain requirements should be fulfilled. The association with CD should be well documented. A favourable response to the gluten-free diet of the non-gastrointestinal manifestation strongly supports the assumption of a gluten-derived disease. Such manifestations could be treated with gluten-free diet even in patients having normal mucosa, but being genetically susceptible to CD and having intestinal markers of latent CD. However, the direct complications of malabsorption, such as osteomalacia, should not be considered as true extraintestinal manifestations of CD.

What we have learned from dermatitis herpetiformis

Dermatitis herpetiformis (DH), a blistering skin disease, is the classical non-gastrointestinal manifestation of CD. Granular IgA deposits in the dermoepithelial junction are pathognomonic of the disease. Ninety per cent of patients with DH have at least minor villous damage similar to that in CD (Reunala et al., 1984). The disease can, however, evolve without small bowel villous damage, or clinical malabsorption. DH and CD share a common HLA association, and they both can occur in one family (Reunala & Mäki, 1993). It has been shown that DH patients with normal small bowel mucosa do have a latent form of CD (Weinstein, 1974). An agressive gluten load in these patients results in villous atrophy (Ferguson et al., 1987). DH patients also have minor alterations in their jejunal mucosa such as markers of CD latency (Savilahti et al., 1992). The skin lesions in DH respond to strict gluten-free diet (Reunala et al., 1984). It is obvious that ingested gliadin is harmful to the skin, regardless of the mucosal morphology.

Other possible extraintestinal manifestations of CD

Dental enamel defects

With careful examination, typical enamel defects can be found in the permanent teeth of most CD patients (Aine et al., 1990), and these defects are gluten-induced (Aine, 1986) (Fig. 1). The enamel damage is also found in patients without malabsorption or jejunal atrophy (Aine et al., 1991). These defects have been shown even in the relatives of CD patients having a genetic predisposition to coeliac disease, but normal jejunal mucosa (Mäki et al., 1991a). Recently, Mariani et al. (1994) showed that coeliac-type enamel defects are associated in CD patients with HLA DR3, but not with DR5,7. The pathogenetic mechanisms of these lesions are not known, but may be due to immunological factors.

Neurological complications: epilepsy and brain atrophy

The neurologic complications are described elsewhere in this book. However, epilepsy with cerebral calcifications (Gobbi et al., 1992), and brain atrophy (Collin et al., 1991) have been described to occur concomitantly with CD. Both diseases are connected with HLA DR3. We have identified one patient with insulin-dependent diabetes mellitus, whose small bowel was initially normal, but who later developed brain atrophy and small bowel villous atrophy compatible with CD (see page 281).

IgA glomerulonephritis

The association between IgA glomerulonephritis and CD has been shown mostly in case reports (DeCoteau et al., 1973; Helin et al., 1983). Pasternack et al. (1990) have shown that 32 per cent of patients with newly diagnosed CD have renal findings compatible with IgA glomerulonephritis but they do not have manifest nephropathy. In animal models, experimental IgA glomerulonephritis has

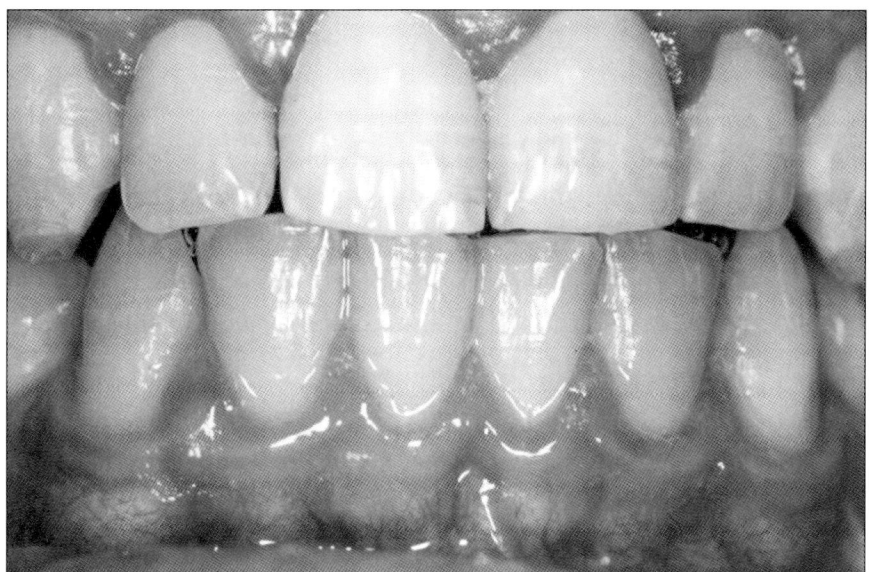

Fig. 1. Gluten-induced permanent-tooth enamel defects in a patient with clinically silent coeliac disease. Typical mild grade II horizontal grooves are seen on examination.

been induced by oral immunization with gliadin (Emancipator *et al.*, 1987) or gluten (Coppo *et al.*, 1989). There is a case report of IgA nephropathy and severe nephrotic syndrome. The patient was found to have CD, and the nephrotic syndrome resolved subsequently on a gluten-free diet (Woodrow *et al.*, 1993). On the other hand, IgA nephropathy does not seem to be associated with the HLA DR3 haplotype (Moore, 1991). Moreover, we could not find any coeliac-type changes in the small bowel mucosa of 20 consecutive patients with IgA nephropathy (Rantala *et al.*, 1994).

Liver diseases

The liver may be affected by CD. Hagander *et al.* (1977) showed that 29 (39 per cent) of 74 coeliac patients had raised serum aspartate-aminotransferase levels. Twelve of them had liver injury, including four cases of chronic active hepatitis. In the study of Jacobsen *et al.* (1990), 62 (47 per cent) of 171 adult patients with CD had some elevated liver enzyme values. In both studies, the enzyme levels decreased after introduction of the gluten-free diet. It has not been studied whether such enzyme abnormalities occur in the silent and latent forms of CD as well.

Connective tissue disorders

According to earlier studies, connective tissue disorders are frequently found in patients with CD. In some, but not in all cases the arthritis improved on a gluten-free diet (Parke *et al.*, 1984; Bourne *et al.*, 1985). We have reported 26 patients with CD detected due to their joint manifestations (Mäki *et al.*, 1988; Collin *et al.*, 1992). This observation has been confirmed in later studies (Unsworth & Brown, 1994). It now seems that arthritis and arthralgia, but not rheumatoid arthritis, are mono-symptomatic forms of CD. As many as 10 per cent of patients with Sjögren's syndrome can have concomitant silent CD (Collin *et al.*, 1992). Both diseases are associated with the HLA DR3 haplotype, commonly observed in autoimmune diseases.

Malignant diseases

Gough *et al.* (1962) were the first to propose that the mucosal lesion in CD can be a premalignant condition. This observation has later been verified both in CD (Holmes *et al.*, 1976) and DH (Leonard *et al.*, 1983). The malignancies occur mainly in the gastrointestinal tract. The development of malignancy in CD can be prevented by a gluten-free diet (Holmes *et al.*, 1989). Interestingly, Freeman and Chiu (1986) have described a patient who developed a malignant lymphoma despite normal jejunal mucosal morphology, but who afterwards showed mucosal deterioration upon gluten challenge. In other words, the maligancy developed at the latent stage of CD.

Other putative extraintestinal manifestations – possibly coincidental

Women with coeliac disease may suffer from relative infertility. This can be due to a shortened reproductive period, as the patients have menarche later and menopause earlier than control subjects (Ferguson *et al.*, 1982; Molteni *et al.*, 1990). The risk for spontaneuous abortions is also increased according to some small study series. It is unclear whether the infertility is caused by malabsorption or malnutrition. Reversible infertility in male coeliac patients has been described as well (Baker & Read, 1975).

Some patients with CD have developed lung cavities (Stevens *et al.*, 1990). Their aetiology remains unknown so far.

There are three previous reports on pericarditis and CD. Dawes and Atherton (1981) described two patients, Faizallah *et al.* (1982) three, and Laine and Holt (1984) one patient with recurrent pericarditis and CD. In all these reports, a gluten-free diet appeared to prevent further attacks of pericarditis. We have seen a 56-year-old previously healthy woman with an abundant pericardial effusion. She had positive reticulin and gliadin antibodies and subsequently was found to have small bowel villous atrophy. The mucosal response to a gluten-free diet was good. In contrast to previously published cases, the pericarditis recurred once during a 10-year follow-up; the pericardial effusion was not as abundant as during the first attack. The pathogenesis of pericarditis in patients with CD remains obscure, but immune complex formations cannot be excluded. CD should be excluded in patients with pericarditis of unknown aetiology.

Table 1. Diseases described in association with coeliac disease (Collin & Mäki, 1994)

Several reports	Some reports
Insulin-dependent diabetes mellitus	Sjögren's syndrome
Selective IgA deficiency	Autoimmune thyroid diseases
Lymphoma	Addison's disease
Small intestine cancer	Pharyngeal and esophageal cancer
Epilepsy with cerebral calcifications	Pancreatic insufficiency
	Dementia
	Asthma and atopy

With permission from *Scand. J. Gastroenterol.* 1994; **29**: 769–775.

Related disorders

Several conditions have been described in association with CD but most of them are probably coincidental. There is however increasing evidence that many endocrinological diseases and auto-immune disorders are occurring with CD more than by chance (Collin & Mäki, 1994). Some of the associated diseases are listed in Table 1. Many of these diseases share the HLA DR3 haplotype. It remains unknown, whether the genetic background alone can explain this association.

References

Aine, L. (1986): Dental enamel defects and dental maturity in children and adolescents with coeliac disease. *Proceedings of the Finnish Dental Society* **82 (suppl 3),** 1–77.

Aine, L., Mäki, M., Collin, P. & Keyriläinen, O. (1990): Dental enamel defects in celiac disease. *J. Oral. Pathol. Med.* **19,** 241–245.

Aine, L., Reunala, T. & Mäki, M. (1991): Dental enamel defects in children with dermatitis herpetiformis. *J. Pediatr.* **337,** 763–764.

Baker, P.G. & Read, A.E. (1975): Reversible infertility in male coeliac patients. *BMJ* **2,** 316–317.

Bourne, J.T., Kumar, P., Huskisson, E.C., Mageed, R., Unsworth, D.J. & Wojtulewski, J.A. (1985): Arthritis and coeliac disease. *Ann. Rheum. Dis.* **44,** 592–598.

Collin, P., Pirttilä, T., Nurmikko, T., Somer, H., Erilä, T. & Keyriläinen, O. (1991): Celiac disease, brain atrophy and dementia. *Neurology* **41,** 372–375.

Collin, P., Korpela, M., Hällström, O., Viander, M., Keyriläinen, O. & Mäki, M. (1992): Rheumatic complaints as a presenting symptom in patients with coeliac disease. *Scand. J. Rheumatol.* **21,** 20–23.

Collin, P. & Mäki, M. (1994): Coeliac disease and associated disorders. Clinical aspects. *Scand. J. Gastroenterol.* **29,** 769–775.

Coppo, R., Mazzucco, G., Martina, G. Roccatello, D., Amore, A., Novara, A., Bargoni, A.,Piccoli, G. & Sena, L.M. (1989): Gluten-induced experimental IgA glomerulopathy. *Lab. Invest.* **60,** 499–506.

Dawes, P.T. & Atherton, S.T. (1981): Coeliac disease presenting as recurrent pericarditis. *Lancet* **i,** 1021–1022.

DeCoteau, W.E., Gerrard, J.W. & Cunningham, T.A. (1973): Glomerulitis in dermatitis herpetiformis. *Lancet* **2** 679–680.

Dicke, W.K. (1950): Coeliakie. Doctoral Thesis, University of Utrecht.

Emancipator, S.N., Ovary, Z. & Lamm, M.E. (1987): The role of mesangial complement in the hematuria of experimental IgA nephropathy. *Lab. Invest.* **57,** 269–276.

Faizallah, R., Costello, F.C., Lee, F.I. & Walker, R. (1982): Adult celiac disease and recurrent pericarditis. *Dig. Dis. Sci.* **27,** 728–730.

Ferguson, A., Blackwell, J.N. & Barnetson, R.St.C. (1987): Effects of additional dietary gluten on the small-intestinal mucosa of volunteers and of patients with dermatitis herpetiformis. *Scand. J. Gastroenterol.* **22,** 543–549.

Ferguson, A., Arranz, E. & O'Mahony, S. (1993): Clinical and pathological spectrum of coeliac disase – active, silent, latent, potential. *Gut* **34,** 150–151.

Ferguson, R., Holmes, G.K.T. & Cooke, W.T. (1982): Coeliac disease, fertility and pregnancy. *Scand. J. Gastroenterol.* **17,** 65–68.

Freeman, H.J. & Chiu, B.K. (1986): Multifocal small bowel lymphoma and latent celiac sprue. *Gastroenterology* **90,** 1992–1997.

Gobbi, G., Bouquet, F., Greco, L., Lambertini, A., Tassinari C.A., Ventura, A. & Zaniboni M.G. (1992): Coeliac disease, epilepsy, and cerebral calcifications. *Lancet* **340,** 439–443.

Gough, K.R., Read, A.E. & Naish, J.M. (1962): Intestinal reticulosis as a complication of idiopathic steatorrhoea. *Gut* **3,** 232–239.

Hagander, B., Berg, N.O., Brandt, L., Norden, Å., Sjölund, K. & Stenstam, M. (1977): Hepatic injury in adult coeliac disease. *Lancet 1,* 270–272.

Helin, H., Mustonen, J., Reunala, T. & Pasternack, A. (1983): IgA nephropathy associated with celiac disease and dermatitis herpetiformis. *Arch. Pathol. Lab. Med.* **107,** 324–327.

Holmes, G.K.T., Stokes, P.L., Sorahan, T.M., Prior P., Waterhouse, J.A.H. & Cooke W.T. (1976): Coeliac disease, gluten-free diet and malignancy. *Gut* **17,** 612–619.

Holmes, G.K.T., Prior, P., Lane, M.R., Pope, D. & Allan, R.N. (1989): Malignancy in coeliac disease – effect of a gluten free diet. *Gut* **30,** 333–338.

Jacobsen, M.B., Fausa, O., Elgjo, K. & Schrumpf, E. (1990): Hepatic lesions in adult coeliac disease. *Scand. J. Gastroenterol.* **25,** 656–662.

Laine, L.A. & Holt, K.M. (1984): Recurrent pericarditis and celiac disease. *JAMA* **252,** 3168.

Leonard, J.N., Tucker, W.F.G., Fry, J.S. *et al.* (1983): Increased incidence of malignancy in dermatitis herpetiformis. *BMJ* **286,** 16–18.

Mäki, M., Hällström, O., Verronen, P., Reunala, T., Lähdeaho, M-L., Holm, K. & Visakorpi, J.K. (1988): Reticulin antibody, arthritis, and coeliac disease in children. *Lancet* **i,** 479–480.

Mäki, M., Aine, L., Lipsanen, V. & Koskimies, S. (1991a): Dental enamel defects in first-degree relatives of coeliac disease patients. *Lancet* **337,** 763–764.

Mäki, M., Holm, K., Collin, P. & Savilahti, E. (1991b): Increase in gamma delta T cell receptor bearing lymphocytes in normal small bowel mucosa in latent coeliac disease. *Gut* **21,** 1412–1414.

Mariani, P., Mazzilli, M.C., Margutti, G., Lionetti, P., Triglione, P., Petronzelli, F., Ferrante, E. & Bonamico, M. (1994): Coeliac disease, enamel defects and HLA typing. *Acta Paediatr.* **83,** 1272–1275.

Molteni, N., Bardella, M.T. & Bianchi, P.A. (1990): Obstetric and gynecological problems in women with untreated celiac sprue. *J. Clin. Gastroenterol.* **12,** 37–39.

Moore, R. (1991): Immunogenetics of IgA nephropathy. *J. Nephrol.* **1,** 1–6.

Parke, A.L., Fagan, E.A., Chadwick, V.S. & Hughes, G.R.V. (1984): Coeliac disease and rheumatoid arthritis. *Ann. Rheum. Dis.* **43,** 378–80.

Pasternack, A., Collin, P., Mustonen, J., Reunala, T., Rantala, I., Laurila K. & Teppo, A-M. (1990): Glomerular IgA deposits in patients with celiac disease. *Clin. Nephrol.* **34,** 56–60.

Rantala, I., Holm, K., Mustonen, J., Collin, P., Kainulainen H. & Mäki, M. (1994): Immunohistochemical quantitation of jejunal T cells, HLA-DR antigen, and human groEL stress protein homologue in IgA nephropathy. IgA Nephropathy International Symposium, Adelaide, Australia.

Reunala, T., Kosnai, I., Karpati, S., Kuitunen, P., Török, E. & Savilahti, E. (1984): Dermatitis herpetiformis: jejunal findings and skin response to gluten-free diet. *Arch. Dis. Child* **59,** 517–522.

Reunala, T. & Mäki, M. (1993): Dermatitis herpetiformis: A genetic disease. *Eur. J. Dermatol.* **3,** 519–526.

Savilahti, E., Reunala, T. & Mäki, M. (1992): Increase of lymphocytes bearing the gamma/delta T cell receptor in the jejunum of patients with dermatitis herpetiformis. *Gut* **33,** 206–211.

Scott, B.B. & Losowsky, M.S. (1975): Coeliac disease: a cause of various associated diseases. *Lancet* **ii,** 956–957.

Sollid, L.M., Markussen, G., Ek, J., Gjerde, H., Vartdal, F. & Thorsby, E. (1989): Evidence for a primary association of celiac disease to a particular HLA-DQ alfa/beta heterodimer. *J. Exp. Med.* **169,** 345–350.

Stevens, F.M., Connolly, C.E., Murray, J.P. & McCarthy, C.F. (1990): Lung cavities in patients with coeliac disease. *Digestion* **46,** 72–80.

Unsworth, D.J. & Brown, D.L. (1994): Serological screening suggests that adult coeliac disease is underdiagnosed in the UK and increases the incidence up to 12 per cent. *Gut* **35,** 61–64.

Weinstein, W.M. (1974): Latent coeliac sprue. *Gastroenterology* **66,** 489–493.

Woodrow, G., Innes, A., Boyd, M. & Burden, R.P. (1993): A case of IgA nephropathy with coeliac disease responding to a gluten-free diet. *Nephrol. Dial. Transplant* **8,** 1382–1383.

Epilepsy and other neurological disorders in coeliac disease, edited by G. Gobbi *et al.*
© 1997 John Libbey & Company Ltd, pp. 19–25.

Chapter 3

From the neolithic revolution to gluten intolerance: benefits and problems associated with the cultivation of wheat

Luigi Greco

Department of Pediatrics, University of Naples, Italy

Extent of gluten intolerance

We have recently reported (Gobbi *et al.*, 1992) a consistent cohort of patients affected by drug-resistant epilepsy with cerebral calcifications, half of whom were improved by a gluten-free diet. All had an atrophic jejunal mucosa, which reverted on this diet. Gluten intolerance is now a recognized cause of brain calcifications and epilepsy, of dementia, of psychiatric disturbances: many researchers believe that in genetically predisposed subjects gluten is not healthy for brain function.

Even after 25 years of extensive experience with gluten intolerance it is hard to imagine that the single most common food intolerance to the single most common staple food in our environment might provoke such a variety of adverse immuno-mediated reactions in any part of the human body. The list is endless, but malignancies, adverse pregnancy outcome and impaired brain function are indeed complications which exceed the tolerable threshold of this food intolerance. On the other hand, today we know that the majority (as many as 9 : 1) of gluten-intolerant subjects, identified by familial or population screening, do not have any complaints, although they do have a flat intestinal mucosa (Catassi *et al.*, 1994).

In conclusion a sizeable proportion of our population (from 0.3 to 1 per cent) is gluten-intolerant and displays a wide spectrum ranging from the asymptomatic to severe life-threatening diseases.

This intolerance is strongly linked to specific genetic markers which have required thousands of years to develop while changes in the environment and in the food we eat require centuries or less.

Hunters, fishers and gatherers

Human beings have been on Earth for over 3 million years, but *Homo Sapiens Sapiens*, our nearest ancestor, is only 100,000 years old. For 90,000 years he conducted a nomadic life getting food by hunting, fishing and collecting fruits, seeds, herbs and vegetables.

Only quite recently (about 10,000 years ago) did some wandering tribes start settlements because they developed the ability to gather enough food to be stored. The cultivation of wild seeds had begun.

Around 10,000 years ago the last glacial period came to an end: a neo-thermal period ensued which marked the passage from the paleolithic to the neolithic age. Ice melted gradually from the equator to the poles over several thousands of years: when new fertile and humid lands were uncovered in South East Asia all of Europe was still covered with ice and northern countries had to wait up to 4000 years more to emerge from a frozen environment.

The great revolution: the first farmers

The discovery in the neolithic age of ways to produce and store food has been the greatest revolution mankind ever experienced. Passage from collection to production led to a system in which human labour produces income for long periods of time. The principle of property was consolidated and fortifications to protect the land and food stores were developed.

Archaeological findings suggest that this revolution was not initiated by man the hunter and warrior, but by the intelligent observations made by woman. The woman carried the daily burden of collecting seeds, herbs, roots and tubers. Most probably she used a stick to dig up roots and tubers and during her work she observed the falling of grain seeds to the ground and their penetration into the soil aided by the rain. She may have been surprised to find new plants growing, and made the final connection between the fallen seeds and new 'cultivated' plants. She was, for thousands of years, the leader in farming practices and provided a more and more important complement to the scanty provender obtained by man the hunter (Heichelheim, 1970).

To the best of our knowledge, the origin of farming practices began in the 'Fertile Crescent': the wide belt of South East Asia which includes Southern Turkey, Palestine, Lebanon and North Iraq. In the highlands abundant rainfall was caused by the neo-thermal switch. In all of this area there existed a wide variety of wild cereals, sometimes in natural extended fields, induced by the rainfall. *Triticum Dicoccoides* (wheat) and *Hordeum Spontaneum* (barley) were common and routinely collected by the inhabitants. The wild cereals had very few seeds (Gobbi, 1995; Catassi *et al.*, 1994; Furon, 1958) and these fell easily to the ground on maturation.

The people from the Uadi el-Natuf Tell of South East Asia (7800 B.C.) provided the first traces of the gradual shift from hunters to grain cultivators. Their economy was based on hunting the gazelle, but their diet also included collected grain seeds. These gradually came to form a substantial proportion of their energy input, as cultivation practices developed. There were no grinding stones or mills and it was most probable that gathering yielded more than cultivation. But during the Proto-Neolithic superior a cuneiform mortar appeared. One thousand to two thousand years later (5000 B.C.) wild animals, more rare due to incoming drought, formed only 5 per cent of the daily diet, while cereals and farmed animals became a sizeable part of it (Furon, 1958).

Stable settlements were founded: the village of Catal-Huyuk in Southern Turkey had a population of 5000 inhabitants in 9000 years B.C. In that area a collection of sickles was found with inserted obsidian blades, smoothed by the routine contact with the siliceous stalk of cereals. The sickles indicate that it was possible to collect seeds not only from the ground, but also by cutting stems of plants which were capable of retaining the seed in an ear (Cambel & Braidwood, 1970).

'Mesopotamic' farming populations, developed a great civilization with large cities and powerful armies to defend their land property and food stores.

In Egypt a civilization based on farming practices developed in the fifth millennium: they became specialists in the cultivation of wheat, barley (to produce beer) and flax.

The expansion of the farmers

While in South East Asia progressive drought made hunting difficult and encouraged farming, in Europe the paleolithic culture of hunters and gatherers persisted for 5000 more years, gradually evolving into the mesolithic age.

In the 'Fertile Crescent' the availability of food stores and the gradual development of animal farming stimulated an unprecedented demographic explosion. The nuclear family was small for hundreds of thousands of years: the birth rate had been limited by nomadic life. In transmigrations the mother had been able to carry one infant, while the others had been obliged to walk on their own. Small babies in between had less chance of surviving. Thus the population remained stable for long periods.

Farmers, on the other hand, were settlers who possessed food stores and took advantage of more hands in the family to help with the farmwork. In this manner family size exploded and, as a result, a progressive continuous need to gain more land ensued.

The farmers' expansion lasted from 9000 B.C. up to 4000 B.C. when they reached Ireland, Denmark and Sweden, settling most cultivable lands in Europe. The expansions followed the waterways of Mediterranean and Danube basins throughout the time of the Egyptians, Phoenicians, Greeks and Romans (Cavalli-Sforza, 1993).

The farmers' expansion was not limited to the diffusion of agricultural practices, but was a 'demic' expansion: that substantially replaced the local dwellers, the mesolithic populations of Europe, by the neolithic people from South East Asia. More than two-thirds of our actual genetic inheritance originated from this new population, while the native genetic background has been progressively lost or confined to isolated geographic areas.

The genetic replacement of the native European population is marked by the B8 specificity of the HLA system. Cavalli-Sforza and coworkers showed that the migration of farmers is parallelled by the diffusion of B8. The frequency of B8 is inversely proportional to the time length of wheat cultivation. In practice B8 appears to be less frequent in populations that have lived on wheat for a longer time, as it is caused by a negative genetic selection in wheat cultivators (Cavalli-Sforza, 1993). We are aware that in Ireland, where wheat cultivation came only 3000 years B.C., a very high frequency of gluten intolerance has been reported.

The revolution of cereals

The early wild cereals, of the *Triticum* (wheat) and *Hordeum* (barley) species were genetically diploid and carried few seeds, which usually fell on the ground at maturation, making harvest very difficult. Chromosomes in single couples (diploidicity) allowed for wide genetic and phenotypic heterogeneity with remarkable variations in the content of protein and starches. Polyploid plants occasionally originated in nature, but they had few chances to survive without artificial (cultivation) practices and were usually lost (Raven *et al.*, 1986).

The beginning of farming, with the use of irrigation, allowed the survival and the expansion of polyploid grains. But these new polyploid grains had substantially reduced genetic variations (since each gene is represented in several copies) and more frequently self-pollinate, causing remarkable increase in genetic uniformity. The first stable formation of polyploid grains is dated around 6000 years B.C.: the genetic uniformity caused a considerable rise in stability and yield, convincing the early farmer to induce a progressive and rapid replacement of the wild species.

Genetic variability of grains was essential in order to adapt the plant to the very different environmental conditions of different areas, but the yield was generally low (Feldmand & Sears, 1981). *Triticum turgide dicoccoides* was crossed with *Triticum fanschii* to originate the *Triticum aestivum*, which is the progenitor of all our present-day wheat. The *aestivum* is an esaploid wheat with 42 chromosomes, versus the 14 of the *T. monococcum*. Such powerful grain replaced all existing varieties to the point where genetic variability is nowadays lost: all over the world we now have 20,000 cultivated species of the same unique *T. aestivum* wheat.

Triticum turgidum dicoccoides, progenitor of the present-day 'durum' wheat with which pasta is made, had just a few seeds encapsulated into a pointed and twilled kernel: at maturation the seeds fell to the ground where penetration was eased by the arrow-shaped structure of the kernel. Ten thousand years ago it was difficult to pick them up: hence the attempt, made by the neolithic people, to select varieties which could retain the seed longer, in order to allow for harvest.

Genetic variability was already substantially reduced in Roman times: 'farrum' (*T. dicoccoides*) and 'Siligo' (*T. vulgaris*) were the common grains. Siligo was used for making bread and contained a certain amount of gluten, while farrum, used mainly for soups, was poorer in gluten content (Giunio, 1977).

Cultivation of wheat and barley was not started or developed in the whole world: only a small geographic area (South East Asia) developed gluten-containing cereals. In Asia rice was the culti-vated species, while in America maize prevailed and in Africa sorghum and millet. All these plants were present in nature and were gradually cultivated in their places of origin (Cavalli-Sforza, 1993). In Europe grains had for centuries been selected in order to improve their homogeneity and productivity, but soon another desirable quality was preferred: the ability to stick, so important in bread making. Early bread making activities tended towards grains that contained greater amounts of a structural protein which greatly facilitated bread making: the gluten.

Gluten was not chosen because of its nutritional characteristics, since it is a protein with relatively low nutritional value, but rather for its commercial qualities. Rice, maize, sorghum and millet do not contain gluten: no leavened bread was prepared with them so the majority of mankind never lived on bread, as we know it.

Over the last 200 years of active genetic selection, and actual genetic manipulation, have changed the aspect of the original Triticale enormously: from few grains and little gluten to great wheat harvests enriched in gluten (50 per cent of the protein content), well adapted to cultivation practices and ready to be handled by enormous threshing machines.

The rise of gluten intolerance

Did everybody adapt to such profound changes in basic nutrition over such a short period of time? South Eastern populations, presumably well adapted to the new foods, largely replaced the existing mesolithic European dwellers who still lived by hunting and gathering. But a proportion of the local populations (or, rather, of their successors) persisted beside the invaders. The changes in eating habits were not well tolerated by everybody.

Lactose intolerance provides an example: populations that have more recently adapted to milk consumption, still lack the genetic ability to digest lactose during infancy. Environment has changed many centuries before any changes in inheritance have been possible. Similarly a considerable proportion of the hunters and gatherers of the pre-neolithic ages have not fully adapted to the great changes induced by the cultivation of wheat.

These people could not recognize gluten as a 'tolerable' protein available for digestion and absorp-tion: they may not have had any problem or complaint for centuries, since the content of gluten in grains was very low, but when 'industrial' quantities of gluten were induced by selection of wheat in order to improve bread making, they were exposed to intolerable quantities of protein or peptide.

This population, genetically identifiable today by their specific HLA pattern, did not recognize, through their HLA system, the gluten peptide as a tolerable item, but because of the similarity of some sequences of gliadin peptides with several pathogenic viruses, they generate a complex defence mechanism (an immuno-response) which does not eventually identify the specific pathogen to destroy, and most probably activates an auto-immune response which ultimately is the origin of the damage to their intestine and other organs.

These descendants of hunters and fishermen, exposed to this subtle challenge, could not develop tolerance and, in the attempt to fight the unknown, they ultimately develop a disease due to excess defence. For centuries they underwent a negative selection pressure, with less chance to survive (Simoons, 1982).

In the last millennium gluten-intolerant children mostly had a difficult start in life: after weaning, malabsorption and malnutrition were the underlying causes of poor defence to infections during infancy and early childhood. Acute infectious diarrhoea was the main killer of infants up to 50 years ago in Europe and up to 15 babies in every thousand died from this condition. In the suburbs of Naples, only 25 years ago, infectious diarrhoea was the main killer (25 per cent of an infant mortality rate of 100 per thousand live births) (Greco, 1976). The vast majority of cases of gluten intolerance occurred among these poor infants.

Why then, with such a poor prognosis for children surviving to adulthood, has gluten intolerance not become extinct, as was in fact the case with several other pathogenic conditions? The intolerant individuals most probably had some selective advantage which counterbalanced the gluten intolerance: it is possible to suggest that it was their very effective HLA Class II system that gave them a selective advantage against infections, which compensated for the disadvantage due to gluten intolerance.

When, in the last 50 years, infantile infections greatly diminished, the descendents of the hunters and gatherers with very active immune defensces, 'over reacted' more frequently to the gluten than to their ordinary illnesses. Hence the rise of the cohort that now appears to manifest, in different ways, gluten intolerance.

However, not all populations of the world were ever exposed to such a nasty protein: the vast majority of mankind, after the development of agriculture, lived on maize, rice, sorghum, millet and tubers: all gluten free. None of them underwent the selective pressure of gluten intolerance and they may in fact have been the reservoir of wild genes.

Finally, breast feeding most probably played a major role in preserving some children from the fatal infections of infancy (Greco *et al.*, 1985). The capacity of breast milk to protect against viral and bacterial attack, the protection given by maternal antibodies and the delaying effect on the manifestation of symptoms of gluten intolerance (in predisposed subjects) may all have protected the hunters and gatherers, who in this manner avoided the development of fatal symptoms and managed to survive and transmit their genes to our population.

Hints on the epidemiology of gluten intolerance

Since the cohort of those suffering from coeliac disease born before World War II had few chances to survive infancy, we nowadays have few adult cases and few long-term complications. Where the intolerance is still manifested mainly in the classical way (infants and small children, malabsorption, diarrhoea, often switched on by an infection) we do not frequent encounter 'atypical' presentations and adult cases or long-term complications. The epidemiological calculations made by gastroenterologists on observed cases may be in great contrast with those made by paediatricians. On the other hand the rarity of 'classical' cases, which has been used as proof of the 'disappearance' of gluten intolerance, is counterbalanced by the presence of atypical and late diagnosis, where active investigations are carried out.

Finally, nutritional attitudes have played a major role with regard to the chances for hunters to manifest gluten intolerance in different age groups: the example of Sweden as compared to Denmark or Finland is a case in point (Maki *et al.*, 1992). As shown by Maki *et al.*, the ability to identify atypical cases may completely change the observed epidemiological pattern in a given region. Hence the reason for the 'iceberg': most cases are still to be discovered (Maki *et al.*, 1988).

Similarly, population-based screening program uncover more 'silent' than overt cases (Catassi *et al.,* 1994).

Nevertheless, the 'cohort effect', regional differences and so on, have up to now failed to overcome the limits of numbers. When local incidence rates are compared with other regions' rates, the 95 per cent confidence intervals of these rates are very often so wide as to contain all the observed rates. No clearcut statistical difference has clearly been shown in the incidence of gluten intolerance in Europe (Greco *et al.,* 1992).

Wherever extensive studies on symptomatic cases have been carried out an incidence of one case per 1000 live births has been reached, but very often the incidence has been much lower: up to one case per 250 live births. Population screening studies invariably conclude to an incidence rate of one every 250. This is very close to the rate predicted by age-adjusted incidence density studies (Magazzu *et al.,* 1994).

Gluten 'sensitive' *vs.* gluten intolerant

The epidemiology of gluten intolerance, which entails tracing a group of our ancestors, may completely change once we consider the increasing knowledge of 'gluten-sensitive' individuals. Six to 10 per cent of first degree relatives of known cases are themselves gluten intolerant and have a flat intestinal mucosa (these are silent cases), but up to 30 per cent of siblings of cases, when challenged with a dose of gluten, activate a specific mucosal immuno-response (with increase in intraepithelial infiltration and activation of T-cells), without having any sign of mucosal damage (Troncone *et al.,* 1995).

We may, in the near future, identify a substantial group of individuals who do not activate, in the presence of gluten, a 'pathogenic' immuno-response (auto-immunity), but who recognize gluten as a 'suspect' protein in the same way as their apparantly tolerant peers.

Finally gluten intolerance is indeed linked to a specific genetic predisposition: most probably at least three genetic loci are involved in the risk of intolerance.

Certainly more than 5 per cent of the current population carry some specific genetic risk.

In conclusion we have a wide population of 'gluten-reactors' in the European Community:

- at least 1 million cases of total intolerance to gluten

- an estimated similar amount of 'gluten sensitive' people

- 10–15 times more 'carriers' of the risk of becoming gluten intolerant.

Thus we have found our ancestral hunters and gatherers: they constitute a substantial proportion of our actual community and do deserve a 'gluten-free' alternative not only as therapy, but as an option in daily life.

References

Cambel, H. & Braidwood, R.J. (1970): An old farmer's village in Turkey. *Le Scienze* **22,** 96–103.

Catassi, C., Ratsch, I.M., Fabiani, E., Rossini, M., Bordicchia, F., Candela, F., Coppa, G.V. & Giorgi, P.L. (1994): Coeliac Disease in the year 2000: exploring the iceberg. *Lancet* **343,** 200–203.

Cavalli-Sforza, L. (1993): (Who we are). Mondadori, Milano.

Feldman, M. & Sears, E.R. (1981): The wild gene resources of wheat. *Scientific American* 98–109.

Furon, R. (1958): Manuel de Prehistoire Generale. Payot, Paris.

Giulio Lucio Moderato Columella (1977): 'Libri rei rusticae' Anni 60–65 dopo Cristo. Ed. Einaudi.

Gobbi, G., Bouquet, F., Greco, L., Lambertini, A., Tassinari, C.A., Ventura, A. & Zaniboni, M.G. (1992): Coeliac disease, epilepsy and cerebral calcifications. *Lancet* **340,** 8817, 439–443.

Greco, L. (1976): Malnutrizione di classe a Napoli *Inchiesta* **24,** 53–63.

Greco, L., Maki, M., Di Donato, F. & Visakorpi, J.K. (1992): Epidemiology of Coeliac Disease in Europe and the Mediterranean area. A summary report on the Multicentric study by the European Society of Paediatric Gastroenterology and Nutrition. In: *Common food intolerances 1: epidemiology of coeliac disease,* eds. S. Auricchio & J.K. Visakorpi, pp. 14–24, Basel: Karger.

Greco, L., Mayer, M., Grimaldi, M., Follo, D., De Ritis, G. & Auricchio, S. (1985): The effect of early feeding on the onset of sympthoms in coeliac disease *J. Pediat. Gastroenterol. Nutr.* **4,** 52–55.

Heichelheim, F. (1970): An ancient economic history, ed A.W. Sijthoff, Leiden.

Magazzù Bottaro, G., Cataldo, F., Iacono, G., Di Donato, F., Patane, R., Cavataio, F., Maltese, I., Romano, C., Arco, A., Totolo, N., Bragion, E., Traverso, G. & Greco, L. (1994): Increasing Incidence of childhood celiac disease in Sicily: results of a multicentric study. *Acta Paediatr.* **83,** 1065–1069.

Maki, M., Holm, K., Ascher, H. & Greco, L. (1992): Factors affecting clinical presentation of coeliac disease: role of type and amount of gluten containing cereals in the diet. In: *Common food intolerances 1: epidemiology of coeliac disease*, eds. S, Auricchio & J.K. Visakorpi, pp. 76–83. Basel: Karger.

Maki, M., Kallonen, K., Landeaho, M.L. & Visakorpi, J.K. (1988): Changing pattern of childhood coeliac disease in Finland. *Acta Paediatr. Scand.* 77, 408–412.

Raven, P.H., Evert, R.F. & Eichorn, S. (1986): *Biology of plants*, 4th ed. New York: Worth Publ. Inc.

Simoons, F.J. (1982): Coeliac disease as a geographic problem. *Food, nutrition and evolution*, pp. 179–199.

Troncone, R., Greco, L., Mayer, M., Mazzarella, G., Maiuri, L., Congia, M., Frau, F., De Virgiliis, S. & Auricchio, S. (1996): Rectal gluten challenge reveals gluten sensitization not restricted to coeliac HLA in siblings of children with coeliac disease: *Gastroenterology,* **111,** 318-324.

Epilepsy and other neurological disorders in coeliac disease, edited by G. Gobbi *et al.*
© 1997 John Libbey & Company Ltd, pp. 27–30.

Chapter 4

Is coeliac disease rare in South India?

D. Nagaraja, P.N. Jaya Kumar[*] and M.H. Suprabha

*Department of Neurology and [*]Neuroradiology, National Institute of Mental Health and Neurosciences
(NIMHANS), Bangalore, 560 029, India*

C oeliac disease (CD), mainly a disorder of children, is relatively rare in India. There are no documented cases of CD from South India which extends from 8° to 18° latitude. However, since wheat and wheat products are not the staple diet of this population, it is not clear whether the disease does not exist or does not manifest. Reports of adult coeliac disease and atypical forms with variable clinical expression suggest that one should look for atypical forms of the disease in areas where the disease is considered rare (Logan *et al.* 1983). Association of CD and neurological diseases, especially epilepsy is well known (Chapman *et al.* 1978, Laidlow *et al.* 1977). Association of epilepsy, cerebral calcification and CD has been well documented (Della Cella *et al.* 1991, Gobbi *et al.* 1988, Sammaritano *et al.* 1988). Gobbi *et al.* (1992) suggested to screen all epilepsy patients with unexplained cerebral calcification for CD. The prevalence of unexplained cerebral calcification and epilepsy in this part of the country has not been reported. Here, we are attempting to look for the prevalence of cerebral calcification, to look for the clinical profile of such patients and to identify any possible CD in them.

Table 1. Profile of calcifications

Total no. of CT with calcifications	103
Single	64
Double	13
3 and above	26
Calcified cysticercus	61
Tumour/granuloma	8
Combination of above	5
Dystrophie calcifications	8
Others	11
(unexplained cortical	4
SWD - 6)	6

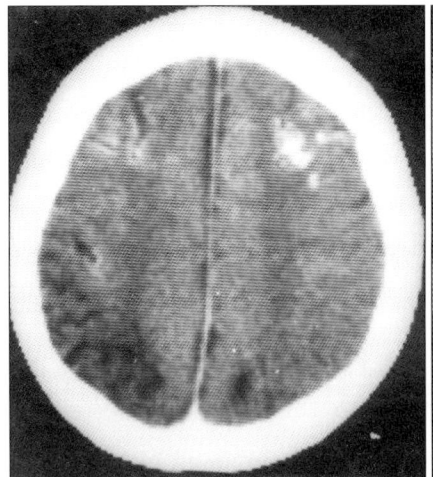

Fig. 1. CT Scan of the head showing bilateral frontal gyral calcifications.

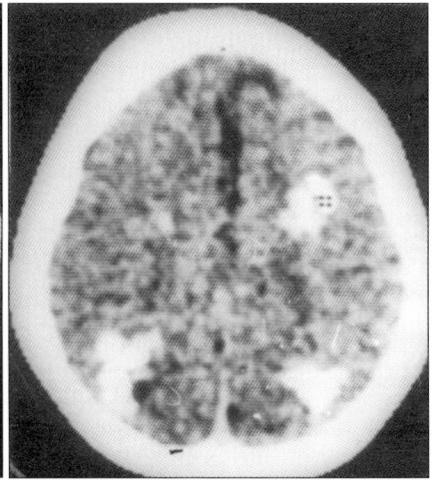

Fig. 2. CT Scan of the head showing multiple gyral calcifications.

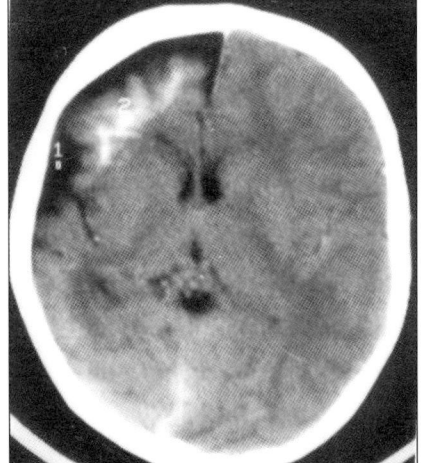

Fig. 3. CT Scan of the head showing right frontal gyral calcification.

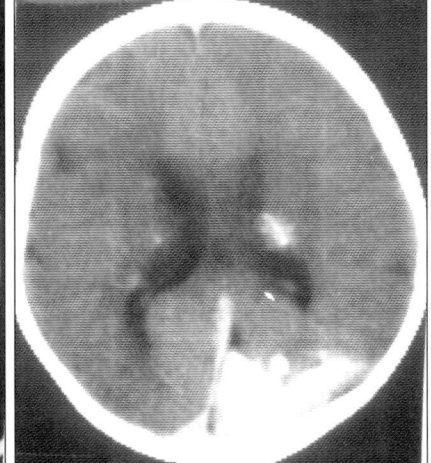

Fig. 4. CT Scan of the head showing left occipital gyral calcification with periventricular specs of calcification.

Methods and results

Personal enquiries with the paediatricians, neurologists and four gastroenterologists practising in the city of Bangalore with a population of over 5.5 million did not reveal any proven documented case of CD. All cranial computerized tomography (CT) scans done over a period of three years (1991–93) at our institute (NIMHANS) were reviewed by two of us. There were 103 scans showing cerebral calcification out of 16,506 CT scans reviewed (0.62 per cent). Fifty of them were males. Thirty patients were below the age of 12 years. Calcifications were single in 64, double in 13, multiple in 36. Calcified cysticercosis accounted for the majority 61 per cent (Table 1). There were 11 patients with gyral calcification of which six showed evidence of Sturge–Weber–Dimitri disease.

In four patients there were no obvious causes for the cortical calcification (Figs. 1–4). The clinical profile of these patients and a similar case seen previously are given in Table 2.

Table 2. Summary of the cases

Clinical	Patient 1	Patient 2	Patient 3	Patient 4	Patient 5
Consanguinity	Present	Present	Present	Absent	Present
Birth history	Normal	Asphyxia	Normal	Normal	Normal
Age at onset	18 months	7 months	1 month	2 months	18 months
Convulsion	Absent	Motor-gen	Motor-gen	Motor-gen	CPS*
Control of seizures	–	Good	Poor	Poor	Poor
Myoclonic jerk	Absent	Present	Absent	Absent	Absent
Milestones	Delayed	Delayed	Delayed	Delayed	Delayed
Motor power	Normal	Normal	Normal	Weakness	Normal
Calcification	Bilateral	Unilat	Bilateral	Unilat	Bilateral
Location	Frontal	Occipital	Frontal	Frontal	Occipital & Frontal
Exposure to gluten	No	No	Rarely	No	Rare

*Complex partial seizures.

Discussion

Bangalore is the capital of the state of Karnataka in South India, having a population of over 5.5 million. The National Institute of Mental Health and Neurosciences (NIMHANS) is the postgraduate institute in the field of mental health and neurosciences. On an average over 10,000 patients are treated every year, one-fifth of them as inpatients. Epilepsy is an important neurological disease accounting for over 2900 cases per year. There was no documented case of CD at this institute. Literature search also failed to show any case from south India. However, wheat and wheat products are not the staple diet in this part of the country. Only migrant population from the north and a small number of persons in the cities use wheat products in the form of chapattis and bread made of wheat flour. Hence, it is not clear whether CD is rare or is not expressed due to non-exposure of the population to wheat products. Estimation of antigliadin, anti-endomysial antibodies, or jejunal biopsy (with typical flat mucosa) may not be useful in identifying cases of CD in this population. If a genetic predisposition exists, it could be in the form of latent or potential CD. Hence it may be worthwhile to look for extraintestinal manifestations of CD, such as idiopathic macrocytic anaemia, alopecia areata responsive to a gluten-free diet, and dermatitis herpetiformis, which are known to occur before the development of classical CD (Auricchio *et al.*, 1988). HLA studies, endothelial cell culture and challenges with gluten are also useful. Anecdotal cases of epilepsy, cerebral calcification and coeliac disease are documented (Della Cella *et al.*, 1991, Molteni *et al.*, 1988). Gobbi *et al.* (1992) in their study of 43 patients demonstrated the association to be more than a chance occurrence and suggested to screen all cases of unexplained cerebral calcification and epilepsy for evidence of CD. In our five cases of unexplained cerebral calcification only four patients had epilepsy. Only two had occasional exposure to a gluten-containing diet. In two, the calcification was unilateral. The location was occipital in two while in the rest it was frontal. Gobbi *et al.* observed the majority of that calcifications in their series were occipital and occipital epilepsy was thought to be a characteristic feature of CD with cerebral calcification. Only one patient in the present series had gastrointestinal symptoms and features of vitamin deficiency during the course of this illness. However, a xylose absorption test done in the other two did not show evidence of malabsorption. It is noteworthy that in the series of Gobbi *et al.* (1992) only two of 31 patients at the time of biopsy had symptoms of GI disturbance and most of them had features suggestive of CD only in the first three years of life. Similarly, of 102 cases of adult CD diagnosed at Edinburgh only 13 had gastrointestinal symptoms (Logan *et al.*, 1983). Hence it may be necessary to evolve provocative tests to diagnose CD in areas where wheat and wheat products are not routinely used as a staple diet.

References

Auricchio, S., Mazzacca, G., Tosi, R., Visakorpi, J.K., Maki, M. & Polanco, I. (1988): Coeliac disease as a familial condition: identification of asymptomatic coeliac patients within family groups. *Gastroenterol. Int.* **1,** 25–31.

Chapman, R.G., Laidlow, J.M., Colin Jones, D.G., Eade, O.E. & Smith, C.L. (1978): Increased prevalence of epilepsy in coeliac disease. *BMJ* **2,** 250–251.

Della Cella, G., Beluchi, C. & Cipollina, F. (1991): Intracranial calcifications – epilepsy – celiac disease: description of a case. *Med. Surg. Pediatr.* **13,** 427–430.

Gobbi, G., Sorrenti, G., Santucci, M. *et al.* (1988): Epilepsy with bilateral occipital calcifications: a benign onset with progressive severity. *Neurology* **38,** 913–920.

Gobbi, G., Bouquest, F., Greco, L., Lambertini, A., Tassinari, C.A, Ventura, A. & Zanboni, M.G. (1992): Coeliac disease, epilepsy and cerebral calcifications. *Lancet* **340,** 439–443.

Laidlow, J.M., Chapman, R.G., Colin Jones, D.G., Eade, O. & Smith, C.L. (1977): Increased prevalence of epilepsy in Coeliac disease. *Gut* **18,** A943.

Logan, R.F.A., Tucker, G., Rifkind, E.A., Heading, R.C. & Ferguson, A. (1983): Changes in clinical features of coeliac disease in adults in Edinburgh and the Lothians 1960–79. *BMJ* **286,** 95–97.

Molteni, N., Bardella, M.T., Baldassarri, A.R. & Bianchi, P.A. (1988): Celiac disease associated with epilepsy and intracranial calcifications: report of two patients. *Am. J. Gastroenterol* **83,** 992–994.

Sammaritano, M., Andermann, F., Melanson, D., Guberman, A., Tinuper, P. & Gastaut, H. (1988): The syndrome of intractable epilepsy, bilateral occipital calcifications and folic acid deficiency. *Neurology* **38,** (Supp 1), 239.

Epilepsy and other neurological disorders in coeliac disease, edited by G. Gobbi *et al.*
© 1997 John Libbey & Company Ltd, pp. 31–34.

Chapter 5a

Prevalence of coeliac disease in the Republic of San Marino: AGA and EMA determinations as screening tests for coeliac disease in children

Susanna Alessandrini, Giovanni Iwanejko, A. Zani[*], F. Muccioli[*] and L. Zanotti[*]

Dipartimento di Pediatria, Ospedale di Stato,Via La Toscana 3, Borgo Maggiore, Republic of San Marino;
[*]Laboratorio Analisi, Ospedale di Stato, Via La Toscana 3, Borgo Maggiore, Republic of San Marino

Introduction

Coeliac disease, in the absence of gastrointestinal symptoms, often presents atypically and is consequently underestimated in comparison with the actual incidence in the population (Auricchio *et al.*, 1988; Auricchio *et al.*, 1990; Cacciari, Salardi & Volta, 1985; Fry, Seah & Hoffbrand, 1974; Molteni, Bardella & Bianchi, 1990; Sher & Mayberry, 1994).

Nowadays, easily performed serological tests (AGA, IgG and IgA, and EMA) are available: their positivity has allowed, in many cases, simplifying the diagnostic process of the disease, which, not long ago, included the performance of complicated tests (including xylose loading, iron loading, chemical test of the faeces) before the patients underwent an intestinal biopsy (Chan *et al.*, 1994; Meeuwisse, 1970; Walker-Smith *et al.*, 1990). Moreover, by monitoring the antigliadin antibodies, it is possible to avoid the three intestinal biopsies required before coeliac disease is definitively diagnosed (ESPGAN) (Bod *et al.*, 1993; McMillan *et al.*, 1991).

From re-examination of our survey over the period from 1977 to 1993 it emerges that, during these sixteen years, coeliac disease has been diagnosed in eight subjects of paediatric age and only four of them presented a 'typical form' at the onset of the disease.

In agreement with the international literature (Collin *et al.*, 1990; Maki *et al.*, 1988; Maki, Koskimies & Visakorpi, 1988; Unsworth & Brown, 1994), our survey also shows that half the subjects presented an 'atypical' symptomatology. These observations persuaded us to join the multicentre study, proposed by SIGEP, concerning AGA screening for coeliac disease.

Table 1. Survey of the period from 1977 to 1993

Subjects	Sex	Age at diagnosis (yr)	Clinical manifestation	HLA
(1) G.S.	F	1.4	Coeliac sprue	DR3
(2) B.F.	F	2	Coeliac sprue	DR11
(3) M.I.	F	4	Coeliac sprue	DR11
(4) T.S.	F	3	Dermatitis herpetiformis	DR7
(5) G.I.	F	1.6	Coeliac sprue	DR3
(6) R.S.	M	5	Anaemia	DR3/7
(7) F.A.	M	6	Constipation	DR7/11
(8) B.F.	M	2	Growth retardation	DR11

Patients and methods

On 31 December 1994 the resident population of the Republic of San Marino was of 24,707, of which 3658 were in the 0–14 age-group: 1,904 males and 1754 females. Our study, carried out from September 1993 to March 1995, examined children coming from the nine 'castles' of our Republic (the nine administative towns of the region), during the periodic check-ups prescribed by the medical advisors to the school system.

The examined groups of school-age children were attending that year, respectively, the first and the the fifth grade of primary school and the third grade of secondary school. The sample was made up of 1448 schoolchildren ranging in age from 5.8 to 14.2 years (mean 10.1). Of these 1424 or 98.3% participated in the study. The selected population contained only one known subject with coeliac disease who did not undergo the screening.

Table 2. Screened subjects

Mean age (yr)	Male	Female	Total
6.5	245	205	450
10.9	256	233	489
13.9	260	225	485
Total	761	663	1424

Blood was taken for the assay of AGA, IgA and IgG and for the assay of serum IgA (Burgin-Wolff *et al.*, 1989; Burgin-Wolff *et al.*, 1991). If IgG and/or IgA values were above the cut-off values (30 i.u./ml and 15 i.u./ml, respectively) we proceeded with the assay for EMA (antiendomysial antibodies). The assay for AGA was carried out by enzyme-linked immunabsorbent assay (ELISA), while for EMA it was carried out by indirect immunofluorescence testing (Troncone & Ferguson, 1991).

(a) Subjects with positive IgG and/or IgA and negative EMA were considered healthy.

(b) Subjects with positive EMA were referred to the second level of examination.

Second level tests included the performance of a full blood test, and jejunal endoscopy with sampling for HLA typing (Ascher *et al.*, 1993; Beutner *et al.*, 1989).

Results and conclusions

Out of 1424 screened subjects, 276 presented an AGA IgG value and 20 an AGA IgA value above the cut-off value (19.3 per cent and 1.4 per cent, respectively). All subjects underwent the assay for serum IgA and only one subject showed a selective IgA deficiency, showing, however, AGA IgG values within the normal range. EMA were positive in 5 subjects, who were referred to the second level of examination.

Three of the biopsied subjects presented a flat mucosa, one subject presented an apparently normal mucosa, which may be considered to represent latent coeliac disease, according to present standards and the fifth subject had partial atrophy with increase in intraepithelial lymphocytes counts.

Table 3. Profile of positive subjects

Subject	Sex	Age (yrs)	IgG	IgA	EMA	Biopsy	Symptoms	HLA
(1) P.C.	F	14.3	+	+	+	–	n.s.[*]	DR3
(2) S.M.	M	6.1	+	+	+	+	n.s.[*]	DR7/11
(3) S.L.	M	7	+	+	+	+	n.s.[*]	DR3/7
(4) T.E.	F	10.5	+	+	+	+	n.s.[*]	n.d.[***]
(5) T.A.	F	13.8	+	+	+	+	A.d.[**]	n.d.[***]

[*]No symptoms; [**]Atopic dermatitis; [***]not done.

The subjects diagnosed by screening were 5 of 1448 children showing a prevalence of 1/289.

Our data, compared with those reported by other authors, confirm that the actual incidence of coeliac disease is underestimated. Table 4 reports the prevalence of a study (Grodzinsky *et al.* 1991) carried out in 1991 in Sweden on 1866 blood donors (between the ages of 18 and 64) where the prevalence was 1/256 and the prevalence in a study carried out in 1994 in Italy by Catassi *et al* (1994) was 1/305 in a population of 3351 schoolchildren between the ages of 11 and 14 years old.

Table 4. Comparison of prevalence in three different countries

1866 healthy blood donors	(age 18–64 years)	1: 256
	(E. Grodzinsky, 1991, Sweden)	
3315 school children	(age 11–15 years)	1: 305
	(C. Catassi, 1994, Italy)	
1424 school children	(age 6–15 years)	1: 289
	(G Iwanejko, 1995, Rep. of S. Marino)	

In conclusion, the analysis of our results confirms the validity of screening in coeliac disease. In particular, although this experience was limited to our small Republic, it arouses interest concerning the clinical picture of coeliac disease which is becoming more and more uncommon in its 'typical' form whereas atypical forms, so called 'silent' or 'latent' cases usually with late onset are increasingly recognized.

Acknowledgement

The authors would like to thank the Gastroenterology Department staff of the State Hospital of San Marino who contributed to this work.

References

Ascher, A., Holm, K., Kristiansson, B. & Maki, M. (1993): Different features of coeliac disease in two neighbouring countries. *Arch. Dis. Child* **69**, 375–380.

Auricchio, S., Greco, L. & Troncone, R. (1990): What is the true prevalence of coeliac disease? *Gastroenterol. Intl.* **3**, 140–142.

Auricchio, S., Mazzacca, S., Tosi, G., Visakorpi, M., Maki, M. & Polanco, I. (1988): Coeliac disease as a familial condition: identification of asymptomatic coeliac patients within family groups. *Gastroenterol. Intl.* **1**, 25–31.

Beutner, E.H., Kumar, V., Chorzelski, T.P. & Szaflarska-Czerwionka, M. (1989): IgG endomysial antibodies in IgA-deficient patients with coeliac disease. *Lancet* **i,** 1261–1262.

Bod, S., Weile, B., Krasilnikoff, P.A. & Gudmand-Hoyer, E. (1993): The diagnostic value of the gliadin antibody test in coeliac disease in children: a prospective study. *J. Pediatr. Gastroenterol. Nutr.* **17,** 260–264.

Burgin-Wolff, A., Berger, R., Gaze, H., Huber, H., Lentze, M.J. & Nussl, D. (1989): IgG, IgA and IgE gliadin antibody determinations as screening test for untreated coeliac disease in children; a multicentre study. *Eur. J. Pediatr.* **148,** 496–502.

Burgin-Wolff, A., Gaze, H., Hadziselimovic, F., Huber, H., Lentze, M.J., Nussl, D. & Reymond-Berthet, C. (1991): Antigliadin and antiendomysium antibody determination for coeliac disease. *Arch. Dis. Child* **66,** 941–947.

Cacciari, E., Salardi, S. & Volta, U. (1985): Can anti-gliadin antibodies detect symptomless celiac disease in children with short stature? *Lancet* **i,** 1469–471.

Catassi, C., Ratsch, I.M., Fabiani, E., Rossini, M., Bordicchia, F., Candela, F. *et al.* (1994): Coeliac disease in the year 2000: exploring the iceberg. *Lancet* **383,** 270–273.

Chan, K.N., Phillips, A.D., Mirakian, R. & Walker-Smith, J.A. (1994): Endomysial antibody screening in children. *J. Pediatr. Gastroenterol. Nutr.* **18,** 316–320.

Collin, P., Hällstrom, O., Maki, M., Viander, M. & Keyrilainen, O. (1990): Atypical coeliac disease found with serological screening. *Scand. J. Gastroenterol.* **25,** 245–250.

Fry, L., Seah, P.P. & Hoffbrand, A.V. (1974): Dermatitis herpetiformis. *Clin. Gastroenterol.* **3,** 145–147.

Grodzinsky, E., Franzen, L. & Strm, M. (1991): High prevalence of coeliac disease in healthy adults revealed by antigliadin antibodies. *Ann. All.* **69,** 66–70.

Maki, M., Kallonen, K., Lhdeaho, M. L. & Visakorpi, J.K. (1988): Changing pattern of childhood coeliac disease in Finland. *Acta Paediatr. Scand.* **77,** 408–412.

Maki, M., Koskimies, S. & Visakorpi, J.K. (1988): Latent coeliac disease. International Coeliac Symposium, London, September 4th–6th.

Mc Millan, S., Haughton, D.J., Biggart, J.D. *et al.* (1991): Predictive value for coeliac disease of antibodies to gliadin, endomysium, and jejunum in patients attending for jejunal biopsy. *BMJ* **303,** 1163–1165.

Meeuwisse, G.W. (1970): Diagnostic criteria in coeliac disease. *Acta Paediatr. Scand.* **59,** 461–463.

Molteni, N., Bardella, M.T. & Bianchi, P.A. (1990): Obstetric and gynaecological problems in women with untreated coeliac sprue. *J. Clin. Gastroeneterol.* **12,** 37–39.

Sher, K.S. & Mayberry J.F. (1994): Female fertility, obstetric and gynaecological history in coeliac disease. *Digestion* **55,** 243–246.

Troncone, R. & Ferguson A. (1991): Anti-gliadin antibodies. *J. Pediatr. Gastroenterol. Nutr.* **12,** 150–158.

Unsworth, D.J. & Brown, D.L. (1994): Serological screening suggests that adult coeliac disease is underdiagnosed in the UK and increases the incidence by up to 12 per cent. *Gut* **35,** 61–64.

Walker-Smith, J.A., Gaundalini, S., Schmitz, J., Shmerling, D.H. & Visakorpi, J.K. (1990): Revised criteria for diagnosis of coeliac disease. *Arch. Dis. Child.* **65,** 909–911.

Epilepsy and other neurological disorders in coeliac disease, edited by G. Gobbi *et al.*
© 1997 John Libbey & Company Ltd, pp. 35–36.

Chapter 5b

Prevalence of coeliac disease in epileptic patients of the Republic of San Marino

S. Naccarato*, F. Casali**, S. Giuliani*, G. Gobbi*, S. Guttmann*, F. Muccioli** and M. Volpini*

*Centro Epilessie, Ospedale di Stato, Republic of San Marino; **Laboratorio Analisi, Ospedale di Stato, Republic of San Marino*

Introduction

The Republic of San Marino is the oldest independent republic in the world. It is situated in the centre of Italy. Nowadays it is populated by approximately 24,000 inhabitants and is served by a Social Security Institute which is responsible for sanitation and offers free health services.

Our neurologic service works inside the State Hospital and there are an average of 2000 patient visits per year. The Epilepsy Centre cares for about 100 patients, all citizens or residents.

A connection between coeliac disease, epilepsy and cerebral calcifications has been recently drawn (Gobbi *et al.*, 1992a,b; Bye & Andermann, 1993; Gobbi *et al.*, 1992). Nevertheless, there are no controlled epidemiologic studies on the prevalence of coeliac disease in epileptic patients.

Methods

We investigated the possible association between coeliac disease, epilepsy and cerebral calcifications according to Gobbi's description in 1992 (Gobbi *et al.*, 1992b), in the epileptic patients seen on our service from January to December 1994. In this period, we evaluated 45 subjects (23 M and 22 F; mean age 31 years; range 5–84), 28 of them with generalized epilepsy and 17 with partial epilepsy.

Twenty-six patients (14 M and 12 F) underwent full laboratory tests for coeliac disease (antigliadin IgG and IgA, antiendomysium antibodies) (McNeish *et al.*, 1979; Burgin-Wolff *et al.*, 1991), Eighteen of them refused to take part in the research; four were excluded because they had an epileptic encephalopathy and one had post-traumatic epilepsy.

Results

Antigliadin IgG and IgA and antiendomysium antibodies were positive for coeliac disease only in one male subject out of 45[*] (3.8 per cent). He had generalized epilepsy with grand mal seizures. The EEG showed generalized spike and wave abnormalities. Seizures disappeared many years ago, nevertheless he is still receiving therapy with PB and PHT.

The Terman-Merrill neuropsychological test showed, at the age of sixteen, borderline intelligence (QI 75).

The following investigations were carried out:

    – jejunal biopsy, showed villous atrophy compatible with coeliac disease

    – HLA typing showed the DQ2 and DR7 phenotypes, that seem to be characteristic of coeliac disease (Corazza *et al.*, 1985)

    – CT scan, negative for cerebral calcifications, and normal MRI.

Conclusions

Laboratory tests for coeliac disease, were carried out in 26 of 45 epileptic patients observed in one year. Only one subject was positive, giving a prevalence of 3.8 per cent. This subject belongs to Group 2 described by Gobbi *et al.*, (1992b).

The value of our observation is limited by the fact that it only documents the association of two very common diseases. As coeliac disease has elevated incidence in the Italian peninsula and the incidence of epilepsy in the normal population is evaluated at about 0.5 per cent, this association in our patient may be a chance finding as suggested by the Italian Working Group (Gobbi *et al.*, 1992b).

On the other hand, considering that epilepsy is a multifactorial disease, it is possible that, in our case, it could have been facilitated by the presence of coeliac disease.

References

Burgin-Wolff, A., Gaze, H., Hadziselimovic, F. *et al.* (1991): Antigliadin and antiendomysium antibody determination for coeliac disease. *Arch. Dis. Child* **66**, 941–947.

Bye, A.M. & Andermann, F. *et al.* (1993): Cortical vascular abnormalities in the syndrome of coeliac disease, epilepsy, bilateral occipital calcifications and folate deficiency *Ann. Neurol.* **34**, 399–403.

Corazza, G.R., Tabacchi, P., Frisoni, M., Prati, C. & Gasbarrini, G. (1985): DR and non-DR Ia allotypes are associated with susceptibility to coeliac disease. *Gut* **26**, 1210–1213.

Gobbi, G., Ambrosetto, P. *et al.* (1992a): Coeliac disease, posterior calcifications and epilepsy. *Brain Dev.* **14**, 23–29.

Gobbi, G., Bouquet, F. *et al.* (1992b): Coeliac disease, epilepsy and cerebral calcifications. *Lancet* **340**, 439–443.

McNeish, A.S. & Harms, H.K. (1979): The diagnosis of coeliac disease. *Arch. Dis. Child* **54**, 783–786.

Part II

Pathophysiological basis of neurological disorders in coeliac disease

Epilepsy and other neurological disorders in coeliac disease, edited by G. Gobbi *et al.*
© 1997 John Libbey & Company Ltd, pp. 39–45.

Chapter 6

The roles of folate and vitamin B$_{12}$ in the central nervous system: lessons from inborn errors

Benedicte Christensen and David S. Rosenblatt

Departments of Human Genetics, Medicine, Pediatrics and Biology, McGill University, Montreal, Quebec, Canada

Introduction

Folate and vitamin B$_{12}$ (cobalamin, Cbl) play a role in areas as diverse as vascular disease and neural tube defects. In North America and Europe Cbl deficiency is almost always due to malabsorption, except for the Cbl deficiency seen in individuals on a strict vegan diet. Pernicious anaemia accounts for 80 per cent of the cases, with the others being due to food-cobalamin malabsorption, jejunal diverticula, tropical sprue, or resection of the stomach or ileum (Savage & Lindenbaum, 1995). Folate deficiency is also mainly due to impaired intestinal absorption or insufficient intake.

The original observation of a progressive myelopathy occurring in association with pernicious anaemia was made more than 100 years ago, and the term subacute combined degeneration of the spinal cord was established by the turn of the century. More recently subtle Cbl deficiency states and their role in a broad range of associated neurological and psychiatric disorders have been highlighted (Lindenbaum *et al.*, 1988).

Even though it is well established that macrocytic anaemia and megaloblastic bone marrow changes may be due to both folate and Cbl deficiency, the presence of neurological symptoms was for a long time considered diagnostic for Cbl deficiency. Increasing attention has been paid to the association of folate deficiency with a variety of neuropsychiatric and neurological disorders, including subacute combined degeneration of the spinal cord (Parry, 1994). Abnormalities of the nervous system have been reported in two-thirds of folate-deficient and in two-fifths to two-thirds of Cbl-deficient patients (Savage & Lindenbaum, 1995; Shorvon *et al.*, 1980).

Impaired folate and Cbl metabolism in early pregnancy have been identified as risk factors for certain birth defects, even in the absence of macrocytosis. For both vitamins it can be speculated that the levels which are sufficient for normal haematopoiesis may not be sufficient for neurological development (Reynolds, 1976).

Biochemistry

Folate polyglutamates in the diet must be hydrolysed to monoglutamates prior to absorption (Halsted, 1980). Reduced folates participate in single carbon transfers that are important in purine and pyrimidine biosynthesis and in the metabolism of histidine, glycine, serine, and methionine (Rosenblatt, 1995).

Cbl bound to intrinsic factor is absorbed in the distal ileum. Newly absorbed Cbl is bound to transcobalamin II (TCII) in the blood (Fenton & Rosenberg, 1995). Although TCII is the physiologically active Cbl transporter, most Cbl in blood is bound to R binders (TCI and TCIII) which may play a role in the removal of toxic Cbl analogues (Kanazawa *et al.*, 1983). The TCII-Cbl complex is endocytosed, and following release of Cbl its trivalent cobalt is reduced (Fenton & Rosenberg, 1995; Pezacka, 1993). Cbl is subsequently converted to adenosylcobalamin (AdoCbl) in the mitochondria and to methylcobalamin (MeCbl) in the cytoplasm. AdoCbl is the cofactor for the mitochondrial methylmalonyl CoA mutase and MeCbl is the cofactor for the cytoplasmic methionine synthase. Methionine synthase requires S-adenosylmethionine, MeCbl, and methyltetrahydrofolate (MeTHF) as cofactors and generates methionine and tetrahydrofolate (THF) as products. This reaction brings together both Cbl and folate metabolism, so that in Cbl deficiency MeTHF accumulates and there is a deficiency of THF.

The study of the inborn errors of folate and Cbl metabolism is useful in understanding the function of these vitamins in the nervous system, and provides important clues to the pathogenesis of the abnormalities seen in the more common vitamin deficiencies.

Inborn errors of folate metabolism

Hereditary folate malabsorption

There have been 15 reported patients with hereditary folate malabsorption, 12 in females (Rosenblatt, 1995). Consanguinity has been seen in four families and several of the patients had undiagnosed siblings who died. Patients with hereditary folate malabsorption have had megaloblastic anaemia, diarrhoea, mouth ulcers, failure to thrive and neurological findings. The latter have included seizures and cerebral calcifications. At times, folate treatment has made seizures worse rather than better. Hereditary folate malabsorption provides the best evidence for a specific transport system for folate at the level of both the intestine and the blood–brain barrier. Often it is possible to correct the haematological findings but not the neurological findings probably because of difficulty in getting sufficient folate into the cerebrospinal fluid.

The cerebral calcification seen in some patients with hereditary folate malabsorption may provide clues to the cause of the calcification in those patients with epilepsy, intracerebral calcification, coeliac disease and folate deficiency (Gobbi *et al.*, 1992). The pathological findings in the latter are similar to the occipital calcifications seen in children treated for leukaemia with antifolates and radiation (Borns and Rancier, 1974; Young *et al.*, 1977), and to the cerebral calcifications seen in Sturge–Weber syndrome (Bye *et al.*, 1993). In most cases the triad of epilepsy, coeliac disease and cerebral calcifications is sporadic and treatment of the coeliac disease has led to increases in serum folate levels and a decrease in seizure frequency (Gobbi *et al.*, 1992; Ventura *et al.*, 1991).

Methylenetetrahydrofolate reductase (MTHFR) deficiency

MTHFR deficiency is an autosomal recessive disease associated with increased homocystine levels in blood and urine and normal or decreased methionine levels (Erbe, 1986). Decreased MTHFR results in decreased MeTHF and thus lack of the folate form required for methionine synthesis.

Patients with severe MTHFR deficiency usually are ill in the first year of life with developmental delay, microcephaly, seizures, and breathing disorders. They do not have megaloblastic anaemia as purine and pyrimidine metabolism are unaffected. Some patients present later with motor and gait abnormalities, peripheral neuropathy and some have had psychiatric disease (Rosenblatt, 1995). Other patients have had recurrent strokes in adulthood. The gene for MTHFR on chromosome 1 has been cloned and 14 mutations described (Goyette *et al.*, 1994; Goyette *et al.*, 1995, 1996).

Aside from patients with severe MTHFR deficiency, there has been recent speculation that a thermolabile MTHFR enzyme is a cause of mild elevations of total plasma homocysteine which is a risk factor for vascular disease (Kang *et al.*, 1988; Kang *et al.*, 1991; Engbersen *et al.*, 1995). An alanine to valine substitution in the MTHFR gene has been identified as the cause of the thermolability and of the resultant elevated total homocysteine levels (Frosst *et al.*, 1995; Christensen *et al.*, 1997).

Glutamate formiminotransferase deficiency

Glutamate formiminotransferase deficiency is associated with excretion of formiminoglutamic acid (FIGLU), but it is uncertain as to whether there is a consistent clinical phenotype. The original Japanese patients had mental retardation, dilatation of cerebral ventricles, cortical atrophy and macrocytic anaemia (Arakawa, 1970). Later patients showed speech abnormalities, no mental retardation and greater FIGLU excretion (Erbe, 1986). Because glutamate formiminotransferase is not expressed in most cultured cells, definitive understanding of the genetics of this disease awaits the cloning of the gene.

Inborn errors of cobalamin metabolism

Disorders of cobalamin absorption and transport

R binder (TCI) deficiency (Shevell & Rosenblatt, 1992) has been reported in only six patients. There have not been any consistent neurological findings and in one patient those found may have been related to alcohol abuse, and in another to cerebrovascular disease. The postulated role of R binders in the removal of potentially toxic cobalamin analogues has been suggested as a mechanism for neurotoxicity.

Defective intrinsic factor (IF) results in megaloblastic anaemia, global developmental delay and myelopathy. The defect can be corrected by normal gastric juice as a source of intrinsic factor.

Defective transport of cobalamin by enterocytes is associated with a specific inability to transport cobalamin. The defect is not corrected by normal gastric juice and is due to defects in the Cbl-IF receptor, receptor internalization, or the transfer of cobalamin to TCII. Clinical features include onset after the first year of life, megaloblastic anaemia, global developmental delay, myelopathy and proteinuria.

Transcobalamin II (TCII) deficiency presents in early infancy with megaloblastic anaemia, failure to thrive and global delay. With inadequate treatment or extended illness, surviving patients have developed mental retardation and neurologic manifestations including myelopathic features resembling subacute combined degeneration of the spinal cord. Mutations identified to date include nonsense mutations and deletions (Li *et al.*, 1994a, b).

Treatment of the inborn errors of cobalamin transport requires the injection of adequate cobalamin. The reversal of neurological deficits depends on the duration of symptoms before treatment.

Defects of cobalamin utilization

These diseases result in the failure to synthesize one or both of the two cofactors MeCbl or AdoCbl. They result in more severe metabolic disease than that seen in the transport disorders. Patients excrete homocystine and methylmalonic acid, either alone or in combination. Seven distinct complementation groups have been identified by means of biochemical and somatic cell genetic studies of cultured fibroblasts (Fenton & Rosenberg, 1995; Shevell & Rosenblatt, 1992).

Combined deficiency of MeCbl and AdoCbl

Three complementation classes present with both homocystinuria and methylmalonic aciduria: cblC, cblD, and cblF. There are more than 90 patients known with cblC whereas cblD represents only two brothers and cblF represents five patients.

Most cblC patients are sick in the first year of life with global developmental delay, seizures, microcephaly, megaloblastic anaemia, failure to thrive, feeding difficulties, and lethargy. Early onset multiorgan failure and thrombotic microangiopathy may be seen. Some cblC patients have a pigmentary retinopathy with perimacular degeneration. Although most cblC patients present in the first year of life, others show a later onset in childhood or adolescence, and present with delirium, psychosis, and spasticity.

Only a pair of brothers has been reported with cblD. One had behavioural problems and mild mental retardation. Cerebrovascular disease due to thrombi was found at age 18 years.

Failure to thrive is found in most of the cblF patients. Other findings include hypotonia, abnormal movements, seizures, anaemia, glossitis, arthritis and skin rash. The cblF patients have abnormal cobalamin absorption.

The defect in cblC, cblD, and cblF occur after endocytosis of TCII-cobalamin, after hydrolysis of the TCII-cobalamin complex, but before MeCbl and AdoCbl are synthesized. The defect in cblF has been localized to the lysosome and may be due to a failure to transport free cobalamin across the lysosomal membrane. In cblC and cblD there is a defect of cobalamin reduction and partial deficiencies of cyanocobalamin β-ligand transferase and of microsomal cob(III)alamin reductase have been described (Pezacka & Rosenblatt, 1994).

Methylcobalamin deficiency

This group includes cblE and cblG complementation groups and is characterized by isolated homocystinuria. Most patients have megaloblastic anaemia, homocystinuria, low or normal methionine levels and no methylmalonic aciduria. Neurologic features are common with psychomotor delay, hypotonia and frequent seizures. Magnetic resonance imaging has demonstrated delayed myelination. One adult patient with cblG had a spastic gait disturbance that began in the third decade of life and which was initially diagnosed as multiple sclerosis. The defect in cblE lies in a reducing system associated with methionine synthase whereas the defect in cblG probably lies in the methionine synthase enzyme itself. The gene for methionine synthase on chromasome 1 has recently been cloned and the first mutations described (Leclerc *et al.*, 1996; Gulati *et al.*, 1996; Li *et al.*, 1996). Treatment of these disorders is with hydroxycobalamin. Prenatal diagnosis and treatment of a cblE patient has resulted in a good outcome. The prognosis appears to be worse for cblG than for cblE.

Adenosylcobalamin deficiency

Patients with adenosylcobalamin deficiency fall into either the cblA or the cblB complementation group and are characterized by cobalamin-responsive methylmalonic aciduria. They have neither megaloblastic anaemia, nor homocystinuria. These patients tend to become ill later than patients with methylmalonyl CoA mutase apoenzyme defects. The defect in cblA is thought to lie in the intramitochondrial reduction of cobalamin whereas the defect in cblB is in the adenosyltransferase enzyme which is the last step in the synthesis of AdoCbl. It is thought that the neurological findings in these patients are secondary to acidosis, but some patients with methylmalonic aciduria have had some developmental delay in the absence of documented acidosis.

All the inborn errors of folate and cobalamin transport and metabolism are thought to be inherited as autosomal recessive diseases.

The role of folate and cobalamin deficiency in neural tube defects

The administration of folic acid has been shown to reduce both the occurrence and recurrence of neural tube defects (Czeizel & Dudas, 1992; Laurence *et al.*, 1981; MRC Vitamin Study Research Group, 1991). The mechanism by which a relative or absolute folate deficiency causes teratogenic effects on the central nervous system is not known. As described above, the alanine to valine substitution in the MTHFR gene (Frosst *et al.*, 1995) recently has been found to be associated with a thermolabile MTHFR enzyme. Enzyme determinations suggest that the frequency of the thermolabile MTHFR is increased in mothers of children with neural tube defect and may represent a genetic risk factor for neural tube defects (Put *et al.*, 1995).

Folate and Cbl deficiency in pregnant women have been identified as independent risk factors for neural tube defects (Kirke *et al.*, 1993). Both elevated levels of homocysteine (Steegers-Theunissen *et al.*, 1994, Mills *et al.*, 1995) and methylmalonic acid (Adams *et al.*, 1995) in serum are associated with an increased risk of having a child with a neural tube defect. Altered Cbl metabolism leading to impaired function of methionine synthase has been suggested as a possible basis for the responsible metabolic defect (Mills *et al.*, 1995).

Neurologic impairment due to drug-induced inhibition of folate or cobalamin metabolism

Nitrous oxide has been shown to cause specific and irreversible inhibition of the Cbl-dependent methionine synthase (Frasca *et al.*, 1986). The occupational and recreational (Gillman, 1992) exposure to nitrous oxide is associated with haematologic and neurologic effects, the latter including peripheral neuropathies and subacute degeneration of the spinal cord (Nunn, 1987).

Aminopterin and methotrexate are potent inhibitors of dihydrofolate reductase and are known to cause both abortion and embryopathy. In two patients with childhood leukaemia in remission, the calcification of cerebral vessels and epilepsy were observed after the combination of radiotherapy and intrathecal methotrexate chemotherapy. An induced folate deficiency is also thought to be responsible for the teratogenic effect of certain antiepileptic drugs such as valproic acid, phenytoin, phenobarbital and primidone (Dansky *et al.*, 1992). The use of valproic acid is associated with a five to twenty-fold increase in the incidence of neural tube defects in man (Wegner & Nau, 1992). The foetal hydantoin syndrome includes mental retardation, craniofacial abnormalities, prenatal and postnatal growth retardation, and limb defects (Hansen & Billings, 1985). In mice, this drug is shown to interfere with folate metabolism by causing a redistribution of folates and a decreased activity of hepatic MTHFR (Billings, 1984).

Acknowledgements

David Rosenblatt is a Principal Investigator in the Medical Research Council of Canada Genetics Group at McGill University. Benedicte Christensen is the holder of the Renouf Fellowship of the Royal Victoria Hospital Research Institute.

References

Adams, M.J., Khoury, M.J., Scanlon, K.S., Stevenson, R.E., Knight, G.J., Haddow, J.E., Sylvester, G.C., Cheek, J.E., Henry, J.P., Stabler, S.P. & Allen, R.H. (1995): Elevated midtrimester serum methylmalonic acid levels as a risk factor for neural tube defects. *Teratology* **51**, 311–317.

Arakawa, T. (1970): Congenital defects in folate utilization. *Am. J. Med.* **48**, 594–598.

Billings, R.E. (1984): Decreased hepatic 5,10-methylenetetrahydrofolate reductase activity in mice after chronic phenytoin treatment. *Mol. Pharmacol.* **25**, 459–466.

Borns, P.F. & Rancier, L.F. (1974): Cerebral calcifications in childhood leukaemia mimicking Sturge–Weber syndrome. *Am. J. Roentgenol. Radium. Ther. Nucl. Med.* **122**, 52–55.

Bye, A.M.E., Andermann, F., Robitaille, Y. *et al.* (1993): Cortical vascular abnormalities in the syndrome of celiac disease, epilepsy, bilateral occipital calcifications, and folate deficiency. *Ann. Neurol.* **34**, 399–403.

Cristensen, B., Frosst, P., Lussier-Cacan, S. *et al.* (1997): Correlation of a common mutation in the methylenetetrahydrofolate reductase (MTHFR) gene with plasma homocysteine in patients with premature coronary artery disease. *Arter. Thromb. Vasc. Biol.* **17**, 569–573.

Czeizel, A.E. & Dudas, I. (1992): Prevention of the first occurrence of neural-tube defects by periconceptional vitamin supplementation. *N. Engl. J. Med.* **327**, 1832–1835.

Dansky, L.V., Rosenblatt, D.S. & Andermann, E. (1992): Mechanisms of teratogenesis: folic acid and antiepileptic therapy. *Neurology* **42**, 32–42.

Engbersen, A.M.T., Franken, D.G., Boers, G.H.J. & Stevens, E.M.B. (1995): Thermolabile 5, 10-methylenetetrahydrofolate reductase as a cause of mild hyperhomocysteinemia. *Am. J. Hum. Genet.* **56**, 142–150.

Erbe, R.W. (1986): Inborn errors of folate metabolism. In *Folates and pterins, vol 3: Nutritional, pharmacological and physiological aspects,* eds. R.L. Whitehead & V.M. Blakley, pp. 413–465. New York: John Wiley and Sons.

Fenton, W.A. & Rosenberg, L.E. (1995): Inherited disorders of cobalamin transport and metabolism. In *The metabolic and molecular bases of inherited disease,* eds. C.R. Scriver, A.L. Beaudet, W.S. Sly & D. Valle, pp. 3129–3150. New York: McGraw-Hill, Inc.

Frasca, V., Riazza, B.S. & Matthews, R.G. (1986): *In vitro* inactivation of methionine synthase by nitrous oxide. *J. Biol Chem.* **261**, 15823–15827.

Frosst, P., Blom, H.J., Milos, R., Goyette, P., Sheppard, C.A., Matthews, R.G., Boers, G.J.H., den Heijer, M., Kluijtmans, L.A.J., van den Heuvel, L.P. & Rozen, R. (1995): A candidate genetic risk factor for vascular disease: a common methylenetetrhydrofolate reductase mutation causes thermoinstability. *Nat. Genet.* **10**, 111–113.

Gillman, M.A. (1992): Nitrous oxide abuse in perspective. *Clin. Neuropharmacology* **15**, 297–306.

Gobbi, G., Ambrosetto, P., Zaniboni, M.G. *et al.* (1992): Celiac disease, posterior cerebral calcifications and epilepsy. *Brain Dev.* **14**, 23–29.

Goyette, P., Christensen, B., Rosenblatt, D.S., & Rozen, R. (1996): Severe and mild mutations in CIS for the methylenetetrahydrofolate reductate (MTHFR) gene and description of 5 novel mutations in MTHFR. *Amer. J. Hum. Genet.* **59**, 1268–1275

Goyette, P., Frosst, P., Rosenblatt, D.S. & Rozen, R. (1995): Seven novel mutations in the methylenetetrahydrofolate reductase gene and genotype/phenotype correlations in severe methylenetetrahydrofolate reductase deficiency. *Amer. J. Hum. Genet.* **56**, 1052–1059.

Goyette, P., Milos, R., Ducan, A.M., Rosenblatt, D.S., Matthews, R.G. & Rozen, R. (1994): Human methylenetetrahydrofolate reductase: isolation of cDNA, mapping and mutation identification. *Nat. Genet.* **7**, 195–200.

Gulati, S., Baker, P., Li, Y.N. *et al.* (1996): Defects in human methionine synthase in cbIG patients. *Hum. Molec. Genet.* **5**, 1859–1865

Halsted, C.H. (1980): Intestinal absorption and malabsorption of folates. *Annu. Rev. Med.* **31**, 79–87.

Hansen, D.K. & Billings, R.E. (1985): Phenytoin teratogenicity and effects on embryonic and maternal folate metabolism. *Teratology* **31**, 363–371.

Kanazawa, S., Herbert, V., Herzlick, B., Drivas, G. & Manusselis, C. (1983): Removal of cobalamin analogue in bile by enterohepatic circulation of vitamin B_{12}. *Lancet* **i**, 707–708.

Kang, S.S., Wong, P.W.K., Susmano, A., Sora, J., Norusis, M. & Ruggie, N. (1991): Thermolabile methylenetetrahydrofolate reductase: An inherited risk factor for coronary artery disease. *Am. J. Hum. Genet.* **48**, 536–545.

Kang, S.S., Zhou, J., Wong, P.W.K., Kowalisyn, J. & Strokosch, G. (1988): Intermediate Homocysteinemia: A Thermolabile Variant of Methylenetetrahydrofolate Reductase. *Amer. J. Hum. Genet.* **43**, 414–421.

Kirke, P.N., Molloy, A.M., Daly, L.E., Burke, H., Weir, D.G. & Scott, J.M. (1993): Maternal plasma folate and vitamin B12 are independent risk factors for neural tube defects. *Quart. J. Med.* **86**, 703–708.

Laurence, K.M., James, N., Miller, M.H., *et al.* (1981): Double-blind randomized controlled trial of folate treatment before conception to prevent recurrence of neural-tube defects. *BMJ* **282**, 1509–1511.

Leclerc, D., Campeau, E., Goyette, P. *et al.* (1996): Human methionine synthase: cDNA cloning and identification of mutations in patients of the cbIG complementation group of folate/cobalamin disorders. *Hum. Molec. Genet.* **5**, 1867–1874

Li, N., Rosenblatt, D.S., Kamen, B.A., Seetharam, S. & Seetharam, B. (1994a): Identification of two mutant alleles of transcobalamin II in an affected family. *Hum. Molec. Genet.* **3**, 1835–1840.

Li, N., Rosenblatt, D.S. & Seetharam, B. (1994b): Nonsense mutations in human transcobalamin II deficiency. *Biochem. Biophys. Res. Comm.* **204,** 1111–1118.

Li, Y.N., Gulati, S., Baker, P.J. *et al.* (1996): Cloning, mapping and RNA analysis of the human methionine synthase gene. *Hum. Molec. Genet.* **5,** 1851–1858.

Lindenbaum, J., Healton, E.B., Savage, D.G., Brust, J.C., Garrett, T.J., Podell, E.R., Marcell, P.D., Stabler, S.P. & Allen, R.H. (1988): Neuropsychiatric disorders caused by cobalamin deficiency in the absence of anemia or macrocytosis. *N. Engl. J. Med.* **318,** 1720–1728.

Mills, J.L., McPartlin, J.M., Kirke, P.N., Lee, Y.J., Conley, M.R., Weir, D.G. & Scott, J.M. (1995): Homocysteine metabolism in pregnancies complicated by neural-tube defects. *Lancet* **345,** 149–151.

MRC Vitamin Study Research Group, (1991): Prevention of neural tube defects: results of the Medical Research Council Vitamin Study. *Lancet* **338,** 131–137.

Nunn, J.F. (1987): Clinical aspects of the interaction between nitrous oxide and vitamin B₁₂. *Br. J. Anaesth.* **59,** 3–13.

Parry, T.E. (1994): Folate responsive neuropathy. *Presse. Med.* **23,** 131–137.

Pezacka, E.H. (1993): Identification and characterization of two enzymes involved in the intracellular metabolism of cobalamin. Cyanocobalamin beta-ligand transferase and microsomal cob(III)alamin reductase. *Biochim. Biophys. Acta.* **1157** (2), 167–177.

Pezacka, E.H. & Rosenblatt, D.S. (1994): Intracellular metabolism of cobalamin. Altered activities of β-axial-ligand transferase and microsomal cob(III)alamin reductase in cblC and cblD fibroblasts. In *Advances in Thomas Addison's diseases,* eds. H.R. Bhatt, V.H.T. James, G.M. Besser, G.F. Bottazzo, & H. Keen, pp. 315–323. Bristol, London: Journal of Endocrinology.

Put, Nvd., Steegers-Theunissen, R., Eskes, T. *et al.* (1995): A common mutation in the 5,10-methylenetetrahydrofolate reductase (MTHFR) gene as a risk factor for neural tube defects. *Ir. J. Med. Sci.* **164** Suppl. 15, 22.

Reynolds, E.H. (1976): Neurology of vitamin B₁₂ deficiency. *Lancet* **ii,** 832–833.

Rosenblatt, D.S. (1995): Inherited disorders of folate transport and metabolism. In: *The metabolic and molecular bases of inherited disease,* eds. C.R. Scriver, A.L. Beaudet, W.S. Sly & D. Valle, pp. 3011–3128. New York: McGraw-Hill.

Savage, D. & Lindenbaum, J. (1995): Neurological complications of acquired cobalamin deficiency: clinical aspects. In: *Megaloblastic anaemias,* ed. S. Wickramasinghe. London: Baillière Tindall.

Shevell, M.I. & Rosenblatt, D.S. (1992): The neurology of cobalamin. *Can. J. Neur. Sci.* **19,** 472–486.

Shorvon, S.D., Carney, M.W.P., Chanarin, I. & Reynolds, E.H. (1980): The neuropsychiatry of megaloblastic anemia. *BMJ* **281,** 1036–1038.

Steegers-Theunissen, R.P.M., Boers, G.H.J., Trijbels, J.M.F. *et al.* (1994): Maternal hyperhomocysteinemia: a risk factor for neural tube defects. *Metabolism* **43,** 1475–1480.

Ventura, A., Bouquet, F., Sartorelli, C., *et al.* (1991): Coeliac disease, folic acid deficiency and epilepsy with cerebral calcifications. *Acta Paediatr. Scand* **80,** 559–562.

Wegner, C. & Nau, H. (1992): Alteration of embryonic folate metabolism by valproic acid during organogenesis: implications for mechanism of teratogenesis. *Neurology.* **42 (suppl. 5),** 17–24.

Young, L.W., Jequier, S. & O'Gorman, A.M. (1977): Intracerebral calcifications in treated leukemia in a child. *Am. J. Dis. Child.* **131,** 1283–1285.

Epilepsy and other neurological disorders in coeliac disease, edited by G. Gobbi *et al.*
© 1997 John Libbey & Company Ltd, pp. 47–54.

Chapter 7

Immunological aspects of coeliac disease: some systemic perturbations

P.D. Howdle

St. James's University Hospital, Leeds LS9 7TF, UK

P.D. Howdle

St. James's University Hospital, Leeds LS9 7TF, UK

There is no doubt that coeliac disease is a disease of the small intestinal mucosa, indeed a mucosal abnormality is part of the definition of the disease and the diagnosis is dependent upon small intestinal mucosal biopsies (Booth, 1974; Trier, 1991; Howdle & Losowsky, 1992).

Nevertheless, there are many well known non-gastrointestinal associations of coeliac disease which have been reported over the years (Cooke & Holmes, 1984; Howdle & Losowsky, 1992) and these are likely to be reported more frequently with an increasing awareness of the more subtle presentations of coeliac disease (Corazza & Gasbarrini, 1995). Such an awareness was behind the reported relationship of coeliac disease, epilepsy and cerebral calcifications (Gobbi *et al.*, 1992) which prompted the writing of the present volume.

Since coeliac disease is a relatively common and life-long condition, as are some of the associated diseases, it is highly likely that some of these associations may occur by chance. However, there is evidence that several associations are more than coincidental, e.g. diabetes mellitus and thyroid disease (Corazza & Gasbarrini, 1995). Such significant associations may be due to major histocompatibility complex similarities, and an activated immune system, allowing genetically predisposed individuals to react immunologically to either gliadin-related or autoantigens. There is thus the suggestion that the immune activation believed to be responsible for the pathogenesis of coeliac disease produces systemic effects and that such systemic perturbations may contribute to the development of non-gastrointestinal manifestations of the disease.

The immunological theory of the pathogenesis of coeliac disease has always had two fundamental questions to answer: which part of gliadin is responsible for the disease and how does that protein produce the pathological changes? The answers to these questions are emerging and the evidence for an immunological pathogenesis of coeliac disease is very strong.

There has been a lot of recent work into the structure of gliadin and a search for that part of gliadin, and therefore presumably the antigenic epitope, which is responsible for the disease. Gliadin is a term referring to the prolamin content of wheat. It is the alcohol-soluble component of the protein mixture termed gluten. There are different prolamins in the other cereals involved in coeliac disease,

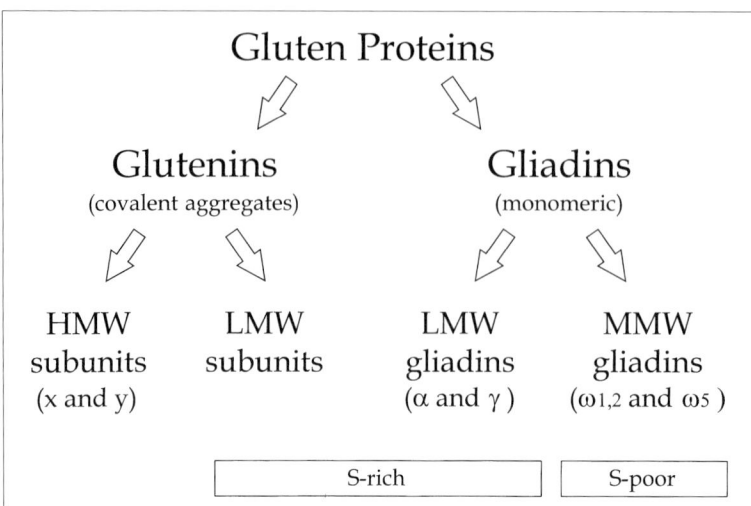

Fig. 1. The classification and nomenclature of wheat gluten proteins, into three groups: HMW, MMW, LMW (high, medium and low molecular weight). MMW and LMW are respectively poor and rich in sulphur-containing amino acids.

i.e. rye, barley and oats; for a comprehensive discussion of cereal chemistry in relation to coeliac disease see Shewry *et al.* (1992) and Wieser (1995). In this chapter only gliadin will be considered. In recent years the gluten proteins in general have been reclassified into three groups, on the basis of highly efficient separation techniques (Wieser 1995) (see Fig. 1). The three different groups are characterized by their molecular mass and the different proportions of constituent amino acids. The primary structures of many of these proteins e.g. α-type gliadin (Kasarda *et al.*, 1984) have now been described.

The search for the gliadin peptide and therefore the possible antigenic epitope responsible for coeliac disease has involved the *in vivo* and *in vitro* testing of a variety of peptides produced by a variety of means. For example, Howdle *et al.* (1984) and Ciclitira *et al.* (1984) showed that all the major gliadin subgroups (α, β, γ and ω-gliadins defined by their electrophoretic mobility) produced detrimental effects on coeliac mucosa using both *in vitro* and *in vivo* techniques. Other workers produced small peptides for *in vitro* testing. Wieser *et al.* (1983, 1984, 1986) isolated pure peptides from a peptic-tryptic digest of gliadin. They ultimately produced two peptides, 22 (residues 3–24) and 31 (residues 25–55) amino acids in length respectively of α-type gliadins. Both these peptides were detrimental to coeliac mucosa in vitro. There were two common sequences to both peptides wherein it was proposed their coeliac activity could lie, i.e. -Pro-Ser-Gln-Gln- and -Gln-Gln-Gln-Pro-. These findings were confirmed by De Ritis *et al.* (1988). More recently other workers have produced synthetic peptides, including these tetra-peptides, and tested them in a variety of systems. Obviously there is great variability between techniques, but there is a consensus that at least these tetra-peptides have some coeliac-like activity (Wieser, 1995). It is highly likely that there are other active peptides and also that, since it is believed their activity lies in initiating an immunological reaction, these tetra-peptides will form a part of slightly larger molecules (e.g. 12–20 amino acids in length) which could potentially be antigenic epitopes.

The second question posed initially was: how does the gliadin protein produce the coeliac mucosal lesion? It has already been suggested that such pathology is a result of an immunological reaction to a particular peptide(s).

There is certainly considerable evidence for immunological activation in coeliac disease. First, there is the predisposition, or genetic susceptibility of the individual who develops the disease. The genetics of coeliac disease are still not fully understood, but there is no doubt about the strong association with the genes of the major histocompatibility complex on chromosome 6. In 1972 the association with the class I allele HLA-B8 was described (Stokes *et al.,* 1972) but the stronger association with the class II allele DR3 was recognized soon afterwards (Keuning *et al.,* 1976). It is now generally accepted that certain specific class II D region genes are present in all coeliac patients, and it has been proposed that particular DQ2 alleles (i.e. DQA1*0501 and DQB1*0201) are the primary HLA susceptibility genes in coeliac disease (Sollid *et al.,* 1989; Tighe & Ciclitira, 1995). These particular alleles are present in 98 per cent of northern European and 92 per cent of southern European coeliac individuals.

The association between coeliac disease and the HLA-B8, DR3, DQ2 haplotype does not fully explain the genetic susceptibility for coeliac disease, since there are many normal individuals with this haplotype who do not have the disease. Nevertheless, this haplotype or one closely associated is always necessary for the disease to develop. This is possibly related to the fact that the class II gene products, i.e. the DQα and β chains, are necessary for presentation of a specific gliadin peptide(s) to the T cell receptor of CD4 lymphocytes (so-called T helper cells). One can thus propose that the immunological basis for the development of the mucosal pathology in coeliac disease is one where a particular gliadin peptide is presented by disease-specific class II molecules on antigen-presenting cells in the mucosa to the lymphocyte clones with T cell receptors specific for the disease initiating epitope of the gliadin. The lymphocytes, particularly CD4 positive (helper) cells then initiate an immunological response, leading to the activation of pro-inflammatory cytokines, complement and immunoglobulin-producing plasma cells (Trejdosiewicz & Howdle, 1995). Evidence for such immunological events is emerging; for example Lundin *et al.* (1993) isolated activated CD4 T cells from coeliac mucosa and showed they were reactive to specific gliadin peptides only when the epitopes were presented by the DQ heterodimer (α1*0501-β1*0201). These data demonstrate that antigen-specific T helper cells exist in the coeliac mucosa and are MHC Class II restricted.

Apart from evidence of immunological activity at the molecular level, there is also morphological evidence of lymphocytic involvement. In a long series of elegant studies, Marsh (Marsh, 1992; Marsh & Crowe, 1995) demonstrated that epithelial lymphocytes in coeliac patients respond in a dose-dependent fashion to gluten challenge. Lymphocytic infiltration and blast formation are early pathological signs occurring before major architectural changes occur with larger and more prolonged gluten loads. These studies therefore support the hypothesis that lymphocyte activation is a precursor of pathological change in the coeliac mucosa.

As the small intestinal pathology develops in coeliac disease, there are also many other immunological abnormalities to be noted, for example not only do epithelial but also lamina propria lymphocytes undergo activation (Trejdosiewicz & Howdle, 1995). These populations are predominantly CD8+ or CD4+ respectively (Trejdosiewicz & Howdle, 1995). The epithelial lymphocytes also show an increased expression of the $\gamma\delta$ form of the T cell receptor, the significance of which is unknown (Halstensen *et al.,* 1989; Trejdosiewicz *et al.,* 1991). Plasma cell numbers for most immunoglobulin classes are increased (Brandtzaeg & Baklien, 1976; Scott *et al.,* 1984; Wood *et al.,* 1987). Concomitantly, there is increased *in vitro* immunoglobulin production (Wood *et al.,* 1986, 1987) including specific antibodies (Ciclitira *et al.,* 1986). More recently, similar observations have been made in intestinal secretions (O'Mahony *et al.,* 1990, 1991). There are some old observations demonstrating immunoglobulin and complement deposition in coeliac mucosa (Doe *et al.,* 1974; Scott *et al.,* 1977) and some very recent observations of the transcription profiles of cytokine genes after gluten challenge (Kontakon *et al.,* 1995).

There is thus abundant evidence of immunological activation and involvement in the pathogenesis of the mucosal lesion of coeliac disease. A simplified model for immunologically mediated mucosal damage in coeliac disease is shown in Fig. 2.

As expected, however, bearing in mind the lymphocyte traffic associated with the gut-associated

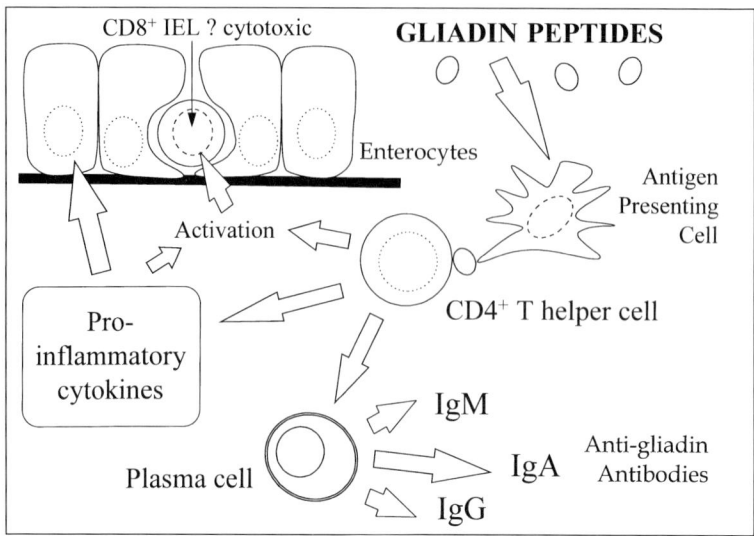

Fig. 2. A diagrammatic model of the mucosal immunological reaction in coeliac disease.

lymphoid tissue, there are systemic perturbations of the immune system in coeliac disease. Some of these were described some time ago, for example the total number of circulating lymphocytes is reduced (O'Donoghue *et al.*, 1976; Bullen & Losowsky, 1978a) although the CD4: CD8 balance is unaltered (Corazza *et al.*, 1983). Several groups have examined peripheral suppressor cell activity in coeliac disease, reporting both increases (Robertson *et al.*, 1982; O'Farrelly *et al.*, 1984a, b) and decreases (Corazza *et al.*, 1986; Sollid *et al.*, 1986). O'Farrelly *et al.* (1984a) suggested that increased helper cell numbers in the small intestinal mucosa, together with increased peripheral suppressor cell activity, may reflect a redistribution of T cell subsets in coeliac disease. This hypothesis is supported by the finding of an inverse relationship between peripheral and mucosal leucocyte migration inhibition factor production, this being related to the gluten content of the diet, suggesting that in the untreated state gluten-sensitive lymphocytes are more likely to be in the mucosa, at the site of gluten presentation, rather than in the periphery (Howdle *et al.*, 1986). Such findings are supported by the observation that a migration inhibition factor is produced in response to gluten peptides by peripheral blood leucocytes, particularly from treated coeliac patients (Bullen & Losowsky, 1978b; Karagiannis *et al.*, 1987; Mantzaris *et al.*, 1990). Leucocyte migration inhibition is not, however, exclusively mediated by T cell factors and could be due to antibody or immune complexes, both of which are present in the circulation of coeliac patients (Corazza *et al.*, 1989; Simpson *et al.*, 1983).

The macrophage procoagulant assay has been suggested as a more specific test of cell-mediated immunity. Devery and colleagues (1990, 1991) showed responses to gluten peptides in peripheral blood of coeliac but not control patients. A related observation from our laboratory is that an increase in serum soluble IL2 receptor in coeliac patients is related to the gluten content of the diet (Crabtree *et al.*, 1989). Since soluble IL2 receptor is principally shed by activated T cells, this is evidence of gluten-related T cell activation in coeliac disease.

Another important observation in the peripheral blood of coeliac disease comes from Gjertsen *et al.* (1994) who isolated and cloned a gluten-specific T cell line from the peripheral blood of a coeliac patient. This clone was also HLA-DQ restricted in its response.

Apart from the changes related to cell-mediated immunity, there are many observations concerning humoral immunity in the peripheral blood in coeliac disease. Early studies reported varying changes in the levels of serum immunoglobulins (Howdle & Losowsky, 1987), although IgA and secretory IgA are usually raised in untreated patients. More recently investigators have measured the levels of isotype anti-gliadin antibodies. These are raised in untreated coeliac patients and are widely used as screening tests for the disease (Troncone & Ferguson, 1991). There is a wide variety of methods, and varying degrees of sensitivity and specificity have been reported (Maki, 1995). Apart from anti-gliadin antibodies, various tissue autoantibodies have also been measured and such assays are also used as screening tests for coeliac disease (Maki, 1995). IgA anti-reticulin antibodies are valuable in the early recognition of coeliac disease (Unsworth & Brown, 1994). The anti-endomysial antibody test has gained popularity in recent years as it gives almost 100 per cent sensitivity and specificity as a screening test for coeliac disease (Maki, 1995). These tissue autoantibodies, although present in the serum, are directed against fibroblast-derived extracellular matrix proteins. Their role in the pathogenesis of coeliac disease is unclear, but it is possible that some of the pathological findings could be the result of autoimmune mechanisms. Apart from the findings related to serum antibody levels in coeliac disease, investigators have also estimated the complement levels and looked for evidence of circulating immune complexes. In general, complement levels are low and immune complexes are present in untreated patients (Howdle & Losowsky, 1987), these observations being in accord with those of complement and immunoglobulin deposition in the mucosa (see above).

Table 1. Some reported systemic diseases associated with coeliac disease

Skin	CNS	Haematological
vasculitis	spinocerebellar degeneration	thrombocytopenic purpura
	epilepsy*	haemolytic anaemia
	Down's syndrome*	hyposplenism*
Lung	Psychiatric	Gastrointestinal
fibrosing alveolitis	schizophrenia	pancreatic insufficiency
bird fancier's lung*	depression	Crohn's disease*
	autism	
Liver	Connective tissue disorders	
primary biliary cirrhosis*	rheumatoid arthritis*	
primary sclerosing cholangitis*	systemic lupus erythematosis	
	sarcoidosis*	
Heart	Endocrine	
recurrent pericarditis*	insulin-dependent diabetes*	
	thyroid disorders*	
Renal	Oral	
IgA nephropathy*	recurrent ulcers*	
glomerulonephritis	dental enamel hypoplasia*	

*Evidence exists of an association which is more than coincidental (Corazza & Gasbarrini, 1995).

From the foregoing summary, it is obvious that there are many immunological perturbations in coeliac disease which occur outside the gastrointestinal tract.

The implication of this review is that coeliac disease is primarily a disease of the small intestinal mucosa caused by an immune reaction to a gliadin peptide in genetically predisposed individuals. The many systemic perturbations described are therefore probably secondary phenomena resulting from the immunological activity in the gut.

The question could be asked: do these systemic perturbations have any clinical significance? There is no simple answer to that question but there are several systemic diseases associated with coeliac disease, where the basis of the association could be immunological. A list of some of these associated diseases is shown in Table 1 (see also Cooke & Holmes, 1984; Howdle & Losowsky, 1992; Corazza & Gasbarrini, 1995). Although such associations may be fortuitous and are probably reported simply because coeliac disease is a fairly common and life-long condition, there are certainly some diseases for which the association is more than coincidental (see Table 1). Such associations may be due to MHC similarities, secondary crossing of antigens through a damaged small intestinal mucosa, deposition of immune complexes in target organs, a reduction in immune surveillance or an activated immune system.

References

Booth, C.C. (1974): Definition of adult coeliac disease. In: *Coeliac disease,* eds. W.T.J.M. Hekkens & A.S. Pena, pp. 17–22. Leiden: Stenfert Kroese.

Brandtzaeg, P. & Baklien. K. (1976): Immunoglobulin-producing cells in the intestine in health and disease. *Clin. Gastroenterol.* **5,** 251–269.

Bullen, A.W & Losowsky, M.S. (1978a): Lymphocyte subpopulations in adult coeliac disease. *Gut* **19,** 892–897.

Bullen, A.W. & Losowsky, M.S. (1978b): Cell mediated immunity to gluten fraction III in adult coeliac disease. *Gut* **19,** 126–131.

Ciclitira, P.J., Evans, D.J., Fagg, N.L.K. *et al.* (1984): Clinical testing of gliadin fractions in coeliac patients. *Clin. Sci.* **66,** 357–364.

Ciclitira, P.J., Ellis, H.J., Wood, G.M., Howdle, P.D. & Losowsky, M.S. (1986): Secretion of gliadin antibody by coeliac jejunal mucosal biopsies cultured *in vitro. Clin. Exp. Immunol.* **64,** 119–124.

Cooke, W.T. & Holmes, G.K.T. (1984): *Coeliac disease.* pp. 225–246. Edinburgh: Churchill Livingstone.

Corazza, G.R., Tabacchi, P., Frisoni, M. *et al.* (1983): T-lymphocyte subsets in adult coeliac disease. *Clin. Sci.* **65,** 89–90.

Corazza, G.R., Sardinelli, P., Londei, M. *et al.* (1986): Gluten specific suppressor T cell dysfunction in coeliac disease. *Gut* **27,** 392–398.

Corazza G.R., Frisoni, M., Mule, P. *et al.* (1989): Cytophilic antibodies cause leucocyte migration inhibition in coeliac disease. *J. Lab. Clin. Med.* **28,** 79–83.

Corazza GR, Gasbarrini G (1995): Coeliac disease in adults. In: *Coeliac disease,* Bailliere's Clinical Gastroenterology, Vol. 9, ed. P.D. Howdle, pp. 329–350. London: Bailliere Tindall.

Crabtree J.E., Heatley, R.V., Juby, L.D. *et al.* (1989): Serum interleukin 2 receptor in coeliac disease: response to treatment and gluten challenge. *Clin. Exp. Immunol.* **77,** 345–348.

De Ritis, G., Auricchio, S., Jones, H.W. *et al.* (1988): *In vitro* (organ culture) studies of the toxicity of specific A-gliadin peptides in celiac disease. *Gastroenterology* **94,** 41–49.

Devery, J.M., Ceczy, C.L., de Carle, D.J. *et al.* (1990): Macrophage procoagulant activity as an assay of cellular hypersensitivity to gluten peptides in coeliac disease. *Clin. Exp. Immunol.* **82,** 333–337.

Devery, J.M., Bender, V., Pentilla, I. & Skerritt, J.H. (1991): Identification of reactive synthetic gliadin peptides specific for coeliac disease. *Int. Arch. Allergy Appl. Immunol.* **95,** 356–362.

Doe, W.F., Henry, K. & Booth, C.C. (1974): Complement in coeliac disease. In: *Coeliac disease,* eds. W.T.J.M. Hekkens & A.S. Pena, pp. 189–196. Leiden: Stenfert Kroese.

Gjertsen, H., Lundin, K., Sollid, L., Eriksen, J. & Thorsby, E. (1994): T-cells recognise a peptide derived from α-gliadin presented by the coeliac disease associated HLA-DQ (α1*0501, β1*0201) heterodimer. *Hum. Immunol.* **39,** 243–252.

Gobbi, G., Bouquet, F., Greco, L. *et al.* (1992): Coeliac disease, epilepsy and cerebral calcifications. *Lancet* **340,** 439–443.

Halstensen, T.S., Scott, H. & Brandtzaeg, P. (1989): Intraepithelial T cells of the TcR γ/δ+ CD8-Vδ1/Jδ1+ phenotypes are increased in coeliac disease. *Scand. J. Immunol.* **30,** 665–672.

Howdle, P.D., Ciclitira, P.J., Simpson, F.G. & Losowsky, M.S. (1984): Are all gliadins toxic in coeliac disease? An *in vitro* study of α, β, γ and ω-gliadins. *Scand. J. Gastroenterol.* **19,** 41–47.

Howdle, P.D., Simpson, F.G. & Losowsky, M.S. (1986): The distribution of gluten-sensitive lymphocytes in coeliac patients – is it related to dietary gluten? *Clin. Exp. Immunol.* **66,** 393–398.

Howdle, P.D. & Losowsky, M.S. (1987): The immunology of coeliac disease. In: *Gastrointestinal and liver immunology*, Bailliere's Clinical Gastroenterology, Vol. 1, eds. R. Wright & H.J.P. Hodgson, pp. 507–529. London: Bailliére Tindall.

Howdle, P.D. & Losowsky, M.S. (1992): Coeliac disease in adults. In: *Coeliac disease*, eds. M.N. Marsh, pp. 49–80. Oxford: Blackwell.

Karagiannis, J.A., Priddle, J.D. & Jewell, D.P. (1987): Cell-mediated immunity to a synthetic gliadin peptide resembling a sequence from adenovirus 12. *Lancet* **i,** 884–886.

Kasarda, D.D., Okita, T.W., Bernadin, J.E. *et al.* (1984): Nucleic acid and amino acid sequences of α-type gliadins from wheat. Proceedings of the National Academy of Sciences of the USA, **81,** 4712–4716.

Keuning, J., Pena, A.S., Van Leeuwen, A. *et al.* (1976): HLA-Dw3 associated with coeliac disease. *Lancet* **i,** 506–507.

Kontakon, M., Przemioslo, R.T., Sturgess, R.P., Limb, G.A., Ellis, H.J., Day, P. & Ciclitira, P.J. (1995): Cytokine mRNA expression in the mucosa of treated coeliac patients after wheat peptide challenge. *Gut* **37,** 52–57.

Lundin, K.E.A., Scott, H., Hansen, T. *et al.* (1993): Gliadin-specific HLA-DQ (α1*0501, (β1*0201) restricted T cells isolated from the small intestinal mucosa of celiac disease patients. *J. Exp. Med.* **178,** 187–196.

Maki, M. (1995): The humoral immune system in coeliac disease. In: *Coeliac disease*, Baillière's Clinical Gastroenterology, Vol. 9, eds. P.D. Howdle, pp. 231–249. London: Bailliere Tindall.

Mantzaris, G.J., Karagiannis, J.A., Priddle, J.D. & Jewell, D.P. (1990): Cellular hypersensitivity to a synthetic dodecapeptide derived from human adenovirus 12 which resembles a sequence of A-gliadin in patients with coeliac disease. *Gut* **31,** 668–673.

Marsh, M.N. (1992): Mucosal pathology in gluten sensitivity. In *Coeliac disease*, ed. M.N. Marsh, pp. 136–191. Oxford, Blackwell,

Marsh, M.N. & Crowe, P.T. (1995): Morphology of the mucosal lesion in gluten sensitivity. In: *Coeliac disease*, Bailliere's Clinical Gastroenterology, Vol. 9, ed. P.D. Howdle, pp. 273–293. London: Bailliere Tindall.

O'Donoghue, D.P., Lancaster-Smith, M., Laviniere, P. & Kumar, P.J. (1976): T cell depletion in untreated adult coeliac disease. *Gut* **17,** 328–331.

O'Farrelly, C., Feighery, C.F., Whelan, C.A. & Weir, D.G. (1984a): Suppressor cell activity in coeliac disease induced by α-gliadin. *Lancet* **ii,** 1305–1307.

O'Farrelly, C., McKeever, V., Feighery, C.F. & Weir, D.G. (1984b): Increased conconavalin A-induced suppression in treated and untreated coeliac disease. *Gut* **25,** 644–648.

O'Mahony, S, Vestey, J.P. & Ferguson, A. (1990): Similarities in intestinal humoral immunity in dermatitis herpetiformis without enteropathy and in coeliac disease. *Lancet* **335,** 1487–1490.

O'Mahony, S., Arranz. E., Barton, J.R. & Ferguson, A. (1991): Dissociation between systemic and mucosal humoral immune responses in coeliac disease. *Gut* **32,** 29–35.

Robertson, D.A.F., Bullen, A.W., Field, H.P. *et al.* (1982): Suppressor cell activity, splenic function and HLA-B8 status in man. *J. Clin. Lab. Immunol.* **9,** 133–138.

Scott, B.B., Scott, D.G. & Losowsky, M.S. (1977): Jejunal mucosal immunoglobulins and complement in untreated coeliac disease. *J. Pathol.* **121,** 219–223.

Scott, B.B., Goodall, A., Stephenson, P. & Jenkins, D. (1984): Small intestinal plasma cells in coeliac disease. *Gut* **25,** 41–46.

Shewry, P.R., Tatham, A.S. & Kasarda, D.D. (1992): Cereal proteins and coeliac disease. In: *Coeliac disease*, ed. M.N. Marsh, pp. 304–348. Oxford: Blackwell.

Simpson, F.G., Field, H.P., Howdle, P.D. *et al.* (1983): Leucocyte migration inhibition test in coeliac disease – a reappraisal. *Gut* **24,** 311–317.

Sollid, L.M., Brusend, O., Ganderneck, G. & Thorsby, E. (1986): The role of the CD8 positive subset of T cells in proliferative responses to soluble antigens. *Scand. J. Immunol.* **23,** 461–467.

Sollid, L., Markussen, G. & Ek, J. (1989): Evidence for a primary association of coeliac disease to a particular HLA-DQ α/β heterodimer. *J. Exp. Med.* **169,** 345–350.

Stokes, P., Asquith, P., Holmes, G.K.T. *et al.* (1972): Histocompatibility antigens associated with adult coeliac disease. *Lancet* **ii,** 162–164.

Tighe, M.R. & Ciclitira, P.J. (1995): The gluten-host interaction. In: *Coeliac disease*, Baillière's Clinical Gastroenterology, Vol. 9, ed. P.D. Howdle, pp. 211–230. London: Bailliere Tindall.

Trejdosiewicz, L.K., Calabrese, A., Smart, C.J. *et al.* (1991): γ/δ T cell receptor-positive cells of the human gastrointestinal mucosa: occurrence and V region gene expression in *H. pylori*-associated gastritis, coeliac disease and inflammatory bowel disease. *Clin. Exp. Immunol.* **84,** 440–444.

Trejdosiewicz, L.K. & Howdle, P.D. (1995): T cell responses and cellular immunity in coeliac disease. In *Coeliac disease,* Bailliere's Clinical Gastroenterology, Vol. 9, ed. P.D. Howdle, pp. 251–272. London: Bailliere Tindall.

Trier, J.S. (1991): Celiac Sprue. *N. Engl. J. Med.* **325,** 1709–1719.

Troncone, R. & Ferguson, A (1991): Anti-gliadin antibodies. *J. Pediatr. Gastroenterol. Nutr.* **12,** 150–158.

Unsworth, D.J. & Brown, D.I. (1994): Serological screening suggests that adult coeliac disease is underdiagnosed in the UK and increases the incidence by up to 12 per cent. *Gut* **35,** 61–64.

Wieser, H. (1995): The precipitating factor in coeliac disease. In *Coeliac disease,* Bailliere's Clinical Gastroenterology, Vol. 9, ed. P.D. Howdle, pp. 191–207. London: Bailliere Tindall.

Wieser, H., Beltz, H-D., Ashkenazi, A. & Idar, D. (1983): Isolation of coeliac-active peptide fractions from gliadin. *Zeit. Lebens-Unters. Forschung,* **176,** 85–94.

Wieser, H., Beltz, H-D., Ashkenazi, A. & Idar, D. (1984): Amino acid sequence of the coeliac active peptide BB142. *Zeit. Lebens-Unters. Forschung* **179,** 371–376.

Wieser, H., Beltz, H-D., Idar, D. & Ashkenazi, A. (1986): Coeliac activity of the gliadin peptides CT-1 and CT-2. *Zeit. Lebens-Unters. Forschung,* **182,** 115–117.

Wood, G., Shires, S., Howdle, P.D. & Losowsky, M.S. (1986): Immunoglobulin production by coeliac biopsies in organ culture. *Gut* **27,** 1151–1160.

Wood, G.M., Howdle, P.D., Trejdosiewicz, L.K. & Losowsky, M.S. (1987): Jejunal plasma cells and in vitro immunoglobulin production in adult coeliac disease. *Clin. Exp. Immunol.* **69,** 123–132.

Epilepsy and other neurological disorders in coeliac disease, edited by G. Gobbi *et al.*
© 1997 John Libbey & Company Ltd, pp. 55–58.

Chapter 8

Role of the HLA class II molecules in the pathogenesis of coeliac disease

Maria Cristina Mazzilli and Margherita Bonamico

Departments of Experimental Medicine and Paediatrics, University of Rome, 'La Sapienza', Italy

Introduction

Coeliac disease (CD), also known as gluten sensitive enteropathy (GSE), is a malabsorptive disorder precipitated in susceptible individuals by the ingestion of gluten proteins.

The earliest evidence that genetic factors are of significance in the susceptibility to CD consisted of isolated reports of multiple cases occurring within families. Subsequently, family studies clearly demonstrated that CD occurred more frequently in the relatives of patients than in the general population (Ellis *et al.*, 1981). In addition, the high rate of concordance for the disorder among monozygotic twins (71 per cent), emphasized the importance of genetic factors (Polanco *et al.*, 1984.

Despite these observations, the mode of inheritance remained unclear: CD belongs to the group of complex genetic diseases that have a tendency to cluster in families but show no discernible inheritance pattern. Family members share most of their genes but also their environment: both factors can cause familial clustering of the disease and it is not easy to discern between them. The discovery that coeliac disease was more frequent among subjects carrying particular histocompatibility antigens represented a major advance. Indeed, HLA appeared to be the main genetic factors in the susceptibility to CD.

The human major histocompatibility complex

HLA

The HLA molecules (Germain, 1994) are encoded by genes located within the major histocompatibility complex (MHC). Cytogenetic studies have mapped the MHC region to the p21.3 band on the short arm of chromosome 6, where it spans approximately four million base pairs of DNA. This complex region contains more than 100 expressed or non-expressed genes arranged in three major gene clusters named class I, class II and class III.

Class I

The class I region contains genes which encode the classical transplantation antigens HLA-A, -B and -C and the other non-classical ones, including HLA-E, -F and -G. HLA class I antigens which are heterodimeric membrane-bound glycoproteins made up of a highly polymorphic heavy chain of 45 kD. This is non-covalently associated with a non-polymorphic β2-microglobulin (β2m), a 123 kD serum protein encoded by a gene on chromosome 15.

Class II

The HLA-D region contains genes encoding three major types of human class II molecules, designated HLA-DR, DQ and DP and coded by three distinct subregions. Class II molecules are heterodimeric membrane-bound glycoproteins which consist of an α (or heavy) chain of 35 kD, and a β (light) chain of 28 kD. The two chains are non-covalently associated. Each subregion contains characteristic α and β chain genes; in the current nomenclature, the protein product is denoted by α or β, and their respective genes by the suffix A or B. The HLA-DR a chain is therefore encoded by the HLA-DRA gene. There is one DRA and multiple DRB genes in the DR subregion. The DRA gene shows very little polymorphism, indeed only one aminoacid substitution has been found from the sequencing of multiple genes. By contrast, the DRB genes are extremely polymorphic. There are individual variations in the number of DRB loci within the subregion, in the number of loci expressed, and the type of alleles at each individual locus. To date, nine DRB loci have been described: DRB1–9, of which all but DRBI, 3, 4 and 5 are pseudogenes. The DRB1 gene is expressed in all haplotypes but the second expressed DRB locus differs according to the haplotype. For DR4, DR7 and DR9 it is DRB4; for DR2 it is DRB5 and for the remainder it is DRB3. At present 60 DRB1 alleles are known, four DRB3 alleles, one DRB4 and four DRB5 alleles.

Two pairs of DQA and DQB genes are present in all haplotypes studied. The DQA1 and B1 genes are expressed and give rise to a well-characterized protein product. Although the DQA2 and B2 genes (previously also known as DX genes) are transcribed, no protein product from these loci has been defined. When DQ $\alpha\beta$ dimers were first identified by alloantisera, they were referred to as DC molecules; DC was reclassified as DQ in 1984. In contrast to DR, there is polymorphism of both the DQA and DQB gene. By DNA sequence, 14 DQA1 and 19 DRB1 alleles are now defined.

There are two sets of HLA-DP genes within the subregion although only the DPA1 and DPB1 genes are expressed as a product; the DPA2 and B2 genes are non-functional pseudogenes, because of several deleterious mutations in the coding sequences. Sequencing studies have revealed 8 DPA1 and 38 DPB1 alleles.

Class III

The class III region contains a heterogeneous collection of over 30 genes, including those that encode the complement proteins Factor B, C2 and C4, the enzyme 21-OH hydroxylase, the heat shock protein HSP70 and tumour necrosis factor (TNF-A and -B).

Polymorphism, haplotypes and linkage-disequilibrium

As mentioned above, one of the hallmarks of the HLA gene products is its high degree of polymorphism. Each genetic region contains several related genes at different loci and there are multiple alleles at each locus. Serological methods remain an important tool for the detection of polymorphism and, in addition to polyclonal antisera which continue to be the mainstay of HLA-typing, monoclonal reagents against HLA class I and class II antigens are now widely available. In the last ten years sophisticated molecular methods have been developed that provided further information on the fine structure of HLA molecules and the complexity of the polymorphic variations. The use of the polymerase chain reaction to amplify specific DNA sequences has greatly facilitated the analysis of HLA polymorphism and the structural basis of allelic variation.

Because of their close linkage, the combination of alleles at each locus on a single chromosome is usually inherited as a unit named haplotype. By simple Mendelian rules, 25 per cent, 50 per cent and 25 per cent of sib pairs will share 2, 1 and no haplotypes respectively.

In spite of this co-segregation within families, at population level the expected frequency of finding a given allele at an HLA locus with a given allele at a second HLA locus should be the product of the frequencies of these two alleles. On the contrary some of the HLA haplotypic combinations are over-represented: alleles at two different loci on the same chromosome occur together more frequently than would be expected by chance. The difference between the observed and expected frequencies is termed 'linkage disequilibrium' (LD). The HLA system shows a high degree of LD between alleles at different loci. LD has been observed between class I, class II, and class III alleles; within the HLA-D subregion, LD between DR and DQ alleles is very strong.

Function of HLA molecules

The principal biological function of HLA molecules is to bind peptide fragments of processed protein antigens and present them to T cells. Class I molecules mainly bind peptide fragments of endogenous proteins, while class II molecules bind peptide fragments of exogenous proteins. Recently, genes involved in antigen processing, TAP, LMP and DM genes, have also been mapped to the class II region of the complex. From analysis of antigen-specific T-cell clones, the minimal length of a peptide fragment which retains T-cell stimulatory proprieties can be deduced. For class I-restricted antigens, the minimum length is nine amino acids, while for class II-restricted antigens, the peptides vary in length, usually between 10 to 20 amino acids in length. Recently, the structural proprieties of a number of these peptide antigens have become clearer, as a result of crystallographic data and aminoacid sequencing of peptides eluted from MHC molecules. These studies have also revealed that different HLA alleles favour the binding of peptides with characteristic sequence motifs. This immune response to different etiopathogenic factors will depend upon the HLA typing of the subject. The comprehension of this biological function of HLA molecules gave reasons for the evolution of HLA polymorphism and its association with autoimmune disease.

HLA and coeliac disease associations

Coeliac disease was first found to be associated with the HLA class I molecule B8. Later on, a stronger association to the class II molecule DR3 was described. The reported associations have been derived from comparison of the distribution of HLA antigens among patients and random controls. The frequency of HLA-B8 and -DR3 (which are in linkage disequilibrium with each other) is increased in CD patients in all populations studied.

DR7 has also been reported to be associated with CD but not in all populations. DR3 and DR7 are in strong LD with DQ2, so that DQ2 has resulted as being the best marker of the disease. These studies are extensively reviewed in Sollid and Thorsby (1993).

We have reported that in an Italian paediatric CD group, living in Rome, the DR7 association was almost completely due to the DR5,7 combination. Similar results have been described in Spanish and in Latin American populations. The high frequency of DR5,7 heterozygotes, significantly higher than that expected by chance, suggested that, besides DQ2, an additional predisposing gene to CD should be carried in the HLA region, closely associated with DR5. DQ2 is a serological determinant of the β chain coded by the DQB1*0201 allele in disequilibrium with DR3 and DR7. Furthermore, DQA1*0501 is associated with DR3 and DR5, so that DR3,x and DR5,7 subjects share the DQA1*0501 and B1*0201 alleles. inherited in cis with DR3 or in trans with DR5 (α chain) and with DR7 (β chain) haplotypes. Different studies confirmed a primary HLA association of CD to the DQ(α1*0501,β1*0201) heterodimer encoded in *cis* or in *trans* position. The immunopathogenic importance of this association is documented by the finding that, in the small intestine, the CD-associated DQ heterodimer represents the main gluten-presenting molecule.

In the examined group of Roman children, we have reported that 92 per cent of CD patients (50 per cent DR3 and 42 per cent DR5,7) carried the DQα/β dimer at risk (Mazzilli et al. 1992). In accordance with previous studies, most of the dimer negative patients typed as DR4, DQ8.

Investigations in HLA and disease associations have made increasing use of family studies. One particularly fruitful approach to the elucidation of the genetics of HLA susceptibility genes has been to examine the segregation of parental HLA haplotypes in sibships containing two or more affected individuals. Affected sib pairs will share the genes causing the disease over the frequencies expected at random in siblings.

We carried out the oligotyping for DRB1, DQA1 and DQB1 genes in 18 affected sib pairs using standard methods. All the families belong to the Italian population except for one. The diagnosis was based on the ESPGAN criteria. The significant distortion of the expected numbers of sib pairs sharing 2,1,0 haplotypes (55 per cent, 33 per cent, 11 per cent vs. 25 per cent, 50 per cent and 25 per cent expected) still confirmed the role of HLA in the pathogenesis of CD.

In a study on 325 first-degree relatives, we estimated the prevalence of CD to be approximately 8.3 per cent. This result is in agreement with the value of 8.7 per cent previously reported (Auricchio et al., 1988). However, when parents and siblings were considered separately, the risks in the two groups were significantly different, being 3 per cent and 18 per cent respectively. As a statistical difference was detected between siblings and parents carrying HLA molecules at risk (79 per cent vs. 59 per cent, $P = 2.1 \times 10^{-3}$), the number of affected siblings over those at risk (30 per cent) was much higher than the number of affected parents over parents at risk (2.2 per cent).

Acknowledgement

This work was partially supported by P.F. Ingegneria Genetica, CNR.

References

Auricchio, S., Mazzacca, G., Tosi, R., Visakorpi, J., Maki, M. & Polanco, I. (1988): Coeliac disease as a familial condition: identification of asymptomatic coeliac patients within family groups. *Gastroenterol. Int.* **1**, 25–31.

Ellis, A. (1981): Coeliac disease: previous family studies. In: *The genetics of coeliac disease,* ed. R.B. McConnel, pp. 197–200. Lancaster: MTP Press.

Germain, R.N. (1994): MHC-dependent antigen processing and peptide presentation: providing ligands for T lymphocyte activation. *Cell* **76**, 287–299.

Mazzilli, M.C., Ferrante, P., Mariani, P., Martone, E., Petronzelli, F., Triglione, P. & Bonamico, M. (1992): A study of Italian pediatric celiac disease patients confirms that the primary HLA association is to the DQ(α1*0501,β1*0201) heterodimer. *Hum. Immunol.* **33**, 133–139.

Polanco, I., Biemond, I., van Leecuwen, A., Schreuder, I., Meera, Khan, P.M., Guerrero, J., D'Amaro, J., Vazquez, C., van Rood, J.J. & Pena, A.S. (1981): Gluten sensitive enteropathy in Spain: genetic and environmental factors. In: *The genetics of coeliac disease*, ed. R.B McConnel, pp 211–231. Lancaster: MTP Press.

Sollid, L.M. & Thorsby, E. (1993): HLA susceptibility genes in celiac disease: genetic mapping and role in pathogenesis. *Gastroenterology* **105**, 910–922.

Epilepsy and other neurological disorders in coeliac disease, edited by G. Gobbi *et al.*
© 1997 John Libbey & Company Ltd, pp. 59–62.

Chapter 9

The significance of HLA association in neurological diseases

Maria Giovanna Marrosu

Cattedra di Neuropsichiatria Infantile II, Università di Cagliari, Via Ospedale 119, 09124 Cagliari, Italy

Introduction

The HLA system consists of many different subregions located on the short arm of chromosome 6. The majority of HLA-disease associations are concerned with class II genes, key participants in triggering activation of autoimmunity, which also occurs in the normal immune response. The HLA-class II region encompasses approximately 1000 kb of DNA and is divided into three major subregions known as DP, DQ and DR. Each of these subregions contains at least one pair of expressed genes encoding a pair of functionally expressed α and β chains. For example, the DQ region contains DQA1 and DQB1 genes, which code for DQα and DQβ chains respectively. The α and β chains form an α-β heterodimer expressed on the surface of the antigen-presenting cell restricted to helper or suppressor T lymphocytes. Some haplotypes contain up to 14 class II loci, but limitation in the expression of permissive α-β dimers restricts the expressed repertoire to four class II molecules for haplotype: DPα-β, DQα-β, DRα-β1, DRα β3,4,5. Each class II haplotype includes DPα-β, DQα-β, DRα-β1, DRα-β3 or 4 or 5, the latter being determined by the haplotype considered.

Whereas DRα chains are essentially invariant, DRβ, DQα, DQβ, DPα and DPβ chains exhibit sequence variants that are responsible for polymorphisms of the class II region characteristic of these molecules. This polymorphism is determined by the germline genetic repertoire of the class II region with multiple alleles at most class II loci. For this reason, it is of paramount importance to know the exact sequence of the class II alleles. Initially, the nomenclature of HLA was referred to on the basis of serologic specificity, such as DR2, DR3, DR4 etc. This specificity is not able to distinguish the sequence of alleles. On the contrary, molecular analysis provides a high degree of gene-specific and haplotype-specific information.

The polymorphism of class II alleles is crucial to immune activation events; it essentially acts in two ways. Initially, polymorphic amino acids determine whether or not specific antigenic peptides will bind and be presented on the surface of antigen-presenting cells to T lymphocytes. Secondly, the polymorphism regulates the developmental selection of T-cell receptor specificities during the process of T-cell differentiation and maturation in the thymus.

The primary sequence of the amino-terminal polymorphic domain is critical for the proper presentation of the antigen to T-cell receptor. Both α and β chains contain two external domains; the membrane external domain is the major site of variation. The foundation for genetic restriction of foreign antigen recognition lies in the formation of a peptide binding groove, the structure of which has been hypothesized by analogy with the class I crystallographic structure. As a similarity, the amino terminal domains of both the α and β chains contribute to α-helices which line the sides and to anti-parallel sheets which line the floor of the peptide binding groove (Brown *et al.*, 1993). Polymorphic amino acids are localized in regions lining the sides and the floor of the peptide binding groove. The peptide is likely to be oriented with its amino terminus at the left-hand end of the binding cleft and its carboxy terminus at the right hand end, as in class I molecules. The left-hand end of the cleft is composed mainly of residues contributed by the non-polymorphic DRα chain (Brown *et al.*, 1993).

Differences among HLA-DR molecules have been defined within three major regions of hypervariability and two regions of more limited variability. Some regions exhibit a hydrophobic pocket; the existence of a diallelic polymorphism of residue 86, as in DR β (G or V in different alleles) may affect this pocket, and could well contribute to the size of the pocket; in turn, this might permit the possibility of accomodating a large hydrophobic residue or an aromatic residue of the foreign peptide in this region (Krieger *et al.*, 1991). It should therefore be borne in mind that the stability of class II molecules requires peptide binding, but the precise class II molecule–peptide contacts that provide this energy have not yet been well defined (Chicz *et al.*, 1993). Identification of naturally processed peptides extracted and sequenced from class II molecules revealed that the bound peptides have 13–25 residues nested at the amino and/or carboxy-terminal ends, suggesting that the peptide binding groove is open at both ends (Krieger *et al.*, 1991). It has been demonstrated that the endogenous peptides can bind multiple DR alleles and this capability must be dependent on the composition and location of several key amino acids within the primary structure (Chicz *et al.*, 1993).

Diseases and HLA class II associations

Numerous studies have documented the presence of an association between certain HLA class II alleles and specific diseases, mainly autoimmune diseases (Nepom & Erlich, 1991). With the introduction of molecular biology techniques, we have been able to discriminate specific alleles associated to diseases (Bell *et al.*, 1989) and to examine the sequence of such alleles (Marsh & Bodmer, 1991). Since molecules encoding within the class II region of the HLA function as genetic restriction elements in the recognition of foreign Ag by CD4$^+$ T cells, the research challenge afforded in the field of HLA-disease association should be directed towards identification of specific key sequences determinant in immunoactivation.

A crucial point of HLA-disease association studies is the finding of allelic variations (amino acid residue polymorphism) which confer susceptibility or resistance to a given disease. Functionally these variations may act by virtue of specific peptide binding or, alternatively, by their role in establishing a T-cell receptor repertoire. For some diseases, a peripheral antigen-presentation function of the susceptibility molecules may be critical, whereas for other diseases the thymic selection role may predominate. In general, there are no specific rules for determinants of class II associated diseases.

A second problem of considerable importance is posed by the so-called linkage-disequilibrium: some DR and DQ alleles are inherited together on a chromosome as a single genetic unit termed a haplotype (haploid genotype). In this case, when a particular HLA gene is associated with a disease, it is not immediately obvious whether the gene itself or some linked gene on the same haplotype is primarily responsible for the disease association. For example, a single gene such as DQB1*0201 may be found in different haplotypes, associated with different DQA and DRB genes. Only through analysis of the extended haplotypes can a type of crude genetic mapping be obtained, which may then be exploited to pinpoint locus-specific and allele-specific contributions to susceptibility.

It is not surprising that many diseases involving immunologic dysfunction, particularly autoimmune diseases, are associated with certain polymorphic HLA alleles.

With regard to neurological diseases associated with HLA alleles, we should consider diseases where an autoimmune component is suspected, such as myasthenia gravis and multiple sclerosis (Tiwari & Terasaki, 1985), as well as other diseases in which autoimmunity is not necessarily involved, such as juvenile myoclonic epilepsy (Greenberg *et al.*, 1988) and narcolepsy (Tiwari & Terasaki, 1985). In the latter diseases, it may be hypothesized that one or more genes, which are strictly linked to HLA system, may confer an apparent association with HLA alleles. Linkage studies in multiplex families and new methodologies, such as linkage with microsatellites, may aid the further understanding of these associations.

The molecular genetic approach to matters concerning HLA and disease associations would involve:

  – first, identification of susceptible haplotype(s),

  – second, identification by analysis of polymorphic linked loci of individual genes in those haplotypes (in cis) or in other haplotypes (in trans) responsible for the association,

  – the third step would then be to identify those specific structural features of the candidate gene itself which could account for disease susceptibility.

The latter objective is greatly aided by the high degree of polymorphism of class II molecules, meaning by this, the variation of sequence occurring between closely related class II alleles.

To demonstrate the above, 2 DR2 splits can be observed, one of which is positively associated to multiple sclerosis, that is DRB1*1501, DQA1*0102, DQB1*0602 haplotype (Hillert & Olerup, 1993), the other DRB1*1601, DQA1*0102, DQB1*0502, negatively associated to MS (Marrosu *et al.*, 1992, 1993). Thus, for any candidate susceptibility gene there is a closely related allelic 'neighbour' not associated with disease. The latter affords the opportunity to compare sequences between the allelic 'nearest neighbours' to gain insight into specific amino acid polymorphisms that account for the susceptibility trait. Such a step bridges the gap between the strictly genetic analysis and the more functional questions of peptide binding and antigen presentation, providing a model of events which trigger autoimmune diseases.

References

Bell, J.I., Todd, J.A. & McDevitt, H.O. (1989): The molecular basis of HLA disease association. In: *Advances in human genetics,* eds. H. Harris, & K. Hirschorn, pp. 10–17. London: Plenum Press.

Brown, J.H., Jardetzky, T.S., Gorga, J.C., Stern, L.J., Urban, R.G., Strominger, J.L. & Wiley, D.C. (1993): Three-dimensional structure of the human class II histocompatibility antigen HLA-DR1. *Nature* **364,** 33–39.

Chicz, R.M., Urban, R.G., Gorga. J.C., Vignali, D.A.A., Lane, W.S. & Strominger, J.L. (1993): Specificity and promiscuity among naturally processed peptides bound to HLA-DR alleles. *J. Exp. Med.* **178,** 27–47.

Greenberg, D.A., Delgado- Escueta, A.V., Widlitz, H., Sparkes, R.S., Treiman, L. & Maldonado, H.M. (1988): Juvenile myoclonic epilepsy may be linked to the BF and HLA loci on human chromosome 6. *Am. J. Med. Genet.* **31,** 185–192.

Hillert, J. & Olerup, O. (1993): Multiple sclerosis is associated with genes within or close to the HLA-DR-DQ subregion on a normal DR15, DQ6, Dw2 haplotype. *Neurology* **43,** 163–168.

Krieger, J.I., Karr, R.W., Grey, H.M., Yu, W.-Y, O'Sullivan, D., Batovsky, L., Zheng, Z.-L., Colon, S.M., Gaeta, F.C.A., Sidney, J., Albertson, M., Del Guercio, M.-F., Chesnut, R.W. & Sette, A. (1991): Single amino acid changes in DR and antigen define residues crucial for peptide-MHC binding and T cell recognition. *J. Immunol.* **146,** 2331–2338.

Marrosu, M.G., Muntoni, F., Murru, M.R., Costa, G., Pischedda, M.P., Pirastu, M., Sotgiu, S., Rosati, G. & Cianchetti, C. (1992): HLA-DQB1 genotype in Sardinian multiple sclerosis: evidence for a key role of DQB1*0201 and *0302 alleles. *Neurology* **42,** 883–886.

Marrosu, M.G., Muntoni, F., Murru, M.R., Costa, G., Congia, M., Marrosu, G., Aiello, I., Pirastu, M. & Cianchetti, C. (1993): Role of predisposing and protective HLA-DQA and DQB alleles in Sardinian multiple sclerosis. *Arch. Neurol.* **50,** 256–260.

Marsh, S.G.E. & Bodmer, G. (1991): HLA class II nucleotide sequences, 1991. *Tissue Antigens* **37,** 181–189.

Nepom, G.T. & Erlich, H. (1991): MHC class II molecules and autoimmunity. *Annu. Rev. Immunol.* **9,** 443–525.

Tiwari, J. & Terasaki, P. (1985): HLA and disease association. New York: Springer-Verlag.

Part III
Epilepsy and coeliac disease

Epilepsy and other neurological disorders in coeliac disease, edited by G. Gobbi *et al.*
© 1997 John Libbey & Company Ltd, pp. 65–79.

Chapter 10

Coeliac disease and epilepsy

Giuseppe Gobbi*, Gianna Bertani* and the Italian Working Group (IWG)[1]
on Coeliac Disease and Epilepsy

Servizio di Neuropsichiatria Infantile, Arcispedale Santa Maria Nuova, Viale Risorgimento 80, 42100 Reggio Emilia, Italy

Introduction

Coeliac disease (CD) is a syndrome consisting of a permanent intolerance to gluten protein. The different clinical findings (active, silent and latent or potential CD) are largely reported in other chapters of this book (*see* Introduction and Chapters 1 and 2). The neurological symptoms of this disorder have already been extensively examined in the past (Cooke & Smith, 1966, Morris *et al.*, 1970; Cooke, 1976; Cooke & Holmes, 1984), and are largely reviewed in other parts of this book (*see* Chapters 33–40). The incidence of epilepsy in patients with coeliac disease and in patients with low folic acid levels has been reported in a number of studies (Grant *et al.*, 1965; Dennis & Taylor, 1969; Norris & Pratt, 1971; Reynolds, 1973; Garwicz & Mortensson, 1976; Laidlow *et al.*, 1977, Chapman *et al.*, 1978). A more recent review of this topic is reported in Chapters 15–17.

In 1988 we reported a severe type of progressive epilepsy in patients with bioccipital corticosubcortical calcifications resembling those found in the Sturge–Weber syndrome without a port-wine facial naevus (Gobbi *et al.*, 1988), and reviewed similar cases reported in the neurological literature

[1] **A. Ambrosetto and P. Ambrosetto**, *Clinica Neurologica, Universita' Bologna;* **F. Balli and V. Galli**, *Clinica Pediatrica, Universita' Modena;* **P. A. Battistella, C. Boniver and F. Donzelli**, *Dipartimento Pediatria, Universita' Padova;* **P. A. Bianchi, N. Molteni and M. T. Bardella**, *Patologia Medica III, Universita' Milano;* **F. Bouquet**, *Divisione di Neuropsichiatria Infantile, Istituto per l'Infanzia, Università Trieste;* **G. Capizzi**, *Istituto di Neuropsichiatria Infantile, Università Torino;* **A. Cernibori**, *Divisione di Neuropsichitria Infantile, Azienda Ospedaliera Sondrio;* **G. R. Corazza**, *Policlinico S. Orsola, Università Bologna;* **G. Della Cella and S. Babbini**, *Divisione di Pediatria, Ospedali Riuniti Chiavari;* **P. G. Garofalo, C. Durisotti and C. Filati**, *Divisione di Neurologia, Ospedale Civile Vicenza;* **A. M. Giunta**, *Clinica Pediatrica II, Università Milano;* **G. Gobbi, G. Bertani and A. Pini**, *Servizio di Neuropsichiatria Infantile, Arcispedale Santa Maria Nuova, Reggio Emilia;* **L. Greco, E. Del Giudice and F. Correale**, *Clinica Pediatrica, Universita' Napoli;* **A. Lambertini and M. G. Zaniboni**, *Divisione di Pediatria, Ospedale Maggiore Bologna;* **A. Miano**, *Divisione di Pediatria, Ospedale Bufalini Cesena;* **A. Parmeggiani and M. Santucci**, *Servizio di Neuropsichiatria Infantile, Università Bologna;* **A. Pascotto and G. Coppola**, *Istituto di Neuropsichiatria Infantile, Universita' Napoli;* **L. Piattella and N. Zamponi**, *Divisione di Neuropsichiatria Infantile, Ospedale Salesi Ancona;* **T. Sacquegna**, *Divisione di Neurologia, Ospedale Maggiore Bologna;* **P. Santanelli**, *Clinica Neurologica, Universita' Napoli;* **C. A. Tassinari**, *Divisione di Neurologia, Ospedale Bellaria, Universita' Bologna;* **C. Tiacci**, *Unità organica di Neurofisiopatologia, Ospedale Policlinico Perugia;* **E. Veneselli**, *Divisione di Neuropsichiatria Infantile, Istituto Gaslini, Universita' Genova;* **A. Ventura**, *Clinica Pediatrica, Istituto per l'Infanzia, Universita' Trieste;* **F. Viani, A. Romeo and A.Van Lierde**, *Centro Regionale Studio Epilessia, Milano.*

(Ambrosetto *et al.*, 1983; Del Giudice *et al.*, 1984; Sammaritano *et al.*, 1985; Tateno *et al.*, 1986; Pagani *et al.*, 1986; Battistella *et al.*, 1986; Piattella *et al.*, 1986; Taly *et al.* 1987). An unexpected series of cases of epilepsy with similar cerebral calcifications, in which CD was casually observed (Garwicz & Mortensson, 1976; Ciccarone *et al.*, 1987; Molteni *et al.*, 1988; Sammaritano *et al.*, 1988; Zaniboni *et al.*, 1989; Della Cella *et al.*, 1991; Ventura *et al.*, 1991; Gobbi *et al.*, 1992a), prompted the organization of an Italian Multicentric Study by neurologists and gastroenterologists to determine the association between CD and Epilepsy. The results of this study showed that 77.4 per cent of patients with epilepsy and cerebral calcifications were affected by CD, demonstrating that the association between CD and Epilepsy is not casual (Gobbi *et al.*, 1992b). Three groups of patients were also identified: (1) patients with CD, epilepsy and cerebral calcifications; (2) patients with CD and epilepsy without cerebral calcifications; (3) patients with epilepsy and cerebral calcifications without CD. In this last group it is still questionable whether these patients are affected by a latent form of CD (*see* Chapter 12).

The aims of this chapter are two-fold: a census of cases with epilepsy and CD up to 1996; and to describe the clinical findings and the outcome of epilepsy in patients with CD, comparing these data with others reported in the literature.

Material and methods

Sixty-three patients (23 males and 40 females) were identified by members of the Italian Working Group (IWG).The patients were collected from two different series: (1) patients with epilepsy and cerebral calcifications of unexplained origin; (2) patients with confirmed CD (according to the 1979 ESPGAN criteria, Mc Neish *et al.*, 1979) and epilepsy. No patient with other known causes of cerebral calcifications was included (namely, encephalitis, purulent meningitis, ossifying mening-oencephalitis, leukemia and chemotherapy, neonatal haemorrhage, congenital infections – TORCH group diseases – or calcium and phosphorus metabolism disturbances). Tuberous Sclerosis and Sturge–Weber Syndrome with port wine facial naevus were also excluded, but three patients with complete Sturge–Weber Syndrome underwent intestinal biopsy as control cases.

Small bowel biopsy was performed with a Watson-Crosby capsule at the Treitz ligament. Morpho-logical evaluation was scored according to Dunnill & Whitehead's criteria (1972). Crypt hyperpla-sia and unequivocal flat mucosa were accepted as markers of CD. Antigliadin IgG and IgA antibodies, antiendomysium antibodies (EmA), xylose load test, serum folic acid and HLA typing were also studied.

Cerebral CT scan was performed according to standard techniques: images were reassessed by a Peer-Review Committee of the IWG.

EEG recordings were carried out according to the 10–20 International System. Psychomotor devel-opment was assessed by the Wechsler Scale for Children or Adults, or other methods (i.e. Brunet Lezine adapted for age test), as appropriate to the age of the subject. Epilepsy was classified according to the 1981 and 1989 ILAE Commission criteria.

The results were compared to those of the existing literature, in order to verify the clinical and outcome of epilepsy in patients with CD.

Written informed consent was obtained before studying the patients or their parents.

Results

The 63 patients (23 males, 40 females) collected by the IWG were divided into three groups:
– Group 1: (42 cases) coeliac disease, epilepsy and cerebral calcifications (CEC);
– Group 2: (12 cases) coeliac disease and epilepsy without cerebral calcifications;
– Group 3: (9 cases) epilepsy and cerebral calcifications without coeliac disease.

From the review of the literature 192 cases were collected and grouped as follows:

– Group 1: (101 cases) coeliac disease, epilepsy and cerebral calcifications (CEC);

– Group 2: (57 cases) coeliac disease and epilepsy without cerebral calcifications;

– Group 3: (24 cases) epilepsy and cerebral calcifications without coeliac disease;

– Group 4: (10 cases) coeliac disease and cerebral calcifcations without epilepsy.

The names of the authors, the number of patients and their geographic distribution and ethnic origin are reported respectively in Tables 1, 2, 3 and 4 for each group.

Table 1. Census of cases of coeliac disease, epilepsy and cerebral calcifications

Authors	Geographic distribution and ethnic origin							
	Cases	Italian	Argentine	Spanish	Swedish	Australian	Canadian (Jewish)	Israeli
Aldao del Rosario, 1992	2		2					
Arroyo et al., 1997	22	6*	16					
Baiges et al., 1994	1			1				
Baquero et al., 1997	1			1				
Benigno et al., 1993	1	1						
Bye et al., 1993	1					1		
Caceres et al., 1992	1		1					
Cesari et al., 1994	2	2						
Cirillo et al., 1997	6	6						
D'Amato et al., 1997	1	1						
De Angelis et al., 1997	1	1						
De Maria et al., 1997	3	3						
Fois et al., 1994	3	3						
Vascotto et al., 1997	23	23						
Garwicz et al., 1976	1				1			
Giaretto et al., 1997	1	1						
Guerrini et al. 1997	1	1						
Hernandez et al., 1994	1			1				
Incorpora et al., 1997	1	1						
Magaudda et al., 1993–7	9	7	2**					
Martinelli et al., 1997	1	1						
Monton et al., 1992	1			1				
Perniola et al., 1997	2	2						
Pinilla et al., 1995	1			1				
Pinto et al., 1997	3	3						
Sammaritano et al., 1988	1						1	
Sfaello, 1996	4		4					
Taddeucci et al., 1997	1	1						
Tanganelli et al.., 1997	1	1						
Tinuper, 1997	1	1						
Vignolo et al.., 1997	1	1						
Volpi et al.., 1995	1	1						
Zelnik, 1996	1							1
IWG – Gobbi & Bertani, 1997	42	42						
Total	143	109	25	5	1	1	1	1

* Grandparents of Italian origin
** Grandparents of Argentine origin

Table 2. Census of cases of coeliac disease and epilepsy without cerebral calcifications

Authors	Cases	Geographic distribution and ethnic origin				
		Italian	Argentinian	Spanish	English	French
Arroyo, 1995	14		14			
Bardella et al., 1994	1	1				
Bathia & Marsden 1997	4				4	
Bermejo et al., 1997	9			9		
Cesari et al., 1994	2	2				
De Maria et al., 1997	2	2				
Elia et al., 1996	2	2				
Fois et al., 1994	7	7				
Guerrini et al., 1997	2	2				
Incorpora et al., 1997	2	2				
Lu et al., 1986	2				2	
Magaudda et al., 1993–97	4	4				
Naccarato et al., 1997*	1	1				
Pinto et al., 1997	3	3				
Tison et al., 1989	1					1
Tozzi et al., 1997	1	1				
IWG – Gobbi & Bertani, 1997	12	12				
Total	69	39	14	9	6	1

*See Alessandrini et al., Chapter 5 of this book.

Table 3. Census of cases of epilepsy and cerebral calcifications without coeliac disease

Authors	Cases	Geographic distribution and ethnic origin				
		Italian	Argentinian	French	Canadian	Brazilian
Gaggero et al., 1996	1	1				
Gizoud et al., 1990	3			3		
Magaudda et al., 1997	13	10	3*			
Masson et al., 1988	1			1		
Nunes et al., 1995	1					1
Sammaritamo et al., 1988	2				2	
Sfaello, 1996	3		3			
IWG – Gobbi & Bertani, 1997	9	9**				
Total	33	20	6	4	2	1

*Grandparents of Argentine origin; **Coeliac disease has been demonstrated in two cases (*see* Chapter 12).

Collecting both the literature and IWG cases, up to now 255 cases have been reported:

– Group 1: (143 cases) coeliac disease, epilepsy and cerebral calcifications (CEC)

– Group 2: (69 cases) coeliac disease and epilepsy without cerebral calcifications;

– Group 3: (33 cases) epilepsy and cerebral calcifications without coeliac disease;

– Group 4: (10 cases) coeliac disease and cerebral calcifications without epilepsy.

Table 4. Census of cases of coeliac disease and cerebral calcifications without epilepsy

Authors	Cases	Geographic distribution and ethnic origin		
		Italian	Argentinian	Spanish
Baquero *et al.*, 1997	1			1
Magaudda *et al.*, 1997	1	1		
Parmeggiani *et al.*, 1997	1	1		
Pinto *et al.*, 1997	1	1		
Rebaudengo *et al.*, 1997	5	5		
Sfaello, 1996	1		1	
Total	10	8	1	1

Analysis of group 1 (CEC)

The Italian Working Group

The IWG CEC group comprises 42 cases (15 males and 27 females) aged between 9 and 34 years (mean age 21.98 years; SD 6.49).

Cerebral calcifications

Clearcut calcifications on CT scan were identified in all cases at a mean age of 12.38 years (range 4–28; SD 6.18). They were located in the parieto-occipital regions in all patients and were bilateral in 36 cases and unilateral in six. In five cases they extended to the frontal region (four bilateral, one unilateral). In two cases (patients 3 and 12) the number of calcifications increased during the evolution before starting the gluten free diet (GFD). The typical neuroimaging pattern of calcifications is reported in Chapter 25.

Coeliac disease

Age at diagnosis of CD ranged between 4 and 30 years (mean 15.73; SD 6.62). In eight cases CD was investigated because of gut complaints presented by the patients. In the remaining 34 cases CD was investigated and diagnosed because of epilepsy and cerebral calcifications. Among these, in 11 cases the diagnosis of CD had been clearly suggested in infancy, but a GFD was not followed or was discontinued after a short period.

Gastrointestinal symptoms, and the results of xylose load test, serum folic acid, HLA typing, antigliadin IgG and IgA antibodies, antiendomysium antibodies (EmA), and jejunal biopsy have been reported and discussed in Chapter 11.

In the three complete SWS patients the intestinal biopsy showed a normal mucosa, and no gastrointestinal complaints were present.

Epilepsy

Age at onset of epilepsy ranged between 1 and 28 years (mean 6.64; SD 5.45). Thirteen children had epilepsy before the age of 3, 25 from 4 to 13 years, and only in four cases did epilepsy start in adulthood. In all but three CEC patients, epilepsy started before the diagnosis of CD. In these three cases (patients 5, 13, 37) epilepsy started 1–2 years after the beginning of a GFD.

All patients had localization-related epilepsy. On the basis of clinical and EEG findings and evolution, the epilepsy was classified as occipital in 36 patients, while the remaining six showed other varieties of partial epilepsies (Table 5). Three patients with onset of epilepsy during a GFD had a symptomatic drug-resistant occipital epilepsy. One of them had reading reflex seizures. The evolution of the occipital epilepsy was benign in 11 cases and drug-resistant in 17. A progressive evolution toward an epileptic encephalopathy (Gobbi *et al.*, 1988) was found in eight cases. In the cases with other types of localization-related epilepsies, the seizures disappeared in one case and were drug-resistant in five.

Table 5. Types of epilepsy and evolution in the IWG CEC Group (42 cases)

Type of epilepsy	Total cases	Age at onset (years)		
		0–3	4–13	> 14
Occipital lobe	**36**	**12**	**23**	**1**
Benign evolution	11	3	8	0
Drug-resistant	17	6	10	1
Severe epileptic encephalopathy	8	3	5	0
Other localization related	**6**	**1**	**2**	**3**
Temporal	4	1	1	2
Central	1	0	1	0
Not specified	1	0	0	1

At the onset of epilepsy, 26 of 42 cases showed focal abnormalities on the EEG and 11 generalized abnormalities. Focal abnormalities were occipital spike waves in 18 cases and occipital slow waves in four. Only in four cases were focal abnormalities found outside the occipital regions. EEG was normal in five cases. Focal abnormalities, when not present at onset, appeared during the evolution in four cases. Bilateral slow spike and wave activity occurred in fourteen cases, eight of them with occipital epilepsy with a progressive evolution towards an epileptic encephalopathy. During the evolution EEGs normalized in three of 12 patients, in whom the seizures have disappeared.

Table 6. Types of epilepsy and evolution in the CEC Group from the literature (99 cases)

Type of epilepsy		Total Cases
Localization-relation		**63**
Occipital epilepsy	30	
Occipital epilepsy with evolution to epileptic encephalopathy	10	
Other localization-related	23	
Complex seizures	*7*	
Partial motor seizures	*8*	
PSG	*7*	
Progressive myoclonic epilepsy	*1*	
Generalized		**9**
Occasional seizures (febrile convulsions)		**1**
Not specified		**26**
Evolution		
Benign	9	
Drug-resistant	29	
Not specified	60	

At the beginning of the epilepsy, mental development was normal in 36 patients, delayed in three and unknown in three, and neurological signs were not detected on clinical examination. At a later phase of the evolution, mental development was normal in 21 cases and delayed in 15 (unknown in six cases). Evolution after gluten-free diet is reported and discussed in Chapter 13.

Literature review

One hundred and one cases were found in the literature, but only 99 are available for clinical analysis. The results of a review of the literature concerning the type and evolution of epilepsy are summarized in Table 6. Calcifications were found in the occipital regions in 67 cases and were bilateral in 61. In twelve cases calcifications progressively increased before the onset of a GFD (Aldao del Rosario M., 1992; Caceres *et al.*, 1992; Bye *et al.*, 1993; Fois *et al.*, 1994; Arroyo *et al.*, 1997; Martinelli *et al.*, 1997). In 32 cases the site of the calcifications was not reported. The histopathological findings of brain lesions, which were reported in two cases, are described and discussed in Chapter 23.

Analysis of Group 2 (coeliac disease and epilepsy, without cerebral calcifications)

The Italian Working Group

Group 2 comprised 12 cases (4 males and 8 females) with a mean age of 10.68 years. No abnormality was documented at CT scan. Coeliac disease was diagnosed at a mean age of 4.5 years (range 1–12) and was confirmed by jejunal mucosal biopsy. At the time of the study, all patients were on a GFD and had no clinical gastroenterological signs.

Epilepsy started at a mean age of 4.8 years. In five of these cases seizures started before the diagnosis of CD. Epileptic seizures were generalized in six cases: four of them had absence seizures and two had tonic–clonic seizures. The remaining six patients had localization-related epilepsy, four of them with occipital seizures. The evolution of the seizures was benign in eight cases and drug resistant in two. In the two patients with occipital epilepsy there was a progressive outcome towards an epileptic encephalopathy.

Mental development was normal in five patients and compromised in seven.

Literature review

Fifty seven cases were found in the literature, but only 55 were available for clinical study. The results of this review, concerning the type and evolution of epilepsy, are summarized in Table 7.

Analysis of Group 3 (epilepsy and cerebral calcifications, without coeliac disease)

The Italian Working Group

Group 3 comprised nine cases (four males and five females). In all cases the CT scan disclosed impressive cortical-subcortical serpiginous calcifications. They were located in the parieto-occipital region in all cases and were bilateral in six and unilateral in three. Cerebral calcifications were diagnosed at an average age of 9.9 years.

A detailed analysis of gastrointestinal symptoms and jejunal mucosal biopsy is reported in Chapter 12. Here it is important to emphasize that seven out of nine patients proved HLA DQW2 and DR3 positive. Folic acid levels were low in four out of eight cases.

Epilepsy started at a mean age of 5.9 years. Two cases had generalized epilepsy with tonic-clonic seizures, while seven patients had localization-related epilepsy. Four of them had occipital epilepsy. At onset of epilepsy the seizure frequency was variable. The EEG findings showed generalized abnormalities in two cases and focal abnormalities in six. In one case the EEG was normal. The evolution of epilepsy was variable: it was benign in three patients, while the seizures were drug-resistant in four, and worsened towards an epileptic encephalopathy in two. Psychomotor development deteriorated in these last two cases.

Table 7. Types of epilepsy and evolution in the Literature Group 2 (55 cases)

Type of epilepsy		Total Cases
Localization related		**42**
Occipital epilepsy	15	
Occipital epilepsy with evolution to epileptic encephalopathy	4	
Other localization related	23	
Complex seizures	*5*	
Partial motor seizures	*6*	
PSG	*2*	
Progressive myoclonic epilepsy	*7*	
Not specified	*3*	
Generalized		**8**
Occasional seizures (Febrile convulsions)		**4**
Not specified		**1**
Evolution		
Benign		10
Drug-resistant		11
Not specified		29

Literature review

Twenty-four patients were collected from the literature, but only twenty-one are available for clinical analysis. Cortical-subcortical calcifications were found in all cases. They were bilateral in all cases but one, and were located in the parieto-occipital regions. In one case the calcifications increased during evolution (Giroud *et al.,* 1990). The results of the review of the literature concerning the type and evolution of the epilepsy are summarized in Table 8.

Table 8. Types of epilepsy and evolution in Literature Group 3 (21 cases)

Types of epilepsy		Total Cases
Localization related		**17**
Occipital epilepsy	14	
Other localization related	3	
Complex seizures	*2*	
PSG	*1*	
Generalized		**1**
Not specified		**3**
Evolution		
Benign	1	
Drug-resistant	2	
Not reported	1	

Analysis of Group 4 (Coeliac disease and cerebral calcifications, without epilepsy)

In this group, ten anecdotal CD patients were collected, who had cerebral calcifications of otherwise unknown origin. The calcifications are quite similar to the occipital calcifications of CEC patients and in five cases they were bilateral and located in the parieto-occipital regions. In four cases they involved the basal ganglia. Eight of them are reported by Italian authors, while the other two are respectively from Argentina and Spain (see Table 4).

Discussion

The results of the study of the IWG and the CEC cases in the literature suggest that, although clinically heterogeneous, epilepsy in these patients is usually localization-related, originating from the occipital lobe, and the course is usually drug-resistant. It is frequently characterized by an early and apparently benign initial phase followed by an epileptic encephalopathy after a seizure-free interval, as described by Gobbi *et al.* (1988) and Giroud *et al.* (1990). As already demonstrated (Gobbi *et al.*, 1992 (b), a GFD seems to control the seizures if started near the onset of epilepsy and early in childhood, confirming the hypothesis of a relation between CD and epilepsy in these patients. Nevertheless, in twenty cases the evolution was benign. In 9 out of the 11 IGW benign cases the outcome of occipital epilepsy was similar to that of early and/or late onset benign childhood epilepsy with occipital paroxysms (CEOP) (Gastaut, 1982; Panayiotopoulos, 1989). As this type of epilepsy tends to be considered an idiopathic form of localization-related epilepsy (Panayiotopoulos, 1993), and thus genetically determined, we might speculate that in these cases the evolution of the seizures is CD-independent, and that the epilepsy and CD association is casual or genetically linked.

Whether the association between CD and epilepsy is merely a coincidence or an association due to a 'linkage disequilibrium' between genes correlated to the two diseases, or whether the epilepsy is a consequence of an untreated CD, is still under discussion. On the one hand, the syndrome of epilepsy and cerebral calcifications might be considered to represent a separate genetically determined entity, a type of Sturge–Weber phacomatosis (Tiacci *et al.*, 1993). In fact, in all these cases the calcifications are located in the parieto-occipital regions and the epilepsy is mainly occipital (65 per cent of cases) while only a few differences have been found in the histopathological findings between the Sturge–Weber Syndrome (SWS) and the two CEC cases who underwent surgery (see Chapter 23 of this book). In this way, the frequent association with coeliac disease might be due to a genetic linkage. On the other hand, there are a number of arguments supporting the hypothesis that gluten intolerance (GI) may cause epilepsy and cerebral calcifications in predisposed subjects. First, the high number of cases with CD and epilepsy observed during the last few years. Up to now, collecting the literature and IWG cases, we have found that 211 cases of epilepsy and CD have already been observed. Moreover, the frequency of CD in patients with cerebral calcifications and epilepsy was much higher than expected: 82 per cent of cases in the IWG series. As there is no reason for a higher frequency of CD in subjects with cerebral calcifications than in the normal population, it cannot be coincidental that 82 per cent of patients with epilepsy and cerebral calcifications had CD. The control of seizures with a GFD immediately following the onset of epilepsy or early in childhood (Gobbi *et al.*, 1992b) and the progressive growth of cerebral calcifications or their late occurrence during evolution before the adoption of a GFD, as reported in two cases in the IWG series and in 12 cases in the literature (Aldao del Rosario, 1992; Caceres *et al.*, 1992; Bye *et al.*, 1993; Fois *et al.*, 1994; Arroyo *et al.*, 1997; Martinelli *et al.*, 1997), clearly suggest that gluten intolerance may cause epilepsy and cerebral calcifications. In a recent epidemiological study, Vascotto & Fois (see Chapter 15) found that the prevalence of epilepsy and cerebral calcifications increases from 0.79 per cent of cases with typical CD diagnosed at a mean age of 5.9 years to 3.5 per cent of cases with silent CD diagnosed at a mean age of 10 years, suggesting that epilepsy and cerebral calcifications may depend on untreated CD.

The pathogenic relationship between CD and cerebral calcifications is also questionable. The calcifications could be due to unrecognized chronic folic acid deficiency due to CD. In fact, some cases have already been reported in the literature in which posterior calcifications were detected in patients with a folic acid deficiency: in one case it was due to a congenital condition (Lanzkowsky,

1970), and, in others, to methotrexate therapy (Young *et al.*, 1977) or radiotherapy (Numaguchi *et al.*, 1975). Chronic folic acid deficiency could also depend on the effect of antiepileptic drugs (Reynolds, 1973). Drug influence, however, seems less probable, since antiepileptic-induced folate deficiency is rare, and in some of our cases therapy was started after the discovery of the calcifications. However, since, in some cases, epilepsy started after the onset of a GFD, and since, in some patients, folic acid levels were within the normal range in patients with a GFD, other causes could be investigated to determine the origin of the cerebral calcifications. In this way, as CD may be associated with different auto-immune disorders and/or auto-antibodies (Copper *et al.*, 1978; Burgin-Wolff *et al.*, 1991; Maki *et al.*, 1991), it could be hypothesized that cerebral calcifications depend on chronic auto-immune or immune-complex-related endothelial inflammation (Gobbi *et al.*, 1992b). The preliminary results of the study by Signore *et al.* (see Chapter 20), who found a significant brain uptake of radio-labelled-IL2 in the occipital lobe of two of three CEC patients, might support this hypothesis. Preferential involvement of the occipital lobe remains unexplained.

There is much discussion as to whether this syndrome is ethnically correlated with the Italian origin of patients, or whether the high incidence of CEC cases in the Italian population is due to the diet, which is especially rich in gluten. Moreover, as a large part of the Argentinian population is of Italian origin, we supposed that the majority of the Argentinian cases were of Italian origin. Census study with ethnic investigation clearly demonstrates that this syndrome, although most widespread in Italy, is found all over the world and that Argentinian CEC patients and the other cases reported outside Italy do not necessarily have an Italian origin. Consequently, we feel that on the one hand the high incidence of CEC cases in Italy is due to the high prevalence of CD in our country, but on the other hand it maybe due, at least in part to the attention paid to this pathology in the clinical practice of our country. In fact, since the article published in the *Lancet* in 1992 (Gobbi *et al.* 1992b) several CEC cases, outside Italy, have been reported.

Two other groups of patients were identified. The first one comprised patients with CD and epilepsy without cerebral calcifications (Group 2). In the IWG patients the CD was diagnosed early, so that they were put on a GFD almost immediately, at a mean age of 4.5 years. As progressive increase in size of cerebral calcifications or their late occurrence before the onset of a GFD, has already been reported only in CEC cases (Aldao del Rosario, 1992; Caceres *et al.*, 1992; Bye *et al.*, 1993; Fois *et al.*, 1994; Arroyo *et al.*, 1997; Martinelli *et al.*, 1997), we cannot exclude that there is some correlation between a prompt GFD and the absence of calcifications in these IWG Group 2 cases. Gobbi *et al.* (1992b) suggested that the association between epilepsy and CD in Group 2 cases was fortuitous, because only generalized seizures, similar to those of idiopathic generalized epilepsies starting in childhood have been found. On the contrary, during recent years a lot of cases with CD and epilepsy without cerebral calcifications have been published (*see* Table 7). These cases clearly demonstrated that localization-related epilepsies are more frequent than generalized ones (42/55 and 8/55, respectively) and, in particular, that cases of occipital epilepsy are especially frequent (19/42), some of which evolve into epileptic encephalopathy. Similar results were obtained in a more recent re-evaluation of the IWG Group's second series. Considering the apparently specific involvement of the occipital lobe in patients with an untreated CD, in agreement with Ambrosetto *et al.* (1992), we suggest careful investigation of CD in all patients with occipital epilepsy of unknown aetiology.

In this group (2) of patients, there are also CD cases affected by a progressive myoclonic ataxia syndrome with cortical myoclonus. This topic is discussed by Bhatia & Marsden in Chapter 36, and by Baquero and co-workers (Addendum).

Group 3 comprises nine patients affected by epilepsy with cerebral calcifications without a flat mucosa. In the literature we found 24 similar cases. All these patients had several similarities with the CEC group: CT scan demonstrated impressive cortico-subcortical calcifications located in the posterior regions and the epilepsy was localization-related in 24 (seven from the IWG and 17 from the literature). Eighteen of these were characterized by partial occipital seizures with evolution towards an epileptic encephalopathy in two. Moreover, among the IWG cases, seven out of nine cases were characterized by the same genetic marker as CD (these patients, in fact, presented some class II HLA antigens, such as DR3 and DQ2, allowing patients with CD to be identified (*see* Chapter 18), and three out of six tested cases had low serum folic acid levels, once again suggesting a diagnosis of CD, and, in particular, a diagnosis of 'Latent CD' with mucosal patchiness (Maki *et al.*, 1990).

Additionally, as reported by Lambertini *et al.* (*see* Chapter 12), the diagnosis of latent CD in two cases seems to have been confirmed by the presence of specific markers such as serum EmA, in one case, and an increased density of intraepithelial gamma/delta receptor lymphocytes in a second intestinal biopsy in the other. Consequently, we speculate that some of these patients could be affected by CD in spite of having a normal intestinal biopsy. We suggest that the syndrome consisting of epilepsy and cerebral calcifications of unexplained origin, especially when this epilepsy is characterized by occipital seizures and the calcifications are located in the posterior regions, may be a gluten-dependent symptom which can occur before and/or without intestinal lesions in patients with HLA characteristics of CD, such as in the case of dermatitis herpetiformis (Ferguson *et al.*, 1992).

In conclusion, the CD and epilepsy association is not only an Italian condition, but has been reported all over the world. The evolution of epilepsy in these patients is usually severe, frequently evolving into epileptic encephalopathy. An early GFD seems to be effective in controlling the epileptic seizures in some of the cases. Since CD may be silent, latent or potential, with possible asymptomatic cases in children, teenagers and young adults, since gastrointestinal signs are often lacking, and since in the CEC IWG cases and in a large number of the CEC cases elsewhere reported, CD was diagnosed only because of epilepsy and cerebral calcifications, we believe that child neurologists may be the only specialists in a position to discover CD in these patients. Child neurologists should be urged to test at least AGA and EmA for CD in all cases of epilepsy with occipital seizures, with or without cerebral calcifications. The role of malabsorption in the pathogenesis of epilepsy and posterior cerebral calcifications and the effectiveness of a GFD in the therapy for epilepsy has yet to be established, although there is no doubt that an appropriate diet may prevent long-term health risks for unrecognized CD (Holmes, 1992) and generally leads to overall physical improvement.

References

Aldao del Rosario, M. (1992): Oligosymptomatic coeliac disease and progressive cerebral calcifications with seizures. *Pediatr. Neurol.* **8** (5), 392.

Alessandrini, S., Iwanejko, G., Zani, A., Muccioli, F., Zanotti, L., Naccarato, S., Casali, F., Giuliani, S., Guttmann, S. & Volpini, M. (1997): Prevalence of coeliac disease in epileptic patients of Republic of San Marino. This book: Chapter 5.

Ambrosetto, G., Antonini, L. & Tassinari, C.A. (1992): Occipital lobe seizures related to clinically asymptomatic celiac disease in adulthood. *Epilepsia* 33, 476–481.

Ambrosetto, P., Ambrosetto, G., Michelucci, R., Bacci, A.(1983): Sturge–Weber syndrome without port-wine facial nevus: report of two cases studied by CT. *Child's Brain* **10**, 387–392.

Arroyo, H.A. (1995): Personal comunication

Arroyo, H., De Rosa, S., & Fejerman, N. (1997): Epilepsy, cerebral calcifications and celiac disease: Argentine multicenter experience. This book: Chapter 14.

Baiges, J., Giné, J.J., Viedma, P., Alfani, O. & Mercé, J. (1994): Epilepsia, calcificaciones cerebrales y celiaquia. *Neurologia* (*Barcelona*) **9**, 485.

Baquero, M., Vichez, J.J., Dominguez, F.J. & Garcia Fernandez, M. (1997): Biooccipital calcifications and coeliac disease with late onset. This book: Addendum.

Bardella, M.T., Molteni, N., Prampolini, L., Giunta, A.M., Baldassarri, A.R., Morganti, D. & Bianchi, P.A. (1994): Need for follow up in coeliac disease. *Arch. Dis. Child.* **70**, 210–213.

Bathia, K.P. & Marsden, C.D. (1997): Progressive myoclonic ataxia associated with coeliac disease. This book: Chapter 35.

Battistella, P.A., Casara, G.L., Carollo, C., Cattelan, C., Condini, C. & Pardatscher, K. (1986): Calcificazioni cerebrali senza angiomatosi cutanea: forma atipica della malattia di Sturge–Weber. *Riv. Ital. Ped.* IJP **12**, 417–418.

Benigno, V., Curto Pelle, M.G., Alabrese, L., Giordano, G. & Mogavero, S. (1993): Calcificazioni cerebrali, epilessia, e malattia celiaca. Osservazione di un caso. *Abstract Book of* Ist Congresso Nazionale SIGEP, 11–13 November 1993, Carbone Edizioni, Palermo Italy, p.40.

Bermejo, A.M., Polanco, I., Castroviejo, I.P., Lopez Martin, V. (1997): Neurological disorders in Spanish children with coeliac disease. This book : Addendum.

Burgin-Wolff, A., Gaze, H., Hadziselimovic, F. *et al.* (1991): Antigliadin and antiendomysium antibody determination for coeliac disease. *Arch. Dis. Child.* **66**, 941–947.

Bye, A.M.E., Andermann, F., Robitaille, I., Bohane, T., Oliver, M. & Anderamann, E. (1993): Cortical vascular abnormalities in the syndrome of celiac disease, epilepsy, bilateral occipital calcification, and folate deficiency. *Ann. Neurol.* **34**, 399–403.

Caceres, L.P., Cervetto, J.L., Del, C. & Toca, Y.M. (1992): Case report: cerebral calcifications, epilepsy and coeliac disease. *Pediatr. Neurol.* 8 (5), 401.

Cesari, P., Pascarella, A., De Maria, G., Lanzani, G., Buffoli, F. & Graffeo, M. (1994): Epilepsie et maladie coeliaque symptomatique,une association à évoquer. *La Presse Médicale* **23**, (16), 764.

Chapman, R.W.G., Laidlow, J.L., Colin-Jones, D.G., Eade, O., Smith, C.L. (1978): Increased prevalence of epilepsy in coeliac disease. *BMJ.* **2**, 250-251.

Ciccarone, V., Rozzi, N., Balli, F. & Galli, V. (1987): Calcificazioni endocraniche simulanti la malattia di Sturge-Weber in una bambina con malattia celiaca. *Riv. Ital. Ped.* **13** (suppl.1), 186.

Cirillo, B., Buono, S., Della Rotonda, G.M., Grimaldi, G., De Prosperis, A., Viotti, L. & Abate, M. (1997): Epilessia e celiachia.Considerazioni su sei casi. This book: Addendum.

Commission on Classification and Terminology of the International League Against Epilepsy. Proposals for revised clinical and electroencephalographic classification of epileptic seizures (1981): *Epilepsia* **22**, 489–501.

Commission on Classification and Terminology of the International League Against Epilepsy. Proposals for revised classification of epilepsies and epileptic syndromes (1989): *Epilepsia* **30**, 389–399.

Cooke, W.T. & Smith, T. (1966): Neurological disorders associated with celiac disease. *Brain* **86**, 683–722.

Cooke, W.T. (1976): Neurological manifestations of malabsorption. In: Handbook of clinical neurology, eds. P.J.Vinken & G.W. Bruyn, vol. 28, pp. 225–241. Amsterdam-New York-Oxford: Elsevier.

Cooke, W.T. & Holmes, G.K.T. (1984): Neurological and psychiatric complications. In: *Coeliac disease,* eds. W.T. Cooke & G.K. T. Holmes, pp. 202–220. Edinburgh: Churchill Livingstone.

Copper, B.T., Holmes, G.K.T. & Cooke, W.T. (1978): Coeliac disease and immunologic disorders. *Br. Med. J.* **1**, 537–542.

D'Amato, L., Maffini, I., Silva, E., Todeschini, A. & Bassanetti, F. (1993): Nuovi aspetti di una vecchia malattia: descrizione di un caso di Celiachia. Abstract Book of Ist Congresso Nazionale SIGEP ed. 11–13 November 1993, Carbone Edizioni, Palermo Italy, p.210.

De Angelis, G.L., Corna, M., Street, M.E., Romanini, E., Capone, C., Sasso, E. & Faienza, C. (1997): Neurological findings in adults with unknow coeliac disease. This book: Addendum.

De Maria, G., Gorno, M.L., Cappa, S.F., Guarneri, B. and Antonini, L. (1997): Neuropsychological evaluation of posterior areas function in coeliac patients with or without epilepsy. This book: Addendum.

Della Cella, G., Beluschi, C., Cipollina, F. (1991): Intracranial Calcifications-Epilepsy-Celiac disease: description of a case. *Med. Surg. Ped.* **13**, 427–430.

Del Giudice, E., Pelosi, L., Romano, A. *et al.* (1984): Unexplained bilateral occipital calcifications and reduced vision. *Neuropediatrics* **15**, 218–219.

De Marco, P. (1996): Personal comunication.

Dennis, J., & Taylor, D.C. (1969): Epilepsy and folate deficiency. *BMJ* **4**, 807–808.

Dunnill, M.S., Whitehead, R. (1972): A method for the quantification of small intestinal biopsy specimen. *J. Clin. Pathol.* **25**, 243–245.

Elia, M., Musumeci, S.A., Failla, P., Ferri, R., Greco, D., Scuderi, C., Castone, A. & Stefanini, M.C. (1996): Celiachia ed epilessia in assenza di calcificazioni cerebrali: a proposito di due nuovi casi. *Boll. Lega It. Epil.* 91/92, in press**.**

Ferguson, A., Arranz, E. and O'Mahony, S. (1992): Definitions and diagnostic criteria of latent and potential coeliac disease. In: *Common food intolerances1: epidemiology of coeliac disease*, eds. S. Auricchio and J.K. Visakorpi, **vol 2**, pp.119–127. Basel: Karger.

Fois, A., Vascotto, M., Di Bartolo, M.R. & Di Marco, V. (1994): Coeliac disease and epilepsy in pediatric patients. *Child's. Nerv. Syst.* **10**, 450–454.

Gaggero, R. (1996): Personal comunication.

Garwicz, S. & Mortensson, W. (1976): Intracranial calcification mimicking the Sturge–Weber syndrome (a consequence of cerebral folic acid deficiency ?). *Pediat. Radiol.* **5**, 5–9.

Gastaut, H. (1982): A new tpe of epilepsy: benign partial epilepsy of children with occipital spike focus. *Clin. Electroencephalogr.* **13**, 13–22.

Giaretto, G., Romani, G., Oderda, G., Malorgio, E. & Ansaldi, N. (1995): Epilessia, calcificazioni intracraniche, malattia celiaca. Descrizione di un caso *Rivista Italiana di Pediatria* **21(5), 7**36–738.

Giroud, M., Borsotti, J.P., Michiels, R., Tommasi, M. & Dumas, R.(1990): Epilepsie et calcifications occipitales bilatérales: 3 cas. *Rev. Neurol.* **4**, 288–292.

Gobbi, G., Sorrenti, G., Santucci, M., Giovanardi Rossi, P., Ambrosetto, P., Michelucci, R. & Tassinari, C.A. (1988): Epilepsy with bilateral occipital calcifications: a benign onset with progressive severity. *Neurology* **38**, 913–920.

Gobbi, G., Ambrosetto, P., Zaniboni, M.G., Lambertini, A., Ambrosioni, G. & Tassinari, C.A. (1992a): Coeliac disease, posterior cerebral calcifications and epilepsy. *Brain. Dev.* **14**, 23–29.

Gobbi, G., Bouquet, F., Greco, L., Lambertini, A., Tassinari, C.A., Ventura, A. & Zaniboni, M.G. (1992b): Coeliac disease, epilepsy and cerebral calcifications. *Lancet* **340**, 439–443.

Grant, H.C., Hoffbrand, A.V., Wells, D.G. (1965): Folate deficiency and neurological disease. *The Lancet* **2**, 763–767.

Guerrini, R., Battini, R., Ughi, C., Chiravalloti ,G., Belmonte, A, Canapicchi, R. & Taddeucci ,G (1997): Prevalence of epilepsy and seizure types in coeliac disease and prevalence of unrecognized coeliac disease in children with neurologic and psychiatric disorders. This book: Chapter16.

Hernandez, M.A., De la Colina, G., Ortigosa, L., Togores, J. M., Flores, J. & Urriza, J. (1994): Epilepsia, calcificaciones bioccipitales y anticuerpos antiendomisio. *Rev. Neurol. (Barcelona)* **22**, 727.

Holmes, G.K.T. (1992): Long-term health risks for unrecognized coeliac patients. In *Common food intolerances1: Epidemiology of coeliac disease*, eds. S. Auricchio & J.K.Visakorpi, **vol 2**, pp.105–118. Basel: Karger.

Incorpora, G., Cocuzzo, R , Bianchini, R., Rotolo, R., Spina, M. & Bottaro, G. (1997): Prevalence of coeliac disease in subjects affected by drug - resistant epilepsy. This book: Addendum.

Laidlow, J.L., Chapman, R.G., Colin-Jones, D.G., Eade, O. & Smith, C.L. (1977): Increased prevalence of epilepsy in coeliac disease. *Gut* **18**, A943.

Lambertini, A., Zaniboni, M.G., Mayer, M., Città, A., and Ventura, A. (1997): Epilepsy and cerebral calcifications with normal jejunal mucosa; latent coeliac disease. This book: chapter 12.

Lanzkowsky, P. (1970): Congenital malabsorption of folate. *Am. J. Med.* **48**, 580–583.

Lu, C.S., Thompson, P.D., Quinn, N. P., Parkes, J .D. & Marsden, C.D. (1986): Ramsey Hunt syndrome and coeliac disease: a new association? *Movement Disorders* **1**, 209–219.

Mc Neish, A.S., Harms, H.K., Rey, J., Shmerling, D.H., Visakorpi, J.K. & Walker Smith, J.A. (1979): The diagnosis of celiac disease. *Arch. Dis.Child.* **54**, 783–786.

Magaudda, A., Dalla Bernardina, B., De Marco, P., Sfaello, Z.M., Longo, M., Colamaria,V., Daniele, O., Tortorella, G., Tata, M .A., Di Perri ,R. & Meduri, M. (1993): Bilateral occipital calcifications, epilepsy and coeliac disease: clinical and neuroimaging features of a new syndrome. *J. Neurol. Neurosurg. Psych.* **56**, 885–889.

Magaudda, A., Dalla Bernardina, B., Magazzu', G., Longo, M., De Marco, P. & Meduri, M (1997): Frequency of occipital bilateral calcifications and epilepsy in coeliac patients. This book: Chapter 17.

Maki, M., Holm, K., Kosmies, S., Hallstrom, O. & Visakorpi, J.K. (1990): Normal small bowel biopsy followed by coeliac disease. *Arch. Dis.Child.* **65**, 1137–1141.

Maki, M., Hallstrom, O., Marttinen, A. (1991): Reaction of human non-collagenous polypeptides with coeliac disease autoantibodies. *Lancet* **338**, 724–725.

Martinelli, O., Tiberti, A., Valseriati, D. & Gobbi, G. (1997): Epilepsy and coeliac disease in a case with cerebral calcifications at follow up. This book: Addendum.

Masson, C., Gallet, J.P., Cheron, F., Masson, M. & Cambier, J. (1988): Epilepsie avec calcifications corticales bilatérales: discussion d'un deficit post-critique durable. *Rev. Neurol.* **144**, 499–502.

Molteni, N., Bardella, M.T., Baldassarri, A.R., Bianchi, P.A. (1988): Celiac disease associated with epilepsy and intracranial calcifications: report of two patients. *Am. J. Gastroent.* **83**, 992–994.

Monton, F., Pérez Senas, M.T., Pérez, J., Zurita, A. & Manas, S. (1992): Epilepsia, calcificaciones occipitales y enfermedad celiaca *Neurologia (Barcelona)* **7**, 350–35.

Morris, J.S., Ajdukiewicz, A.B. & Read, A.E. (1970): Neurological disorders and adult coeliac disease. *Gut* **11**, 549–554.

Norris, J.W., Pratt, R.F. (1971): A controlled study of folic acid in epilepsy. *Neurology* **21**, 659–664.

Numaguchi, Y., Hoffman, I.C., Sones, I.P. (1975): Basal ganglia calcifications as a late radiation effect. *Am. J. Rad.* **123**, 27–28.

Nunes, M.L., Costa da Costa, J., Severini, M.H. (1995): Early onset bilateral calcifications and epilepsy. *Pediatr. Neurol.* **13**, 80–82.

Pagani, M., Arietto, V., Benvenuti, C., Lanfranchi, V. & Valseriati, D. (1986): Un caso atipico di Sturge-Weber Krabbe con calcificazioni intracraniche bilaterali in assenza di angiomatosi cutanea. In: *Atti del VII Convegno di Neurologia Infantile*, eds. P. Benedetti, P. Curatolo & S. Ottaviano., p. 110. Rome: Sigma-Tau.

Panayiotopoulos, C.P. (1989): Benign childhood epilepsy with occipital paroxysms: a 15 year prospective study. *Ann. Neurol.* **26**, 51–56.

Panayiotopoulos, C.P. (1993): Benign childhood epilepsy with occipital paroxysms. In: *Occipital seizures and epilepsies in children*, eds. F. Andermann, A. Beaumanoir, L. Mira, J. Roger & C.A. Tassinari., pp. 151–164. London, Paris, Rome: John Libbey.

Parmeggiani, A., Bertani, G., Santucci, M., Lolli, G., Zaniboni, M.G., Gobbi, G., Pini, A. and Giovanardi, Rossi, P. (1997): Coeliac disease, mental retardation and macrocephaly: two affected sisters. This book: Addendum.

Perniola, T., Margari, L., De Iaco, M.G., Buttiglione, M., Figliolia, B., Polito, A., De Giacomo, A. & Simone, I. (1996): Migraine in the bilateral occipital calcification - epilepsy -coeliac disease syndrome. This book: Addendum.

Piattella, L., Zamponi, N., Cenci, L., Rossi, R. & Papa, O. (1986): Calcificazioni biooccipitali ed epilessia: malattia di Sturge-Weber atipica o nuova sindrome. *Boll. Lega. Ital. Epil.* **54/55**, 139–142.

Pinilla Moraza, J., Gil Pujades, A., Labarga Echevarria, P. & Astiazaran, F. (1995): Epilepsia, calcificaciones cerebrales y celiaqia. Un nuevo caso. *Neurologia (Barcelona)* **10**, 214–215.

Pinto, P., Agostinis, C., Defanti, C.A. (1997): The triad of epilepsy, coeliac disease and cerebral calcifications: in search of the missing item. This book: Addendum.

Rebaudengo, N., Pignatta , P., Liboni, W., Sategna Guidetti, C., Bruno, M. & Grosso, S. (1996): Epilepsy and neurological findings in adults coeliac patients. This book: Addendum.

Reynolds, E.H. (1973): Anticonvulsants, folic acid and epilepsy. *Lancet* **1**, 1376–1378.

Sammaritano, M., Andermann, F., Melanson, D., Guberman, A., Tinuper, P. & Gastaut, H. (1985): The syndrome of epilepsy and bilateral occipital cortical calcifications. *Epilepsia* **26**, 532.

Sammaritano, M., Andermann, F., Melanson, D., Guberman, A., Tinuper, P. & Gastaut, H.(1988): The syndrome of intractable epilepsy, bilateral occipital calcifications and folic acid deficiency. *Neurology* **38** (suppl.1), 239.

Sfaello, Z. M., (1996): Personal comunication.

Taddeucci, G., Chiaravalloti, G., Di Gangi, G., Ciulli, L., Fierabracci, M., Balsano, L. & Ughi, C. (1997): Manifestazioni neurologiche e calcificazioni endocraniche in un caso di celiachia atipica. This book: Addendum.

Taly, A.B., Nagaraja, D., Das, S., Shankar, S.K. & Pratibha, N.G. (1987): Sturge-Weber-Dimitri disease without facial nevus. *Neurology* **37**, 1063–1064.

Tanganelli, P., Malfatto, L., Beluschi, C., Babbini, S., Gianbartolomei, G. & Regesta, G. (1997): Coeliac disease, epilepsy, and cerebral calcifications: Report of a typical case with long term follow-up. This book: Addendum.

Tateno, A., Matsui, A., Sakuragawa, N., Nonaka, I. & Arima, M. (1985): Two siblings with multiple intracranial haemangiomatosis with calcifications. *J. Neurol.* **232**, 112–114.

Tiacci, C., D'Alessandro, P., Cantisani, T.A., Piccirilli, M., Signorini, E., Pelli, M.A., Cavalletti, M.L., Castellucci, G., Palmeri, S., Battisti, C. & Federico, A. (1993): Epilepsy with bilateral occipital calcifications: Sturge–Weber variant or a different encephalopathy? *Epilepsia* **34**, 528–539.

Tinuper, P. (1997): Pathological findings of coeliac disease, epilepsy and cerebral calcifications. This book: Chapter 23.

Tison, F., Arne, P. & Henry, P. (1989): Myoclonus and adult coeliac disease. *J. Neurol.* **236**, 307–308.

Tozzi, E., Gentile, T., Angelini, R., Meucci , M. V., Pace, F., Tobia, L., Marrelli, A., Aloisi, P., Papola, F., Cervelli, C., & De Matteis, F. (1997): Coeliac disease, headache and epilepsy: report of seven cases. This book: Addendum.

Vascotto, M., Fois, A. (1997): Epilepsy and coeliac disease. A collaborative study. This book: Chapter 15.

Ventura, A., Bouquet, F., Sartorelli, C., Barbi, E., Torre, G., Tommasini, G. (1991): Coeliac disease, folic acid deficiency and epilepsy with cerebral calcifications. *Acta. Paediatr. Scand.* **80**, 559–562.

Vignolo, M., Naselli, A., Biancheri, R., Grazia, P. & Veneselli, E. (1997): Report of a case of CEC with onset of epilepsy after one year of gluten free diet. This book: Addendum.

Volpi, L., Migliore, M.R., Moscano, F.C. & Franzoni, E. (1991): Rapporti tra dieta priva di glutine e terapia dell'epilessia: segnalazione di un caso. *Abstract Book of Convegno pediatrico SIP- Sez.Emiliano Romagnola*, 19 October 1991. Humana Centro Studi e Ricerche, Milan, Italy, p.143.

Young, L.W., Jequier, S. & O'Gorman, A.M. (1977): Intracerebral calcifications in treated leukemia in a child. *Am. J. Dis. Child.* **131**,1283–1285.

Zaniboni, M.G., Lambertini, A., Gobbi, G., Romeo R., Conti,G., Ambrosioni, G., Ambrosetto P., Santucci, M., Michelucci, R. & Tassinari C.A. (1989): Celiac disease and epilepsy with occipital calcifications: an uncasual association. In: *Proceedings of the 1st British Italian Paediatric Gastroenterology Meeting,* 22–23 September 1989, eds. G. Banchini, S. Guandalini, G.L. De Angelis & J.A. Walker-Smith., p. 54, Parma.

Zelnik, N. (1996): Personal comunication.

Epilepsy and other neurological disorders in coeliac disease, edited by G. Gobbi *et al.*
© 1997 John Libbey & Company Ltd, pp. 81–82.

Chapter 11

Gastrointestinal symptoms in coeliac disease, epilepsy and cerebral calcifications

A. Lambertini, M.G. Zaniboni and G.Banchini*

*Department of Paediatrics, Azienda Ospedaliera di Bologna e *Reggio Emilia, Italy*

Introduction

It is now clear that coeliac disease (CD) can appear with different clinical manifestations and different incidence depending on the geographic area (Greco *et al.*, 1992). This could be due to various factors such as, for example, the genetic background of the population, quality and quantity of gluten, the age at gluten introduction and breast feeding.

The symptoms are often moderate at the beginning of the disease, and therefore it is not diagnosed correctly. Subsequently, the concurrent appearance of other more obvious symptoms concerning different systems prevents or delays correct diagnosis.

Such a delay frequently occurs in the cerebral calcification (CEC) triad, as can be seen in the majority of cases found in the international literature (Gobbi *et al.*, 1992).

Patients and method

The ethiopathogenic aspects, the extraintestinal symptoms and the radiologic findings of CEC are discussed in depth in other chapters of this book. Here we will discuss the intestinal symptoms and the main laboratory findings of patients affected by CEC who underwent observation of the Italian Working Group from 1990 to 1994.

The subjects were 42 patients divided in to two groups: the first consisted of 37 patients affected by epilepsy and cerebral calcifications in whom it was subsequently possible to diagnose the presence of CD; the second group was made up of five patients with epilepsy and CD who later developed cerebral calcifications.

The diagnosis of CD was made in all patients according to the most recent ESPGAN criteria (Walker-Smith *et al.*, 1990).

Table 1. The main GI clinical and laboratory data

No of patients = 42	Mean age at diagnosis of CD = 15.7 ± 6.6 years
Male = 16	
Female = 26	Current mean age = 21.9 ± 6.4 years

Anamnesis: GI symptoms suggesting CD in early childhood

Abdominal distention 22/42
Vomiting 6/42
Diarrhoea 28/42
Recurrent aphthous stomatitis 4/42
Iron deficiency anaemia 9/42
Short stature 4/42

Previous clinical diagnosis of CD = 14/42
Out of these 14 subjects, 10 underwent gluten-free diet for a mean period of 3 years; the diet was then abandoned by the family.

Genetics:
HLA = 26/42   DQ2 = 23/26
Heterodimer = 20/42   Positive = 18/20

Antibodies:
Gliadin antibodies IgA or IgG = 33/42   Positive = 26/33
EmA = 6/42   Positive = 6/6

Serum folic acid = 28/42   Low = 23/28

Conclusions

The present study suggests that:

(1) CD can appear at any time during life when it is not promptly diagnosed, it can evolve in silent or paucisymptomatic forms with modification of the clinical picture according to age;

(2) the GI symptoms are usually present in the first years of life but their absence does not rule out the possibility of CD;

(3) it is possible that, in the case of epilepsy, the presence of other specific symptoms such as short stature, iron deficiency anaemia and mild GI symptoms is underestimated;

(4) other specialists, such as paediatric neurologists and neuropsychiatrists, need to understand the heterogeneous nature of CD. Screening for CD must always be carried out in order to identify those affected as soon as possible.

References

Greco, L., Maki, M., Di Donato, F. & Visakorpi, K. (1992): Epidemiology of coeliac disease in Europe and the Mediterranean area. In: *Common food intolerances 1: epidemiology of coeliac disease*, eds. S. Auricchio & J.K. Visakorpi, pp. 25–56. Basel: Karger.

Gobbi, G., Bouquet, F., Greco, L., Lambertini, A., Tassinari, C.A., Ventura, A. & Zaniboni, M.G. (1992): Coeliac disease, epilepsy and cerebral calcifications. *Lancet* **340,** 439–443.

Walker-Smith, J.A., Guandalini, S., Schmitz, J., Shmerling, D.H. & Visakorpi, J.K. (1990): Revised criteria for diagnosis of coeliac disease. *Arch. Dis. Child* **65,** 909–911.

Epilepsy and other neurological disorders in coeliac disease, edited by G. Gobbi *et al.*
© 1997 John Libbey & Company Ltd, pp. 83–87.

Chapter 12

Epilepsy and cerebral calcifications with normal jejunal mucosa: latent coeliac disease?

Andrea Lambertini, Maria Gilda Zaniboni, Marina Mayer*, Angelo Città** and Alessandro Ventura***

*Divisione di Pediatria, Ospedale Maggiore, Bologna, Italy; *Istituto di Clinica Pediatrica, 2° Policlinico, Università di Napoli, Italy; **Laboratorio di Immunoistochimica, Istituto per l'Infanzia, Trieste, Italy; ***Istituto di Clinica Pediatrica, Università di Pisa, Italy*

Introduction

There have been various reports in the last few years of a significant association between epilepsy with occipital cerebral calcifications (EBOC) and coeliac disease (CD) (Sammaritano *et al.*, 1988; Molteni *et al.*, 1988; Ventura *et al.*, 1991; Gobbi *et al.*, 1992a; Tortorella *et al.*, 1993). In particular, in the recently updated Italian Working Group (IWG) study, 42 out of 51 (82 per cent) subjects with EBOC systematically investigated with intestinal biopsy were diagnosed as having CD due to the presence of classic subatrophy of the intestinal mucosa (Gobbi *et al.*, 1992b; Gobbi, 1995). The number of cases of EBOC with atrophic mucosa was slightly lower than reported by the IWG, but was in any case always higher than 50 per cent, in the subsequent reports in the literature (Magaudda *et al.*, 1993); Tiacci *et al.*, 1993). To date there are still no elements by which it can be established with certainty whether the correlation between EBOC and CD indicates merely an association due to a 'linkage disequilibrium' between the genes involved in the two diseases or whether it is in fact the unrecognized (and thus untreated) gluten intolerance that favours the onset of EBOC in genetically predisposed subjects. This second hypothesis would seem to be supported by the observation, confirmed several times (Ventura *et al.*, 1991; Gobbi *et al.*, 1992b; Guerrini *et al.*, 1997; Tanganelli *et al.*, 1997), that gluten-free diet (GFD) can help control the epilepsy in subjects with EBOC, at least when it is started at an early stage. Even if a causal relationship between untreated CD and EBOC is thought to exist, cases of EBOC in which CD was ruled out due to normal intestinal mucosa still require an explanation.

In the series collected by the IWG, nine subjects with EBOC fall within this category. Increasing attention has recently focussed on the well documented condition defined as latent coeliac disease (Weinstein, 1974; Ferguson *et al.*, 1992). These are cases in which, despite a pathological, biological or clinical response to eating gluten, the classic atrophy of the intestinal mucosa is not present, but will subsequently develop ('Finnish' model, which refers to the cases described by Maki (1990)). It may also have occurred previously and did not subsequently reappear even after inclusion of gluten in the diet ('French' model, which refers to the cases described by Schmitz (1984)). In practice, therefore, the definition of latent coeliac disease can be applied to those subjects who fulfill the following two conditions: normal biopsy with free diet containing gluten, who will present, or have presented at another time in their life, gluten-dependent atrophy of the intestinal mucosa (Ferguson *et al.*, 1992).

Cases with latent CD suggest that in subjects with gluten intolerance environmental factors are necessary to render the disease overt at the intestinal level. At the same time, the existence of cases of latent CD demonstrates how mucosal atrophy can no longer be considered an absolute and necessary criterion for the diagnosis of CD.

It is currently believed that latent CD is closely though not absolutely correlated with the isolated or associated presence of certain biological markers of a genetic-type (DQ2 antigen of the HLA system and, markedly, a particular α/β heterodimer coded by the DQA1*0501 and DQB1*0201 alleles). Immunological (high titres of antigluten antibodies in the serum and in the duodenal secretions, high serum titres of antiendomysium antibodies – EmA), histological (increase in intraepithelial lymphocytes in the intestinal mucosa, reduction in the villi/crypt ratio, evaluated with classic morphometric or computerized techniques) or immunohistological (increase in intraepithelial lymphocytes with γ/δ receptor in the intestinal mucosa), findings suggest this to be the case.

In this study we aim to verify the hypothesis that cases of EBOC with apparently normal intestinal mucosa are in effect cases of latent CD.

Patients and methods

The study included nine subjects with EBOC (five females and four males aged between 14 and 23 years) in whom the intestinal biopsy, examined with an optic microscope, appeared normal.

HLA typing for class II antigens was performed in all cases and a search for the DQA1*0501 and DQB1*0201 heterodimer was made in two.

Seven of nine biopsies were re-examined with computerized morphometric analysis.

Five out of nine patients agreed to undergo an additional test for EmA dosage and 2/9 to a further intestinal biopsy 3–6 years after the previous normal result. In these two cases, in addition to the classic histological examination, the density of the intraepethelial γ/δ receptor lymphocytes was also determined.

Serological tissue typing for HLA class II DR and DQ antigens was performed by using the standard microcytoxicity assay (Terasaki & McClelland, 1964). HLA genotype was determined according to the workshop protocol (Sasazuki & Kimura, 1991).

Antigliadin IgG and IgA were assessed by enzyme-linked immunosorbent assay (Alfa-gliatest, Eurospital, Trieste, Italy).

Antiendomysium antibodies were assessed by immunosorbent assay (Antiendomysium Eurospital, Trieste, Italy).

Morphometric analysis (Ferguson *et al*, 1971; Troncone *et al*, 1995) allowed us to evaluate villous height, crypt depth, villous/crypt depth ratio and intraepithelial lymphocytes (IEL) count.

Intraepithelial γ/δ T-cell-receptor lymphocytes were determined according to Savilhati (1992).

Results

Morphometry on retrospective histological samples

None of the seven biopsies re-examined after a period of time showed significant morphometric alterations.

HLA

Seven of nine subjects proved DR3 DQ2 positive. In two cases a search was made for the DQA1*0501 and DQB1*0201 heterodimer and one case proved positive.

EmA

In one of the five subjects in whom it was possible to check the presence of EmA in the serum, these proved positive (while a previous dosage, 18 months earlier, had been negative). The family of this girl did not give consent to a second intestinal biopsy.

New biopsies and γ/δ lymphocyte density

Villous atrophy or crypt hypertrophy was not present in either of the two cases who underwent a second intestinal biopsy, but in one case a significant increase in intraepithelial γ/δ receptor lymphocytes was observed ($11/mm^3$, mean of healthy controls and other intestinal diseases: 2.1; range: 0–3)

Overall, therefore, 7/9 subjects with EBOC and morphologically normal intestinal biopsy were characterized by the same genetic markers as CD and in two cases the diagnosis of latent CD seemed to be confirmed by the presence of specific markers such as serum EmA or the increased density of intræpithelial γ/δ receptor lymphocytes.

Discussion

The results obtained, though based on a small number of subjects studied (and limited due to the reticence of the families to give their consent to repeat blood or histological tests), do not allow us to reply conclusively to the question of whether cases of EBOC with normal intestinal mucosa can in fact be classified as latent CD. However, several factors emerged from our study which support this possibility.

In the majority of cases (7/9) in our study, as in most of the cases reported in the literature (Magaudda *et al.*, 1993; Tortorella *et al.*, 1993), the HLA DQ2 phenotype is present, which characterizes the great majority of coeliacs, with or without EBOC. Moreover, in one of the two cases the DQA1*0501 – DQB1*0201 heterodimer, considered to be an even more specific marker of coeliac disease, was identified. In the same case, a significant increase was observed in the number of γ/δ lymphocytes in the intestinal mucosa, an event which is currently considered to be one of the most specific markers of latent CD (Troncone *et al.*, 1995). The case in which the EmA (negative at the time of the first biopsy) became positive after a period of time is particularly significant. In a series of diabetic subjects, Maki recently (1995) reported the possibility of the subsequent appearance of EmA in previously negative subjects and documented its high predictive value compared with the onset of subtotal villous atrophy in previously normal mucosa. Antibodies to endomysium represent, as a matter of fact, a strong marker of latent CD. In a recent study, 28 per cent of patients with positive reticulin antibodies and normal small bowel villous architecture developed villous atrophy during the following five years (Holm *et al.*, 1994). Moreover, all five cases of of an Italian study with positive EmA and first normal biopsy developed the typical subtotal villous atrophy in the following two years (during which their diet contained a normal quantity of gluten).

The possibility that gluten-dependent symptoms in subjects with the HLA characteristics of coeliac disease occur before and/or without intestinal lesions is well-known, the most representative model being dermatitis herpetiformis (Weinstein, 1974; Ferguson et al., 1987; Chorzelski et al., 1988).

Epilepsy, in EBOC, is to a certain degree reversible by GFD, apparently correlated with the starting time (Ventura et al., 1991; Gobbi et al., 1992b; Guerrini et al., 1997; Tanganelli et al., 1997). This occurrence is per se a strong indication that EBOC is, at least in genetically predisposed subjects, favoured by the inclusion of gluten in the diet. Current knowledge about latent CD and our data support the hypothesis that at least some subjects with EBOC with normal intestinal mucosa fall in this category and can in fact benefit from GFD. On the other hand, a history of malabsorption documented with specific tests, or even a previous diagnosis of coeliac disease (subsequently refuted), as with the presence of indirect signs of malabsorption (low blood level of folic acid) are reported in the literature (Gobbi et al., 1992b; Magaudda et al., 1993; Tiacci et al., 1993), thus assuming for these cases a 'French' type model of latent CD ('the atrophy that heals').

Two sisters with EBOC and normal intestinal mucosa have been described (Tortorella et al., 1993) and are per se evidence of genetic predisposition to the disease. The study of latent CD markers in these two sisters (DQA1*0501 – DQB1*0201 heterodimer, antiendomysium antibodies repeated after a period of time, computerized morphometry, intraepithelial gamma/delta receptor lymphocytes) and an attempt to follow a gluten-free diet could provide valuable information in clarifying whether EBOC and CD are genetically determined diseases, statistically associated because they share some genetic markers in linkage disequilibrium or, whether a causal relationship exists between the two conditions even in the absence of alterations of the intestinal mucosa.

References

Chorzelski, T.P., Rosinska, D., Beutner, E.H., Sulej, J. & Kumar V. (1988): Aggressive gluten challenge of dermatitis herpetiformis cases converts them from seronegative to seropositive for IgA-class endomysial antibodies. *J. Am. Acad. Dermatol.* **18,** 672–678.

Ferguson, A. & Murray, D. (1971): Quantitation of intraepithelial lymphocytes in human jejunum. *Gut* **12,** 988–994.

Ferguson, A., Blackwell, J.N. & Barnetson, R.S.C. (1987): Effects of additional dietary gluten on small-intestinal mucosa of volunteers and of patients with dermatitis herpetiformis. *Scand. J. Gastroenterol.* **22,** 543–549.

Ferguson, A., Arranz, E. & O'Mahony, S. (1992): Definitions and diagnostic criteria of latent and potential coeliac disease. In: *Common food intolerances 1: epidemiology of coeliac disease,* eds. S. Auricchio & J.K. Visakorpi, pp. 119–127. Basel: Karger.

Gobbi, G., Ambrosetto, P., Zaniboni, M.G., Lambertini, A., Ambrosioni, G. & Tassinari, C.A. (1992): Celiac disease, posterior cerebral calcifications and epilepsy. *Brain Dev.* **14,** 23–29.

Gobbi, G., Bouquet, F., Greco, L., Lambertini, A., Tassinari, C.A., Ventura, A. & Zaniboni, M.G. (1992): Coeliac disease, epilepsy, and cerebral calcifications. *Lancet* **340,** 439–443.

Gobbi, G. (1995): Coeliac disease, epilepsy and cerebral calcifications. Proceedings of the International Meeting *Epilepsy and other neurological disorders in coeliac disease,* Republic of S. Marino, April 10–12, 1995.

Guerrini, R., Ughi, C., Battini, R., Chiaravacoti, G., Dal Monte, A., Carapicchi, R. & Taddeucci, G. (1997): (Prevelance of epilepsy and seizures types in coeliac disease and prevelance of unrecognised coeliac disease in children with neuroligic and psychiatric disorders. In: *Epilepsy and other neurological disorders in coeliac disea*se. This volume, chapter 16, Ed. G. Gobbi et al. London: John Libbey.

Holm, K., Savilhati, E., Koskimies, S., Lipsanen, V. & Maki, M. (1994): Immunohistochemical changes in the jejunum in first degree relatives of patients with coeliac disease and the coeliac disease marker DQ genes HLA class II antigen expression, interleukin-2 receptor positive cells and dividing crypt cells. *Gut* **35,** 55–60.

Magaudda, A., Dalla Bernardina, B., De Marco, P., Sfaello, Z., Longo, M., Colamaria, V., Daniele, O., Tortorella, G., Tata, M.A., Di Perri, R. & Meduri, M. (1993): Bilateral occipital calcification, epilepsy and coeliac disease: clinical and neuroimaging features of a new syndrome. *J. Neurol. Neurosurg. Psychiatry* **56,** 885–889.

Maki, M., Holm, K., Koskimies, S., Hallstrom, O. & Visakorpi, J.K. (1990): Normal small bowel biopsy followed by coeliac disease. *Arch. Dis. Child.* **65,** 1137–1141.

Maki, M., Hupponen, T., Holm, K. & Hallstrom O. (1995): Seroconversion of reticulin autoantibodies predicts coeliac disease in insulin dependent diabetes mellitus. *Gut* **36,** 239–242.

Molteni, N., Bardella, M.T., Baldassarri, A.R. & Bianchi P.A. (1988): Celiac disease associated with epilepsy and intracranial calcifications: report of two patients. *Am. J. Gastroenterol.* **83,** 992–994.

Sammaritano, M., Andermann, F., Melanson, D., Guberman, A., Tinuper, P. & Gastaut H. (1988): The syndrome of intractable epilepsy, bilateral occipital calcifications and folic acid deficiency. *Neurology* **38,** 239.

Sasazuki, T. & Kimura, A. (1992): *HLA 1991*, vol. 1. Oxford: Oxford University Press.

Savilhati, E., Maki, M., Holm, K., Koskimies, S., Lipsanen, V., Reunala, T. & Klemola, T. (1992): Immunological markers of latent coeliac disease. In *Common food intolerances 1: epidemiology of coeliac disease*, eds. S.Auricchio & J.K. Visakorpi, pp. 128–141. Basel: Karger.

Schmitz, J., Arnaud-Battandier, F., Jos, J. & Rey, J. (1984): Long term follow-up of childhood coeliac disease. Is there a natural recovery? *Pediatr. Res.* **18,** 1054 (Abstract).

Tanganelli, P., Malfatto, L., Beluschi, C., Babbini, S., Giambartolomei, G. & Regesta, G. (1997): Coeliac disease, epilepsy and cerebral calcifications. Report of a typical case with long-term follow-up.Proceedings of the International Meeting *Epilepsy and other neurological disorders in coeliac disease,* Republic of S.Marino, April 10–12, 1995..This volume. Addendum. London: John Libbey.

Terasaki, P.I. & Mc Clelland, J.D. (1964): Microdroplet assay for human serum cytotoxins. *Nature* **204,** 998–1000.

Tiacci, C., D'Alessandro, P, Cantisani, T.A., Piccirilli, M., Signorini, E., Pelli, M.A., Cavalletti, M.L., Castellucci, G., Palmeri, S., Battisti, C. & Federico, A. (1993): Epilepsy with bilateral occipital calcifications: Sturge–Weber variant or a different encephalopathy? *Epilepsia* **34,** 528–539.

Tortorella, G., Magaudda, A., Mercuri, E., Longo, M. & Guzzetta, F. (1993): Familial unilateral and bilateral occipital calcifications and epilepsy. *Neuropediatrics* **24,** 341–342.

Troncone,R., for the SIGEP Working Group on Latent Coeliac Disease (1995): Latent coeliac disease in Italy**.** *Acta Paediatr.* **84,** 1252–1257

Ventura, A, Bouquet, F., Sartorelli, C., Barbi, E., Torre, G. & Tommasini, G. (1991): Coeliac disease, folic acid deficiency and epilepsy with cerebral calcifications. *Acta Paediatr. Scand.* **80,** 559–562.

Weinstein, W.M. (1974): Latent celiac sprue. *Gastroenterology* **66,** 489–493.

Epilepsy and other neurological disorders in coeliac disease, edited by G. Gobbi *et al.*
© 1997 John Libbey & Company Ltd, pp. 89–92.

Chapter 13

Gluten-free diet and evolution of the seizures in coeliac disease and epilepsy

E. Del Giudice

Department of Pediatrics, University of Naples Federico II, Via S. Pansini, 5, 80131 Naples, Italy

Introduction

The large Italian multicentre study coordinated by Gobbi *et al.* (Gobbi *et al.*, 1992) has been a fundamental step in understanding of the association between coeliac disease (CD) and epilepsy, even though an apparent increase in the prevalence of epilepsy among patients with CD had already been reported in the literature (Chapman *et al.*, 1978). The study identified two groups of CD patients: one with epilepsy *and* cerebral calcifications and one with epilepsy *only*; a third group of patients with epilepsy and cerebral calcifications *without* clinically manifest CD (but with a HLA phenotype consistent with a diagnosis of CD) was also found.

One of the points raised by the Italian study was related to the factors involved in seizure control. Seizures ceased or were reduced in frequency by at least 50 per cent in a third of patients with the full-blown syndrome (CD, epilepsy and cerebral calcifications) after introduction of a gluten-free diet (GFD); patients whose seizures stopped were younger at onset of the GFD and their epilepsy was of shorter duration.

Another Italian study of patients diagnosed with CD in childhood (Bardella *et al.*, 1994) has suggested, based on retrospective evidence, that early identification and treatment will prevent or reverse the tendency to epilepsy.

As an extension and follow-up of the Italian multicentre study (Gobbi *et al.*, 1992), additional information was gathered to analyse further the relationship between seizure course and the GFD.

Patients and methods

Clinical data from 40 patients (13 male, 27 female; mean (SD) age 21.2 (6.8) years (range 9–37)) from 14 centres widespread all over Italy were collected either directly or by phone calls to the treating doctors.

Epileptic seizures were classified according to the 1981 criteria of the International League Against Epilepsy (Commission on Classification and Terminology, 1981).

EEG abnormalities were defined as follows: (1) Occipital paroxysmal discharges, not otherwise specified; (2) Occipital paroxysmal discharges suppressed by eye opening; (3) Occipital paroxysmal discharges, bilateral but clearly prevalent on one side; (4) Occipital paroxysmal discharges focalized to one side. The frequency of seizures was defined as: 'very frequent' if one/day or more; 'frequent' if one/week or more; 'rare' if one/month or less.

Seizure outcome was defined as 'improved' if seizure frequency either decreased by more than 50 per cent or attacks stopped; 'worse' if seizure frequency increased by more than 50 per cent.

Results

Table 1 part (a) shows the percentage distribution of the initial seizure type in our series: partial seizures, either simple or complex, or secondarily generalized constitute the largest group. Table 1 part (b) shows the distribution of concomitant EEG abnormalities: most patients showed a pattern of posterior paroxysmal discharges sometimes preferentially lateralized or clearly focalized to one side. Considering the possible outcome in relationship to the different type of initial seizure and EEG abnormalities, no significant differences have been found between the different groups.

Table 1. Types of Seizures and EEG before gluten-free diet

(a)	Seizures	Patients	%	(b)	EEG epileptic activity	Patients	%
	Simple partial	11	27.5		Occipital	13	34.2
	Complex partial	7	17.5		Occipital, eye reactive	10	26.3
	Secondarily generalized	8	20		Occipital, lateralized	6	15.8
	Partial + generalized	6	15		Occipital, focalized	8	21.1
	Generalized	8	20		Normal – not available	3	2.6
	Total	40	100			40	100

Figure 1 shows the effect of the gluten load measured in number of years with gluten: there is a definite trend towards better outcome for CD patients with less gluten load.

A direct correlation was found when the number of years with gluten was plotted against the number of years with seizures (Pearson's correlation coefficient $r = 0.657$; $p = 0.0001$).

Next, the age at onset of epilepsy and the number of years with seizures were evaluated in terms of seizure outcome: the chances of seizures stopping or improving after GFD was not related to the age at onset of epilepsy; on the contrary there was a trend towards a better outcome for patients having had fewer years with seizures.

Finally the effect of strictly or loosely adhering to the GFD was examined: good compliance was significantly associated with better outcome when compared with the stable or unchanged group (Fig. 2).

The possible effect on outcome of good compliance with GFD in the group of patients taking antiepileptic drugs (AEDs) has also been studied: from our data no significant differences were found between bad or a good compliance with GFD for patients on AEDs.

Discussion

That epilepsy was more frequent among coeliac patients confirms previous findings. More recent is the recognition of a specific syndrome, first proposed by Sammaritano et al. (1988), which includes intracranial calcifications as well partial seizures.

An important issue coming from the large multicentre Italian Study (Gobbi et al., 1992) is the relationship between gluten-free diet and the evolution of seizures. First of all, a prolonged exposure to gluten renders CD patients prone to develop epilepsy, as also demonstrated in the study of the Milan group (Bardella et al., 1994). On the other hand, in the present study, the number of years

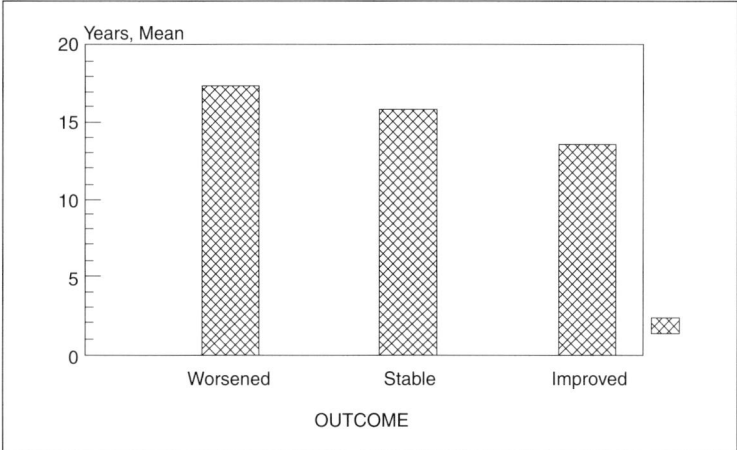

Fig. 1. Impact of the gluten burden on seizure outcome. The three columns indicate the group of patients with a worse, unchanged, or improved seizure frequency, respectively. Bars show the average number of years during which they were exposed to gluten. The chi square for trends was 2.05, p = 0.1.

with gluten, ('the gluten load') strictly correlates with the number of years with seizures: more gluten, more seizures.

Even though some criticism may be proposed by epileptologists in terms of classification issues, we must conclude from our series that the specific types and/or subtypes of seizures correlate poorly with subsequent outcome. This conclusion appears to be confirmed by a recent epidemiologic study (Cockerell *et al.*, 1995).

After introduction of the gluten-free diet patients do better in terms of outcome if they have had less seizures and therefore probably less gluten. In any case patients who strictly adhere to the GFD have a better outcome. The effect of the gluten-free diet appears to be protective and long-lasting.

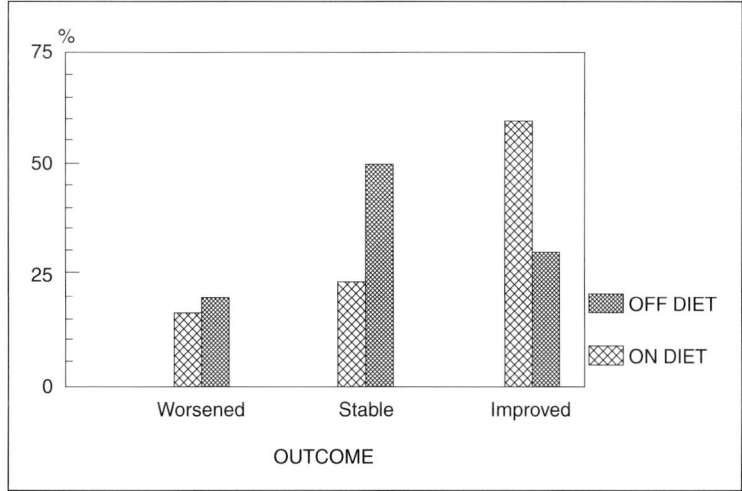

Fig. 2. Seizure outcome according to compliance groups. The percentage distribution of patients who were good compliers to GFD (large squares) compared to poor compliers (small squares) is shown for each outcome group. The chi square was 8.11, p = 0.005.

The apparent inefficacy of good compliance to GFD in patients receiving AEDs is probably due to the degree of already established brain damage caused by the long exposition to gluten.

Epilepsy is a symptom of cerebral dysfunction, even in the case of CD, epilepsy and intracranial calcifications. The aetiology may well turn out to be much more important for classification and prognosis than the type of seizures and of epileptic syndrome.

Acknowledgements

I wish to thank the following colleagues for providing clinical data of their patients: Drs. G. Gobbi, A. Lambertini, C.A. Tassinari, Bologna; V. Galli, Modena; A. Miano, Cesena; L. Piattella, Ancona; C. Filati, Vicenza; N. Molteni, M.T. Bardella, Milan; A. Pascotto, Naples; C. Tiacci, Perugia; G. Capizzi, Torino; E. Veneselli, Genoa; A. Ventura, Trieste, Pisa.

References

Bardella, M.T., Molteni, N., Prampolini, L., Giunta, A.M., Baldassarri, A.R., Morganti, D. & Bianchi, P.A. (1994): Need for follow up in coeliac disease. *Arch. Dis. Child.* **70,** 211–213.

Chapman, R.W.G., Laidlow, J.M., Colin-Jones, D., Eade, O.E. & Smith, C.L. (1978): Increased prevalence of epilepsy in coeliac disease. *BMJ* **ii,** 250–251.

Cockerell, O.C., Johnson, A.L., Sander, J.W.A.S., Hart, Y.M. & Shorvon, S.D. (1995): Remission of epilepsy: results from the national general practice study of epilepsy. *Lancet* **346,** 140–144.

Commission on Classification and Terminology of the International League Against Epilepsy. (1981): Proposal for revised clinical and electroencephalographic classification of epileptic seizures. *Epilepsia* **22,** 489–501.

Gobbi, G., Bouquet, F., Greco, L., Lambertini, A., Tassinari, C.A., Ventura, A. & Zaniboni, G. (1992): Coeliac disease, epilepsy, and cerebral calcifications. *Lancet* **340,** 439–443.

Sammaritano, M., Andermann, F., Melanson, D., Guberman, A., Tinuper, P. & Gastaut, H. (1988): The syndrome of intractable epilepsy, bilateral occipital calcifications and folic acid deficiency. *Neurology* **38** (Suppl. 1), 239.

Epilepsy and other neurological disorders in coeliac disease, edited by G. Gobbi *et al.*
© 1997 John Libbey & Company Ltd, pp. 93–101.

Chapter 14

Epilepsy, cerebral calcifications and coeliac disease: Argentine multicentre experience

Hugo A. Arroyo[*], Susana De Rosa[**], Natalio Fejerman[*] and members of the Working Group and Hospital Filiation[1]

[*]*Neurology Department,* [**]*Gastroenterology Department,* [***]*Pathology Department, Hospital Nacional de Pediatría, 'J. P. Garrahan', Combate de los Pozos 1881, 1405 Buenos Aires, Argentina*

Introduction

Dimitri (1923) published the first description of the gyriform pattern of calcifications, in Sturge–Weber Syndrome (SWS). The term atypical SWS, was used to describe those patients with the characteristic radiological findings but without the portwine facial nevus (Ambrosetto *et al.*, 1983; De Marco & Lorenzin, 1990; Giroud *et al.*, 1990; Gobbi *et al.*, 1988; Tali *et al.*, 1987; Tardieu *et al.*, 1966).

Some of the patients with atypical SWS had meningeal angiomatosis (De Chiro & Lindgren, 1951), but the 'double tram sign' thought to be specific of SWS was later also found associated with: cerebral glioma (Lindgren, 1939, cited in De Chiro & Lindgren, 1951), purulent meningitis (Adeloye & Bohrer, 1971), encephalitis (Williams & Fowler, 1972), ossifying meningoencephalopathy (Wackenheim, 1973), leukaemia and/or intrathecal methrotexate or skull irradiation (Borns & Rancier, 1974).

Garwicz & Mortensson (1976) described two patients with intracranial calcifications mimicking SWS, epilepsy and coeliac disease (CD) in one of them. Folic acid deficiency was postulated as the cause of central nervous system involvement. An increased prevalence of epilepsy in patients with CD was later confirmed (Chapman & Laidlow, 1978).

Several authors, most of them Italian, reported the association of epilepsy and cerebral calcifications, similar to SWS, in patients with oligosymptomatic CD (Ambrosetto *et al.*, 1992; Crosato & Senter, 1992; Della-Cella *et al.*, 1991; Fois *et al.*, 1993; Gobbi *et al.*, 1992; Magaudda *et al.*, 1991; Molteni *et al.*, 1988; Piatella *et al.*, 1993; Sammaritano *et al.*, 1988; Tiacci *et al.*, 1993; Ventura *et*

---

1   *Hospital Nacional de Pediatría 'J.P. Garrahan' – H.A. Arroyo[*], S. De Rosa[**], N. Fejerman[*], V. Ruggieri[*], M. Massaro[*], R. Caraballo[*], E. Guastavino[**], M.T. Dávila[***]; Hospital Italiano de Buenos Aires – R. Benavente[*], P. Kenny[*]; Hospital de Niños 'R. Gutierrez' – J. Di Memo[*], J. Grippo[*], N. Castagnino[**], E. Mavromatopulos[**]; Hospital de Niños de Rosario – M. Aldao[*]; Hospital de San Isidro – M. Mora[*]; Policlínico Posadas – M. Toca[**], L. Cáceres[*].*

al., 1991). Gobbi *et al.* (1992) and Magaudda *et al.* (1993) published results of studies on the largest series of patients with epilepsy, cerebral calcifications and CD, defining the epileptic aspects of this new syndrome.

We recently reported nine patients with the triad of the syndrome (Arroyo *et al.*, 1992) and drew attention to the hypodense areas around the calcifications seen on CT scans. The aim of this investigation was to confirm the presence of this association in Argentina, a country with a large number of Italian immigrants, and the presence of the hypodense areas around the calcifications. We also tried to establish a relationship between the diet and evolution of the epilepsy.

Patients

Twenty-two patients, 14 females and eight males, with ages ranging from 4.2 to 18 years (mean: 10 years), had epilepsy associated with cerebral occipital calcification of unknown origin. A protocol was prepared to detect coeliac disease in these cases, excluding patients with cerebral calcifications due to: tuberous sclerosis, complete Sturge–Weber disease, congenital infections, encephalitis, purulent meningitis, leukemia, chemotherapy, radiotherapy and alterations in calcium-phosphate metabolism. Patients with epilepsy and CD without cerebral occipital calcifications were not included.

There was no history of consanguinity. Ethnic background was traced, and six families were of Italian origin. Two families were Argentine for three generations. All the other children had Argentine parents but no data could be obtained about their ancestors.

Methods

All patients had a detailed clinical gastroenterological evaluation and a jejunal biopsy with Crosby–Kugler or Watson capsules.

Hollander-fixed, paraffin embedded tissues from jejunal biopsies were examined for measurements of villous and crypt length and non-mitotic intraepithelial lymphocytes (ILEs) (normal < 40/100 enterocytes) on sections stained with haematoxylin and eosin (Garcia de Davila *et al.*, 1993, Marsh, 1982). Distribution and immunoreactivity of T-cells were studied using monoclonal antibodies CD 43 and CD 45 RO (Clonab and Dako). Immunostaining was performed by the immunoperoxidase technique employing the avidin–biotin peroxidase system.

Antigliadin IgG antibodies (AGA) were assessed by ELISA and antiendomysium antibodies (AEA), by immunofluorescent indirect test (De Rosa *et al.*, 1993).

When a diagnosis of CD was unequivocal, patients were put on gluten-free diet (GFD) and followed by the gastroenterology departments.

Parents and siblings also underwent detailed clinical gastroenterological evaluations, AGA and AEA. Jejunal biopsy was carried out whenever CD was suspected.

The epileptic seizures and syndromes were classified according to 1981 and 1989 criteria of the International League Against Epilepsy (Commission, 1981, 1989). Mental level or psychomotor development was assessed by the Wechsler scale.

All patients had several EEGs during wakefulness and sleep with electrode placement according to the 10–20 International System (Jasper 1958). Cerebral CT scanning and MRI were performed according to standard techniques. The Mann–Whitney statistical method was used with a significance of $P < 0.05$.

Results

Gastroenterological findings

The 22 cases studied were diagnosed for CD by intestinal biopsy. Chronic diarrhoea and abdominal distension were present in all patients. They started at a mean age of 2.2 years (range 4 months to 5 years), preceding the onset of seizures in all cases. One patient was on a strict GFD when epilepsy relapsed.

At the time of the diagnosis of CD only two patients showed failure to thrive and one had short stature, while the others did not present symptoms and signs of malabsorption. The diagnosis of CD was suspected in 21 patients because of the known association of epilepsy and cerebral occipital calcification with CD. Four patients had first degree family members with CD. Follow up since CD diagnosis was a mean of 2.2 years (6 months–10 years).

AGA and AEA antibodies were positive in 12 and nine of the patients evaluated, respectively.

Jejunal biopsy

Jejunal biopsy samples had the features of subtotal and severe partial villous atrophy in 20 patients. Another two children showed moderate partial villous atrophy with marked increase of ILEs (> 40/ 100 enterocytes). Twelve biopsies studied showed a marked increase in the number of mucosal T-cells and predominance in villous epithelium. T-lymphocytes were strongly positive with both monoclonal antibodies.

Epilepsy and EEG findings

The mean age of onset of epilepsy was 4.9 years (range 1–16 years). At onset, 21 patients (95 per cent) had partial seizures with or without secondary generalization. Only one (5 per cent) had generalized tonic clonic seizures; 18 patients had partial seizures with motor signs and 17 with visual symptoms; eight had episodes of amaurosis, two complained of visual illusions and 11 of migraine-like episodes with elementary visual hallucinations, headache and vomiting. The frequency of seizures was between twice a week to less than one per year. Family history of epilepsy was only present in two patients but there was no association with cerebral calcification or CD.

EEG was normal at onset of epilepsy in 12 patients. In the remaining 10, occipital spikes and/or posterior slow wave activities were found.

All patients received anticonvulsants after the first or second seizure. Mean follow up was 7.4 years (range 2–16 years). In the majority of patients (86 per cent) epilepsy had a relatively benign evolution. Two patients, with partial seizures at onset, developed a severe form of epilepsy with atonic, atypical absence and generalized tonic-clonic seizures.

The evolution of the EEG (2 to 16 years of follow up) was also relatively benign. The last EEG was normal in 13 of the 22 patients; nine of them had a normal EEG throughout the evolution. In the remaining nine cases, posterior slow waves were found in five, occipital spikes in two and generalized spike-waves complexes in two. The latter two EEGs belonged to those patients who developed an epileptic encephalopathy.

Neurological evaluation and mental level

Neurological examination was normal in all but three patients: two were microcephalic and one had cortical blindness; five patients had moderate or slight mental retardation, two of whom deteriorated over time; six had normal IQ but severe learning disabilities; 11 children (50 per cent) had a normal IQ.

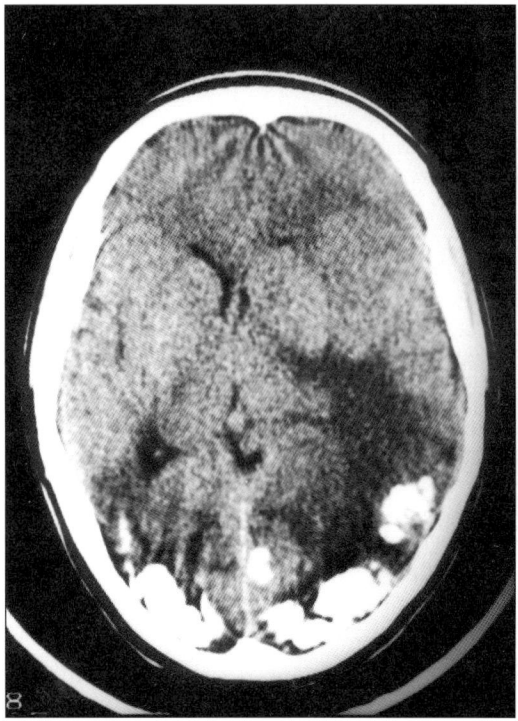 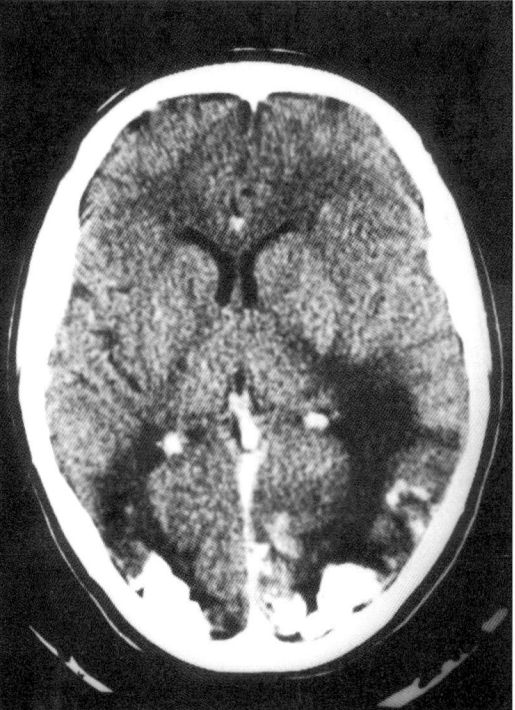

Fig. 1a. Enhanced brain CT scan. Bilateral occipito-parieto calcifications, with surrounding hypodensity, left more than right, with mass effect.

Fig. 1b. The same patient one week after steroid treatment.

Neuroradiological findings

Cerebral CT scanning was carried out several times throughout the evolution in most of the patients. The revisions of previous CT scans, before entry into the study, had been normal in six patients at epilepsy onset. In 11 cases, cortico-subcortical bilateral parieto-occipital calcifications with flocculo-nodular appearance were already present at epilepsy onset. In another five patients, calcifications were more extensive spreading to the temporal and frontal region. The CT of one girl (2 years after onset of epilepsy) showed a decrease in white matter density around the ventricles and corona radiata.

After a mean period of one year, the six patients with normal CTs at the onset of the epilepsy, developed bilateral occipital calcifications. An increase in size of cerebral calcification was seen in four patients and in three other cases, new CT scans showed significant extension of the calcifications spreading to temporal frontal regions and cerebellum.

The CT scans of five cases revealed a decrease in white matter density around the calcifications, without enhancement after injection of contrast. One of these patients was admitted to the hospital with signs of intracranial hypertension and the CT scan showed a large hypodense area around the calcifications with shift of the midline and compression of the lateral ventricle, which improved with the administration of steroids (Fig. 1). In another patient there was a marked reduction of the hypodense areas after one year of GFD.

A total of 10 patients were examined by MRI; five showed in the TI weighted sequence a decreased signal and in the T2 weighted sequence an increased signal, in the parieto-occipital region, around the calcifications (Fig. 2). These findings coincided with the CT images. In other five patients, MRI

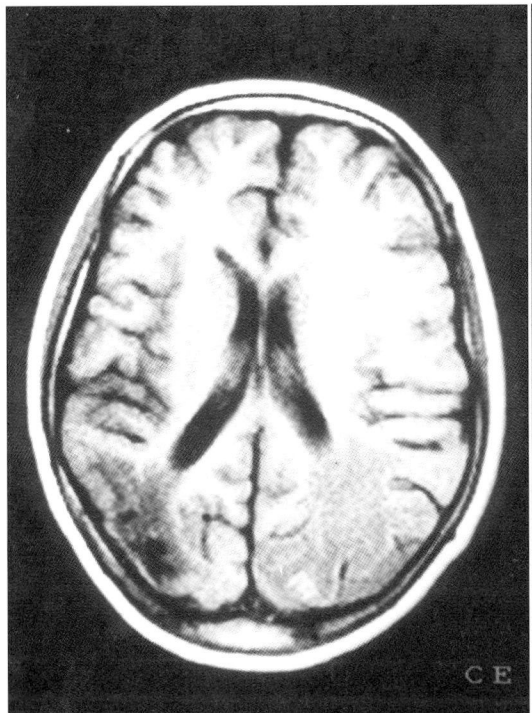 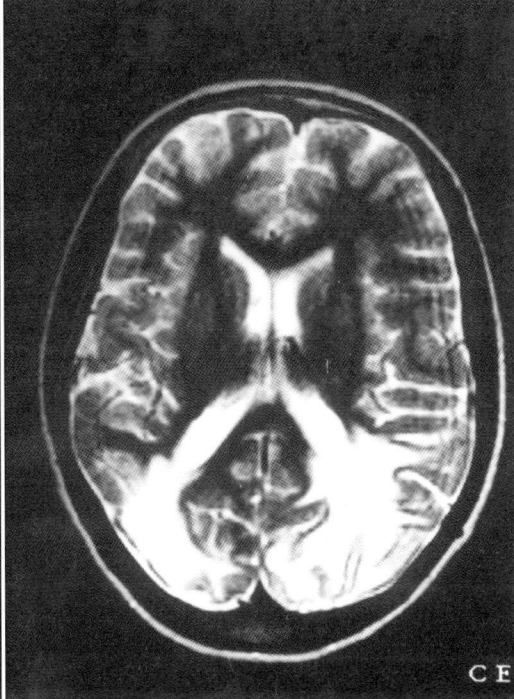

Fig. 2a. Brain MRI. Hypointense occipito-parieto images in T1 weighted sequence. Void cortical signal corresponding to calcifications.

Fig. 2b. Hyperintense signal in the same areas in T2 weighted sequence.

did not show any differences from the CT scan. No sign of leptomeningeal angiomatosis was found even after injection of gadolinium.

Prognosis of epilepsy; the correlation with GFD and other variables

No significant correlation was found with: sex, age at onset of epilepsy, type of seizures at onset, neuroradiological findings and their evolution, first EEG and mental level.

Considering the evolution of the epilepsy, three groups of patients were identified (Fig. 3):

– *Group 1*: (7 patients). Epilepsy was controlled after a period of 4 years with antiepileptic drugs, suggesting a relatively benign evolution of their epilepsy.

– *Group 2*: (5 patients). These kept having seizures while on antiepileptic drugs before coeliac disease was diagnosed. Epilepsy was controlled after the introduction of GFD.

– *Group 3:* (3 patients). Neither drugs nor GFD stopped the encephalopathic type of evolution of their epilepsy.

Duration of epilepsy up to the onset of GFD was compared among the three groups and there was a significant difference ($P < 0.05$) between groups 2 and 3. Therefore a shorter latency (time between onset of seizures and onset of GFD) increased the probability of seizure control.

Discussion

Reports of patients with epilepsy and cerebral calcifications associated with CD have been increas-

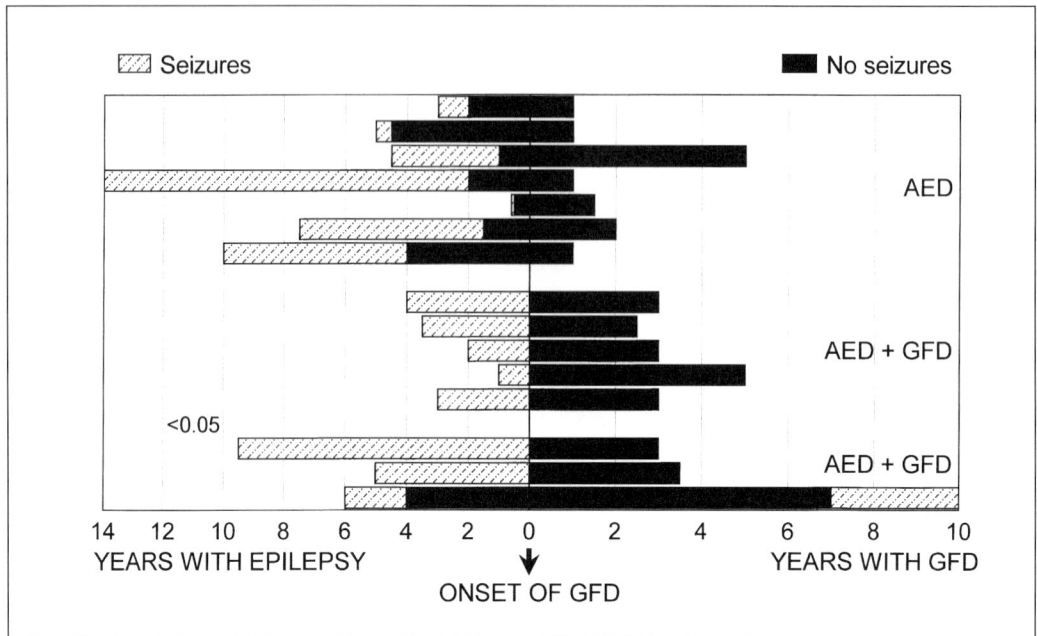

Fig. 3. Evolution of epilepsy: its relationship with antiepileptic drugs (AEDs) and gluten free diet (GFD).

ingly published during recent years. The two largest series, with 29 and eight patients with the complete triad (Gobbi *et al.*, 1992; Magaudda *et al.*, 1993), are patients of Italian origin.

Some of our results are similar to those of others but there are some differences and here we report neuroradiological findings which have been seldom described.

The absence of gastrointestinal symptoms at the time of CD diagnosis and the antecedent of chronic diarrhoea and abdominal distension during the first years of life, were common characteristics of the majority of patients (Gobbi *et al.*, 1992; Magaudda *et al.*, 1993). This type of CD patient could suffer from a silent or latent variant (Ferguson *et al.*, 1993). With one exception, the diagnosis of CD was suspected in all patients, because of its known association with epilepsy and cerebral calcifications.

Partial seizures were the most common type found in this study (95 per cent). Most of the patients had symptoms (amaurosis, visual illusions, simple visual hallucinations) related to an origin in the occipital lobe. Similar findings have been published (Ambrosetto *et al.*, 1992; Gobbi *et al.*, 1992; Magaudda *et al.*, 1993; Ventura *et al.*, 1991), so that this type of seizure seems to be a common feature of this syndrome.

In spite of large parieto-occipital calcifications, permanent visual deficits have been scarcely reported (Crosato & Senter, 1992). One of the patients in this series developed cortical blindness. We are planning to investigate vision in these patients in detail.

Patients with this syndrome seem to have a variable outcome, but there is a tendency to suggest progressive severity (Gobbi *et al.*, 1988; Gobbi *et al.*, 1992; Magaudda *et al.*, 1993; Tiacci *et al.*, 1993). Only three cases (13 per cent) of the present series had drug resistant epilepsy and two developed an epileptic encephalopathy with concomitant intellectual deterioration after a mean follow up of 7.4 years.

Is there a role of GFD in the evolution of epilepsy in this syndrome? We have shown that there is an inverse statistical correlation between the length of epilepsy before GFD and its evolution in some patients. Gobbi *et al.* (1992) arrived at the same conclusion. Bardella *et al.* (1994) found that four patients, out of 128 with CD diagnosed in the first year of life, had epilepsy and cerebral calcifications. They belonged to a group with poor diet compliance. On the other hand, we found that in some patients the evolution of epilepsy had no relation with the diet. Longer follow up, a greater number of patients and, most importantly, earlier diagnosis of CD could clarify the relationship between the evolution of epilepsy and GFD.

The cerebral CT images of parieto-occipital bilateral flocculo nodular cortico-subcortical calcifications are one of the clues for diagnosis. However, as we have mentioned in a previous report (Arroyo *et al.*, 1992), calcifications can appear after the onset of epilepsy. In two out of 18 patients (Magaudda *et al.*, 1993) cerebral calcifications were detected one and three years after seizure onset. Cerebral calcifications are initially located in the occipital region but, after a variable period of time, they grow and spread to other regions such as frontal, or parietal lobes and also to the cerebellum (Aldao, 1992; Fois *et al.*, 1993; Gobbi *et al.*, 1992; Magaudda *et al.*, 1993).

In 1992, Arroyo *et al.*, reported nine patients with this syndrome. Their cerebral CT images showed hypodense areas around the calcifications. They suggested that leukodystrophy-like images were secondary to vascular changes probably related to CD. These findings were again demonstrated in the present series, in five patients. Fois *et al.* (1993) reported a patient with epilepsy and CD with cerebral progressive calcifications and hypodense areas, which on MRI were hyperintense on T2 weighted images. They were located in the white matter of the occipital, temporal and frontal lobes.

What is the significance of these images? Are they areas of oedema or of demyelinization? Probably they are related to vascular changes such as vasculitis, as has been show in a patient with CD and isolated cerebral vasculitis (Rush *et al.*, 1986). The role of CD is also supported by the marked reduction of the cerebral CT hypodense areas following a year of GFD. In favour of demyelinization but against vasculitis, are the pathological changes reported in an excised occipital lobe (Bye *et al.*, 1993). The role of folic acid deficiency in the pathogenesis of cerebral calcification or hypodense areas seems very unlikely in view of the high frequency of low folate in CD patients and the uncommon association with cerebral calcifications.

The initial confusion of this group of patients with epilepsy, cerebral calcifications and CD with those who have atypical SWS can now be easily avoided on clinical and neuroradiological grounds (Arroyo *et al.*, 1995; Magaudda *et al.*, 1993). No patients with hypodense cerebral areas on cerebral CT and MRI scan have been described with SWS (Marti-Bonmatí *et al.*, 1993). On the other hand, none of the 15 patients with typical SWS which we investigated with AGA and AEA were positive (unpublished results).

The results of this investigation confirm that this association is also present in Argentina as previously reported (Arroyo *et al.*, 1992; Arroyo *et al.*, 1995) and that it is the largest series outside Italy. Due to the large Italian immigration to Argentina and identical HLA of Argentine and Southern European CD patients (Herrera *et al.*, 1994) it can be postulated that this group of patients has a genetic background similar to that of the Italian group.

References

Adeloye, A. & Bohrer, S. (1971): Intracranial 'tram-line' calcification in purulent meningitis. *W. Afr. Med. J.* **20**, 195–196.

Aldao, M.R. (1992): Oligosymptomatic coeliac disease and progressive cerebral calcification with seizures. *Pediatr. Neurol.* **8**, 392.

Ambrosetto, G., Antonini, L. & Tassinari, C.A. (1992): Occipital lobe seizure due to clinically asymptomatic celiac disease in adulthood. *Epilepsia* **33**, 476–481.

Ambrosetto, P., Ambrosetto, G., Michelucci, R. & Bacci. A. (1983): Sturge–Weber syndrome without port wine facial nevus. *Child's Brain* **10**, 387-–392.

Arroyo, H.A., Massaro, M., De Rosa, S., Caraballo, R., Di Blasi, M., Taratuto, A. & Fejerman, N. (1992): Epilepsy, posterior cerebral calcifications and celiac disease. *Pediatr. Neurol.* **8,** 389.

Arroyo, H.A., Avalos, M. & Fejerman, N. (1995): Epilepsia, calcificaciones cerebrales,enfermedad celíaca y síndrome de Sturge–Weber: sus diferencias. *Revista de Neurologia* **23** supl.3, 381.

Arroyo, H.A., De Rosa, S., Ruggieri, V., Massaro, M,, Guastavino, E., Garcia de Davila, M.T., Caraballo, R. & Fejerman, N. (1995): Epilepsia, calcificaciones cerebrales y enfermedad celiaca. *Arch. Arg. Ped.* **93,** 310-316.

Bardella, M.T., Molteni, N., Prampolini, L., Giunta, A.M., Baldassarri, A.R., Morganti, D. & Bianchi, P.A. (1994): Need for follow up in celiac disease. *Arch. Dis. Child.* **70,** 211–213.

Borns, P.F. & Rancier, L.F. (1974): Cerebral calcifications in childhood leukemia mimicking Sturge–Weber syndrome. *Am. J. Roentg.* **122,** 52–55.

Bye, M.T., Andermann, F., Robitaille, Y., Bohane, T., Andermann, E.(1993): Cortical vascular abnormalities in the syndrome of celiac disease, epilepsy, and bilateral occipital calcifications, and folate deficiency. *Ann. Neurol.* **34,** 399–403.

Chapman, R.W.G. & Laidlow, J.M. (1978): Increased prevalence of epilepsy in coeliac disease. *BMJ* **2,** 250–251.

Commission on Classification and Terminology of the International League Against Epilepsy. Proposal for revised classification of epileptic seizures. (1981): *Epilepsia* **22,** 489–501.

Commission on Classification and Terminology of the International League Against Epilepsy. Proposal for revised classification of epilepsies and epileptic syndromes (1989): *Epilepsia* **30,** 389–399.

Crosato, F. & Senter, S. (1992): Cerebral occipital calcifications in celiac disease. *Neuropediatrics* **23,** 214–217.

Della Cella, G., Belucchi, C. & Cipolina, F. (1991): Intracranial calcifications – epilepsy – celiac disease.Description of a case. *Med. Surg. Pediatr.* **13,** 427–430.

De Marco, P. & Lorenzin, G. (1990): Growing bilateral occipital calcifications and epilepsy. *Brain Dev.* **12,** 342–344.

De Rosa, S., Litwin, N., Davila, M.T.G., de, Ruiz, J.A., Guastavino, E., Pini, A. & Querlat, A.M. (1993): Correlación de anticuerpos antigliadina y antiendomisiales clase IgA (AGA-IgA, EMA-IgA) con histología intestinal en la enfermedad celíaca. *Acta Gastroenterol. Latinoamer.* **23,** 19–25.

Di Chiro, G. & Lindgren, E. (1951): Radiographic findings in 14 cases of Sturge–Weber syndrome. *Acta Radiol. Stockh.* **35,** 387–399.

Dimitri, V. (1923): Tumor cerebral congenito.(Angioma Cavernoso) *Rev. Assoc. Med. Arg.* **36,** 1029.

Ferguson, A., Arranz, E. & O'Mahony, S. (1993): Clinical and pathological spetrum of coeliac disease-active, silent, latent, potential. *Gut* **34,** 150–151.

Fois, A., Balestri, P., Vascotto, Farnetani, M.A., Di Bartolo, R. M., Di Marco, V. & Vindigni, C. (1993): Progressive cerebral calcifications, epilepsy, and celiac disease. *Brain Dev.* **15,** 79–82.

Garcia de Dávila, M.T. & De Rosa, S. (1993): Indice mitótico de linfocitos intraepiteliales en niños con enfermedad celíaca. Estudio retrospectivo. *Acta Gastroenterol. Latinoamer.* **23,** 83–85.

Garwicz, S. & Mortensson, W. (1976): Intracianial calcification mimicking the Sturge–Weber syndrome. A consequence of cerebral folic acid deficiency? *Pediat. Radiol.* **5,** 5–9.

Giroud, M., Borsotti, J.P., Michiels, R., Tommasi, M. & Dumas, R. (1990): Epilepsie et calcifications occipitales bilaterales: 3 Cas. *Rev. Neurol.* **146,** 4, 288–292.

Gobbi, G., Sorrenti, G., Santucci, M., Giovanardi Rossi, P., Ambrosetto, P., Michelucci, R. & Tassinari, C.A. (1988): Epilepsy with bilateral occipital calcifications: A benign onset with progressive severity. *Neurology* **38,** 913–920.

Gobbi, G., Bouquet, F., Greco, L., Lambertini, A., Tassinari, C. A., Ventura, A. & Zaniboni, M.G. (1992): Coeliac disease, epilepsy and cerebral calcifications. *Lancet* **340,** 439–443.

Gobbi, G., Ambrosetto, P., Zaniboni, M.G., Lambertini, A., Ambrosioni, G. & Tassinari, C.A. (1992): Cerebral calcifications and epilepsy. *Brain Dev.* **14,** 23–29.

Herrera, M., Theiler, G., Augustovski, F., Chertkoff, L., Fainboim, L., De Rosa, S., Cowan, E.P. & Satz, M.L. (1994): Molecular characterization of HLA class II genes in celiac disease patients of Latin American caucasian origin. *Tiss. Antigens* **39,** 1–5.

Jasper, H. (1958): Report of the committee on method of clinical examination in EEG. *EEG. Clin. Neurophysiol.* **10,** 370–375.

Magaudda, A., Medori, M. & Longo, M. (1991): The syndrome of bilateral occipital calcifications (BOC) epilepsy and celiac disease. Clinical and neuroimaging features of 13 patients. *Epilepsia* **32,** 119–120.

Magaudda, A., Dalla Bernandina, B., De Marco, P., Sfaello, Z., Longo, M., Colamaria, V., Daniele, O., Tortorella, G., Tata, M. A., Di Perri, R. & Meduri, M. (1993): Bilateral occipital calcification, epilepsy and coeliac disease: clinical and neuroimaging features of a new syndrome. *J. Neurol. Neurosurg. Psych.* **56,** 885–889.

Marsh, M.N. (1982): Studies of intestinal lymphoid tissue. The predictive value of raised mitotic indices among jejunal epithelial lymphocytes in the diagnosis of gluten sensitive enteropathy. *J. Clin. Pathol.* **35,** 517–525.

Marti-Bonmatí, L., Menor, F. & Mulas, F. (1993): The Sturge–Weber syndrome: correlation between the clinical status and radiological CT and MRI findings. *Child's Nerv. Syst.* **9,** 107–109.

Molteni, N., Bardella, M.T., Baldassarir, A.R. & Bianchi, P.A. (1988): Celiac disease associated with epilepsy and intracranial calcifications: report of two patients. *Am. J. Gastroenterol.* **83,** 992–994.

Piatella, L., Zamponi, N., Cardinali, C., Porfiri, L. & Tavoni, M.A. (1993): Endocranial calcifications, infantile celiac disease, and epilepsy. *Child's Nerv. Syst.* **9,** 172–175.

Rush, P.J., Inman, R., Bernstein, M., Carlen, P., & Resch, L. (1986): Isolated vasculitis of the central nervous system in a patient with celiac disease. *Am. J. Med.* **81,** 1092–1094.

Sammaritano, M., Andermann, F., Melanson, D., Guberman, A., Tinuper, P. & Gastaut, H. (1988): The syndrome of intractable epilepsy, bilateral occipital calcification and folic acid deficiency. *Neurology* **38,** 992–994.

Tali, A.B., Nagaraja, D., Das, S., Shankar, S.K. & Pratibha, N.G.(1987): Sturge–Weber – Dimitri disease without facial nevus. *Neurology* **37,** 1063–1064.

Tardieu, G., Metzger, J. & Brusset, B.(1966): Calcifications intracraniennes de type Sturge–Weber sans angiome cutané chez un infirme moteur-cérébral. *Revue Neurol.* **114,** 466–469.

Tiacci, C., D'Alessandro, P., Cantisani, T.A., Piccirilli, M., Signorini, E., Pelli, M. A., Cavalletti, M. L., Castellucci, G., Palmeri, S., Battisti, C. & Federico, A. (1993): Epilepsy with bilateral occipital calcifications: Sturge–Weber variant or a different encephalopathy? *Epilepsia* **34,** 528–534.

Ventura, A., Bouquet, F., Sartorelli, C., Barbi, E., Torre, G. & Tommasini, G. (1991): Coeliac disease, folic acid deficiency and epilepsy with cerebral calcifications. *Acta Paediatr. Scand.* **80,** 559–562.

Wackenheim, A. (1973): Meningoencephalopathie ossifiante. *J. Belge. Radiol.* **56,** 373–375.

Williams, J.P. & Fowler, G.W. (1972): Gyriform calcifications following encephalitis. *Neuroradiology* **4,** 57–59.

Part IV

Frequency of epilepsy in coeliac disease and frequency of coeliac disease in epilepsy

Epilepsy and other neurological disorders in coeliac disease, edited by G. Gobbi *et al.*
© 1997 John Libbey & Company Ltd, pp. 105–110.

Chapter 15

Frequency of epilepsy in coeliac disease and vice versa: a collaborative study

M. Vascotto and A. Fois

Clinica Pediatrica, Università di Siena, Via P.A. Mattioli, 10, 53100 Siena, Italy

Introduction

The relationship between epilepsy and coeliac disease is still not clear. Historically, attacks of unconsciousness were described by Cooke in five adult coeliac patients (Cooke & Smith, 1966) and Chapman in 1978 reported a prevalence of 5.5 per cent in coeliac patients, most of them with complex partial seizures (Chapman *et al.*, 1978). The association of epilepsy, coeliac disease (CD) and cerebral calcifications (CC) is now a recognized entity (Sammaritano *et al.*, 1988; Gobbi *et al.*, 1992; Magaudda *et al.*, 1993). Calcifications can be progressive (Fois *et al.*, 1993; Gobbi *et al.*, 1988). In a previous paper we have studied the prevalence of coeliac disease in a group of paediatric patients with different types of epilepsy (Fois *et al.*, 1994). All patients were screened for anti-gliadin IgA and IgG antibodies (AGA IgA and IgG) and more recently with antiendomysial antibodies (AEM Ab) in serum. Indications for CD were found in nine patients and in all of them a jejunal biopsy showed mucosal atrophy. In three of them computer assisted tomography disclosed cerebral calcifications. More recently we have observed a patient with a late diagnosed and treated coeliac disease who died of a cerebral haemorrhage caused by an autoimmune thrombocitopenic purpura with autoimmune anaemia (Toti *et al.*, 1996).

Coeliac disease seems therefore to be associated with cerebral calcifications which can be progressive. Some aspects of this situation are not clarified. First, the incidence of CC in CD has not been determined. Second, the relationship between the beginning of the diet and onset of cerebral calcifications is not clear. The pathogenesis of the CC is also not clarified because the role of folic acid deficiency is not definitively demonstrated and other possibilities have been considered. Multicentre collaborative studies might help to answer the questions regarding the prevalence of epilepsy among coeliac patients, the prevalence of CC among coeliac patients with epilepsy and the possible role of folic acid deficiency in the appearance of CC.

Such a study was therefore proposed and accepted by a number of Italian paediatric institutions caring for patients with CD. The list and the names of contributors are reported at the end of this chapter.

Method of study

A questionnaire was mailed to all the paediatric institutions. Answers were received from 65 of them with information regarding coeliac patients with a minimum follow up of 1.5 years. The questions regarded: (1) the type of clinical presentation of CD; (2) the type and age of onset of seizures; (3) EEG findings; (4) response to anticonvulsant medication; (5) the presence of neurological abnormalities; (6) the presence and localization of cerebral calcifications; (7) the age at diagnosis of CD; (8) the age when coeliac diet was started; (9) compliance with the gluten free diet; (10) if possible, blood folic acid levels in patients with CC.

CD was considered 'classic' when major criteria were present. The presentation was considered to be 'atypical' when diarrhoea was absent. The disease was classified as 'silent' when clinical symptoms were absent and CD was suspected on the basis of significant increase in titer of AGA IgA and AGA IgG and possibly of AEM Ab in the serum followed by jejunal biopsy with a suggestive histological picture. This subclassification was considered useful in order to clarify the relationship between the age at the beginning of the diet and epilepsy with or without CC, since it is reasonable to think that in patients with atypical or silent CD a gluten free diet was started later than in patients with classic CD.

If the answers to these questions were not completely clear, further details were obtained through telephone contacts with the physicians responsible for the compilation of the questionnaire.

Table 1. Clinical and imaging findings in 21 patients with typical CD and epilepsy

Patient	Age (years)	Age at diagnosis of CD (years)	Seizures	Brain imaging
1. A.A.	16	2	CPS + GTCS	Normal
2. B.B.	22	0.5	CPS	Diffuse CC
3. C.M.	14	1	Absence	Normal
4. D.R.	17	12	SPS	Focal CC
5. D.M.	12	1	GTCS	Normal
6. E.M.	14	5	SPS	Focal CC
7. F.E.	16	2	Hallucinatory	Focal CC
8. F.D.	11	2	GTCS	Diffuse CC
9. C.J.	16	11	GTCS	Normal
10. M.C.	20	8	SPS	Diffuse CC
11. N.F.	19	13	CPS	Diffuse CC
12. N.P.	20	12	GTCS	Normal
13. P.A.	21	1	CPS + GTCS	Focal CC
14. P.E.	14	3	GTCS	Normal
15. P.C.	18	?	SPS	Diffuse CC
16. P.R.	11	6	SPS	Diffuse CC
17. P.E.	4	1	GTCS	Normal
18. S.S.	17	12	GTCS	Not performed
19. S.C.	8	1.5	GTCS	Diffuse CC
20. T.A.	15	9.5	SPS + CPS	Focal CC
21. Z.E.	20	16	GTCS	Not performed

CD, coeliac disease; CPS, complex partial seizure; SPS, simplex partial seizure; GTCS, generalized tonic-clonic seizure; CC, cerebral calcification.

Results

A screening programme for CD was started at our institution in 1988. This population differs from that reported in the national survey because the subjects examined were in-patients admitted to our Paediatric Institution which acts as a reference centre, mainly for neurological disorders. The screening procedure consisted of evaluating AGA IgA and IgG in the serum and determining AEM Ab when AGA IgA and/or AGA IgA were positive. The test was repeated and if again found positive a jejunal biopsy was proposed to the parents and performed in all 10 subjects. The histological picture was considered indicative of CD when atrophy of intestinal villi, crypt hyperplasia and infiltration of the lamina propria by lymphocytes and plasma cells were present.

Data on 3969 patients with CD with a minimum follow up of 1.5 years were obtained from paediatric institutions. Afebrile seizures were present in 46 subjects. Seizures were classified according to the 1989 criteria of the International League Against Epilepsy (ILAE): 16 patients had generalized tonic clonic seizures (GTCS), 10 had complex partial seizures (CPS), eight had simple partial seizures (SPS), two had CPS and SPS, five had GTCS and CPS, two had absence seizures, one had SPS and myoclonic seizures, one had hallucinatory seizures, and one had status epilepticus. A brain CT scan was obtained in 41 patients and CC were discovered in 26 children.

Frequency of epilepsy and CC in patients with classic CD

The number of reported patients with classic CD was 2627. Seizures were present in 21 subjects with a prevalence of epilepsy of 0.79 per cent. CC were demonstrated in 12. The mean age at diagnosis of CD was 5.9 years.

Table 2. Clinical and imaging findings in 18 patients with atypical CD and epilepsy

Patients	Age (years)	Age at diagnosis of CD (years)	Seizures	Brain Imaging
1. B.D.	14	6	CPS	Focal CC
2. C.R.	16	10	SPS	Diffuse CC
3. D.A.	12	10.5	CPS + SPS	Diffuse CC
4. D.G.	7	6	GTCS	Diffuse CC
5. D.F.	12	10.5	Absences	Normal
6. F.A.	16	13	GTCS + SPS	Focal CC
7. I.C.	16	9	CPS	Diffuse CC
8. M.A.	3	1	SPS	Normal
9. M.E.	13	13.5	Status epilepticus	Focal CC
10. M.P.	21	18	CPS	Focal CC
11 P M	11	8.5	SPS	Normal
12. P.A.	9	1.5	TCS	Not performed
13. R.M.	20	10.5	CPS	Normal
14. R.R.	21	13	CPS	Diffuse CC
15. S.D.	17	13.5	CPS	Not performed
16. S.G.	18	13	CPS	Focal CC
17. S.A.	16	10	CPS + GTCS	Diffuse CC
18. T.M.	10	1	GTCS	Normal

Frequency of epilepsy and CC in patients with atypical CD

Clinical presentation for CD was considered to be atypical in 993 subjects. Epilepsy was diagnosed in 18 with a prevalence of 1.8 per cent. CC were demonstrated in 11. The mean age at diagnosis was 9.7 years.

Frequency of epilepsy and CC in patients with silent CD

There were 169 of these patients. Seizures were present in six with a prevalence of 3.5 per cent and CC in 3. The mean age at diagnosis was 10 years.

Data regarding these patients are reported in Tables 1, 2 and 3.

Table 3. Clinical and imaging findings in 6 patients with silent CD and epilepsy

Patient	Age (years)	Age at diagnosis of CD (years)	Seizures	Brain Imaging
1. B.G.	10	5	CPS + GTCS	Diffuse CC
2. C.D.	14	11.5	GTCS	Normal
3. C.G.	13	11	CPS	Focal CC
4. K.M.	17	7.5	GTCS	Normal
5. S.A.	30	28	SPS + myoclonic	Focal CC
6. S.D.	3	2.5	GTCS	Normal

Patients diagnosed at the Paediatric Institute of Siena

The total number of patients screened at the Paediatric Institute of Siena was 1210. Different types of epilepsy were present in all. CD was diagnosed in 10 patients: the origin of epilepsy was considered to be cryptogenic in nine and secondary to tuberous sclerosis in one. A CT scan was obtained in all 10 and showed CC in three. In one patient the calcifications were progressive. Another patient (MNM), a 16 year old girl with CC, died after a cerebral haemorrhage which occurred because of an intractable autoimmune trombocytopaenia and anaemia (Fisher Evans Syndrome). This patient is the object of another report (Toti *et al.*, 1996). Data regarding these patients with epilepsy and CD with and without CC are reported on Table 4.

Table 4. Clinical and imaging findings in 10 children with coeliac disease and epilepsy, diagnosed by screening at the Paediatric Institute, University of Siena

Patient	Type of CD	Age at diagnosis (years)	EEG	Seizures	Brain Imaging
1. A.R.	Typical	4	SWs right occipital	CPS, transient blindness	Occipital CC
2. B.D.	Late-onset atypical	9.5	S left temporal	CPS, GTCS	Bilat. diff. CC
3. Z.L.	Late-onset atypical	9.5	S left temporal	CPS, GTCS	Small hypod. area left front
4. R.V.	Silent	5.2	S right parietal	CPS	Normal
5. T.A.	Late-onset atypical	8.4	S left occipital	Atypical absences, GTCS	Normal
6. D.G.C.	Late-onset atypical	9.2	SWs diff.	CPS, transient blindness	Normal
7. M.F.	Late-onset atypical	8	SWs bioccipital	CPS	Normal
8. B.V.	Late-onset atypical	17.6	Minimal SW diff.	CPS	Normal
9. M.M.N.	Late-onset atypical	14	SWs bioccipital	CIPS	Occip. CC
10. B.L.	Silent	8.5	SWs multifocal	CPS	Cerebral haematomas

S, spikes; SWs, spikes and slow waves.

Discussion

This large series of 3969 patients with CD yields data which are worth discussing. We will consider the data obtained from the national survey separately from those obtained from the subjects screened at the Paediatric Institute of Siena. In the data obtained from the national survey the overall prevalence of epilepsy was 1.15 per cent with 50 per cent of the patients showing CC. The overall prevalence of epilepsy therefore appears to be only slightly higher than the prevalence of epilepsy in the general paediatric population, considered to range between 0.5–1 per cent. However, the separate evaluation of the three groups with classic, atypical and silent CD was quite interesting. Among the 2627 subjects with classic type of CD, 21 had epilepsy with a prevalence of 0.79 per cent which is within the prevalence limits of epilepsy in the general population as mentioned before. Cerebral calcifications were present in 12 but in these patients the mean age at diagnosis was 5.5 years in comparison to 4.4 years in patients with CD and epilepsy without CC.

This finding is more evident if we consider the 991 patients with atypical disease. Epilepsy was present in 16 with a prevalence of 1.6 per cent. In this group the mean age at diagnosis of patients with epilepsy without CC was 7.5 years but the mean age at diagnosis was 11 years in the 11 patients with CC. These data are even more significant when we consider the 161 patients with silent CD who have a prevalence of 3.5 per cent of epilepsy; the mean age at diagnosis of CC in this series was 7 years but it was 14.6 years in the three subjects with CC. A trend toward a progressively increasing age at diagnosis seems to be evident considering the three groups, because a definitely higher incidence of epilepsy is present in the silent cases; obviously their diagnosis of CD was secondary to the results of the screening. The length of the period of exposure to gluten seems to be an important variable when CD is associated with epilepsy and in particular when CC are present.

In the series of 1210 subjects diagnosed by screening for CD at the Paediatric Institute of Siena this trend appears to be confirmed since the age at diagnosis for patients with epilepsy and CD was 9.4 years. It may be hypothesized that the pathogenesis of CC may be related to low levels of folic acid in the serum. In our national survey, low folic acid levels in the serum were reported in 14/16 of the subjects in which this was measured. In our patient with epilepsy, CC and Fisher Evans Syndrome the levels of folic acid were low but it is possible that an immune mechanism or a silicate toxicity are to be considered (Toti *et al.*, 1996).

Gobbi *et al.* (1992) reported a group of 29 patients with CD, epilepsy and CC in which the age at diagnosis of CD was 14.8 years in subjects attending various neurological departments and 19.2 years in those attending paediatric and gastrointestinal departments. Moreover they suggest that if a gluten free diet is started early in childhood, it may be effective in controlling seizures.

If the importance of a late diagnosis of CD with regard to the pathogenesis of epilepsy should be confirmed, it's reasonable to consider that early diagnosis could be important in order to prevent neurological as well as other well known complications of CC. Because the incidence of CD in Italy is now considered to be around 3.28:1000 (Catassi *et al.*, 1994) a screening programme in order to detect atypical and silent cases should be considered. Clinical awareness of the sometimes subtle and early clinical symptoms together with the possibility of population screening with AGA and/or EMA determination as proposed by Catassi (Catassi *et al.*, 1994) seems to be important in order to prevent all these complications.

Acknowledgements

Torino Ped. Clin. (Prof. Ansaldi Balocco); Novara Ped. Clin (Prof. Bona); Ped. Dep. of Asti Hospital (Dr. Cavallo); Ped. Dep. of Cuneo Hospital (Prof. Spada); Ped. Dept. of Vercelli Hospital (Prof. Cerruti Mainardi); Ped. Dept. of Savigliano Hospital (Dr. Fusco); Ped. Clin. V. S. Paolo of Milano Hospital (Prof. Principi); Ped. Dept .of Lecco Hospital (Prof. Dodesini); Ped. Dept. of Desenzano Hospital (Prof. Monacelli); Ped. Dept. of Meratti Hospital (Dr. Dellamorte); Ped. Dept. of Manerbio Hospital (Dr. Rovetta); Ped. Dept. of Suzara Hospital (Dr. Bertelli); Brescia Ped. Clin. (Prof. Ugazio); Ped. Dept. of Erba Hospital (Dr. Scaravelli); Verona Ped. Clin. (Prof. Mastella); Ped. Dept of. Belluno Hospital (Prof. Colleselli); Padova Ped. Clin. (Prof. Zacchello); Ped. Dept. of Montebelluna Hospital (Dr. Berziolli); Ped. Dept. of Conegliano Hospital (Dr. Semini); Ped. Dept. of S. Donà del Piave Hospital (Dr. Dianesi); Ped. Dept. of Rovigo Hospital (Dr. Temporin); Ped. Dept. of Gorizia Hospital (Dr. Romitelli); Ped. Dept. of S. Vito al Tagliamento Hospital (Prof. Sartorelli); Ped. Clin. of Genoa Gaslini Hospital (Prof. De Toni); Genoa Inst. of Inf. Neurops. (Dr. Veneselli); Ravenna Ped. Hospital (Dr. Scorza); Bologna Ped. Clin. (Prof. Cacciari); Bologna Ped. Clin. III (Prof. Lazzeri); Piacenza Ped. Dept. (Prof. Basanetti); Bologna Center of Ped. Neur. (Prof. Fransoni); Cagliari Ped. Clin. I (Prof. Corda); Cagliari Microcitemico Hospital (Prof. De Virgilis); Ped. Dept. of Ozieri Hospital (Dr. Fele); Sassari Ped. Clin. (Prof. Meloni); Ped. Dept.of Livorno Hospital (Dr. Vallese); Cecina Ped. Dept. (Dr. Di Bartolo); Pisa Clin.Dept. (Dr. Ughi); Arezzo Ped. Dept. (Dr. Giani); Ped. Dept. of San Sepolcro Hospital (Dr. Bartolomei); Ped. Dept. of Prato Hospital (Dr. Pazzaglia); Ped. Gast. Meyer di Firenze Hospital (Prof. Ciampolini); Ancona Inf. Neurops. (Prof. Piattella); Ped. Clin.

I of Rome University 'La Sapienza' (Prof. Imperato); Ped. Dept. of Teramo Hospital (Dr. Di Battista); Ped. Div. of Campobasso Hospital (Dr. Nebbia); Ped. Dept. of Piedimonti Matesi Hospital (Dr. Cappello); Ped. Dept. of Napoli Hospital SS Annunziata (Prof. Tancredi); Napoli Ped. Clin. II (Prof. Auricchio); Napoli Ped. Clin. III (Prof. Rea); Bari Ped. Clin and Soc. (Prof. Rigillo); Bari Ped. Clin. I (Prof. Schettini); Casarano Ped. Dept. (Dr. Corvaglia); Fasano Ped. Dept. (Dr. Scianaro); Ped. Dept. of San Giovani Rotondo Hospital (Dr. Altilia); Manduria Ped. Dept. (Dr. Cosma);Catanzaro Ped. Clin. (Prof. Guandalini); Ped. Dept. of Catanzaro Hospital 'Pugliese' (Prof. Muscolino); Ped. Dept. of Licata Hospital (Dr. Marrani); Ped. Dept. of Palermo Hospital (Prof. Lo Iacono); Catania Ped. Clin. (Prof. Russo); Ped. Dept. of Messina Hospital (Prof. Macchia).

References

Catassi, C., Rätsch, I.-M., Fabiani, E., Rossini, M., Bordicchia, E., Candela, F., Coppa, G.V. & Giorgi, P.L. (1994): Coeliac disease in the year 2000: exploring the iceberg. *Lancet* **343,** 200–203.

Chapman, R.W.G., Laidlow, J.M., Colin Jones, D., Eade, O.E. & Smith, C. (1978): Increased prevalence of epilepsy in coeliac disease. *BMJ* **ii**, 250–251.

Cooke, W.T. & Smith, W.T. (1966): Neurological disorders associated with adult coeliac disease. *Brain* **89,** 683–722.

Fois, A., Balestri, P., Vascotto, M., Farnetani, M.A., Di Bartolo, R.M, Di Marco, V. & Vindigni, C. (1993): Progressive cerebral calcifications, epilepsy and celiac disease. *Brain Dev.* **15,** 79–82.

Fois, A., Vascotto, M., Di Bartolo, R.M. & Di Marco, V. (1994): Celiac disease and epilepsy in pediatric patients. *Child. Nerv. Sys.* **10,** 450–454.

Gobbi, G., Sorrenti, G., Santucci, M., Giovanardi Rossi, P., Ambrosetto, P., Michelucci, R. & Tassinari, C.A. (1988): Epilepsy with bilateral occipital calcifications: a benign onset with progressive severity. *Neurology* **38,** 913–920.

Gobbi, G., Bouquet, F., Greco, L., Lambertini, A., Tassinari, C.A, Ventura, A. & Zaniboni, M.G. (1992): Coeliac disease, epilepsy and cerebral calcifications. *Lancet* **340,** 439–443.

Magaudda, A., Dalla Bernardina, B., De Marco, P., Sfaello, Z., Longo, M., Colamaria, V., Daniele, O., Tortorella, G., Tata, M.A., Di Perri, R. & Meduri, M. (1993): Bilateral occipital calcification, epilepsy and coeliac disease: clinical and neuroimaging features of a new syndrome. *J. Neurol. Neurosurg. Psychiatr.* **56,** 885–889.

Sammaritano, M., Andermann, F., Melanson, D., Guberman, A., Tinuper, P. & Gastaut, H. (1988): The syndrome of intractable epilepsy, bilateral occipital calcifications and folic acid deficiency. *Neurology* **38,** (suppl) 239.

Toti, P., Balestri, P., Cano, M., Galuzzi, P., Megha, T, Farnetani, M.A., Palmeri, M.L., Vascotto, M., Venturi, C. & Fois, A. (1996). Coeliac Disease with cerebral calcium and silica deposits. X-ray spectroscopic findings. An autopsy study. *Neurology* **46**, 1088-1092.

Epilepsy and other neurological disorders in coeliac disease, edited by G. Gobbi *et al.*
© 1997 John Libbey & Company Ltd, pp. 111–120.

Chapter 16

Prevalence of epilepsy and seizure types in coeliac disease, and unrecognized coeliac disease in children with neurologic and psychiatric disorders

Renzo Guerrini[*], Roberta Battini[*], Claudio Ughi[**], Giuseppina Chiaravalloti[**], Anna Belmonte[*], Raffaello Canapicchi[***] and Grazia Taddeucci[**]

[*]*Istituto di Neuropschiatria e Psicopedagogia dell'Età Evolutiva dell'Università di Pisa, Fondazione Stella Maris, Via dei Giacinti 2, 56018 Calambrone, Pisa, Italy;* [**]*Clinica Pediatrica dell'Università di Pisa, Pisa, Italy;* [***]*Dipartimento di Neuroradiologia, Ospedale Santa Chiara, Pisa, Italy*

Introduction

Coeliac disease is a permanent intolerance to protein gluten and is characterized by three elements: (1) mucosal atrophy, with various degrees of malabsorption and malnutrition (2) clinical and histological improvement after an adequate gluten-free diet period, (3) recurrence of clinical and histological manifestations after the re-introduction of gluten into the diet.

The more widely recognized etiopathogenetic theory refers to a gluten-induced bowel lesion of immunological origin. The protein gluten would therefore be an antigen which in coeliac patients induces an abnormal immunological response at mucosal level (Behrman & Vaughan, 1987). Modern diagnostic methods have highlighted latent forms of coeliac disease, which were formerly misdiagnosed. This has allowed detection of previously unknown clinical presentations, which have been defined as atypical as they did not include diarrhoea. Recognition of these forms has stimulated a thorough revision of epidemiological data. It is now estimated that 1/200 children is affected by coeliac disease (silent, asymptomatic, atypical or typical). This figure has substantially increased compared to that of 1/2000 quoted in the 1970s (Littlewood *et al.*, 1980; Swinson, 1980; Grodzinsky *et al.*, 1992; Catassi *et al.*, 1995). The methods for detection of serum antigliadin antibodies (AGA) (O'Farrelly *et al.*, 1983; Volta *et al.*, 1983) and antiendomysium antibodies (AEA) (Cataldo *et al.*, 1993) have facilitated both confirmation of symptomatic forms and recognition of atypical forms; the latter are now estimated to occur in the majority of patients, while their prevalence was estimated at 11 per cent prior to introduction of AGA (Andreotti *et al.*, 1988; Auricchio *et al.*, 1990; Ceccarelli *et al.*, 1991, 1992; Catassi *et al.*, 1995).

Clinical spectrum of coeliac disease

Presenting symptoms of coeliac disease vary considerably and depend greatly on age of onset. Gastrointestinal symptoms are prominent in the 'classical' form, appearing in the first two years of life. Chronic diarrhoea, weight loss, dystrophic appearance and anorexia occur in all patients, irritability and vomiting in about one third (Behrman & Vaughan, 1987). Atypical forms, which are characterized by non-bowel involvement, are more frequent in children over two years and in adults. In addition to iron-deficiency resistant anaemia (Andreotti *et al.*, 1988; Ceccarelli *et al.*, 1991), short stature and puberty delay (Cacciari *et al.*, 1983), recently reported manifestations include: isolated low weight, recurrent abdominal pain, stypsi, headache, herpetiform dermatitis, psychiatric and neurological disorders, especially epilepsy (Chapman *et al.*, 1978; Sammaritano *et al.*, 1988; Gobbi *et al.*, 1992; Fois *et al.*, 1993).

Coeliac disease may also occur in a silent form, i.e. without any obvious clinical manifestation. For example 10 per cent of parents of coeliac patients present with subtotal asymptomatic villous atrophy (Auricchio *et al.*, 1988).

In 1966 Cooke & Smith noted 'attacks of unexplained loss of consciousness' in 5 out of 16 patients with coeliac disease, all having other neurological disorders. In 1970 Morris *et al.* carried out a case study on 30 coeliac patients, describing two who had seizures: one 'Grand Mal' and the other myoclonic. In 1978, Chapman observed that nine out of 185 coeliac patients had epilepsy, seven of whom had temporal lobe seizures. These data provide evidence of the frequent occurrence of epilepsy in coeliac disease. Sammaritano *et al.* (1988) provided the first report of epilepsy with cerebral calcifications and folic acid deficiency. Brain atrophy and dementia, with or without epileptic seizures, was later identified in five adult patients with coeliac disease. The syndrome proved to be progressive and resistant to gluten-free diet in most of the patients (Collin *et al.*, 1991).

An Italian multi-centre study has recently analysed the association between coeliac disease, epilepsy, and bilateral occipital calcifications similar to those of the Sturge–Weber syndrome, in 43 patients, many of whom had previously been misdiagnosed (Gobbi *et al.*, 1992). The relationship between coeliac disease and epilepsy with or without cerebral calcifications remains an object of debate.

Cerebral calcifications similar to those observed in coeliac disease have also been described in folic acid deficiency, following intrathecal administration of methotrexate associated with skull irradiation (Garwicz & Mortensson, 1976), and in congenital folate malabsorption (Corbeel *et al.*, 1985). Folate deficiency may arise from inadequate intake, defective absorption, which can be isolated or part of a generalized malabsorption syndrome, increased requirements or intake of folic acid antagonists. In all these cases there may be calcifications located in the basal ganglia or in the occipital cortex in association with megaloblastic anaemia and mental retardation. Oral treatment with folic acid may cure the anaemia, diarrhoea and recurrent infections but fail to prevent seizures, mental retardation or cerebral calcifications (Corbeel *et al.*, 1985). Cerebral calcifications in coeliac patients may therefore be correlated with chronic folic acid deficiency (Ventura *et al.*, 1991). Coeliac disease, epilepsy and cerebral calcifications may therefore constitute a new genetic syndrome (Gobbi *et al.*, 1992; Tiacci *et al.*, 1993; Pascotto *et al.*, 1994). Immunological screening has been employed to explore this association.

Seizure types reported in coeliac patients were variable: simple or complex partial seizures, tonic-clonic generalized seizures, absences, myoclonic seizures (Gobbi *et al.*, 1992) and both spontaneous and photic-induced occipital seizures (Ambrosetto *et al.*, 1992; Magaudda *et al.*, 1993). Despite a gluten-free diet, the prognosis of epilepsy is severe in many patients with coeliac disease, epilepsy and cerebral calcifications (Ambrosetto *et al.*, 1992; Tiacci *et al.*, 1993). However gluten-free diet seems to be effective in controlling seizures in some patients if introduced in early childhood, shortly after the onset of epilepsy (Gobbi *et al.*, 1992).

No precise estimation of the prevalence of neurological symptoms, in particular epilepsy, has been made in a coeliac population in follow-up. The frequent atypical forms (Andreotti *et al.*, 1988; Auricchio *et al.*, 1990; Ceccarelli *et al.*, 1991; Catassi *et al.*, 1995) have led to investigation of the possible influence of coeliac disease on cryptogenic pathologies of the central nervous system (CNS). The extent to which latent coeliac disease influences neurological and psychiatric disorders, particularly epilepsy, is largely unknown, despite some estimations (Cupps *et al.*, 1983; Rush *et al.*, 1986).

In an attempt to clarify this point, we studied 263 patients with coeliac disease from the Paediatric Clinic of the University of Pisa and 100 patients with neurological and psychiatric disorders from the Institute of Child Neuropsychiatry of the University of Pisa in whom we carried out screening for coeliac disease.

Table 1. Coeliac disease in 263 patients

	Patients	M/F	Age at follow-up	Age at diagnosis	Follow-up
Atypical forms	127/263	44/82 R = 1/2	Mean: 12 years (2 years 3 months–45 years)	Mean: 11 years 6 months (1 year 3 months – 43 years)	Mean: 8 years (3 months–18 years)
Typical forms	136/263	41/95 R = 1/2	Mean: 3 years 7 months (9 months–18 years 8 months)	Mean: 1 year 9 months (6 months–18 years)	Mean: 10 years (1 month–18 years)

Prevalence of epilepsy and other neuropsychiatric disorders in coeliac disease

Patients and methods

We studied 263 patients with CD (89 boys and 174 girls) aged 6 months–43 years (mean age at diagnosis, 7 years 8 months). In 72 patients the original diagnosis of CD had been made clinically, before methods for detection of serum antigliadin antibodies became available. In 191 patients diagnosis was confirmed by antigliadin IgG and IgA, antiendomysium assessment, and jejunal biopsy (Watson–Crosby capsule at the level of the Treitz ligament). Morphology was scored according to Dunnil criteria (Dunnil & Whitehead, 1972). Marked flattening of the mucosa with subtotal or total villous atrophy were regarded as markers of CD.

Table 2. Atypical forms of coeliac disease. Presenting symptoms in 127 patients

Short stature	48 (37.7%)	Herpetiform Dermatitis	3 (4.7%)
Sideropenic anaemia	26 (20.4%)	Stypsi	3 (4.7%)
Asymptomatic	14 (11%)	**Headache**	3 (4.7%)
Recurrent abdominal pain	8 (6.2%)	Vomiting	3 (4.7%)
Low weight	8 (6.2%)	**Psychiatric/behavioural disorders**	2 (1.5%)
Pubertal delay	7 (5.5%)	**Epilepsy***	2 (1.5%)
Diarrhoea and/or stypsi	7 (5.5%)		(1 with posterior calcifications)
Anorexia	6 (4.7%)	Polyuria/polydipsia	1 (0.7%)
Asthenia	4 (3.1%)	Atopic dermatitis	1 (0.7%)

*Isolated symptom

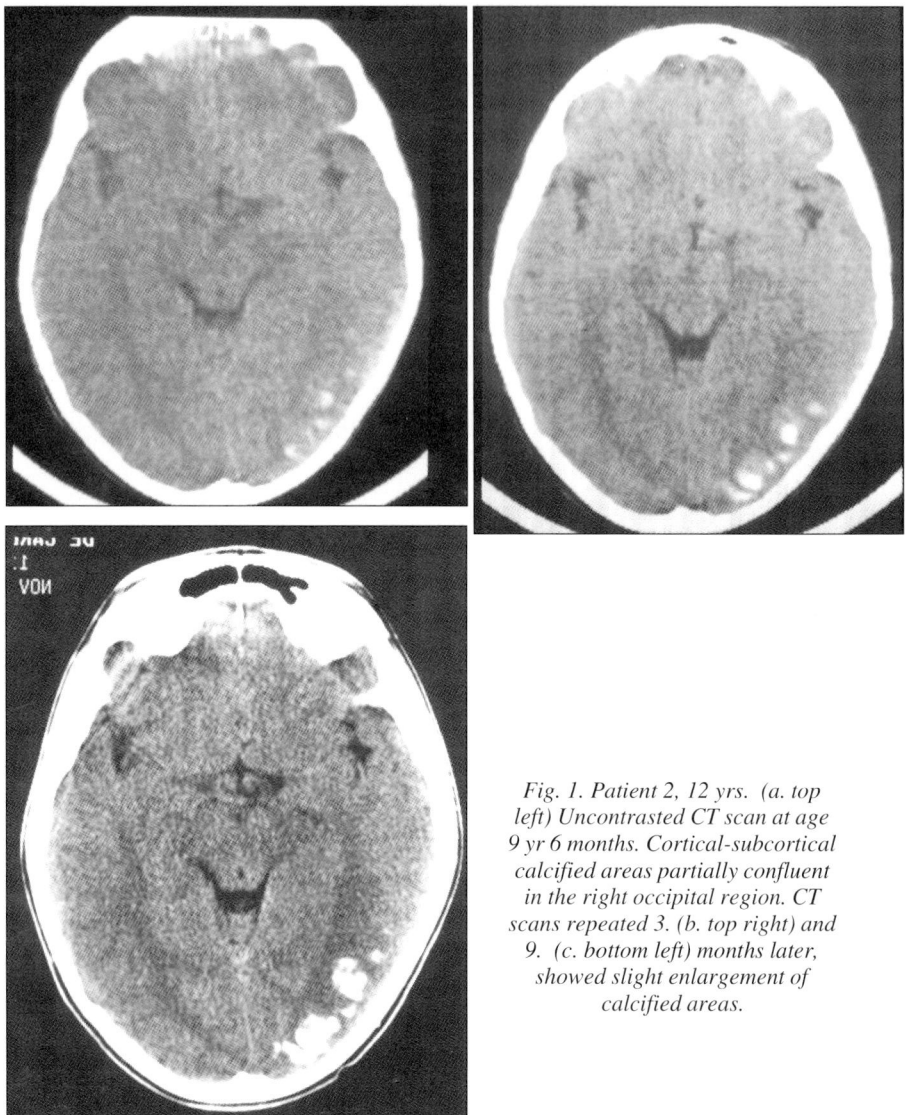

Fig. 1. Patient 2, 12 yrs. (a. top left) Uncontrasted CT scan at age 9 yr 6 months. Cortical-subcortical calcified areas partially confluent in the right occipital region. CT scans repeated 3. (b. top right) and 9. (c. bottom left) months later, showed slight enlargement of calcified areas.

Results

We found 136 typical and 127 atypical forms (Table 1). In atypical forms, presenting symptoms of CD were variable (Table 2). Epilepsy was present in 3 patients: one in whom a typical form of CD had been diagnosed before seizure onset (case 1) and 2 with atypical forms, who were brought to medical attention because of epileptic seizures (cases 2 and 3).

Case reports

Case 1. Female, 24 years

One first degree relative had epilepsy and another CD. She had normal postural development but was moderately mentally retarded. At 8 months, diagnosis of CD was made on a clinical basis,

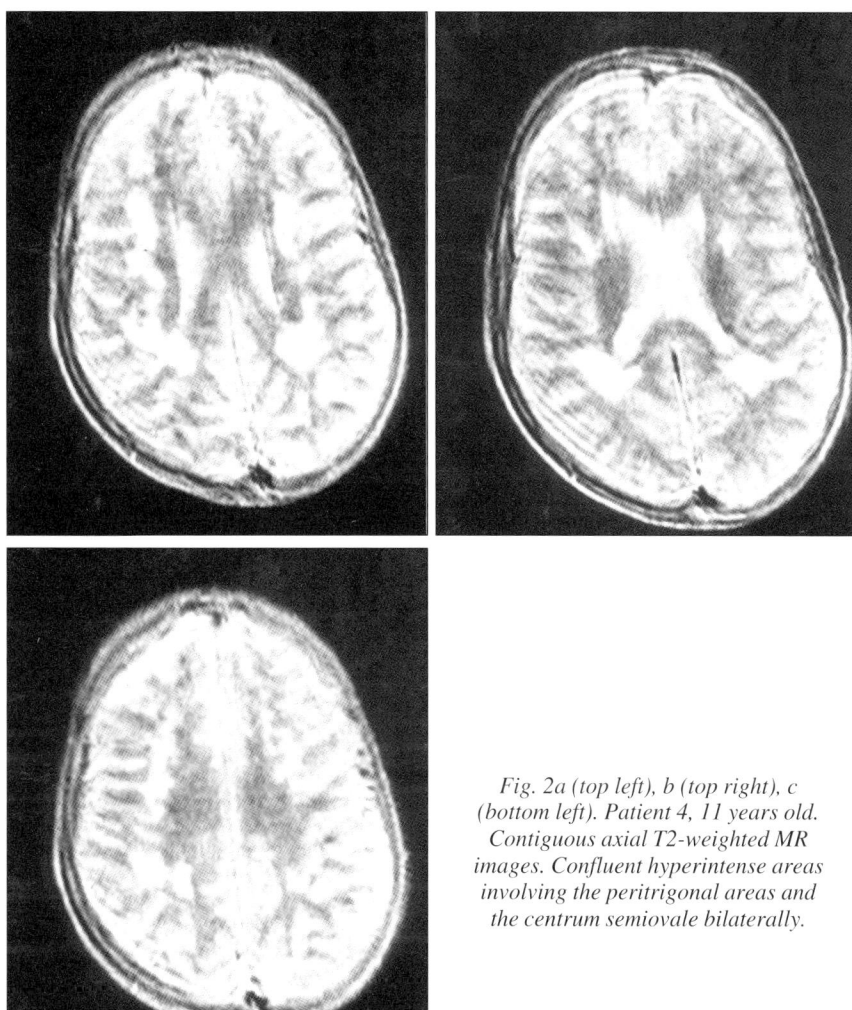

Fig. 2a (top left), b (top right), c (bottom left). Patient 4, 11 years old. Contiguous axial T2-weighted MR images. Confluent hyperintense areas involving the peritrigonal areas and the centrum semiovale bilaterally.

followed by the onset of generalized tonic–clonic seizures. The EEG showed generalized interictal epileptiform abnormalities. In spite of treatment with phenobarbital (PB) and valproate (VPA) she presented several complex partial seizures (CPS) and unilateral seizures per year. She became seizure-free from age 13 on a combination of VPA and benzodiazepines (BDZ). Computed tomography (CT) scan and magnetic resonance imaging (MRI) were normal. She was put on a gluten-free diet at age 23 years.

Case 2. Boy, 12 years

He had normal development. From the age of 7 he showed atopic dermatitis and diarrhoea. From the age of 9 years and 6 months he presented recurrent brief episodes of headache with phosphenes and emesis. The EEG revealed right posterior slow waves and CT scanning showed occipito-posterior-temporal calcifications (Fig. 1a). Gadolinium-MRI was normal. CT scans repeated 3 and 9 months after the first CT examination showed mild worsening (Fig. 1b, c). PB monotherapy failed to control seizures. CD was diagnosed at age 10 years (AGA, AEA and jejunal biopsy). He was put on a gluten-free diet. General improvement was noted 3 months later. No further seizures have occurred in the past 2 years.

Case 3. Boy, 8 years 6 months

Somatic and cognitive development were mildly delayed. At the age of 6 years 8 months, he presented a cluster of generalized tonic–clonic seizures during fever. EEG, CT and MRI scan were normal. Coeliac disease was suspected because of the short stature (3–10 percentile). Diagnosis was confirmed with AGA, AEA and jejunal biopsy. Gluten-free diet and PB therapy were started with no seizure relapse.

Prevalence of coeliac disease in children with neurological or psychiatric disorders

Patients and methods

We selected 100 patients (60 boys, 40 girls) aged 1–25 years (mean age 9 years) to be tested for CD. Patients were investigated for either or both of the following reasons:

   – the aetiology of their neuropsychiatric disorder was unknown, or the clinical expression had atypical features;
   – somatic underdevelopment was part of the clinical phenotype.

Forty-eight children had been diagnosed as suffering from different types of epilepsy: idiopathic generalized epilepsy in five; idiopathic partial epilepsy in 12; cryptogenic generalized epilepsy in two; cryptogenic partial epilepsy in five; symptomatic partial epilepsy in 12; symptomatic generalized epilepsy in eight and epilepsy undetermined whether partial or generalized (severe myoclonic epilepsy) in four.

Fifteen children showed mental retardation associated with dysmorphic features and short stature, 12 showed cognitive impairment alone, 12 autism/psychosis, six cerebral palsy, five behavioural disorders and two chromosomal abnormalities.

Results

The results are summarized in Table 3.

Table 3. Screening for CD in 100 children with neurologic or psychiatric disorders

Presenting symptoms	Epilepsy	Mental retardation + short stature + dysmorphic features	Isolated mental retardation	Autism/ Psychosis	Cerebral palsy	Behavioural disorders	Chromosomal abnormalities
Total number of patients	48	15	12	12	6	5	2
Coeliac disease	–	3	1	1	1	–	–

The following case reports illustrate the clinical findings of the 6 patients with CD.

Case reports

Case 4. Boy, 15 years

This boy had moderate cognitive and statural delay (10 percentile) associated with dysmorphic

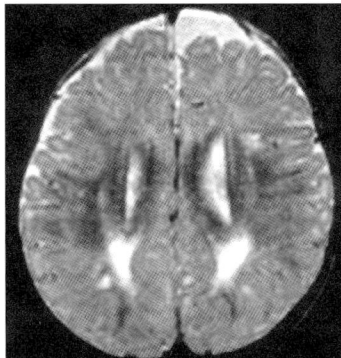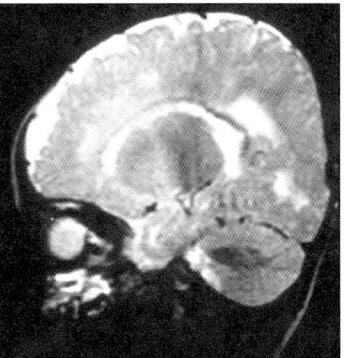

Fig. 3a (top left). Patient 5; 1 year 6 months. Axial T2-weighted MR images. Bilateral periventricular hyperintensity extending into the corona radiata.

Fig. 3b (top right). Patient 5; 1 year 6 months. Sagittal plane (Left). Periventricular confluent hyperintense areas involving the frontal, parietal and occipital lobes.

features: micrognatia, hypertelorism and low set ears. CD was diagnosed at age 10 (AGA, AEA, jejunal biopsy). EEG revealed bilateral occipital epileptiform abnormalities. MRI, performed at age 11, showed hyperintense white matter abnormalities in the centrum semiovale and near the ventricular horns (Fig. 2a–c). There were no brain calcifications on the CT scan.

Case 5. Boy, 2 years 2 months

This boy had severe cognitive and statural delay, microcephaly, low weight (3rd percentile) and dysmorphic features: low frontal hairline, blue sclerae, hypertelorism, epicanthus, short nose, long philtrum and prognatism. CD was diagnosed at age 1 year 6 months. The EEG revealed slow wave activity on both occipital regions. MRI showed high signal intensity lesions in both peritrigonal regions (Fig. 3a, b). There were no brain calcifications on the CT scan.

Case 6. Boy, 4 years 6 months

This boy had mild cognitive delay, short stature (10th–25th percentile) and dysmorphic features: low posterior hairline, broad nasal bridge, cleft- and arched palate, micrognatia, malformed auricles, preauricular tags, 11 ribs, scoliosis and contracted toes. CD was diagnosed at age 1 year 3 months. CT scan was normal.

Case 7. Boy, 2 years

This boy had perinatal hypoxic-ischaemic encephalopathy. At age 8 months he presented some episodes of lateral head deviation accompanied by 'stiffening', which disappeared after ACTH administration. MRI showed diffuse leukodystrophic lesions. Diagnosis of CD was suspected at age 1 year because of chronic diarrhoea, low weight and poor statural growth. Diagnosis of CD was confirmed by AGA and AEA. Jejunal biopsy was not performed. Gastrointestinal improvement occurred soon after the child started the gluten-free diet. At follow-up, 1 year later, there were no apparent clinical changes.

Case 8. Girl, 6 years 6 months

This child was referred because of mild mental retardation. Gastrointestinal symptoms had been present from an early age. AGA and AEA were positive. CD was suspected and confirmed by jejunal biopsy at age 2 years 6 months. The CT-scan was normal. After gluten-free diet was started gastrointestinal symptoms ceased and growth parameters proceeded normally.

Case 9. Boy, 12 years

This child was referred because of psychosis. CD was diagnosed at age 9 years after stunted growth (10 percentile) was noticed. AGA and AEA were repeatedly abnormal, but jejunal biopsy could not be performed and gluten-free diet was refused.

Discussion and conclusions

Epilepsy was found in 3 out of 263 patients with CD (1.14 per cent), a prevalence only slightly higher than that observed in the general population (0.5–1 per cent). Endocranial calcifications were found in only one patient who presented with 'cryptogenic' occipital seizures.

In atypical forms, presenting symptoms were variable. Apart from some abnormalities considered common for the atypical forms (low stature, iron-deficiency anaemia), the prevalence of other atypical presentations, including neurological and psychiatric symptoms (headache, psychiatric and behavioural disorders, epilepsy) ranged between 1.5 per cent and 6.2 per cent (Table 2).

In rare cases, silent CD provoked symptomatic or 'cryptogenic' epilepsy. Seizures, EEG patterns and severity of the clinical picture were not homogeneous. Only one of the three epilepsy patients presented with the typical association of coeliac disease, epilepsy and cerebral calcifications.

Mentally retarded patients and those with dysmorphic features and hyposomia (cases 4, 5 and 6) showed occipital EEG abnormalities, and high intensity signal areas on MRI in the white matter of the semioval centres. Whether these findings represent a mere coincidence or can be correlated to CD remains open to question. A comparable observation was made by A. Federico in a boy with multiple dysmorphic features and mental retardation (personal communication), and by Fois and colleagues (1993) who described a patient with similar signal hyperintensity areas, associated with cerebral calcifications and drug-resistant epilepsy. An autoimmune cerebral vasculitis, akin to that described by Rush et al. (1986), was considered. However this aetiology was to be confirmed since Fois's patient did not show any other sign indicative of vasculitis. Furthermore, this hypothesis seems improbable in our two patients with abnormal white matter signal on MRI (cases 4 and 6), in whom an autoimmune mechanism would have been expected to act very early in life, since such lesions were consistently related to early developmental delay.

The association of coeliac disease, dysmorphic features, hyposomia, mental retardation and areas of white matter attenuation seems worthy of further study. In particular, it appears useful to clarify whether white matter abnormalities may play a role in the genesis and persistence of the cognitive defect and whether they disappear or attenuate after gluten-free diet is started.

Dedication

This paper is dedicated to the memory of Professor Mario Ceccarelli who devoted much of his work to children with coeliac disease.

References

Ambrosetto G., Antonini L. & Tassinari, C.A. (1992): Occipital lobe seizures related to clinically asymptomatic celiac disease in adulthood. *Epilepsia* **33,** 476–481.

Andreotti, G., Deganello, A., Chiesa, M. & Burlina, A.B. (1988): Aspetti atipici della malattia celiaca nell' infanzia. *Acta Paed. Latina* **2,** 189–194.

Auricchio, S., Greco, L. & Troncone, R. (1990): What is the true prevalence in coeliac disease? *Gastroenterol. Int.* **3,** 140–142.

Auricchio, S., Mazzacca, G., Tosi, R., Visakorpi, J., Maki, M., Polanco, I., Ballati, G., Bonamico, M., Picarelli, A. & Viander, M. (1988): Coeliac disease as a familial condition: identification of asymptomatic coeliac patients within family groups. *Gastroenterol. Int.* **1**, 25–31.

Behrman, R.E. & Vaughan, V.C. (1987): *Nelson's Textbook of Pediatrics*, Thirteenth edition, pp. 804–805. Philadelphia: Saunders.

Cacciari, E., Salardi, S. & La Zzari, R. (1983): Short stature and coeliac disease: a relationship to consider even in patients with no gastrointestinal tract symptoms. *J. Pediatr.* **103**, 708–711.

Cataldo, F., Trippiedi, M.A., Marino, V., Maltese, I., Traverso, G., Paternostro, D. & Albeggiani, A. (1993): Anticorpi antiendomisio ed anticorpi antigliadina nella diagnosi e nel follow-up della malattia celiaca. *Minerva. Pediatr.* **45**, 29–33.

Catassi, C., Raetsch, I.M., Fabiani, E. & Ricci, S. (1995): High prevalence of undiagnosed coeliac disease in 5280 Italian students screened by antigliadin antibodies. *Acta Paediatr.* **84**, 672.

Ceccarelli, M., Caiulo, V.A. & Ughi, C. (1991): Changing pattern of coeliac disease in Western Toscana. *Acta Paediatr. Scand.* **80**, 547–548.

Ceccarelli M. & Chiaravalloti G. (1992): Forme atipiche di malattia celiaca. Atti Convegno 'Celiachia 2000: alla scoperta di un iceberg', pp. 45–50. Urbino, 24 Ottobre 1992.

Chapman, R.W.G., Laidlow, J.M., Colin-Jones, D., Eade, O.E. & Smith, C.L. (1978): Increased prevalence of epilepsy in coeliac disease. *BMJ* **2**, 250–251.

Collin, P., Pirttila, T., Nurmikko, T., Somer, H., Erila, T. & Keyrilainen, O. (1991): Celiac disease, brain atrophy, and dementia. *Neurology* **41**, 372–375.

Cooke, W.T. & Smith, W.T. (1966): Neurological disorders associated with adult coeliac disease. *Brain* **89**, 683–722.

Corbeel, L., Van den Berghe, G., Jacken, J., Van Tornout, J. & Eeckels, R. (1985): Congenital folate malabsorption. *Eur. J. Pediatr.* **143**, 284–290.

Cupps, T.R., Moore, P.M. & Fauci, A.S. (1983): Isolated angitis of the central nervous system. *Am. J. Med.* **74**, 97–105.

Dunnil, M.S. & Whitehead, R. (1972): A method for the quantification of small intestinal biopsy specimens. *J. Clin. Pathol.* **25**, 243–245.

Fois, A., Balestri, P., Vascotto, M., Farnetani, M., Di Bartolo, R.M., Di Marco, V. & Vindigni, C. (1993): Progressive cerebral calcifications, epilepsy and celiac disease. *Brain Dev.* **15**, 79–82.

Garwicz, S. & Mortensson, W. (1976): Intracranial calcification mimicking the Sturge–Weber syndrome. A consequence of cerebral folic acid deficiency? *Pediat. Radiol.* **5**, 5–9.

Gobbi, G., Bouquet, F., Greco, L., Lambertini, A., Tassinari, C.A., Ventura, A. & Zaniboni, M.G. (1992): Coeliac disease, epilepsy and cerebral calcifications. *Lancet* **340**, 439–443.

Grodzinsky, E., Franzen, L., Hed, J. & Strom, M. (1992): High prevalence of celiac disease in healthy adults revealed by antigliadin antibodies. *Ann. Allergy* **69**, 66–70.

Littlewood, J.M., Crollik, A.J. & Richards, I.D.G. (1980): Childhood coeliac disease is disappearing. *Lancet* **ii** 1359.

Magaudda, A., Dalla Bernardina, B., De Marco, P., Sfaello, Z., Longo, M., Colamaria, V., Daniele, O., Tortorella, G., Tata, M.A., Di Perri, R. & Meduri, M. (1993): Bilateral occipital calcification, epilepsy and coeliac disease: clinical and neuroimaging features of a new syndrome. *J. Neurol. Neurosurg. Psychiatr.* **56**, 885–889.

Morris, J.S., Ajdukiewiccz, A.B. & Read, A.E. (1970): Neurological disorders and adult coeliac disease. *Gut* **11**, 549–554.

O'Farrelly, C., Kelly, J., Hekkens, W., Bradley, B. & Thompson, A. (1983): Alfa gliadin antibody levels: a serological test for celiac disease. *BMJ* **286**, 2007–2009.

Pascotto, A., Coppola, G., Ecuba, P., Liguori, G. & Guandalini, S. (1994): Epilepsy and occipital calcifications with or without celiac disease: report of four cases. *J. Epilepsy* **7**, 130–136.

Rush, P.J., Inman, R., Bernstein, M., Carlen, P. & Resch, L. (1986): Isolated vasculitis of the cerebral nervous system in a patient with celiac disease. *Am. J. Med.* **81**, 1092–1094.

Sammaritano, M., Andermann, F., Melanson, D., Guberman, A., Tinuper, P. & Gastaut, H. (1988). The syndrome of intractable epilepsy, bilateral occipital calcifications and folic acid deficiency. *Neurology* **38**, 239.

Swinson, C.M. & Levi, A.J. (1980): Is coeliac disease underdiagnosed? *BMJ* **281**, 1258–1260.

Tiacci, C., D'Alessandro, P., Catisani, T.A., Piccirilli, M., Signorini, E., Pelli, M.A., Cavalletti, M.L., Castellucci, G., Palmeri, S., Battisti, C. & Federico, A. (1993): Epilepsy with bilateral occipital calcifications: Sturge–Weber variant or a different encephalopathy? *Epilepsia* **34**, 528–539.

Ventura, A., Bouquet, F., Sartorelli, C., Barbi, E., Torre, G. & Tommasini, G. (1991): Coeliac disease, folic acid deficiency and epilepsy with cerebral calcifications. *Acta Paediatr. Scand.* **80,** 559–562.

Volta U., Lenzi M. & Cassani F. (1983): Gliadin antibodies in coeliac disease. *Lancet* **i**, 1285.

Epilepsy and other neurological disorders in coeliac disease, edited by G. Gobbi *et al.*
© 1997 John Libbey & Company Ltd, pp. 121–132.

Chapter 17

Bilateral occipital calcifications, epilepsy and coeliac disease: Report of 22 cases and prevalence study of calcifications and epilepsy in coeliac disease

Adriana Magaudda[#], Bernardo Dalla Bernardina[#], Giuseppe Magazzù[*], Marcello Longo[**], Mario Meduri[***], Raoul Di Perri and Pasquale De Marco[##]

Departments of Neurology, [*]Pediatrics, [**]Radiology and [***]Psychiatry, University of Messina, Messina, Italy, [#]Institute of Child Neuropsychiatry, University of Verona, Italy, [##]Centro 'Angeli Custodi', Istituti Ospedalieri, Trento, Italy

Introduction

The combination of bilateral occipital calcifications (BOC), epilepsy and coeliac disease (CD) has been recognized as a distinct syndrome since the publication of two extensive case studies (Gobbi *et al.*, 1992b; Magaudda *et al.*, 1991, 1993) underlined the association of the three pathologies in a single individual. Due to the similarities between BOC and the calcifications found in Sturge–Weber syndrome, these patients were initially described as atypical cases of Sturge–Weber (Ambrosetto *et al.*, 1983; Del Giudice *et al.*, 1988; Gugliantini *et al.*, 1980; Pagani *et al.*, 1986; Piattella *et al.*, 1986) because of the absence of nevus flammeus and the consistently bilateral calcifications. Following sporadic case-reports in earlier literature, in which BOC and epilepsy had been found in conjunction with coeliac disease (Garwicz & Mortensson, 1976; Gugliantini *et al.*, 1980; Molteni *et al.*, 1988; Sammaritano *et al.*, 1988; Ventura *et al.*, 1989), BOC patients began to be screened systematically for coeliac disease (Gobbi *et al.*, 1992a), with the result that between 52 per cent (Magaudda *et al.*, 1993) and 77 per cent (Gobbi *et al.*, 1992b) of BOC patients were found to also suffer from CD. The precise relationship between these two pathologies has not yet been clarified and remains the subject of animated debate.

The present chapter is divided into two sections: in the first the characteristic clinical picture and neuroradiological features of patients with BOC are outlined, drawing on case histories, recently amplified, from an Italo-Argentine collaborative study, the results of which have already been published (Magaudda *et al.*, 1993). The second part describes the results of a study presented at the Symposium on Epilepsy and Other Neurological Disorders in Coeliac Disease (Republic of San Marino, 10–12 April 1995), in which we evaluated the frequency of BOC and of epilepsy in a group of patients suffering from CD.

Section I. Clinical picture and neuroradiological features of patients with BOC

Our study group comprised 22 patients, 13 females and nine males, of mean age 14.5 years (range 6–23 years), whose common characteristic was the presence of cryptogenic BOC (i.e. BOC for which all pathologies known as possible causes of endocranial calcifications had been excluded). One patient showed unilateral calcifications, but was nevertheless included in the study because she was the sister of a patient with BOC.

Apart from the two patients just mentioned, family history was irrelevant in all cases. Personal history showed that four patients had suffered from febrile convulsions and that ten had manifested mild symptoms of malabsorption during childhood.

Neurological examination was normal in 20 patients, and remained so during the course of the illness; in one case a bilateral reduction of the visual field was observed and one case had progressive cortical blindness. Intellectual level was normal in 16 patients, while mild deterioration was observed in six cases.

Epilepsy

20 patients (91 per cent of cases) suffered from epilepsy, which is the symptom that most often leads to the performance of a cranial CT scan and so to the discovery of BOC.

One patient was not classified as epileptic because she had experienced a single hemiclonic seizure at four years of age, but had suffered no further attacks.

The remaining patient had been incidentally diagnosed with BOC following a skull X-ray for head trauma. Two types of epilepsy were identified among patients with BOC: partial epilepsy and generalised and partial epilepsy.

Partial epilepsy

16 patients suffered from partial epilepsy, which was occipital in the majority of cases (13 patients). The mean age at seizure onset was 5.7 years (range: 7 months–16 years).

The semeiology of the seizures was variable: versive and/or visual seizures (simple hallucinations, amaurosis); visual seizures followed by complex partial attacks; complex partial seizures without visual symptoms; status epilepticus. The frequency of the seizures was irregular, with a tendency for them to appear in clusters. The course of the epilepsy was variable. In seven patients, now aged between 10 and 16 years, seizures ceased at a mean age of 8.1 years. In four patients, now aged between 6 and 22 years, seizures continued uninterruptedly. In five patients, now aged between 11 and 20 years, a three-phase evolution was observed, consisting of a highly active early phase, with very frequent seizures, sometimes with status epilepticus (four cases), followed by a long seizure-free interval beginning at a mean age of 4.8 years, and then, at a mean age of 10.3 years, by a recurrence of the seizures, which did not correlate with the withdrawal of anti-epileptic therapy. In these patients, the seizures of the third phase were the same as those at the onset of the illness, and renewed treatment with anticonvulsant drugs was generally effective. In one patient, affected by reflex seizures induced by eating, the seizures were drug resistant.

Mild intellectual deterioration was detected in only two patients.

Generalized and partial epilepsy

Four patients had a severe form of epilepsy, characterized in the early phase by the coexistence of

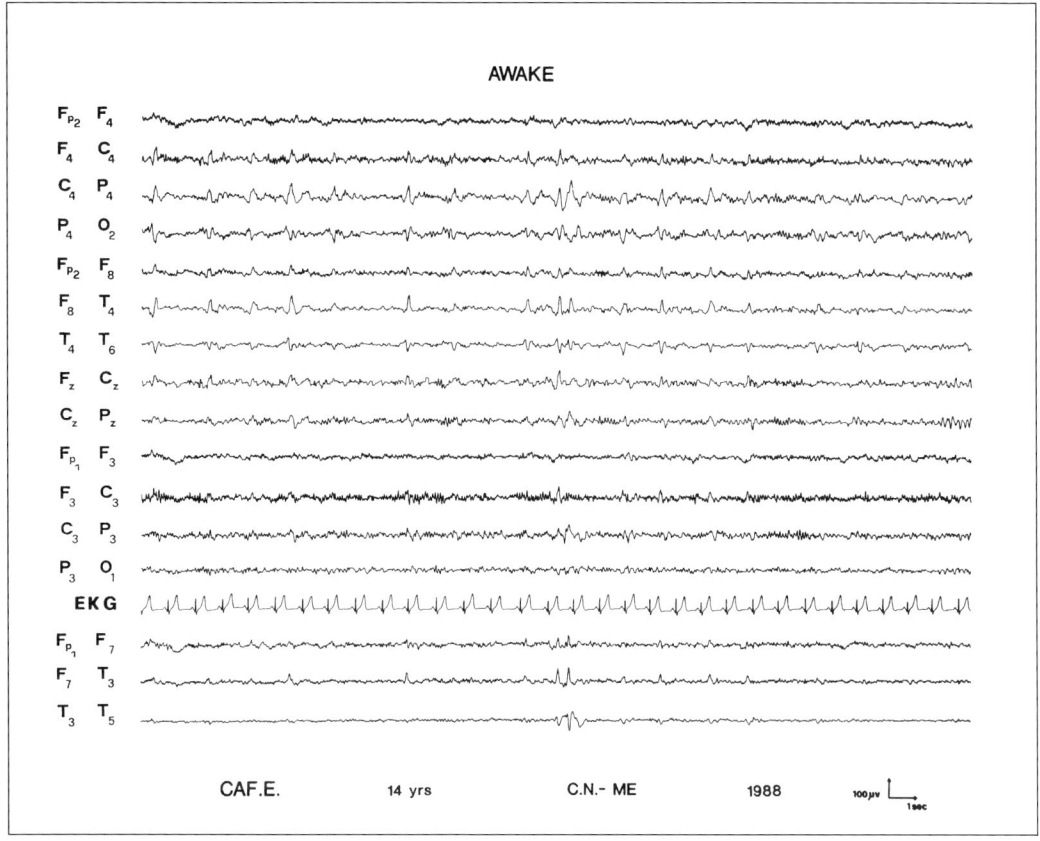

Fig. 1. Pseudoperiodic slow spikes in the right temporo-parieto-occipital regions.

partial seizures (versive and/or visual) with generalized seizures (absences or tonic seizures), which occurred daily or more than once a day. The mean age at seizure onset was 5.2 years (1–9 years).

The seizures continued uninterrupted in two cases, while the other two patients experienced a seizure-free interval of 1 year and 5 years respectively. During the course of the illness a worsening of the symptomatology was observed in all cases, with a clinical picture characterized by very frequent, drug-resistant, polymorphous seizures (atypical absences, partial seizures with falls, visual seizures). Concomitantly, clear intellectual deterioration was observed.

EEG

No typical EEG pattern for BOC patients has been established, since this varies during the course of the illness and from one patient to another. Certain distinct characteristics, however, do emerge from an analysis of the series of EEG performed on our patients:

In the *early stages of the illness*, EEG during wakefulness showed, in most cases, the presence of spikes or spike and wave complexes, localized to one or both occipital regions. For most of these patients, no EEGs during sleep were available in the early phase of the illness.

In the *later stages of the illness*, EEG during wakefulness showed the persistence of paroxysmal abnormalities in all cases, even in those patients who were seizure-free for many years. In those patients with partial epilepsy, EEG during wakefulness showed the presence of focal occipital abnormalities which, in four cases, took the form of pseudo-periodic slow spikes (Fig. 1). In sleep,

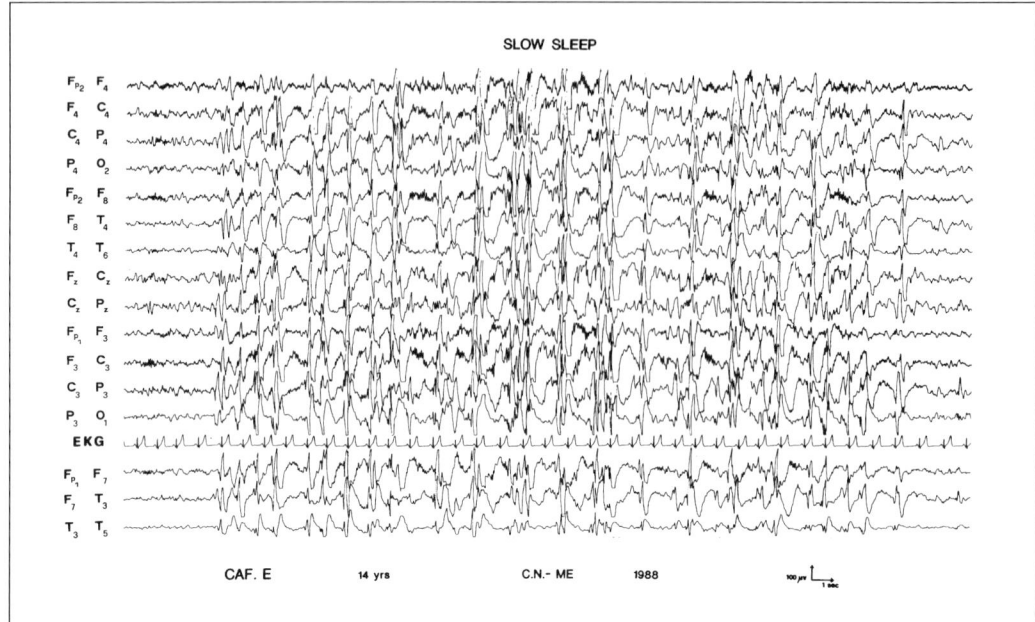

Fig. 2. During sleep, apperance of secondarily diffused slow spike-slow wave complexes, predominant over posterior regions.

there was a bilateral diffusion to anterior regions of these occipital abnormalities (Fig. 2), and diffuse subclinical rapid discharges could appear in the posterior regions.

In those patients with generalized and partial epilepsy, on the other hand, a significant bilateral diffusion of the occipital abnormalities was already visible in the EEG during wakefulness, with the appearance of long bursts of secondarily diffused slow spike–slow wave complexes. During sleep, EEGs took on a 'Lennox-like' aspect, with the appearance of diffuse discharges of fast polyspike –slow wave complexes and diffuse rapid discharges, similar to those associated with the tonic seizures of the Lennox–Gastaut syndrome. These were mainly seen over posterior regions.

Neuroimaging

The most effective means of detecting the presence of BOC is undoubtedly the CT scan. Magnetic Resonance (MR), performed in the standard way, did not show the calcifications at all; skull X-rays were performed in 13 cases but only showed the presence of BOC in four. Cerebral angioscinti-graphy (six cases) and cerebral angiography (four cases) proved to be of no diagnostic value.

In all patients, CT scans showed the presence of bilateral, flocculo-nodular, cortico-subcortical calcifications, of variable size, located in the parieto-occipital regions (Fig. 3).

In only one case were the calcifications unilateral. Frontal calcifications were also present in five of the 22 patients. The administration of contrast medium did not induce enhancement in any instance. The cerebral parenchyma around the calcifications did not show alteration in any of the patients and, in particular, there were no signs of lobar or hemispheric atrophy.

It is difficult to establish when BOC appear, since CT is not usually performed until after the onset of the seizures, when patients are normally 5 or 6 years old. Early CT scans were available for only two of our patients. In these cases the first scan, performed at 2 and 3 years of age respectively, was normal. BOC appeared at 4 years of age in one patient; in the other case, unilateral left parieto-occipital calcifications appeared at 6 years and BOC at 11 years. BOC were monitored in

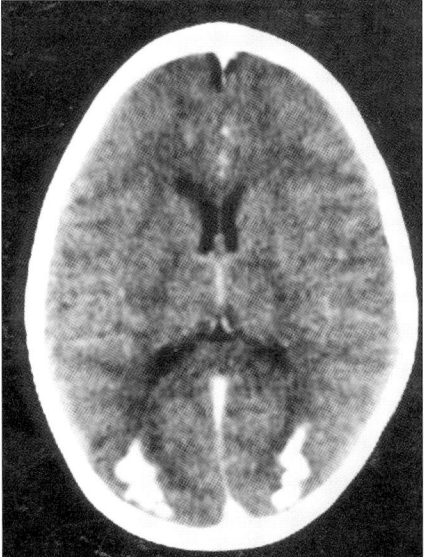

*Fig. 3. Typical CT image of BOC in a 10
year old boy.*

13 cases by the performance of one or more control CT scans. These indicated that the calcifications increase in density and volume during the pre-pubescent phase, while after this the lesions remain stable.

The neuroradiological characteristics of BOC can therefore be clearly differentiated from those of Sturge–Weber syndrome, and may be summarized as follows:

(1) absence of lobar or hemispheric atrophy, which, in contrast, is almost always present in Sturge–Weber syndrome;

(2) consistently bilateral location of the calcifications, found in only 15–19 per cent of Sturge–Weber patients;

(3) cortico-subcortical location of the calcifications, compared to the predominantly cortical location in Sturge–Weber syndrome;

(4) MR is normal in BOC, abnormal in Sturge–Weber syndrome, where it shows lobar or hemispheric atrophy related to the site and size of the angioma.

Coeliac disease and BOC

Nineteen of the 22 patients underwent intestinal biopsy to determine the presence or absence of CD. Atrophy of the intestinal villi compatible with a diagnosis of coeliac disease was found in 10 of the 19 patients (52 per cent). Eight of these 10 patients had suffered from mild symptoms of malabsorption, which had only led to an early diagnosis of coeliac disease in three cases. Two of the nine patients whose intestinal biopsy was normal had also experienced mild malabsorption symptoms.

As regards the influence of a gluten-free diet on epilepsy, reliable information was available for only three of our patients. In one case seizures stopped shortly after the patient started to follow a gluten-free regimen, established 5 years after seizure onset, at 5.5 years of age. In the other two cases, diagnosis of coeliac disease was made at a later stage (when the patients were respectively 8 and 12 years old) and the diet, started 1 and 3 years after the onset of the seizures, did not modify the course of the epilepsy.

HLA

HLA studies were only conducted in four cases. In the two patients from the same family, neither of whom suffered from CD, the typical CD antigens DR7 and DQW2 were found. In another two patients with CD, antigens considered typical of CD were also found: DR3 and DQW2 in one case, and DR7 and DQW2 in the other.

Discussion

From our data and those in the literature, the clinical characteristics of patients with bilateral occipital calcifications emerge quite clearly.

In the majority of patients, the symptom which leads to a diagnosis of BOC is epilepsy. Only one of our patients had never experienced epileptic seizures, while we have found only one example in the literature of BOC without epilepsy: a patient who suffered from cephalalgia (Battistella *et al.*, 1987). The age at onset of the seizures is very variable (the mean is 5–6 years), ranging from the first year of life to 19 years of age (Gobbi *et al.*, 1992b; Magaudda *et al.*, 1993; Tiacci *et al.*, 1993). The electro-clinical symptomatology of the epilepsy also varies. In most cases the epilepsy is partial, and often occipital (Ambrosetto *et al.*, 1992; Gobbi *et al.*, 1992b ; Magaudda *et al.*, 1993; Tiacci *et al.*, 1993), with a variable outcome which ranges from cases that respond well to treatment (Battistella *et al.*, 1987; Crosato and Senter, 1992; Del Giudice *et al.*, 1988; De Marco & Lorenzin, 1990; Garwicz & Mortensson, 1976;) to drug-resistant cases (Bye *et al.*, 1993; Gugliantini *et al.*, 1980; Sammaritano *et al.*, 1988; Tortorella *et al.*, 1993). A particular form of epilepsy was observed in a minority of cases, with seizures of various different types at the onset of the illness and occipital abnormalities on EEG. Subsequently, an electro-clinical picture very similar to that of Lennox–Gastaut syndrome developed, with atypical absences, seizures with falls, partial seizures (both visual and non-visual), while EEGs showed significant secondary diffusion of occipital abnormalities. In these cases there was also marked intellectual deterioration (Gobbi *et al.*, 1988; Gobbi *et al.*, 1992a; Magaudda *et al.*, 1993; Piattella *et al.*, 1986; Tiacci *et al.*, 1993).

A three-phase development of the epilepsy is characteristic, with an early phase which may be very active, and may even include status epilepticus; a seizure-free interval which may last as long as 10 years; and then a recurrence of the seizures, usually during puberty. This three-phase development has been observed both in some patients with partial epilepsy and in some of those patients with a serious, 'Lennox-like' form of epilepsy. Seven cases of generalized epilepsy have also been reported by Gobbi *et al.* (1992b).

The EEG, as mentioned earlier, showed no consistent pattern, but rather one that varied according to the type of epilepsy. The abnormalities most often found were bilateral and asynchronous, located in both occipital regions, and could take the form of spike and wave complexes and/or pseudo-periodic slow spikes (Magaudda *et al.*, 1993; Tiacci *et al.*, 1993). In patients with serious, 'Lennox-like' epilepsy, the EEG, during both wakefulness and sleep, resembled that of Lennox–Gastaut syndrome, although it always showed a clear predominance of paroxysmal abnormalities over posterior regions (Gobbi *et al.*, 1988; Magaudda *et al.*, 1993).

In spite of the extreme variability of the prognosis for epilepsy, the neurological picture is essentially normal for most patients. Rare cases of visual field deficit have been reported (Ciarmatori *et al.*, 1987; Tiacci *et al.* 1993), and there was also one case of this type among our patients. Another of our patients showed progressive cortical blindness.

The fact that neurological examination was normal and that it remained so during the course of the illness differentiates BOC patients from those with Sturge–Weber syndrome. Sturge–Weber patients almost always show signs of focal neurological deficit (Alexander, 1972) and, in bilateral cases, devastating psycho-motor retardation (Boltshauser *et al.*, 1976).

Intellectual deterioration, on the other hand, is always observed in those patients with 'Lennox-like' epilepsy and in some patients with drug-resistant partial epilepsy.

Three cases have been reported (Giroud *et al.*, 1990) where CT scanning shows bilateral occipital calcifications, and in whom the neurological picture is reminiscent of Gerstmann's childhood syndrome (dysgraphia, dyscalculia, disorientation, finger agnosia without aphasia). Associated multidirectional nystagmus, optic ataxia, concentric reduction of the visual field and a static and dynamic cerebellar syndrome were also observed. In that study no reference was made to the presence or absence of coeliac disease.

The authors themselves were unable to offer an explanation for the differences in the progression of the illness in their cases of BOC compared to those reported in the literature.

The neuroimaging features of BOC now seem to have been firmly established (Longo *et al.*, 1992; Magaudda *et al.*, 1990, 1993), and consist of flocculo-nodular, cortico-subcortical, parieto-occipital calcifications, sometimes also present in the frontal lobes. It is important to emphasise that neither CT nor MR showed any alteration of the cerebral parenchyma, either in the vicinity of the calcifications or in other areas. This is the principal characteristic that enables BOC to be distinguished from brain imaging in Sturge–Weber and from other cases, reported in the literature (Fois *et al.*, 1993), in which epilepsy and coeliac disease are associated with progressive cerebral calcifications and widespread damage to the white matter, suggestive of progressive leukoencephalopathy.

The neuroimaging features of BOC, as mentioned above, are generally stable. A slight increase in density and volume of the calcifications is observed in serial CT performed before 10–12 years of age. No further modification of the calcifications is observed after puberty, which correlates well with the stability of the neurological picture.

The most interesting aspect of this new syndrome (BOC, epilepsy and coeliac disease) is the high frequency of CD in patients with BOC and epilepsy. The exact nature of the relationship between BOC and CD, however, remains to be clarified. Some authors have suggested that BOC might be caused by a folic acid deficiency associated with malabsorption (Garwicz and Mortensson, 1976; Gugliantini *et al.*, 1980; Piattella *et al.*, 1990; Sammaritano *et al.*, 1988; Ventura *et al.*, 1989; Zaniboni *et al.*, 1989). This hypothesis was based on reports in the literature concerning cases of acute lymphocytic leukaemia in which endocranial calcifications had appeared following intrathecal methotrexate treatment, together with radiotherapy, which causes inhibition of folic acid metabolism (Borns and Rancier, 1974; Colamaria *et al.*, 1985; Flament-Durant *et al.*, 1975; Mueller *et al.*, 1976; Smith *et al.*, 1980; Spehel *et al.*, 1974; Young *et al.*, 1977).

This hypothesis does not seem plausible to us for the following reasons: coeliac disease is not found in all patients with both BOC and epilepsy; folic acid deficiency is not found in all patients with BOC, epilepsy and CD; the rare reported cases of patients affected by a congenital deficit of the metabolism of folic acid who also had neurological signs did not have intracranial calcifications. These were reported in only one patient (Lanzkowsky, 1970) and they were localized to the basal ganglia and had a punctiform, rather than a flocculo-nodular appearance.

Other neurologic disorders in patients with CD have been reported: (Cooke & Smith, 1966) peripheral neuropathy, (Cooke, 1976; Pallis & Lewis, 1974), cerebellar syndrome (Finelli, 1980; Kristoferitsch & Pointner, 1987), diffuse cerebral and cerebellar atrophy and dementia (Collin *et al.*, 1991; Kinney *et al.*, 1982). No correlation between the neurologic disorder and a nutritional deficiency could be established in any of these cases. As a matter of fact, the character and distribution of the neuropathalogic lesions did not resemble the established patterns of deficiency diseases such as nutritional (alcoholic) cerebellar degeneration, subacute combined degeneration, or pellagra (Kinney *et al.*, 1982). Furthermore, an appropriate diet was not beneficial in any of the cases, not even where an indisputable vitamin B12 or folic acid deficiency had been detected (Collin *et al.*, 1991; Kinney *et al.*, 1982). The authors conclude, therefore, that 'nutritional, toxic, infectious, autoimmune, genetic and therapeutic factors must all be considered' as possible causes of CNS disorders associated with CD, and favour the hypothesis of a common genetic origin for CD and the neurologic disorder.

Pathological findings, though scarce (Bye *et al.*, 1993; Taly *et al.*, 1987; Tateno *et al.*, 1985), suggest that the bilateral occipital calcifications are an expression of a vascular malformation which, as far as we know, is not induced by metabolic changes.

Gobbi *et al.* (1992b) reported the presence of HLA-DR3, DR7 and DQW2 in most patients with BOC, irrespective of the presence or absence of CD. In our familial cases of BOC and epilepsy without CD we found the HLA pattern (DR7, DQW2) usually found in coeliac disease (Tortorella *et al.*, 1993).

These findings strongly suggest that a similar HLA pattern may cause the susceptibility both for CD and BOC.

Section II. Frequency of bilateral occipital calfications and epilepsy in coeliac disease

While it seems clear from the literature (Gobbi *et al.*, 1992b; Magaudda *et al.*, 1993) that a high percentage of patients with bilateral occipital calcifications and epilepsy, ranging from 52 to 77 per cent, are also affected by coeliac disease, the prevalence of bilateral occipital calcifications in patients with coeliac disease without epilepsy has never been investigated. Moreover, the prevalence of epilepsy in patients with coeliac disease has rarely been mentioned, and the increased prevalence of epilepsy in coeliac patients reported by Chapman *et al.* (1978) has not been confirmed.

The aims of our study were to evaluate the prevalence of:

  – BOC in coeliac patients without epilepsy;

  – epilepsy in a large group of patients with coeliac disease.

Patients and methods

Forty-five patients with CD without epilepsy underwent CT scanning in order to evaluate the frequency of BOC. They were selected from 495 coeliac patients followed at the University Hospital of Messina. Their age ranged between 10 and 53 years. In order to verify the hypothesis that a persistent nutritional deficiency is the cause of BOC, we enrolled patients with different lengths of exposure to gluten. They were classified, according to age at diagnosis of CD, in three Groups: < 2 years (16); 18 years (14); > 18 years (15). 130 patients who underwent CT in the same period for head trauma were considered as a control group. We retrospectively evaluated the prevalence of epilepsy in the 495 coeliac patients.

Results

Cranial CT exhibited unilateral cortico-subcortical punctiform calcifications localized in the left occipital lobe in an 18 year old girl diagnosed to have coeliac disease at 10 years of age. In this patient serum calcium, phosphorus, parathormone, calcitonin and TORCH test were normal, excluding some of the causes of intracranial calcifications. No case of BOC was found in the control group. The prevalence of BOC in coeliac patients without epilepsy was, therefore, not different when compared with the control group (1/45 *vs.* 0/130; $P = 0.25$).

Of 495 coeliac patients, six (1.21 per cent) were affected by epilepsy: two had occipital epilepsy symptomatic of BOC; two patients had generalized idiopathic epilepsy; one patient had post-traumatic epilepsy and one had cryptogenic occipital epilepsy. The prevalence of BOC in coeliac patients with epilepsy (2/6) was, therefore, significantly higher ($P < 0.03$) than the prevalence of BOC in coeliac patients without epilepsy (1/45). The prevalence of epilepsy in coeliac patients (6/495 = 1.21 per cent) was higher than that observed in the general population of our region

(25/6887 = 0.36 per cent), $P = 0.015$) but it did not reach statistical significance when the two cases of bilateral occipital calcification were excluded (0.8 per cent; $P = 0.12$).

Discussion

The results of our study demonstrate that the prevalence of bilateral occipital calcifications in coeliac patients without epilepsy is not different from that observed in the control group. On the contrary, the prevalence of bilateral occipital calcification is higher in coeliac patients with epilepsy in comparison to that observed in coeliac patients without epilepsy, suggesting that when bilateral occipital calcifications are present they have clinical significance.

The lack of a high prevalence of bilateral occipital calcifications in patients with coeliac disease, even in those with a long exposure to gluten, seems to be contrary to the hypothesis of a nutritional deficiency as a cause of the calcifications.

The prevalence of epilepsy in patients with CD (1.21 per cent) is higher than that (0.36 per cent) in our general population (Morgante *et al.*, 1990), but when one excludes the patients with BOC it is not statistically different. Furthermore, in three of the four coeliac patients with epilepsy without occipital calcifications epilepsy was clearly independent of coeliac disease: two had generalized idiopathic epilepsy which has a genetic aetiology and in one patient attacks began after head trauma. The fourth patient was similar to other rare cases reported in literature (Ambrosetto *et al.*, 1992) of occipital epilepsy without bilateral occipital calcifications in coeliac patients. In these patients it is not known whether a relationship between epilepsy and coeliac disease exists. Therefore, our data, collected from a very large series of coeliac patients, do not confirm the high prevalence rate (5.5 per cent) of epilepsy in coeliac disease previously reported (Chapman *et al.*, 1978).

In conclusion, coeliac patients without epilepsy do not show an increased prevalence of bilateral occipital calcifications in comparison to the general population. The high prevalence of epilepsy in coeliac disease seems related to the presence of bilateral occipital calcifications. If one excludes this aetiology, the types and frequency of epilepsy in coeliac disease are similar to those found in the general population.

Conclusions

The main points which emerge from our discussion so far are summarized below.

– The combination of BOC, CD and epilepsy constitutes a distinct syndrome.

– This is characterized by epilepsy, which is occipital in most cases, typically develops in three phases, and has a variable outcome (from cases with early remission of the seizures to cases which evolve towards a pattern of epileptic encephalopathy).

– This syndrome is a non-progressive neurologic disorder, as shown by the fact that neurologic examination remains normal during the course of the illness and that brain imaging does not change. Intellectual deterioration is observed only in those cases with severe forms of epilepsy.

– The most prominent neuroimaging characteristic consists of bioccipital, cortico-subcortical, flocculo-nodular calcifications without cerebral atrophy.

– The few available pathological findings suggest that BOC are the expression of a vascular malformation.

– CD is often but not always present. The most plausible current hypothesis is that the association of BOC and CD relates to a common HLA pattern.

– BOC are rarely asymptomatic, as indicated by the lack of any higher prevalence of BOC in CD patients without epilepsy when compared to the general population.

– CD would not seem in itself to be a pathology leading to epilepsy. The higher frequency of epilepsy in patients with CD is closely linked to the presence of cases of BOC, of which epileptic seizures are the clinical expression.

Acknowledgements

The authors thank Miss Elizabeth Mc Ilvanney for the translation of the text and Miss Rita Alfa for her kind cooperation. Members of the collaborative study are: Dr. Zenon SFAELLO, Neuropediatrics Department, Catholic University of Cordoba, Argentina; Dr. Ornella DANIELE, Institute of Neuropsychiatry, University of Palermo, Italy; Prof. Maria Rossana TATA, Department of Neurophysiopathology, University of Naples, Italy; Dr. Vito COLAMARIA, Institute of Child Neuropsychiatry, University of Verona, Italy; Dr. Rodolfo BENAVENTE, Pediatric Department, Italian Hospital, Buenos Aires, Argentina; Dr. Gaetano TORTORELLA, Institute of Child Neuropsychiatry, University of Messina, Italy; Dr. Giuseppe CAPIZZI, Institute of Child Neuropsychiatry, University of Torino, Italy.

References

Alexander, G.L. (1972): Sturge–Weber syndrome. In: *Handbook of clinical neurology*, vol. 14, eds. P.J. Vinken & G.W. Bruyn, pp. 213–240. Amsterdam: North Holland.

Ambrosetto, P., Ambrosetto, G., Michelucci, R. & Bacci, A. (1983): Sturge–Weber syndrome without port-wine facial nevus. *Child's Brain* **10**, 387–392.

Ambrosetto, G., Antonini, L., & Tassinari, C.A. (1992): Occipital lobe seizures related to clinically asymptomatic celiac disease in adulthood. *Epilepsia* **33**, 476–481.

Battistella, P.A., Mattesi, P., Casara, G.L., Carollo, C., Condini, A., Allegri, F. & Rigon, F. (1987): Bilateral cerebral occipital calcifications and migraine-like headache. *Cephalalgia* **7**, 125–128.

Boltshauser, E., Wilson, J. & Hoare, R.D. (1976): Sturge–Weber syndrome with bilateral intracranial calcification. *J. Neurol. Neurosurg. Psychiatr.* **39**, 429–435.

Borns, P.F. & Rancier, L.F. (1974): Cerebral calcification in childhood leukemia mimicking Sturge–Weber syndrome. *Am. J. Roentgenol.* **122**, 52–55.

Bye, A.M.E., Andermann, F., Robitaille, Y., Oliver, M., Bohane, T. & Andermann, E. (1993): Cortical vascular abnormalities in the syndrome of celiac disease, epilepsy, bilateral occipital calcifications and folate deficiency. *Ann. Neurol.* **34**, 399–403.

Chapman, R.W.G., Laidlow, S.M. & Colin-Jones, D. (1978): Increased prevalence of epilepsy in coeliac disease. *BMJ* **2**, 250–251.

Ciarmatori, C., Alesi, C., Michelucci, R. & Tassinari, C.A. (1987): Epilessia e calcificazioni occipitali: un caso con crisi riflesse dislessia. *Boll. Lega It. Epil.* **58/59**, 93–97.

Colamaria, V., Tatò, L., Avanzini, S., Capovilla, G., Paino-Ferrara, F. & Dalla Bernardina, B. (1985): Complicazioni tardive della radioterapia nei tumori cerebrali infantili. *Riv. Ital. Ped.* (IJP) **11**, 406–411.

Collin, P., Pirtilla, T., Nurmikko, T., Somer, H., Erilä, T. & Keyriläinen, O. (1991): Celiac disease, brain atrophy, and dementia. *Neurology* **41**, 372–375.

Cooke, W.T. (1976): Neurologic manifestations of malabsorption. In: *Handbook of clinical neurology*, vol. 28, eds. P.J. Vinken & G.W. Bruyn, pp. 225–241. Amsterdam: North Holland.

Cooke, W.T. & Smith, W.T. (1966): Neurological disorders associated with adult coeliac disease. *Brain* **89**, 683–722.

Crosato, F. & Senter, S. (1992): Cerebral occipital calcifications in celiac disease. *Neuropediatrics* **23**, 214–217.

Del Giudice, E., Romano, A., Pelosi, L., Napolitano, E. & Diano, A. (1988): Bilateral cerebral posterior calcifications and epilepsy: atypical Sturge- Weber or a new nolosogical entity? In *Diagnostic and therapeutic problems in pediatric epileptology*, eds. C. Faienza & G.L. Prati, pp 183–184, Amsterdam: Elsevier Science.

De Marco, P. & Lorenzin, G. (1990): Growing bilateral occipital calcifications and epilepsy. *Brain Dev.* **12**, 342–344.

Finelli, P.F., McEntee, W.J., Ambler, M. & Kenstenbaum, D. (1980): Adult celiac disease presenting as cerebellar syndrome. *Neurology* **30**, 245–249.

Flament Durant, J., Ketelbant-Balasse, P., Maurus, R., Regnier, R. & Spehl, M. (1975): Intracerebral calcifications appearing during the course of acute lymphocitic leukemia treated with methotrexate and X-rays. *Cancer* **35**, 319–325.

Fois, A., Balestri, P., Vascotto, M., Farnetani, A., Di Bartolo, R., Di Marco, V., & Vindigni, C. (1993): Progressive cerebral calcifications, epilepsy, and celiac disease. *Brain Dev.* **15**, 79–82.

Garwicz, S. & Mortensson, W. (1976): Intracranial calcification mimicking the Sturge–Weber syndrome. A consequence of cerebral folic acid deficiency? *Pediat. Radiol.* **5**, 5–9.

Giroud, M., Borsotti, J.P., Michiels, R., Tommasi, M. & Dumas, P. (1990): Epilepsie et calcifications occipitales bilaterales: 3 cas. *Rev. Neurol.* **4**, 288–292.

Gobbi, G., Sorrenti, G., Santucci, M., Giovanardi-Rossi, P., Ambrosetto, P., Michelucci, R. & Tassinari, C.A. (1988): Epilepsy with bilateral occipital calcifications. A benign onset with progressive severity. *Neurology* **38**, 913–920.

Gobbi, G., Ambrosetto, P., Zaniboni, M.G.,Lambertini, A., Ambrosioni, G. & Tassinari, C.A. (1992a): Celiac disease, posterior cerebral calcifications and epilepsy. *Brain Dev.* **14**, 23–29.

Gobbi, G., Bouquet, F., Greco, L., Lambertini, A., Tassinari, C.A., Ventura, A. & Zaniboni, M.G. (1992b): Coeliac disease, epilepsy, and cerebral calcifications. *Lancet* **340**, 439–443.

Gugliantini, P., Carnevale, E., Fariello, G., Rosati, D., Donfrancesco, A., Miano, C. & Sagui, G. (1980): Calcificazioni endocraniche simulanti la sindrome di Sturge–Weber. *Riv. Ital. Ped.* (IJP) **5**, 851–855.

Kinney, H.C., Burger, P.C., Hurwitz, B.J., Hijmans, J.C. & Grant, J.P. (1982): Degeneration of the central nervous system associated with celiac disease. *J. Neurol. Sciences* **53**, 9–22.

Kristoperitsc, W. & Pointner, H. (1987): Progressive cerebellar syndrome in adult coeliac disease. *J. Neurol.* **234**, 116–118.

Lanzkowsky, P. (1970): Congenital malabsorption of folate. *Am. J. Med.* **48**, 580–583.

Longo, M., Magaudda, A., Dalla Bernardina, B., Daniele, O., Capizzi, G., Tortorella, G., Sfaello, Z. & Meduri, M., (1992): Sindrome delle calcificazioni occipitali bilaterali, epilessia e malattia celiaca. Diagnosi differenziale con la Sturge–Weber. Studio multicentrico in 20 casi. In: *Neuroradiologia*, ed. G. Scotti, pp. 109–112. Udine: Ed. del Centauro.

Magaudda, A., Colamaria, V., Narbone, M.C., Capizzi, G., Landre, E., De Domenico, P. & Dalla Bernardina, B. (1990): Calcificazioni occipitali bilaterali senza nevo flammeo: studio di 8 casi. *Boll. Lega It. Epil.* **70/71**, 251–254.

Magaudda, A., Meduri, M., Longo, M., Daniele, O., Tortorella, G. & Dalla Bernardina, B. (1991): The syndrome of bilateral occipital calcifications (BOC) epilepsy and coeliac disease: clinical and neuroimaging features of 13 patients. *Epilepsia* **32** (supp.1), 119–120.

Magaudda, A., Dalla Bernardina, B., De Marco, P., Sfaello, Z., Longo, M., Colamaria, V., Daniele, O., Tortorella, G., Tata, M.R., Di Perri, R. & Meduri, M. (1993): Bilateral occipital calcification, epilepsy and coeliac disease: clinical and neuroimaging feature of a new syndrome. *J. Neurol. Neurosurg. Psych.* **56**, 885–889.

Molteni, N., Bardella, M.T., Baldassari, A.R. & Bianchi, P.A. (1988): Celiac disease associated with epilepsy and intracranial calcifications: report of two patients. *Am. J. Gastroenterol.* **5**, 5–9.

Morgante, L., De Domenico, P. & Coraci, M.A. (1990): A prevalence study of epilepsy: door-to-door survey in a Sicilian community. *Boll. Lega It. Epil.* **70/71**, 321–322.

Mueller, S., Bell, W. & Seibert, J. (1976): Cerebral calcifications associated with intrathecal methotrexate therapy in acute lymphocytic leukemia. *J. Pediatrics* **88**, 650–653.

Pagani, M, Arietti, V., Benvenuti, C., Lonfranchi, V. & Valseriati, D. (1986): Un caso atipico di Sturge–Weber–Krabbe con calcificazioni intracraniche bilaterali in assenza di angiomatosi cutanea. In *Atti del VII Convegno di Neurologia Infantile* eds. P. Benedetti, P. Curatolo & S. Ottaviano, p. 110, Roma: Sigma-Tau.

Pallis, C.R. & Lewis, P.D. (1974): Neurological complications of coeliac disease and tropical sprue. In: *The neurology of gastrointestinal disease*, ed. J. Walton, pp. 138–156. Philadephia, PA: W.B. Sanders Co.

Piattella, L., Zamponi, N., Cenci, L., Rossi, R. & Papa, O. (1986): Calcificazioni bioccipitali ed epilessia: malattia di Sturge–Weber atipica o nuova sindrome? *Boll. Lega It. Epil.* **54/55**, 139–142.

Piattella, L., Zamponi, N. & Porfiri, L. (1990): Calcificazioni cerebrali multiple e celiachia. *Boll. Lega It. Epil.* **70/71**, 263–264.

Sammaritano, M., Andermann, F., Melanson, D., Gubermann, A., Tinuper, P. & Gastaut, H. (1988): The syndrome of intractable epilepsy, bilateral occipital calcifications and folic acid deficiency. *Neurology* **38** (suppl.1), 239.

Smith, D., Bloch, S. & Al-Rashid, R.A. (1980): Basal ganglia calcification on CT scanning in children with acute lymphocytic leukemia. *Neuroradiology* **20**, 91–93.

Spehl, M., Flament, J., Maurus, R., Delalieux, G., Brihaye, J. & Cremer, N. (1974): Calcifications intracraniennes diffuses appairaissant à la suite d'une leucémie aigue. *Ann. Radiol.* **17**, 417–422.

Taly, A.B., Nagaraja, D., Das, S., Shankar, S.K. & Pratibba, N.G. (1987): Sturge–Weber-Dimitri disease without facial nevus. *Neurology* **37**, 1063–1064.

Tateno, A., Matsui, A., Sakuragawa, N., Nonaka, I. & Arima, M. (1985): Two siblings with multiple intracranial hemangiomatosis with calcification. I. *Neurol.* **232,** 112–114.

Tiacci, C., D'Alessandro, P., Cantisani, T.A., Piccirilli, M., Signorini, E., Pelli, M.A., Cavalletti, M.L., Castellucci, G., Palmeri, S., Battisti, C. & Federico, A. (1993): Epilepsy with bilateral occipital calcifications: Sturge–Weber variant or a different encephalopathy? *Epilepsia* **34,** 528–539.

Tortorella, G., Magaudda, A., Mercuri, E., Longo, M. & Guzzetta F. (1993): Familial unilateral and bilateral occipital calcifications and epilepsy. *Neuropediatrics* **24,** 341–342.

Ventura, A., Barbi, E., Bouquet, F., Tommasini, G. & Sartorelli C. (1989): Calcificazioni endocraniche ed epilessia occipitale. Una conseguenza della celiachia? *Proc. XV National Congress of Italian Society of Neuropediatrics,* November, Florence (Italy).

Young, L.W., Jequier, S. & O'Gorman, A.M. (1977): Intracerebral calcifications in treated leukemia in a child. *Am. J. Dis. Child* **131,** 1284–1285.

Zaniboni, M.G., Lambertini, A., Romeo, N., Conti, R. & Ambrosioni, G. (1989): Celiac disease and epilepsy with occipital calcification: an uncasual association. *First British Italian Paediatric Gastroenterology,* Joint Meeting, September, Parma (Italy).

Part V

Aetiopathological basis to correlate epilepsy and coeliac disease

Epilepsy and other neurological disorders in coeliac disease, edited by G. Gobbi *et al.*
© 1997 John Libbey & Company Ltd, pp. 135–142.

Chapter 18

Mechanisms of seizure origin and spread in adults with coeliac disease and bilateral occipital calcifications

Andrea Bernasconi, Neda Ladbon-Bernasconi, François Dubeau, Alan Guberman*, André Olivier and Frederick Andermann

*Montreal Neurological Institute and Hospital, McGill University, Montreal, Quebec, Canada, and
Ottawa General Hospital, Ottawa, Ontario, Canada

Introduction

The reason for the selective vulnerability of the occipital lobe, and the relationship between the cortico-subcortical calcifications and the epileptic seizures in patients with coeliac disease is largely unknown. In the syndrome of coeliac disease, epilepsy and bilateral occipital cerebral calcifications (CEBOC), occipital lobe seizures are frequently encountered (Magaudda *et al.*, 1993; Gobbi *et al.*, 1992; Ambrosetto *et al.*, 1992; Garwicz & Mortensson, 1976; Banerji & Hurwitz, 1971). Secondary generalization with a severe progressive encephalopathy resembling the Lennox-Gastaut syndrome occurs more rarely (Gobbi *et al.*, 1995; Gobbi *et al.*, 1988). Furthermore, other types of partial seizures have also been found in patients who have in addition temporo- parietal and frontal calcifications (Tateno *et al.*, 1985; Tiacci *et al.*, 1993; Gobbi *et al.*, 1992).

In patients with CEBOC, occipital lesions may lead to EEG epileptic discharges in the temporal lobe (Bye *et al.*, 1993; Gobbi *et al.*, 1992; Sammaritano *et al.*, 1985).

The causal relationship between the occurrence of occipital lobe seizures and the occipital lobe calcifications is debated (Ambrosetto *et al.* 1992), but when clear lateralization can be established, resection of the calcifications has been reported to lead to good seizure control (Bye *et al.* 1989; Bye *et al.*, 1993).

We describe the clinical, EEG and radiological findings in three patients with CEBOC previously described in abstract form (Sammaritano *et al.*, 1985; Sammaritano *et al.*, 1988). One of the subjects underwent pre-surgical investigation with stereotactic multiple intracranial depth electrodes implantation (Olivier *et al.*, 1987).

Case histories

Case 1. A 43-year-old Ashkenazi Jewish male was diagnosed to have coeliac disease at the age of one. He developed, at the age of 11, seizures which occurred 6–10 times monthly. During the attacks he suffered loss of consciousness, eye and head deviation toward the left side, walking automatisms and abnormal behavior. He also reported short-lasting episodes of blurred vision, starting usually in the left side of the visual field. He was treated with phenytoin 300 mg, valproate acid 1000 mg and primidone 1000 mg. He was hospitalized in 1981. The neurological examination was normal and he had no naevus flammeus. The CT scan showed tramtrack-like bilateral occipital calcifications. A diagnosis of Sturge–Weber syndrome was suggested by the radiologist. In hospital he had eight seizures characterized by loss of consciousness with head deviation to the left and quick secondary generalization. Unfortunately, none of these seizures was recorded. Prolonged scalp EEG recordings with sphenoidal electrodes showed bi-temporal independent interictal epileptiform discharges with right-sided predominance. The abnormal activity involved the dorso-lateral and mesial regions on the temporal lobe on the right side and was confined to the infero-mesial structures on the left. The lack of clear electroclinical correlation discouraged any surgical intervention. Seizures continued despite high levels of medication. He died 12 years later due to an unrelated cause.

Case 2. A 49-year-old woman was the result of a normal pregnancy and delivery. At the age of 6 months she was diagnosed to have coeliac disease and was then hospitalized several times for treatment of coeliac crises with vomiting, anorexia, lethargy and bulky stools. She had transient growth failure in the first two years of life. Between the ages of 16 months and 3 years, often in relation to an episode of coeliac crisis, she had recurrent prolonged febrile convulsions, more prominent on the right side. Her habitual epileptic seizures began at the age of 3. They were preceded by abdominal pain, nausea, and salivation. Later dizziness and vertigo, as well lightheadedness or bi-occipital headaches were described. This progressed to speech arrest, loss of consciousness associated with swallowing movements, head version to the right, or prolonged blinking, followed by postictal confusion and fatigue. She never had episodes of secondary generalization. Her EEGs showed epileptiform abnormalities over the inferior surface of the left temporal lobe.

She was investigated at the age of 49 because of medically refractory complex partial seizures occurring several times a day. She had no malabsorption symptoms. Her treatment consisted of 5 mg of folate daily and of a gluten-free diet. Duodenal biopsy revealed mild villous atrophy. She had a history of atypical chronic psychosis with schizoaffective features diagnosed at the age of 40, which were treated with a daily dose of 600 mg of lithium. The neurological examination, including the Goldmann visual field perimetry was normal. She had no naevus flammeus. Neuropsychological assessment showed severe verbal and visual spatial memory deficits. On the Wechsler Intelligence Scale for adults-revised (WAIS-R), her full scale IQ was 82 (verbal IQ, 87; and performance IQ, 76). Prolonged video-EEG telemetry recordings with sphenoidal electrodes showed epileptiform abnormalities over both infero-mesial temporal lobes, predominating on the right, and moderate paroxysmal generalized disturbance of the cerebral activity maximal over anterior head regions. Interictal epileptiform abnormalities originated independently from both infero-mesial temporal regions. No seizures were recorded. CT and MRI showed bilateral occipital lobe calcifications. Volumetric study (MRIV) demonstrated significant bilateral mesial temporal atrophy involving both amygdala and hippocampus (right hippocampus: 2954.1 mm^3; left hippocampus: 3039.5 mm^3; right amygdala: 1709.3 mm^3; left amygdala: 1730.2 mm^3). Since one could not lateralize her attacks on the basis of surface recording, surgical treatment could not be advised. Bilateral dual pathology was diagnosed. A depth electrode study was considered, but since it was unlikely to lead to surgery that could render her seizure-free, this was not performed. She was discharged receiving carbamazepine and clobazam.

Case 3. A 32-year-old male was the result of a normal pregnancy and delivery. Early developmental milestones were normal, but he later showed cognitive deficit and since the age of 7 attended a special school. At age 11 he had his first grand-mal seizure. Some of the attacks started with sudden blindness. A CT scan showed bilateral occipital calcifications (Fig. 1) and angiograms were normal. The scalp EEG showed a right occipital focus. Visual fields were intact. He was treated with phenytoin, phenobarbital and carbamazepine and his seizures were not controlled.

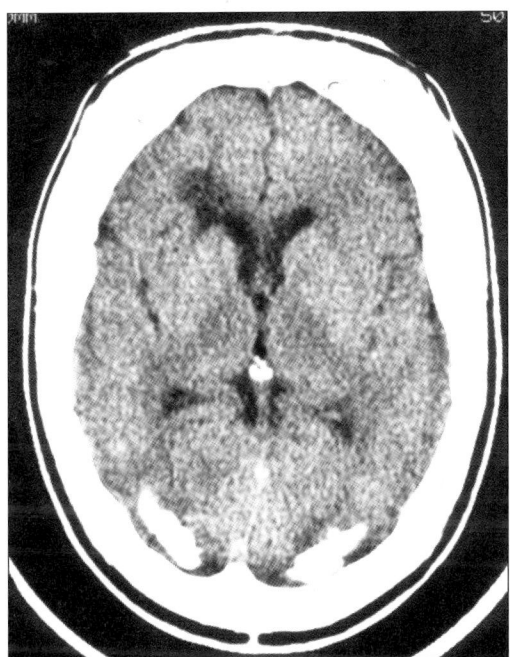

Fig. 1 (Patient 3) CT scan shows bilateral occipital calcifications. Right hypodense lesion over the right frontal horn. Diffusely thickened skull, particularly in both frontal regions (right is left on image).

At age 20, he started to have recurrent episodes of diarrhoea. Duodenal biopsy revealed severe villous atrophy. There was no malabsorption syndrome. A diagnosis of coeliac disease was made, and a gluten-free diet was recommended along with daily treatment with 10 mg of folic acid. He never adhered to the diet. He was investigated at the age of 22. He had generalized tonic–clonic seizures without warning, whereas others were ushered in by visual loss. He also had episodes of unresponsiveness and aggressive behaviour with aimless walking followed by major seizures. Attacks were clustered in one week per month. A seizure was recorded during video-EEG monitoring: His eyes deviated to the right, his right arm elevated and this was followed by secondary generalization. EEG onset was generalized followed by predominantly right temporal postictal abnormalities. MRI showed bi-occipital calcifications and a right frontal non-calcified lesion.

He was reinvestigated 10 years later because of increasing seizure frequency. Despite treatment with 40 mg of clobazam, 550 mg of phenytoin, 800 mg of carbamazepine and 3000 mg of valproic acid, he still had episodes of sudden loss of vision lasting less than one minute, sometimes followed by loss of consciousness, chewing and moaning, fumbling movements of the hands and walking automatisms. He also had seizures characterized by motionless stare and angry expression, followed by amnesia. There was frequent secondary generalization. Neurological examination, including the visual fields was normal and he had no skin lesions. Full scale IQ was 73. Serum folic acid, blood count, serum calcium, phosphate and albumin were within the normal ranges. Prolonged video-EEG recordings showed generalized interictal epileptiform abnormalities consisting of bursts of sharp and slow waves at 2–4 Hz, at times predominating over the right hemisphere, particularly the posterior temporal region. In addition, independent epileptic abnormalities were recorded from both temporal regions (equipotentiality at T3-Sp1, Sp2-T4 and C4-T4) with shifting side predominance. Four seizures were recorded. In one, the clinical onset preceded the first electrographic changes which were seen over the left hemisphere, with predominance over infero-mesial temporal lobe structures. In another, the first electrographic changes were recorded from the right temporal region as well as from both parieto-occipital areas; subsequently, a definitive regional accentuation in the left temporal lobe was noticed. The onset of a third seizure was recorded over both centro-temporo-parietal regions, followed by right-sided predominance. Another seizure onset was documented over the right fronto-temporal region. Clinically, these attacks consisted of a motionless stare followed by tonic head deviation to the left, with later head turning to the right, dystonic posture of both arms, some clonic movements of the left side of the face and secondary generalization. There were no convincing clinical lateralizing features. Based on this information, accurate localization of seizure onset was not possible. High resolution MRI again showed the bilateral occipital calcifications and the non calcified right frontal lesion (Fig. 2). Volumetric studies (MRIV) of amygdala and hippocampus were normal.

Considering the discrepancy between the clinical history of transitory visual loss suggesting occipital lobe seizures and the fronto-temporal ictal surface EEG changes, accurate localizing diagnosis was not possible. The right frontal lesion, probably dysplastic, was also suspected to be clinically

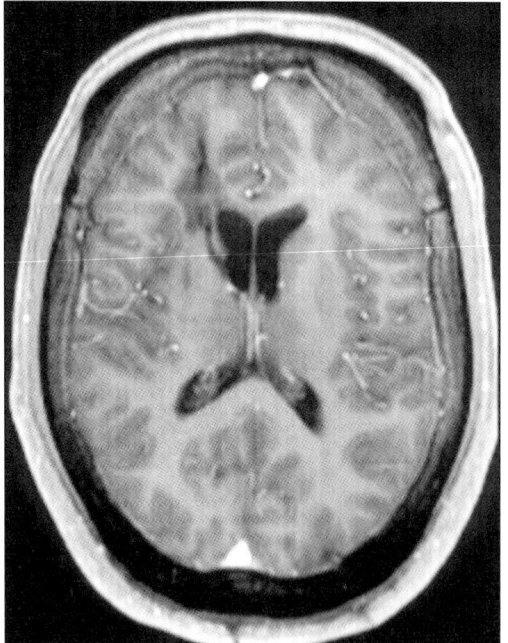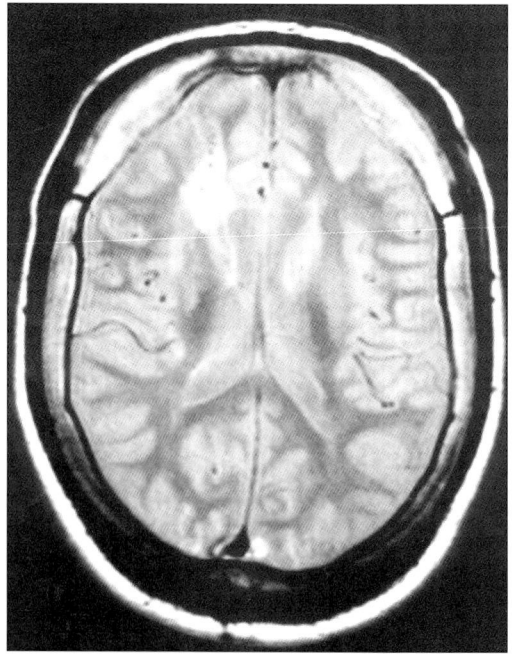

Fig. 2 (Patient 3). (A) Axial T1 MR image with Gadolinium shows abnormal signal intensity extending from the right frontal horn to the cortical surface with multiple areas of signal void. (B) On a proton density image, the lesion shows a hyperintense signal. This may represent dysplastic cortex associated with anomalous venous drainage (right is left on image).

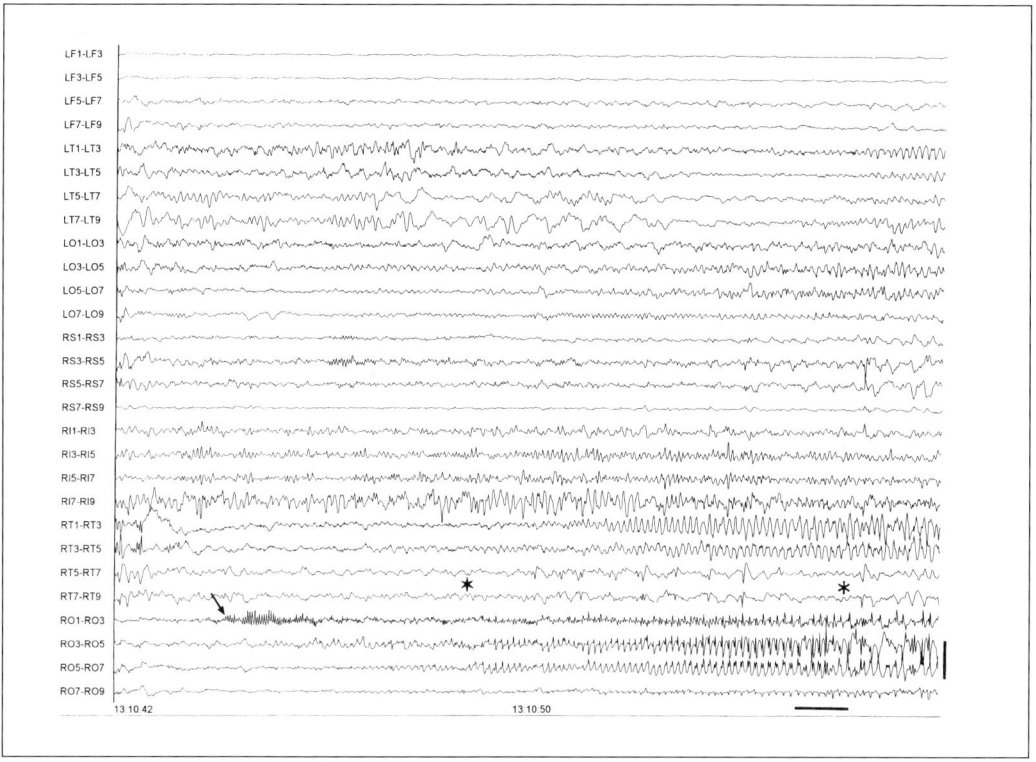

Fig. 3. Ictal depth electrode recording in patient 3. Sixty-four channel bipolar montage (vertical bar: 75 mV ; horizontal bar: 1 second). Depth electrodes were placed horizontally through the second right temporal convolution, the frontal lobe and the lateral occipital cortex. Each electrode had nine contacts separated by 5 mm. Electrodes were aimed at the right anterior hippocampus (RT), the left anterior hippocampus (LT). Contacts 1 and 2 sampled from the mesial structures and the more superficial contacts (6–9) from the neocortical areas. Electrodes were also aimed at the right frontal anterior cingulate gyrus (RS), the right mesio-orbital cortex (RI), the left mesio-orbital cortex (LF), the right occipital (RO) and the left occipital (LO) structures. A total of four epidural electrodes on the right and four on the left (not shown) were inserted aiming at the frontal and centro-parietal areas. (Continued on next page.)

significant in the genesis of some of the attacks. He was therefore readmitted for stereotactic intracranial depth electrodes implantation. Intracerebral depth electrodes were inserted in both frontal, temporal and occipital lobes. Four epidural electrodes were also placed on the left and four on the right side aiming at frontal and centro-parietal areas. Two right parietal electrodes were inserted epidurally to as ground and reference respectively. He underwent video-EEG monitoring for 12 days using a computer-based system to record from 64 channels referentially. Five seizures were recorded starting in the right occipital lobe. Two were pure electrical seizures and remained confined to this structure. In the others seizures there was spread to the temporal and frontal lobes. They showed loss of consciousness associated with early eye and head version to the left, followed by tonic posture of the limbs, predominantly the right arm, and secondary generalization (Fig. 3).

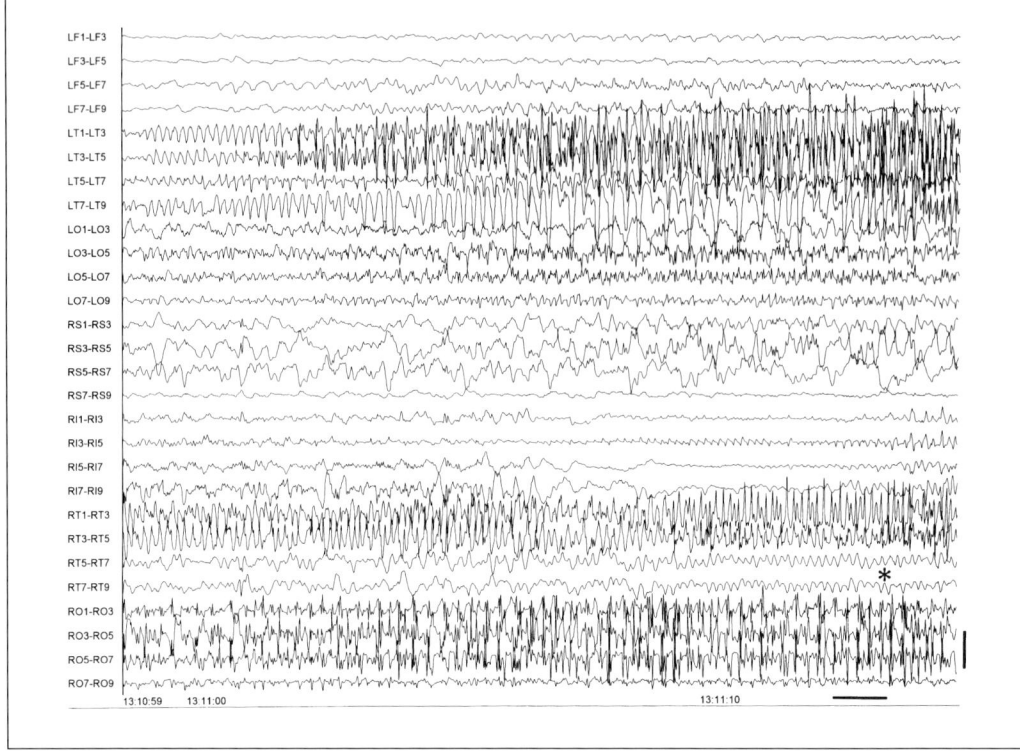

Fig. 3. cont. The seizure onset is characterized by low amplitude polyspike activity at 21 Hz recorded from the deepest contact of the right occipital lobe electrode (RO1-RO3, arrow). Two seconds later the activity evolved into rhythmic 8–10 Hz activity recorded from the more superficial contacts (RO3-RO5, RO5-RO7). Subsequently the seizure spread to the deepest contact of the right temporal lobe electrodes (RT1-RT3, RT3-RT5), and later to the left mesial and superficial temporal region, becoming diffuse over both cerebral hemispheres afterwards. The patient had no warning. He presented with conjugate eye deviation towards the left side (*), followed by tonic head deviation to the left and lip smacking (*). Subsequently, he had jerking of both legs (*). About four seconds later a generalized clonic attack ensued.

Discussion

The three patients presented with intractable epilepsy characterized by complex partial seizures with oroalimentary, ambulatory or gestual automatisms, and adversive symptoms. Two had also simple partial seizures with an aura of loss of vision and frequent secondary generalization. Scalp EEG recordings in all three patients showed epileptiform abnormalities over temporal lobes. In two of them (patients 1 and 2) complex and partial motor manifestations were considered to indicate rapid seizure spread and thus did not contribute to the localization of the primary seizure generator (Palmini *et al.*, 1993). In patient 3, despite the presence of an additional potential epileptogenic lesion in the right frontal area, which was possibly considered to represent focal cortical dysplasia, depth electrodes studies showed that all the seizures originated within the right occipital area and that contralateral adversive movements were related to seizure spread to the fronto-temporal region. The nature of the frontal lesion remains unclear, but it does not seem to be responsible for the attacks. The patient with a history of prolonged febrile convulsions and complex partial seizures of temporal lobe origin with oroalimentary automatisms and a viscero-sensory aura (patient 2), had seizures most likely related to her bilateral hippocampal and amygdalar atrophy as demonstrated on MRIV. Nevertheless, her prolonged episodes of eye-blinking suggested concomitant occipital lobe seizures (Olivier *et al.*, 1982), which were however not demonstrated during the scalp EEG recordings.

In CEBOC, the encephalopathy appears to be caused by a process of primary calcification of the vessel walls as suggested by a SPECT study with ^{99}Tc-H-MPAO demonstrating hypoperfusion in the areas harbouring the calcifications (Tiacci *et al.* 1993). The cerebral cortex shows neuronal loss, reactive gliosis surrounding the cortical microcalcifications and white matter degeneration (Tinuper *et al.*, 1996; Bye *et al.*, 1993). Hypodensity on CT and abnormal MRI signal, usually anterior to the calcifications, have also been described (Bye *et al.*, 1993; Gobbi *et al.*, 1992). Toti *et al.* (1996) reported autopsy results of a patient with calcifications containing silica. They hypothesize that the silica salts were toxic and could lead to the neuronal loss observed in the central part of the lesions and to the seizures.

Our observations support the concept of a causal relationship between the occipital calcifications, the epileptogenicity of the surrounding cortex, and the seizures in patients with CEBOC. Despite the clinical and scalp EEG pattern suggesting a frontal or temporal origin, these symptoms may be explained by rapid anterior spread of seizures generated within the occipital lobes, as demonstrated in case 3 with depth electrode study. The second patient had dual pathology, that is, hippocampal atrophy in both hemispheres in addition to the calcifications. This was probably the result of the early prolonged febrile convulsions triggered by coeliac crises. Based on previous data (Palmini *et al.*, 1993) and the present observations, MRI volumetric studies and intracranial EEG investigation in patients with CEBOC and extra-occipital lesions may permit differentiation between a single occipital generator and multifocal seizure origin.

Even though the occipital calcifications are bilateral the seizures may originate entirely or predominantly in one hemisphere. This has been shown in the patient reported by Bye *et al.* (1993) and suggested by the investigations of our third patient.

Fortunately, the epilepsy in these patients is not always severe to the point where surgical treatment must be considered. The absence of field defect in affected persons is striking, setting them apart from the findings in individuals with Sturge–Weber syndrome. Surgical resection, when unilateral onset can be demonstrated, will lead to hemianopia which may be acceptable to the patient even though there is no preoperative certitude that all seizures will cease after resection. When mesial temporal atrophy coexists, and especially when it is bilateral, surgical planning is further compli cated. As in other patients with dual pathology, the best results may be obtained when both the lesion and the atrophic mesial temporal structures can be resected. This option of course depends on clear demonstration of unilateral rather than bilateral seizure onset.

References

Ambrosetto, G., Antonini, L., Tassinari, C.A. (1992): Occipital lobe seizures related to clinically asymptomatic celiac disease in adulthood. *Epilepsia.* **33**, 476–481.

Banerji, N.K. & Hurwitz, L.J. (1971): Neurological manifestations in adult steatorrhoea (probable gluten enteropathy). *J. Neurol. Sci.* **14**, 125–141.

Bye, A.M., Matheson, J.M. & Mackenzie, R.A. (1989): Epilepsy surgery in Sturge–Weber syndrome. *Aust. Paediatr. J.* **25**, 103–105.

Bye, A.M., Andermann, F., Robitaille, Y., Oliver, M., Bohane, T. & Anderman, E. (1993): Cortical vascular abnormalities in the syndrome of celiac disease, epilepsy, bilateral occipital calcifications, and folate deficiency. *Ann. Neurol.* **34**, 399–403.

Garwicz, S. & Mortensson, W. (1976): Intracranial calcification mimicking the Sturge–Weber syndrome: a consequence of cerebral folic acid deficiency? *Pediat. Radiol.* **5**, 5–9.

Gobbi, G., Sorrenti, G., Santucci, M., Rossi, P.G., Ambrosetto, P., Michelucci, *et al.* (1988): Epilepsy with bilateral occipital calcifications: a benign onset with progressive severity. *Neurology*, **38**, 913–920.

Gobbi, G., Ambrosetto, P., Zaniboni, M.G., Lambertini, A., Ambrosioni, G. & Tassinari, C.A. (1992): Celiac disease, posterior cerebral calcifications and epilepsy. *Brain Dev.* **14**, 23–29.

Gobbi, G., Bertani, G., Pini, A., Lambertini, A., Zaniboni, M.G., Greco, L. *et al.* (1995): The syndrome of coeliac disease, epilepsy and cerebral calcifications. *Epilepsia.* **36**, 156.

Magaudda, A., Dalla Bernardina, B., De Marco, P., Sfaello, Z., Longo, M., Colamaria, V. *et al.* (1993): Bilateral occipital calcification, epilepsy and coeliac disease: clinical and neuroimaging features of a new syndrome. *J. Neurol. Neurosurg. Psychiatry*, **56**, 885–889.

Olivier, A., Gloor, P., Andermann, F. & Ives, J. (1982): Occipitotemporal epilepsy studied with stereotaxically implanted depth electrodes and successfully treated by temporal resection. *Ann. Neurol.* **11**, 428–432.

Oliver, A., Marchand, E., Peters, T. & Tyler, J.L. (1987) Depth electrode implantation at the Montreal Neurological Institute and Hospital. In: *Surgical treatment of the epilepsies.* Ed. J. Engel, Jr. New York: Raven Press, pp. 595–602.

Palmini, A., Andermann, F., Dubeau, F. *et al.* (1993) Occipitotemporal epilepsies: evaluation of selected patients requiring depth electrodes studies and rationale for surgical approaches. *Epilepsia*, **34**, 84–96.

Sammaritano, M., Andermann, F., Melanson, D., Guberman, A., Tinuper, P. & Gastaut, H. (1985): The syndrome of epilepsy and bilateral occipital cortical calcifications. *Epilepsia.* **26**, 532.

Sammaritano, M., Andermann, F., Melanson, D., Guberman, A., Tinuper, P. & Gastaut, H (1988): The syndrome of intractable epilepsy, bilateral occipital calcifications, and folic acid deficiency. *Neurology*, **38**, 239.

Tateno, A., Matsui, A., Sakuragawa, N., Nonaka, I. & Arima, M. (1985): Two siblings with multiple intracranial haemangiomatosis with calcification. *J. Neurol.* **232**, 112–114.

Tiacci, C., D'Alessandro, P., Cantisani, T.A., Piccirilli, M., Signorini, E., Pelli, M.A. *et al.* (1993): Epilepsy with bilateral occipital calcifications: Sturge–Weber variant or a different encephalopathy? *Epilepsia.* **34**, 528–539.

Tinuper, P., Plazzi, G., Provini, F., Cerullo, A., Gambarelli, D., Pellissier, J.F. *et al.* (1996): Celiac disease, epilepsy, and occipital calcifications: histopathological study and clinical outcome. *J. Epilepsy*, **9**, 206–209.

Toti, P., Balestri, P., Cano, M., Galluzzi, P., Megha, T., Farnetani, M.A. *et al.* (1996): Celiac disease with cerebral calcium and silica deposits - x-ray spectroscopic findings, an autopsy case. *Neurology*, **46**, 1088–1092.

Chapter 19

HLA in coeliac disease and epilepsy

Vilma Mantovani, Maria Gilda Zaniboni*, Elisa Collina and Michela Bragliani

Tipizzazione Tissutale Laboratorio Analisi Malpighi, Azienda Policlinico S. Orsola-Malpighi, Bologna, Italy;
*Divisione Pediatria Ospedale Maggiore, Azienda USL, Bologna, Italy

Introduction

HLA class II molecules are membrane-bound glycoproteins that are expressed as heterodimers of α and β chains on the surface of antigen-presenting cells. These molecules interact with antigen peptide fragments and with the T-cell receptor, playing an essential role in the immune response (Korman *et al.*, 1985; Lechler *et al.*, 1990). These highly polymorphic molecules have been involved in the susceptibility to certain immune disorders (Tiwari & Terasaki, 1985).

The genetic predisposition to coeliac disease (CD) is strongly associated with some HLA haplotypes, particularly with the DQ2 allele (Corazza *et al.*, 1985; Tosi *et al.*, 1983). DNA analysis of HLA class II genes has recently suggested that the primary association with CD is the DQα/β heterodimer encoded by the DQA1*0501 and the DQB1*0201 genes located either in *cis* (on the same chromosome) or in *trans* (on different chromosomes) position (Kagnoff, 1990; Mantovani *et al.*, 1993; Sollid *et al.*, 1989).

The association of CD with neurological disorders is well documented, especially with epilepsy (Chapman *et al.*, 1978; Laidlow *et al.*, 1977). Recent data on the relation between CD and epilepsy with cerebral calcifications suggest that this association is not incidental and it could be a genetically determined syndrome (Gobbi *et al.*, 1988; Gobbi *et al.*, 1992; Ventura *et al.*, 1991; Zaniboni *et al.*, 1991).

The present work was undertaken to investigate the HLA involvement in patients with CD, epilepsy and cerebral calcifications, by analysing the HLA polymorphism at phenotypic and genotypic levels.

Material and methods

Patients and controls

Twenty patients with epilepsy, bilateral occipital calcifications and biopsy-proven CD (CEC patients) took part in the study.

Four patients with cerebral calcifications of unexplained origin and epilepsy but without CD (CCE

143

patients), and one patient with CD and epilepsy but without calcifications (CDE patient), were also included in the study. In addition, 351 Italian healthy individuals were studied as controls.

HLA phenotyping

Serological tissue typing for HLA class II DR and DQ antigens was performed in patients and controls by using the standard microcytotoxicity assay (Terasaki & McClelland, 1964).

HLA genotyping

Genomic DNA was extracted from peripheral blood leucocytes of patients and healthy controls (Maniatis *et al.*, 1982) and submitted to polymerase chain reaction (PCR) amplification of the second exon of DQA1 and DQB1 genes (Saiki *et al.*, 1988; Mantovani *et al.*, 1993).

The amplified DNA was denatured, spotted on nylon membranes and hybridized with digoxigenin-labelled oligoprobes specific for DQA1*0501 and DQB1*0201 alleles, according to the Workshop protocol (Sasazuki & Kimura, 1991). The signal of positive hybridization was detected by AMPPD as chemiluminescent substrate for alkaline phosphatase conjugated to antidigoxigenin antibody Fab fragments and autoradiographed.

Statistics

The HLA allele frequencies were compared in patients and controls by the *Chi*-square test with Yates' correction and the *P*-values were corrected by the number of comparisons made (p_c).

The strength of association between alleles and disease susceptibility was estimated for each allele by calculating the relative risk (RR).

Results

In Table 1 are shown the HLA class II serological alleles which were found to be significantly increased in patients when compared to healthy controls. The DQ2 allele was highly associated to the disease in CEC patients (90 per cent in CEC *vs.* 38.7 per cent in controls, $p_c=10^{-4}$), conferring a RR=14.2.

Twelve CEC patients (60 per cent) exhibited the DR3–DQ2 haplotype and five cases (25 per cent) were heterozygous for DR11,DR7–DQ7,DQ2 haplotypes. One CEC patient had DR7, DR8–DQ2,DQ4. The remaining two CEC lacking DQ2 were DR4,DR13–DQ8,DQ1 and DR4,DR11–DQ7.

The DQ2 allele was more frequent as well in CCE patients (75 per cent) compared to controls, though the difference was not statistically significant.

The CDE patient included in the study exhibited the DR4,DR11–DQ7,DQ8 haplotypes.

DNA typing results of HLA-DQ genes are shown in Table 2.

Table 1. *HLA class II serological alleles found to be increased in CEC and CCE patients compared to controls*

HLA alleles	CEC N	CEC %	CCE N	CCE %	Controls N	%
DQ2	18[*]	90.0	3	75.0	136	38.7
DR3–DQ2	12[**]	60.0	2	50.0	69	19.7
DR11,7–DQ2,7	5[***]	25.0	0	0	25	7.1
Total	20		4		351	

[*]$p_c = 10^{-4}$, RR = 14.2; [**]$p_c = 10^{-4}$, RR = 6.1; [***]$p_c = 10^{-2}$, RR = 4.3.

Table 2. DNA typing of HLA-DQ genes in patients and controls

Patients	DQA1 * 0501, DQB1 * 0201	DQA1 * 0501, DQB1 * other	DQA1 * other, DQB1 * 0201	DQA1 8 other, DQB1 * other
CEC n = 20	18* (90.0%)	0	1	1
CCE n = 4	0 0	3	1	1
CDE n = 1	0 0	1	0	0
Controls n = 351	87 (24.8%)	nd	nd	nd

*pc = 10^{-7}; nd, not determined.

Eighteen CEC patients (90 per cent) had the DQA1*0501,DQB1*0201 alleles, whereas one patient had only the DQB1*0201 and one patient lacked both alleles. The frequency of the combination of these alleles was significantly increased in CEC patients compared to controls (p_c=10^{-7}, RR=27.3). None of the four CCE patients presented both alleles, neither did the CDE patient.

Discussion

Our study on the involvement of the HLA complex in susceptibility to the syndrome of epilepsy, bilateral occipital calcifications and CD indicates a positive association with the serological class II DQ2 or, alternatively, DR4 alleles.

In addition, our DNA analysis on the HLA-DQ locus reveals that the strongest association with CEC syndrome is the DQα/β heterodimer encoded by the DQA1*0501 and DQB1*0201 genes. In most CEC patients (60 per cent) these DQ molecules are encoded in *cis* position (those carrying the DR3–DQ2 haplotype). In five cases (25 per cent) the predisposing heterodimer is encoded in *trans* position (patients being DR11,DR7–DQ7,DQ2 heterozygous).

HLA-DQ2 allele and DQ heterodimer are present in 18 among 20 CEC patients (90 per cent), conferring a relative risk of 14.2 and 27.3, respectively. The remaining two cases show the DR4 allele.

The DQ2 allele and the DQα*0501/β*0201 heterodimer are known to be strongly associated with the genetic predisposition to classical CD (Corazza et al., 1985; Kagnoff, 1990; Sollid et al., 1989; Tosi et al., 1983). The rare coeliac patients lacking these HLA markers always exhibit the DR4 allele (Mantovani et al., 1993, Tosi et al., 1986). Our data therefore indicate that the HLA phenotype as well as the HLA genotype predisposing to CEC are the same as those that predispose to CD. These results are also confirmed by the lack of these genetic markers in the four patients with cerebral calcifications and epilepsy, but without CD.

Our study suggests that the genetic contribution of HLA involves CD susceptibility, regardless of the presence or absence of neurological aspects of the disease.

It is conceivable that in individuals with the same immunogenetic background, other genetic or environmental factors are specifically related to the onset of the CEC syndrome.

Although the HLA complex seems unrelated to the neurological aspects in CEC syndrome, the strong association between HLA markers and CD found in our patients suggests that an investigation of the HLA class II should be carried out, before undertaking intestinal biopsy.

In cases of epilepsy and cerebral calcifications of unexplained origin, which are negative to gliadin or endomysium antibody test, the lack of DQ α/β heterodimer or DR4 allele, can rule out CD. On the other hand, the detection of these HLA markers should lead to a search for jejunal mucosal villous atrophy suggestive of CD.

References

Chapman, R.G., Laidlow, J.M., Colin Jones, D.G., Eade, O.E. & Smith, C.L. (1978): Increased prevalence of epilepsy in coeliac disease. *B.M.F.* 2, 250–251.

Corazza, G.R., Tabacchi, P., Frisoni, M., Prati, C. & Gasbarrini, G. (1985): DR and non-DR Ia allotypes are associated with susceptibility to coeliac disease. *Gut* **26,** 1210-1213.

Gobbi, G., Sorrenti, G., Santucci, M., Giovanardi Rossi, P., Ambrosetto, P., Michelucci, R. & Tassinari, C.A. (1988): Epilepsy with bilateral occipital calcification: a benign onset with progressive severity. *Neurology* **38,** 913–920.

Gobbi, G., Bouquet, F., Greco, L., Lambertini, A., Tassinari, C.A., Ventura, A. & Zaniboni, M.G. (1992): Coeliac disease, epilepsy, and cerebral calcifications. *Lancet* **340,** 439–443.

Kagnoff, M.F. (1990): Understanding the molecular basis of coeliac disease. *Gut* **31,** 497–499.

Korman, A.J., Boss, J.M., Spies, T., Sorrentino, R., Okada, K. & Strominger, J.L. (1985): Genetic complexity and expression of human class II histocompatibility antigens. *Immunol. Rev.* **85,** 45–86.

Laidlow, J.M., Chapman, R.G., Colin Jones, D.G., Eade, O. & Smith, C.L. (1977): Increased prevalence of epilepsy in coeliac disease. *Gut* **18,** 943.

Lechler, R.I., Lombardi, G., Batchelor, J.R., Reinsmoen, N. & Bach, F.H. (1990): The molecular basis of alloreactivity. *Immunol. Today* **11,** 83–88.

Maniatis, T., Fritsch, E.F. & Sambrook, J. (1982): Molecular cloning, 14th edn., Cold Spring Harbor: CSH Laboratory.

Mantovani, V., Corazza, G.R., Bragliani, M., Frisoni, M., Zaniboni, M.G. & Gasbarrini, G. (1993): Asp57-negative HLA DQB chain and DQA1*0501 allele are essential for the onset of DQw2-positive and DQw2-negative coeliac disease. *Clin. Exp. Immunol.* **91,** 153–156.

Sasazuki, T. & Kimura, A. (1992): *HLA 1991*, vol. I. Oxford: Oxford University Press.

Sollid, L.M., Markussen, G., Ek, J., Gjierde, H., Vartdal, F. & Thorsby, E. (1989): Evidence for a primary association of coeliac disease to a particular HLA-DQ α-β heterodimer. *J. Exp. Med.* **169,** 345–350.

Terasaki, P.I. & McClelland, J.D. (1964): Microdopplet assay for human serum cytotoxins. *Nature* **204,** 998–1000.

Tiwari, J.L. & Terasaki, P.I. (1985): HLA and disease associations. New York: Springer-Verlag.

Tosi, R., Vismara, V., Tanigaki, N., Ferrara, G.B., Cicimarra, F., Buffolano, W., Follo, D. & Auricchio, S. (1983): Evidence that coeliac disease is primarily associated with a DC locus allelic specificity. *Clin. Immunol. Immunopathol.* **28,** 395–404.

Tosi, R., Tanigaki, N., Polanco, I., De Marchi, M., Woodrow, J.C. & Hetzel, P.A.S. (1986): A radioimmunoassay typing study of non-DQw2-associated celiac disease. *Clin. Immunol. Immunopathol.* **39,** 168–172.

Ventura, A., Bouquet, F., Sartorelli, C., Barbi, E., Torre, G. & Tommasini, G. (1991): Coeliac disease, folic acid deficiency and epilepsy with cerebral calcifications. *Acta Pediatr. Scand.* **80,** 559–562.

Zaniboni, M.G., Ambrosetto, P., Lambertini, A., Parmeggiani, A., Santucci, M., Gobbi, G. & Tassinari, C.A. (1991): Epilessia, calcificazioni endocraniche, malattia celiaca. *Minerva Pediatr.* **43,** 215–218.

Epilepsy and other neurological disorders in coeliac disease, edited by G. Gobbi *et al.*
© 1997 John Libbey & Company Ltd, pp. 147–149.

Chapter 20

Occipital lobe involvement in coeliac disease: an unresolved issue

Giuliano Avanzini

Istituto Nazionale Neurologico C. Besta, Via Celoria 11, 20133 Milano, Italy

Although the association of coeliac disease epilepsy and cerebral calcification is a well recognized clinical entity (Gobbi *et al.*, 1992), its pathogenesis is still incompletely understood.

The cerebral calcifications are typically located in both occipital lobes and have often led to a diagnosis of Sturge–Weber syndrome without nevus flammeus (Ambrosetto *et al.*, 1983; Battistella *et al.*, 1986; Piattella *et al.*, 1986). Accordingly, the seizures are characterized by visual symptomatology suggestive for an occipital origin. The preferential involvement of the occipital lobe in seizure generation is confirmed in 183 patients with coeliac disease (see Chapter 10 of this book) either *with* (108 patients) or *without* (75 patients) bilateral occipital calcification. Indeed it has long been known that occipital seizures may be an early manifestation of cerebral involvement in coeliac disease, with the calcifications developing later (Arroyo *et al.*, 1996; Martinelli *et al.*, 1966). This finding suggests that the coeliac disease-induced dysfunction of the occipital lobe is not directly dependent on the local deposit of calcium, but rather on the pathogenic mechanism itself.

According to Bye *et al.* (1993), this mechanism involves vascular abnormalities with pial angiomatosis and vein fibrosis. The ensuing alteration of blood–brain barrier might hypothetically account for both epileptogenic changes in neuronal function and progressive deposition of calcium salts. Further advances in the understanding of the relationship between epileptogenesis and the calcifications associated with coeliac disease may develop from better knowledge of their pathogenesis. Possible involvement of folate deficiency has been suggested (Sammaritano *et al.*, 1988): interestingly occipital calcifications may occur in leukaemic children treated with antifolate agents (Young *et al.*, 1977).

It must be pointed out that whereas in patients with epilepsy and bilateral occipital calcifications the existence of coeliac disease can be predicted with high probability, the reverse is not true. The occurrence of this epileptic syndrome in coeliac disease is in fact found only in 1.2 per cent of cases (Magaudda *et al.*, 1996; Guerrini *et al.*, 1996). In addition, according to Gobbi & Bertani (1997), 31 cases of epilepsy with occipital calcification have been reported with no evidence of coeliac disease. Therefore the possibility that the cerebral involvement in coeliac disease might be related to an additional pathogenic factor cannot be ruled out at present. Present difficulty in understanding the fundamental mechanism underlying this special type of epilepsy is a major obstacle in trying to interpret the preferential involvement of the occipital lobe. Other neurological epileptogenic disorders ranging from some severe encephalopathies to benign partial epilepsies, show the same predisposition to involve occipital structures. Besides the Sturge–Weber syndrome, Lafora disease (Roger *et al.*, 1983) and mitochondrial disorders (Andermann, 1993) should be mentioned as well as benign childhood epilepsy with occipital paroxism (BCEOP). Notably MELAS syndrome (mitocondrial encephalomyopathy with lactic acidosis and stroke-like episodes) and BCEOP present with migrainous attacks and occipital localizing features and probably account for the majority of cases previously reported under the heading of basilar migraine (Camfield *et al.*, 1978). This raises the question of whether selective susceptibility of the posterior vascular system to different pathogenic factors may account for the localized occipital expression of these neurological disorders. Although attractive, the attempt to correlate such an hypothetical vascular vulnerability with the posterior localization of the vascular changes found both in Sturge–Weber Syndrome and in coeliac disease with epilepsy and occipital calcification is not sufficiently supported by the available data. What is shown by SPET and PET studies is that the occipital lobe has a particularly high perfusion (Spreafico *et al.*, 1988) and metabolic (Phelps & Mazziotta, 1985) requirements compared to other cortical areas. It can therefore be expected that mitocondrial abnormalities affecting various components of the respiratory chain may selectively impair the occipital regions, giving rise to clinical signs of occipital dysfunction.

The finding of mitochondrial abnormalities in some cases of migraine with occipital auras (Montagna *et al.*, 1988) might support this view. Whether this hypothesis can be extended to other encephalopathies presumably related to metabolic disturbances such as Lafora disease is a matter of speculation. In conclusion the preferential involvement of the occipital lobe in 1.2 per cent of patients with coeliac disease challenges any hypothetical explanation based on the available information. Further progress in understanding the anatomo-functional organization of the occipital lobe on the one hand and the pathogenesis of this peculiar syndrome on the other, may clarify the issue.

References

Ambrosetto, P., Ambrosetto, G. & Michelucci, R. *et al.* (1983): Sturge–Weber syndrome without port-wine facial nevus: report of two cases studied by C.T. *Child Brain* **10,** 387–392.

Andermann, F. (1993): Occipital epileptic abnormalities in mitochondrial disorders – preferential involvement, illustrations of clinical patterns, current progress in neurobiology and a hypothesis. In: *Occipital seizures and epilepsies in children*, eds. F. Andermann, A. Beaumanoir, L. Mira, J. Roger & C.A. Tassinari, pp. 111–120. London: John Libbey.

Arroyo, H., De Rosa, S. & Fejerman, N. (1996): Epilepsy, cerebral calcifications and celiac disease: Argentine multicentre experience. This book, chapter 14.

Battistella, P.A., Casara, G.L. & Carollo, C. *et al.* (1986): Calcificazioni cerebrali senza angiomatosi cutanea: forma atipica della malattia di Sturge–Weber. *Riv. Ital. Pediatr.* **12,** 417–418.

Bye, A.M.E., Andermann, F., Robitaille, Y., Oliver, M., Bohane, T. & Andermann, E. (1993): Cortical vascular abnormalities in the syndrome of celiac disease, epilepsy, bilateral occipital calcifications, and folate deficiency. *Ann. Neurol.* **34,** 399–403.

Camfield, P., Metrakos, K. & Andermann, F. (1978): Basilar migraine, seizures and severe epileptiform EEG abnormalities. *Neurology* **28,** 584–588.

Gobbi, G. & Bertani, G. (1997): Census of patients with epilepsy and coeliac disease with their geographic distribution and ethnic origin. This book, Chapter 10.

Gobbi, G., Bouquet, F. & Greco, L., *et al.* (1992): Coeliac disease, epilepsy, and cerebral calcifications. *Lancet* **340,** 439–443.

Guerrini, R., Battini, R., Ughi, C., Chiravalloti ,G., Belmonte, A., Canapicchi, R. & Taddeucci, G. (1996): Prevalence of epilepsy and seizure types in coeliac disease and prevalence of unrecognized coeliac disease in children with neurologic and psychiatric disorders. This book, Chapter 16.

Magaudda, A., Dalla Bernardina, B., Magazzu', G., Longo, M.,De Marco, P. & Meduri, M. (1996): Frequency of occipital bilateral calcifications and epilepsy in coeliac patients. This book, chapter 17.

Martinelli, O., Tiberti, A., Valseriati, D. & Gobbi, G. (1996): Epilepsy and coeliac disease in a case with cerebral calcifications at follow up. This book, Addenda.

Phelps, M.E. & Mazziotta, J.C. (1985): Positron emission tomography: human brain function and biochemistry. *Science* **228,** 799–809.

Piattella, L., Zamponi, N., Cenci, L., *et al.* (1986): Calcificazioni bioccipitali ed epilessia: malattia di Sturge–Weber atipica o nuova sindrome. *Boll. Lega. It. Epil.* **54/55,** 139–142.

Roger, J., Pellissier, J.F., Bureau, M., Dravet, C., Revol, M. & Tinuper, P. (1983): Le diagnostic precoce de la maladie de Lafora: importance des manifestations paroxystiques visuelles et interet de la biopsie cutanèe. *Rev. Neurol.* **139,** 115–124.

Sammaritano, M., Andermann, F. & Melanson, D. *et al.* (1988): The syndrome of intractable epilepsy, bilateral occipital calcifications, and folic acid deficiency. *Neurology* **38,** (suppl. 1), 239.

Spreafico, G., Cammelli, F., Gadola, G. (1988): Tomografia ad emissione in medicine nucleare. La SPECT nello studio del flusso ematico cerebrale. p. 38. Brescia: New Elscint Technologies.

Young, L.W., Jequier, S. & O'Gorman, A.M. (1977): Intracerebral calcifications in treated leukemia in a child. *Am. J. Dis. Child* **133,** 1283–1285.

Epilepsy and other neurological disorders in coeliac disease, edited by G. Gobbi *et al.*
© 1997 John Libbey & Company Ltd, pp. 151–157.

Chapter 21

Imaging of autoimmune phenomena in patients with coeliac disease and associated neurological disorders

Alberto Signore, Marco Chianelli, Luigi Maiuri[*], Elisabetta Ferretti, Raffaella Barone, Enrica Procaccini, Marco Greco, Alessio Annovazzi, Giuseppe Ronga, Paolo Pozzilli and Antonio Picarelli

Institute of Clinica Medica II, University of Rome 'La Sapienza', and [*]Institute of Paediatrics, University of Naples, Italy

Introduction

The possibility of detecting chronic inflammatory sites *in vivo* is an important objective for diagnostic and therapeutic purposes. Nuclear medicine techniques may allow achievement of this goal. Many different approaches have been described including the injection of ^{111}In-labelled autologous lymphocytes (Issekutz *et al.*, 1980, Peters *et al.*, 1983), ^{99m}Tc-labelled nanocolloids (De Schrijver *et al.*, 1987; Streule *et al.*, 1988) and, more recently, radiolabelled monoclonal antibodies (MoAb) directed against specific lymphocyte antigens (Linda *et al.*, 1990) or radiolabelled polyclonal human IgG (Fischman *et al.*, 1990; Block *et al.*, 1990; Oyen *et al.*, 1990).

All these techniques, although successful in many cases, are characterized by low specificity and sensitivity and have some disadvantages which stimulate the development of new radiopharmaceuticals. In the last few years, attention has been focused on biologically active peptides that mediate their action by specific receptors expressed on target cells. These proteins have great potential as radiopharmaceuticals for imaging cells and tissues to which they bind, with particular regard to acute inflammations and infections. Interleukin-2 (IL2), a lymphocyte growth factor that binds mainly to activated T-lymphocytes (Robb *et al.*, 1981), could be of particular interest as a radiopharmaceutical for *in vivo* detection of chronic inflammations characterized by a mononuclear cell type of infiltration in target tissue. Immunohistochemical studies of tissue biopsies in several immune-mediated conditions have revealed that 10 to 30 per cent of tissue infiltrating mononuclear cells (mainly T-lymphocytes) express interleukin-2 receptors (IL2R) as a sign of cell activation (Hanafusa *et al.*, 1990; Itoh *et al.*, 1993; Foulis *et al.*, 1986). We therefore labelled IL2 with ^{123}I and investigated its specificity for *in vivo* detection of mononuclear cell infiltration in animal models (Signore *et al.*, 1987; Signore *et al.*, 1992; Signore *et al.*, 1994). In this study we describe the use of ^{123}I-IL2 scintigraphy for the non-invasive evaluation of disease activity in patients with coeliac disease in which it has been possible to correlate the results obtained *in vivo* with histological findings obtained by jejunal biopsy.

Patients and methods

The following subjects were studied:

(a) *10 patients with newly discovered coeliac disease* diagnosed by jejunal biopsy and by the presence of anti-gliadin (AGA, IgG and IgA) and/or anti-endomysium (EMA) antibodies (2M and OF, mean age 31.1 years ± 11.6 SD). Seven patients (2 M and 5 F) were investigated a second time after 12–19 months of gluten-free diet, and a second jejunal biopsy was performed, by measurement of AGA, EMA and ^{123}I-IL2 scintigraphy. The presence of IL2R+ cells in the intestinal mucosa was investigated by immunohistochemical staining on cryostat sections of biopsy specimens using an anti-CD25 monoclonal antibody (2A3, Becton Dickinson).

(b) *3 patients with long-standing coeliac disease and associated epilepsy.* These patients were on gluten-free diet and taking anti-epileptic drugs. Previously performed brain CT scans showed the presence of occipital calcifications as described by Gobbi *et al.* (1992).

(c) *10 normal subjects* (6M and 4F, mean age 28.6 years ± 14.0 SD), AGA and EMA negative.

Ethical approval was obtained by the local Committee (University of Rome 'La Sapienza') and each individual participating in the study gave his/her informed consent.

Labelling of IL2 and HPLC purification of ^{123}I-IL2

Human recombinant IL2 (EuroCetus, The Netherlands) was labelled using an enzymatic method as previously described (Signore *et al.*, 1992).

Gamma camera imaging and data analysis

Subjects investigated with ^{123}I-IL2 were fasting for at least 8 h and received 400 mg of $KClO_4$ orally 20 min before the study to prevent stomach and thyroid uptake of free [123]I. Approximately 2mCi of ^{123}I-IL2 (< 5 µg IL2) were administered i.v. and images were acquired with a single head Elscint SP4 γ camera fitted with a low energy and medium resolution collimator. Planar anteroposterior images (collected in a 256 × 256 pixel matrix) and tomographic (SPET) images (collected in a 64 × 64 pixel matrix acquiring 60 frames of 20 s each during a 360° rotation) were acquired 1h after injection. Transaxial sections of 10 pixel thickness were reconstructed along the abdomen or the brain. Images were then filtered using a Hanning filter (0.5 cycles) and a pre-attenuation correction (0.125 cm^{-1} attenuation coefficient).

For quantitative analysis of radioactivity, several regions of interest (ROI) were drawn and radioactivity was measured per pixel of area. Bowel/marrow radioactivity ratios (B/M) were also calculated for each intestinal ROI after normalization of counts per ROI area. The scintigraphy was considered positive when at least one B/M ratio was greater than the mean of highest B/M ratios in normal subjects + 2 SD.

Results

No adverse reactions or side effects were observed following the i.v. administration of ^{123}I-IL2 in all cases studied.

In normal subjects ^{123}I-IL2 rapidly clears from plasma by renal metabolism, as described for unlabelled IL2 (Donohue & Rosenberg, 1983; Sands & Loveless, 1989; Konrad *et al.*, 1990) and only low levels of circulating radioactivity are detectable 30 min after injection. No significant gastrointestinal uptake is detectable in normal subjects. We found a variable degree of spleen uptake which can be explained by the physiological presence of IL2R positive mononuclear cells in this tissue. In normal subjects the mean B/M ratio was 1.28 ± 0.3 (range 0.75–1.95).

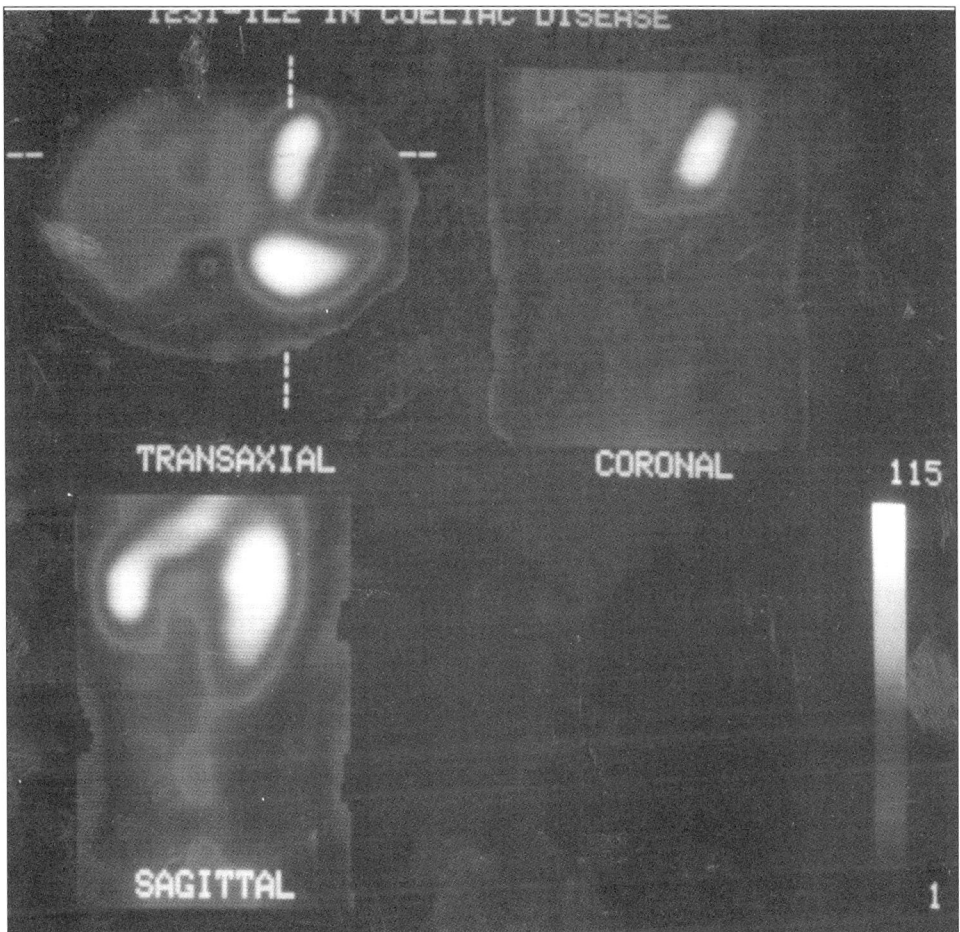

Fig. 1. SPET images obtained in a patient with recently diagnosed coeliac disease 1 h after injection of ^{123}I-IL2. One transaxial, one coronal and one sagittal section are shown. Slice thickness is 3 pixels. A localized accumulation of tracer is detectable in the first tract of the jejunum, anteriorlto the left kidney.

A variable degree and extent of intestinal uptake of radiolabelled IL2 was found in patients with coeliac disease (Fig. 1). ^{123}I-IL2 uptake was significantly higher than in normal subjects in all intestinal ROIs (Table 1). All coeliac disease patients had a positive scintigraphy at time of diagnosis (Table 2).

Immunohistochemical analysis of intestinal biopsies showed that all patients at diagnosis had partial atrophy of intestinal villi and extensive mononuclear cell infiltration. Most infiltrating cells were IL2R+ve (18–75 cells/mm of jejunal mucosa).

Table 1. Target/background radioactivity ratios for different bowel ROIs in patients with coeliac disease and normal subjects 1 h after i.v. injection of ^{123}I-IL2

	Coeliac after diet (n = 7)		Coeliac at diagnosis (n = 10)		Normal subjects (n = 10)
Right up	1.25 ± 0.24	P = 0.03[*]	2.13 ± 0.65	P = 0.001	1.18 ± 0.29
Right down	1.14 ± 0.30	P = n.s.[*]	1.69 ± 0.59	P = 0.003	1.10 ± 0.18
Centre up	1.74 ± 0.13	P = 0.02	2.58 ± 0.74	P = 0.0001	1.54 ± 0.21
Centre down	1.60 ± 0.28	P = 0.03[*]	2.51 ± 0.89	P = 0.002	1.44 ± 0.25
Left up	1.36 ± 0.18	P = 0.02[*]	2.68 ± 0.71	P = 0.0001	1.46 ± 0.29
Left down	1.15 ± 0.02	P = 0.01*	2.25 ± 0.84	P = 0.0001	1.09 ± 0.14

Student's test for [*]paired or unpaired data; n.s. = not significant.

After 12–18 months of gluten free diet patients showed a normal mucosa at biopsy with few infiltrating mononuclear cells of which very few were IL2R+ve (0–4 cells/mm of jejunal mucosa; P <0.0001 vs. patients at diagnosis). A significant reduction of bowel radioactivity was observed in all ROIs (Table 1). AGA titre was also significantly decreased.

A positive correlation was found between the number of IL2R+ve cells per millimetre of jejunal mucosa and the B/M ratio calculated in the jejunal region of interest by ^{123}I-IL2 scintigraphy (r^2 = 0.727; P <0.0001).

Two of the three patients studied with epilepsy showed a significant IL2 uptake in the occipital lobe corresponding to the area where calcifications were found on CT scanning (Fig. 2a,).

Table 2. Results of scintigraphy in patients and normal subjects

	Positive*	Negative
Coeliac patients at diagnosis (bowel)	10/10	0/10
Coeliac patients after gluten-free diet (bowel)	0/7	7/7
Long standing coeliac patients with epilepsy (brain)	2/3	1/3
Normal subjects (bowel)	0/10	10/10
Normal subjects (brain)	0/10	10/10

*Positivity is defined by target/background ratio greater than normal mean + 2 SD.

Discussion

There have been previous attempts in humans and in animal models to detect tissue infiltrating lymphocytes in autoimmune diseases by using autologous ^{111}In-labelled lymphocytes (Kaldany et al., 1982; Gallina et al., 1985). Results of these studies were promising in some cases but overall the technique was not very sensitive, probably because only a small amount of ^{111}In can be used to label lymphocytes in vitro due to their high sensitivity to radiation damage.

In order to overcome the limits and disadvantages of this technique we developed a new approach to label in vivo the activated lymphocytes present in infiltrated tissues, based on the i.v. injection of radiolabelled interleukin-2.

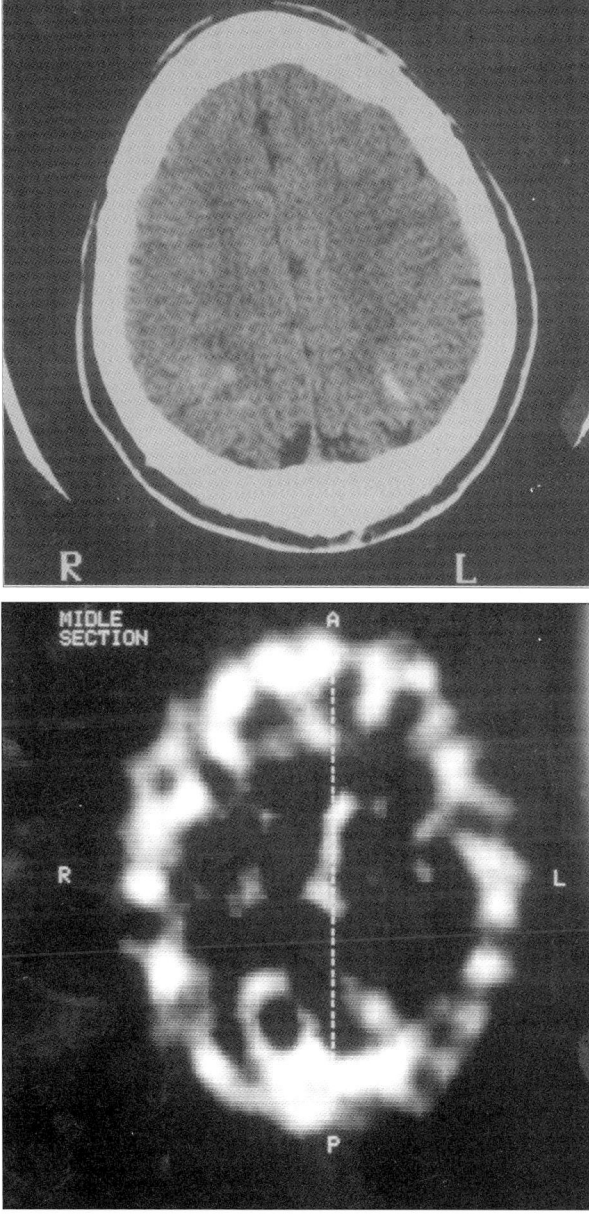

*Fig. 2. Computerized tomography (a. top) and SPET images
(b. bottom) of the brain in a patient with coeliac disease and
epilepsy with occipital calcifications. A focal accumulation of
^{123}I-IL2 is detectable in the occipital lobe corresponding to
the periphery of the calcification.*

Here we validated the use of ^{123}I-IL2 scintigraphy for *in vivo* detection of tissue infiltrating lymphocytes in coeliac disease patients by comparing the scintigraphic results with histopathological findings. Our results showed that ^{123}I-IL2 significantly accumulates in the bowel of all coeliac disease patients and the degree of uptake significantly correlates with the number of IL2R+ve lymphocytes present per millimetre of jejunal mucosa.

These data suggest the use of radiolabelled-IL2 scintigraphy for assessment of disease activity instead of invasive jejunal biopsy, as IL2 scintigraphy provides information on the entire intestinal tract. This method might be applied also in those patients with discordance between the gliadin antibody and the biopsy and to detect associated autoimmune disorders such as type 1 diabetes and thyroiditis. The finding that patients with epilepsy and brain calcifications show significant uptake of radiolabelled-IL2 suggests that these brain lesions may have an autoimmune pathogenesis. Alternatively, the brain uptake of IL2 may be due to binding to glial cells since, following activation, these cells can express surface IL2 receptors (Sakai *et al.*, 1995; Zwain *et al.*, 1994; Benveniste *et al.*, 1987). This may have important implications for diagnosis, prevention and therapy of these disorders.

References

Benveniste, E.N., Herman, P.K. & Whitaker, J.N. (1987): Myelin basic protein-specific RNA levels in interleukin-2-stimulated oligodendrocytes. *J. Neurochem.* **49**, 1274–1279.

Block, D., Ogtrop, M.V., Arndt, J.W. *et al.* (1990): Detection of inflammatory lesions with radiolabelled immunoglobulins. *Eur. J. Nucl. Med.* **16**, 303–305.

De Schrijver, M., Streule, K., Senekowitsch, R. *et al.* (1987): Scintigraphy of inflammation with nanometer-sized colloidal tracers. *Nucl. Med. Comm.* **8**, 895–908.

Donohue, J.H. & Rosenberg, S.A. (1983): The fate of interleukin-2 after *in vivo* administration. *J. Immunol.* **130**, 2203–2208.

Fischman, A.J., Rubin, R.H., White, J.A. *et al.* (1990): Localization of Fc and Fab fragments of non-specific polyclonal IgG at sites of inflammation. *J. Nucl. Med.* **31**, 1199–1205.

Foulis, A.K., Liddle, C.N., Farquharson, M.A., Richmond, J.A. & Weir, R.S. (1986): The histopathology of the pancreas in type 1 (insulin-dependent) diabetes mellitus: a 25-year review of deaths in patients under 20 years of age in the United Kingdom. *Diabetologia* **29**, 267–274.

Gallina, D.L., Pelletier, D., Doherty, P. *et al.*. (1985): [111]Indium-labelled lymphocytes do not image or label the pancreas of BB/W rat. *Diabetologia* **28**, 143–47.

Gobbi, G., Ambrosetto, P., Zaniboni, M.G., Lambertini, A., Ambrosioni, G. & Tassinari, C.A. (1992): Coeliac disease, posterior cerebral calcifications and epilepsy. *Brain Dev.* **14**, 23–29.

Hanafusa, T., Miyazaki, A., Miyagawa, J. *et al.* (1990): Examination of islets in the pancreas biopsy specimens from newly diagnosed type 1 (insulin-dependent) diabetic patients. *Diabetologia* **33**, 105–111.

Issekutz, T., Chin, W. & Hay, J.B. (1980): Measurement of lymphocyte traffic with [111]Indium. *Clin. Exp. Immunol.* **39**, 215–221.

Itoh, N., Hanafusa, T., Miyazaki, A. *et al.* (1993): Mononuclear cell infiltration and its relation to the expression of major histocompatibility complex antigens and adhesion molecules in pancreas biopsy specimens from newly diagnosed insulin-dependent diabetes mellitus patients. *J. Clin. Invest.* **92**, 2313–2322.

Kaldany, A., Hill, T., Wentworth, S. *et al.* (1982): Trapping of peripheral blood lymphocytes in the pancreas of patients with acute-onset insulin-dependent diabetes mellitus. *Diabetes* **31**, 463–466.

Konrad, M.W., Hemstreet, G., Hersh, E.M. *et al.* (1990): Pharmacokinetics of recombinant interleukin-2 in humans. *Cancer Res.* **50**, 2009–2017.

Linda, P., Langsteger, W., Koltringer, P. *et al.* (1990): Immunoscintigraphy of inflammatory processes with a technetium-99m-labelled monoclonal antigranulocyte antibody (MAb BW 250/183). *J. Nucl. Med.* **31**, 417–423.

Oyen, W.J.G., Claessens, R.A.M.J., van Horn, J.R. *et al.* (1990): Scintigraphic detection of bone and joint infections with Indium-111-labelled nonspecific polyclonal human immunoglobulin G. *J. Nucl. Med.* **31**, 403–412.

Peters, A.M., Saverymuttu, S.H., Reafy, H.J. *et al.* (1983): Imaging of inflammation with 111-Indium tropolonate labelled leukocytes. *J. Nucl. Med.* **24**, 39–44.

Robb, R.J., Munck, A. & Smith, K.A. (1981): T-cell growth factor receptors: quantitation, specificity and biological relevance. *J. Exp. Med.* **154**, 1455–1474.

Sakai, N., Kaufman, S. & Milstien, S. (1995): Parallel induction of nitric oxide and tetrahydrobiopterin synthesis by cytokines in rat glial cells. *J. Neurochem.* **65,** 895–902.

Sands, H. & Loveless, S.E. (1989): Biodistribution and pharmacokinetics of recombinant, human ^{125}I-interleukin-2 in mice. *Int. J. Immunopharmacol.* **11,** 411–416.

Signore, A., Chianelli, M., Ferretti, E., Negri, M., Andreani, A. & Pozzilli, P. (1994): A new approach for *in vivo* detection of insulitis: activated lymphocyte targeting with ^{123}I-labelled interleukin-2. *Eur. J. Endocrinol.* **131,** 431–437.

Signore, A., Chianelli, M., Toscano, A., Ronga, G., Monetini, L., Nimmon, C.C., Britton, K.E., Pozzilli, P. & Negri, M. (1992): A radiopharmaceutical for imaging areas of lymphocytic infiltration: ^{123}I-interleukin-2. Labelling procedure and animal studies. *Nucl. Med. Comm.* **13,** 713–722.

Signore, A., Parman, A., Pozzilli, P., Andreani, D. & Beverley, P.C.L. (1987): Detection of activated lymphocytes in endocrine pancreas of BB/W rats by injection of 123-interleukin-2: an early sign of type 1 diabetes. *Lancet* **ii,** 537h540.

Streule, K., De Schrijver, M. & Fridrich, R. (1988): ^{99}Tc-labelled HSA-nanocolloid versus 111-ln oxine-labelled granulocytes in detecting skeletal septic process. *Nucl. Med. Comm.* **9,** 56–67.

Zwain, I.H., Grima, J. & Cheng, C.Y. (1994): Regulation of clusterin secretion and mRNA expression in astrocytes by cytokines. *Mol. Cell. Neurosci.* **5,** 229–237.

Part VI

Other diseases with epilepsy and cerebral calcification: differential diagnosis

Epilepsy and other neurological disorders in coeliac disease, edited by G. Gobbi *et al.*
© 1997 John Libbey & Company Ltd, pp. 161–170.

Chapter 22

Clinical and pathological findings in Sturge–Weber syndrome and other congenital neurological diseases with epilepsy and calcifications

Alexis Arzimanoglou[*] and Philippe Evrard[**]

[*]*Child Neurology Unit and Epilepsy Research Group, Hôpital de la Salpêtrière, Paris, France;*
[**]*Child Neurology Department, Hôpital Robert Debré, Paris, France*

Epileptic seizures and cerebral calcifications are often present in both Sturge–Weber and tuberous sclerosis patients. These entities are usually classified as neurocutaneous syndromes, since both the skin and the nervous system are involved. The cutaneous manifestations may not be present in all cases. Tuberous sclerosis is a dominantly inherited disorder with a variable expression and a high incidence of new mutations. The primary anomaly of tuberous sclerosis is an abnormal differentiation and growth of neuronal and glial cells, associated with migration anomalies and disorganization of the cortical architecture, formation of hamartomas and rarely neoplasia. In contrast to tuberous sclerosis and to the neurofibromatoses, Sturge–Weber (SW) syndrome is usually sporadic and only a handful of doubtful familial cases are on record (Gomez, 1987). It consists of facial, retinal, and cerebral angiomatosis.

Sturge–Weber syndrome

Sturge–Weber (SW) syndrome is classically characterized by the association of a congenital facial capillary angioma with leptomeningeal angiomatosis, almost always ipsilateral to the cutaneous naevus but exceptions to the rule are not infrequent and the correlation between the extent and location of the naevus and that of the pial angioma is poor (Arzimanoglou & Aicardi, 1993; Alexander, 1972; Boltshauser *et al.*, 1976; Gomez & Bebin, 1987). Some children have bilateral naevus with unilateral pial involvement or vice versa. Angiomas may extend beyond the face and involve the neck, trunk or limbs on one or both sides. Though the presence of a pial angioma is a prerequisite for diagnosis, facial angioma may be lacking. We recently evaluated the results of 20 patients with SW syndrome operated on at the Neurosurgery Department at the Hôpital des Enfants Malades in Paris and at the Montreal Neurological Institute (Arzimanoglou *et al,.* 1997). Typical pial angiomatosis was confirmed in all twenty but facial angioma was absent in eight. An identical pial angioma may be present in isolation or in association with choroidal angioma without facial naevus. For all practical purposes, such cases pose the same problems as the complete forms and should be regarded as belonging to the same syndrome (Aicardi, 1992).

The embryologic continuity of the vascular plexus of the skin, eye and telencephalon suggests that an abnormality of the embryologic vascular plexus would explain the simultaneous existence of these separate lesions. The leptomeningeal venous angiomatosis is striking and affects mainly occipital and occipital parietal regions but does not extend into the cortex. The underlying cerebrum contains extensive calcification with or without involvement of the white matter. Some of the calcifications are oriented around blood vessels but most lie in the neuropil, unrelated to obvious vasculature (Wohlwill & Yakovlev, 1957). Despite the extensive calcification, gliosis is surprisingly minimal. The pathogenesis of the calcification is unknown.

Norman and Schoene (1977) have suggested that calcifications of the pial arteries may be related to diminished blood flow in an area which, in turn, may produce stasis, hypoxia and increased capillary permeability. Hypoxic damage may result from the venous congestion secondary to failure of cortical vein development. Calcifications of the adjacent brain cortex are distributed in the molecular layer and the outer zone of the pyramidal cell layer. These mineral deposits contain mostly calcium phosphate and carbonate. They are believed to form as a result of local tissue hypoxia. Repeated seizures are undoubtedly implicated in aggravating prognosis, but their sole responsibility is far from proven. The vasomotor and thrombotic phenomena, or both, may be due to decompensation by the increased metabolic rate resulting from seizures. It deserves special mention that a definite regression of mental abilities runs parallel to the repetition and severity of seizures (Arzimanoglou & Aicardi, 1993) or that, in most patients, hemiplegia first appears following an episode of repeated seizures or status. Some authors (Mc Caughan *et al.*, 1975; Garcia *et al.*, 1981) discuss the role of recurrent thrombotic episodes producing an apparently gradual loss of function and propose the use of antiplatelet agents.

The *clinical diagnosis* of SW syndrome is usually straightforward. Seizures are the major neurological manifestation, occurring in 75–90 per cent of patients (Gilly *et al.*, 1977; Gomez & Bebin, 1987). Acquired hemiplegia occurs in at least one third of the cases. It usually appears after a prolonged seizure. Episodes of postictal transient hemiparesis may precede permanent deficit. Hemiplegic episodes not following an epileptic attack and sometimes accompanied by migraine-like headache and occasionally vomiting are observed in many cases (Gilly *et al.*, 1977; Arzimanoglou & Aicardi, 1993). These episodes may be the consequence of vasomotor disturbances within and around the angioma. Hemianopia is extremely frequent as a result of the usually posterior location of the pial lesion. Glaucoma is found in about 30 per cent of SW patients. Mental subnormality occurs in approximately 60 per cent of patients and is strongly related to the occurrence of seizures.

The *types of seizures* observed are multiple and the course of epilepsy is highly variable (Arzimanoglou & Aicardi, 1993). Several types may be observed in the same patient. They commonly begin in the first two years of life. They are often abrupt and catastrophic in onset and may compromise further development. In the series of Arzimanoglou & Aicardi (1993) 13 of 23 children had their first seizure before age one year and five more before age three. The first seizure was an episode of partial or unilateral status in six patients.

Simple partial seizures, mainly clonic, are frequent. Partial sensory seizures are less frequently reported and a visual aura is surprisingly rare. Complex partial seizures most commonly consist of head rotation or eye deviation to the side opposite the angioma or initial motor phenomena in the limbs followed by loss of consciousness and often hypotonia. Over time they become more frequent and have a tendency to last longer. Secondary generalization is not infrequent. Apparently generalized seizures, usually tonic–clonic in type but, in some, purely tonic or atonic were reported

(Arzimanoglou & Aicardi, 1993). One patient in that series had classical infantile spasms in addition to myoclonic, atonic and clinically partial seizures.

The *EEG* may show reduced background amplitude of tracings on the affected side sometimes with associated paroxysmal abnormalities (Brenner & Sharbrough, 1976) but this may be a late sign. Chevrie *et al.* (1988) reported three cases with unilateral pial angioma who presented bilateral and even synchronous discharges.

Computed tomography is a useful tool for the detection of calcifications which are frequently visible at a few months of age or even in the newborn period. It also permits regular surveillance of an eventual progressive atrophy. Pial angiomatosis is not clearly visible using CT scanning. Enhancement is often observed and involves the adjacent cerebral cortex as a result of blood–brain barrier damage.

Magnetic Resonance Imaging (MRI) with contrast enhancement is a powerful tool for delineating the extent of the pial angioma and for excluding involvement of the opposite hemisphere (Lipski *et al.*, 1990; Elster *et al.*, 1990; Vogl *et al.*, 1993). If the patient is a candidate for surgical intervention for intractable epilepsy, MRI should not be performed in proximity of a convulsive episode to avoid false demarcation due to intracortical leakage following blood–brain barrier alterations. Both short echo and long repetition time (TR)/echo time (TE) studies should be done. In addition, gradient echo (GRE) sequences are helpful to demonstrate the presence of microcalcifications (Kuzniecky & Jackson 1995). Complementary information can be obtained by using functional imaging with positron emission tomography (PET) or single photon emission computed tomography (SPECT) (Chugani *et al.*, 1989; Chiron *et al.*, 1989).

The natural history of patients with SW syndrome is variable and this also applies to the evolution of the seizure profile. Some patients may present an initial cluster of seizures, then remain seizure-free for several months or years, sometimes even without medication. In others, epilepsy is of a rather late onset and seizures may be rare. Remissions – sometimes prolonged for several months – with later recurrence are reported. The variable evolution of epilepsy explains the difficulty in evaluating the rhythm of progression, if present, and consider criteria for surgery (Arzimanoglou, 1997).

The main target of *therapy* in SW syndrome is prevention of epileptic seizures and treatment is clearly indicated from the first seizure. The rules applicable to epilepsies of other causes, especially to refractory cases, should be followed. In a recent series of 23 patients (Arzimanoglou & Aicardi, 1993) treatment was with antiepileptic drugs only in 14 patients, the remaining nine presenting an intractable epilepsy, which necessitated surgical treatment. We most often used carbamazepine, valproate or vigabatrin, but therapy should be individualized according to the patient's response. The use of acetazolamide, when associated to carbamazepine, proved beneficial for three patients. Episodes of status epilepticus should be arrested as soon as possible, using benzodiazepines or intravenous phenytoin, in an effort to prevent the appearance of post convulsive hemiplegia.

It is not unusual to find that medical therapy cannot prevent seizures. In such cases, surgery should be considered early, before irreversible damage has occurred (Aicardi & Arzimanoglou, 1991; Hoffman *et al.*, 1979; Ito *et al.*, 1990; Ogunmekan *et al.*, 1989; Rasmussen *et al.*, 1972; Revol *et al.*, 1984). In fact the therapeutic approach to SW syndrome should be considered as a typical example for dealing with lesional epilepsy surgery. Initially treatment should always be medical (Roach *et al.*, 1994). Parallel to medical treatment trials, all procedures permitting evaluation of the extension of lesions (EEG, MRI, eventually PET or SPECT) should be undertaken and progression of lesions should be carefully monitored. When the clinician has acquired, for a given patient, sufficient data to evaluate the potential benefits and risks of surgery, this solution must be proposed.

A decision is relatively easy to reach in cases of unilateral pial angiomas limited to the occipital lobe, especially if hemianopia is already present, as is often the case. The issue is much more complicated when intractable seizures are associated with no motor deficit and the pial angioma involves the motor strip. Progressive enlargement of existing calcifications, increasing focal atrophy observed in serial CT scans, frequency and duration of transient neurological deficits, aggravation of motor deficits and spasticity that may follow prolonged epileptic attacks, are elements that highly suggest progression (Arzimanoglou, 1997). Timing and type of surgery (hemispherectomy, cortical resection of the abnormal cortex or lobectomy) must be decided on the basis of clinical analysis, EEG and neuroimaging data and performed in centres with age-appropriate facilities for preoperative evaluation, postoperative care, as well as experience in pediatric epilepsy surgery (Roach *et al.*, 1994).

Syndromes related to the Sturge–Weber syndrome

Several other syndromes are characterized by the association of cutaneous abnormalities and vascular malformations of the CNS. Cutaneous involvement may not be a major feature, calcifications are not systematically present, and neurological symptoms may be the presenting feature. Several of these are genetically determined and it is important to make careful enquiries about possible other cases in the lineage (Aicardi, 1992). The exact nosological situation of several of these syndromes is not clear.

A syndrome of *bilateral facial naevi, macrocrania and anomalous venous* return through superficial veins (Shapiro & Shulman, 1976) is probably different from the SW syndrome. The association of Sturge–Weber and Klippel–Trenaunay syndromes is possible (Stephen *et al.*, 1975).

Children with *epilepsy and bilateral occipital calcification*s without cutaneous naevus flammeus have been reported (Di Chiro & Lindgren, 1951; Garwicz & Mortensson, 1976; Sammariatano *et al.*, 1985). Disorders that can produce cerebral calcifications (ossifying meningoencephalopathy, encephalitis, leukaemia, purulent meningitis, prenatal infections, hypoparathyroidism) were excluded in these patients. Gobbi *et al.* (1988) described a common clinical pattern of evolution for an apparently benign occipital epilepsy with calcifications associated with progressive mental deterioration. Seizures become more and more frequent, leading to a rather severe generalized symptomatic epilepsy. The presence of coeliac disease was reported in patients with epilepsy and bilateral occipital calcifications. The question of whether this condition is related to Sturge–Weber syndrome has been raised.

To our knowledge, coeliac disease has never been reported in patients with typical leptomeningeal angiomatosis, which remains the hallmark for the diagnosis of SW syndrome. The typical case of epilepsy with bilateral occipital calcifications reported by Taly (1987), which the authors attributed to SW syndrome, did not show clear presence of leptomeningeal angiomatosis. In our opinion the diagnosis of SW syndrome cannot be retained when a pial angioma is not present. Reports suggest that screening for coeliac disase of patients with SW syndrome is negative and our experience with two patients supports these results. This also applies to SW cases without facial angioma but with other features that permit the diagnosis of typical Sturge–Weber (pial angioma). Furthermore, progressive atrophy often observed in patients with SW syndrome and active epilepsy is not a feature of the cases of epilepsy with bilateral occipital calcifications. In the series reported by the Italian Working Group on coeliac disease and epilepsy (1993), three typical cases of SW syndrome underwent intestinal biopsy as control cases. Mucosa was reported normal and no gastrointestinal complaints were present. Data reported by Tiacci *et al.* (1993) favour the hypothesis that we are not dealing with a SW variant. The authors consider the syndrome of epilepsy with bilateral occipital calcifications as a separate entity of unknown cause, characterized by a remarkably homogeneous neuroradiologic picture and an equally remarkable variability in the clinical picture, frequently associated with coeliac disease. An abnormality of genetic origin is considered.

Tuberous sclerosis

Tuberous sclerosis (TS) is, after NF1, the second most common of the neurocutaneous disorders

(Huttenlocher, 1984; Gomez, 1988). Often, the diagnosis is made at the time of first evaluation for a convulsive disorder. Accurate early diagnosis is important for genetic counselling of this dominantly transmitted disorder with high penetrance and variable expressivity. The genetic disorder has been identified, with the TSC1 and TSC2 genes localized respectively on chromosome 9q 34.3 and chromosome 16p 13.3 (Fryer *et al.*, 1987; Kandt *et al.*, 1992). However, a specific molecular marker has not yet been found and genetic heterogeneity seems likely.

The cause of the disease is unknown. It involves an abnormality of differentiation of embryonic cells, with a tendency to hamartomatous proliferation and a disturbance of the migrational process of CNS cells. The extraneural lesions of this multi-organ disease involve the skin (facial angiofibroma, hypomelanotic maculas, shagreen patch, dermal fibroma, *cafe au fait* spots), the heart (rhabdomyoma), the kidney (angiomyolipomatosis), the lung (lymphangiomatosis), the spleen (haemangiomatosis), the liver (haemangiomatosis), and the bones (fibrous dysplasia). Ungual fibromas (Koenen's tumours) appear at puberty or later. Estimates of the incidence of phakomas (retinal hamartomas) vary widely. It appears that they are found in half the cases, either single or multiple.

In the brain, the characteristic features are cortical tubers, subependymal nodules and giant cell tumours. The *cortical tubers* are identified by their nodular appearance, firm texture, and variability in site, number and size. Microscopically, the tubers consist of subpial gliosis with orientation of the glial processes perpendicular to the pial surface and a retained neuronal lamination with giant multinuceated cells that are not clearly neuronal or astrocytic. The junction between grey and white matter is indistinct and may be partly demyelinated. The cerebral cortex between tubers has normal architecture, both by examination with routine stains and with the Golgi method (Huttenlocher & Wollman, 1980).

Subependymal nodules are small excrescences on the ventricular walls that resemble wax that has dripped down the side of a candle, hence the term 'candle guttering' which is traditionally used. They are protuberant and generally firm and often rock-hard because of dense calcifications. Despite superficial appearance suggesting that these lesions are astrocytic, recent studies indicate that the cells are unique (Nakamure & Becker, 1983). They are frequently negative with antibodies to GFAP using immunoperoxidase methods and, on electron microscopy, they do not contain the bundles of intermediate filaments that can normally be identified in large astrocytes. The subependymal giant cell tumours presumably arise from such cells, which accounts for their characteristic subependymal location. The glial retinal hamartoma (phacoma) looks histologically like the subependymal candle gutterings.

The *clinical manifestations* of TS vary considerably with the extent of involvement and age at onset. The diagnostic criteria outlined in Table 1 concern the different specificity and reliability of the various lesions seen in the TS complex. Our ability to confirm the nature of a given lesion may be limited (Roach *et al.*, 1992).

In infants and children, seizures are the most common presenting symptom. If epilepsy begins during the first months of life, the types of seizure usually observed are partial motor seizures and infantile spasms. The high incidence of infantile spasms and hypsarrhythmia has long been emphasized (Chevrie & Aicardi, 1977). As Curatolo (1994) points out, it is now clear that infants with TS are clinically and electroencephalographically different from those with classical infantile spasms and hypsarrhythmia due to other causes (Dulac *et al.*, 1984). Partial seizures may precede, coexist with, or evolve into infantile spasms. Subtle lateralizing features, such as tonic eye deviation, head turning, subtle clonic phenomena mainly involving the face, are part of the symptoms observed but are often missed by parents or doctors until the infantile spasms occur. Later on, a mixed seizure disorder develops in the large majority of patients. Complex partial seizures were reported in 17 of 25 patients with TS who had spasms and in 11 of 15 children who initially had other types of seizures (Yamamoto *et al.*, 1987). Apparently generalized tonic–clonic seizures, tonic or atonic seizures are also frequently seen.

Table 1. Diagnostic criteria for tuberous sclerosis complex (TSC)

Diagnostic Criteria Committee of the National Tuberous Sclerosis Association (1992)

Definite TSC = Either one primary, two secondary or one secondary plus two tertiary features
Probable TSC = Either one secondary plus one tertiary feature, or 3 tertiary features
Suspect TSC = Either one secondary or two tertiary features

Primary features

Facial angiofibromas[*]
Multiple ungual fibromas[*]
Cortical tuber (histologically confirmed)
Subependymal nodule or giant cell astrocytoma (histologically confirmed)
Multiple calcified subependymal nodules protruding into the ventricle
Multiple renal astrocytomas[*]

Secondary features

Affected first-degree relative
Cardiac rhabdomyoma (histologic or Rx confirmation)
Other retinal hamartoma or achromic patch[*]
Cerebral tubers (imaging confirmation)
Noncalcified subependymal nodules (imaging confirmation)
Shagreen patch[*]
Forehead plaque[*]
Pulmonary lymphoangiomatosis (histologic confirmation)
Renal angiomyolipoma (histologic or radiographic confirmation)
Renal cysts (histologic confirmation)

Tertiary features

Hypomelanotic macules[*]
'Confetti' skin lesions
Renal cysts (radiographic evidence)
Randomly distributed enamel pits in deciduous and/or permanent teeth
Hamartomatous rectal polyps (histologic confirmation)
Bone cysts (radiographic evidence)
Pulmonary lymphangiomatosis
Cerebral white-matter 'migration tracts' or heterotopias (MRI evidence)
Gingival fibromas
Hamartoma of other organs (histologic confirmation)
Infantile spasms

*Histologic confirmation is not required if the lesion is clinically obvious.

Mental retardation is common. It is found only in patients who have had seizures, especially in children with early onset epilepsy (Gomez, 1988). The presence of several types of seizures and of a rather high frequency are additional factors indicating unfavourable prognosis (Curatolo, 1996). That also suggests that both the number and localization of cortical tubers play an important role. In addition to mental subnormality, autistic features or other deviant behaviours such as hyperkinesia or aggressiveness are not infrequently found in patients with TS and a history of infantile spasms (Hunt & Dennis, 1987). Other neurological deficits are rare, with the exception of raised intracranial pressure that can occur following the development of intraventricular giant cell tumours.

The diagnosis of TS is clinically easy when many features of the disorder are present (Table 1). However, in infancy the most characteristic manifestations may be lacking. By far the most characteristic diagnostic tool is neuroimaging by CT and MRI (Aicardi, 1992). The *CT appearance* of subependymal hamartomas changes with the age of the patient. They are rarely calcified in the first year of life and calcified lesions tend to increase in number with age (Kingsley *et al.*, 1986). On the contrary, in infants younger than one year of age, cortical tubers appear on CT as lucencies within broadened cortical gyri but the lucency diminishes with age. This makes cortical hamartomas difficult to identify in older children and adults.

MRI is more accurate than CT in detecting cortical tubers, but their appearance also changes with age. In neonates, they appear as enlarged gyri that are hyperintense compared with the surrounding unmyelinated white matter on T1-weighted images and hypointense on T2-weighted images. As white matter myelinates, the appearance of the cortical tubers changes, to become hyperintense on the T2-weighted images with increasing age. When cortical tubers calcify, they often appear bright on T1-weighted images, presumably because of the T1 shortening caused by the crystals of calcium (Henkelman *et al.*, 1991; Barkovich, 1995). MRI appearance of subependymal nodules will also change as the signal of the surrounding white matter changes. Relatively hyperintense on T1-weighted images and hypointense on T2-weighted initially, they gradually become isointense with the white matter. Larger subependymal nodules manifest a variably low signal intensity on the T2-weighted images, which depends on the extent of calcification (Altman *et al.*, 1988; Martin *et al.*, 1987; Barkovich, 1995). Finally, MRI demonstrates white matter lesions, hyperintense on long TR and isointense or hypointense on short TR images (Canapicchi, 1995). Microscopically, white matter lesions are composed of clusters of dysplastic giant and heterotopic cells, with gliosis and abnormal nerve fibre myelination. As Canapicchi *et al.* (1995) point out, the site, shape, and histopathologic findings of white matter lesions confirm that tuberous sclerosis is a disorder of both histogenesis and cell migration.

The *EEG* is of interest to clarify the type of epilepsy associated with TS (Cusmai *et al.*, 1990; Dulac *et al.*, 1984; Curatolo, 1995). At seizure onset, waking EEGs show multifocal or focal spike discharges and irregular focal slow activity. Abnormalities increase during sleep. Atypical hypsarrhythmia, often asymmetrical, is present in one third of cases. Video-EEG monitoring and analysis of EEG patterns, in patients presenting with partial motor seizures and infantile spasms, may suggest a focal origin of the spasms (Dulac, 1984; Curatolo, 1995). Later in life the EEG abnormalities are similar to what is observed in the Lennox–Gastaut syndrome. They may include multifocal abnormalities associated with bursts of bilateral and more synchronous spike and wave complexes.

Management of patients with TS and severe epilepsy may be difficult. Infantile spasms should immediately be treated with vigabatrin, since all studies showed a high percentage of control (Chiron *et al.*, 1995). In some cases with giant cell tumours which show a tendency to enlarge, a palliative shunt or surgical resection may be necessary. The presence of multiple calcified or uncalcified lesions, even when associated with apparently bilaterally synchronous EEG abnormalities, is not necessarily one exclusion criterion for surgery. Where possible, the epileptogenic area must be localized by appropriate explorations. Criteria for surgery and timing remain to be defined.

Genetic counselling is also an essential part of the management of TS patients. Clinical examination of parents should be careful, with a search for subtle clinical signs. After taking into account the type of genetic counselling demanded, investigations may need to be completed with at least ophthalmological examination and MRI.

In conclusion, Sturge–Weber syndrome with or without facial angioma, is a well defined clinical entity characterized by the presence of a pial angioma and related neurological symptoms. The syndrome of epilepsy with bilateral occipital calcifications cannot be considered as a variant of the Sturge–Weber syndrome. Several other disorders may associate calcifications and epilepsy, the mechanisms involved is apparently rather variable. As for tuberous sclerosis it should be regarded as a primary cell dysplasia resulting from embryonic ectoderm, mesoderm and endoderm anomalies.

References

Aicardi, J. & Arzimanoglou, A. (1991): Sturge–Weber syndrome. *Int. Pediatr.* **6,** (2) 129–134.

Aicardi, J. (1992): *Diseases of the nervous system in childhood*, pp. 862–868. London: Mac Keith Press.

Alexander, G.L. & Norman, R.M. (1960): The Sturge–Weber syndrome. Bristol: John Wright & Sons.

Alexander, G.L. (1972): Sturge–Weber syndrome. In: *Handbook of clinical neurology*, vol. 14, eds. P.J. Vinken & G.W. Bruyn, pp. 223–240. Amsterdam: Elsevier.

Altman, N., Purser, R. & Post, M. (1988): Tuberous sclerosis: characteristics at CT and MRI imaging. *Radiology* **167,** 527–532.

Arzimanoglou, A. & Aicardi, J. (1993): The epilepsy of Sturge–Weber syndrome: clinical features and treatment in 23 patients. *Acta Neurol. Scand.* Suppl. **140,** 18–22.

Arzimanoglou, A. (1997): The treatment of Sturge–Weber syndrome with respect to its clinical spectrum. In: *Paediatric epilepsy syndromes and their surgical treatment*, eds. I. Tuxhorn, H. Holthausen & H.B. Boenigk. London: John Libbey, in press.

Barkovich, A.J. (1995): Disorders of neuronal migration and organization. In: *Magnetic Resonance in epilepsy*, eds. R Kuzniecky & G.D. Jackson, pp. 235–255. New York: Raven Press.

Boltshauser, E., Wilson, J. & Hoare, R.D. (1976): Sturge–Weber syndrome with bilateral intracranial calcification. *J. Neurol. Neurosurg. Psych.* **39,** 429–435.

Brenner, R.P. & Sharbrough, F.W. (1976): Electroencephalographic evaluation in Sturge–Weber syndrome. *Neurology* **26,** 629–632.

Bye, A.M., Matheson, J.M. & Mackenzie, R.A. (1989): Epilepsy surgery in Sturge–Weber syndrome. *Aust. Paediatr. J.* **25,** 103.

Canapicchi, R., Abbruzzese, A., Guerrini, R. *et al.* (1995): Neuroimaging of tuberous sclerosis. In: *Dysplasias of cerebral cortex and epilepsy,* eds. R. Guerrini *et al.*, pp. 151–162. New York: Lippincott-Raven.

Chevrie, J.J. & Aicardi, J. (1977): Convulsive disorders in the first years of life: etiological factors. *Epilepsia* **18,** 489–498.

Chevrie, J.J., Specola, N. & Aicardi, J. (1988): Secondary bilateral synchrony in unilateral pial angiomatosis: successful surgical treatment. *J. Neuro. Neurosurg. Psych.* **51,** 663–670.

Chiron, C., Raynaud, C., Tzourio, N., Diebler, C., Dulac, O., Zibovicius, M. & Syrota, A. (1989): Regional cerebral blood flow by SPECT imaging in Sturge–Weber disease: an aid for diagnosis. *J. Neurol. Neurosurg. Psych.* **52,** 1402–1409.

Chiron, C., Dumas, C., Dulac, O. *et al.* (1995): Vigabatrin versus hydrocortisone as first-line monotherapy in infantile spasms due to tuberous sclerosis. *Epilepsia* **36,** S265.

Chugani, H.T., Mazziotta, J.C. & Phelps, M.E. (1989): Sturge–Weber syndrome: a study of cerebral glucose utilization with positron emission tomography. *J. Pediatr.* **114,** 244–253.

Curatolo, P. (1994): Tuberous sclerosis In: *Infantile spasms and West syndrome*, eds. O. Dulac, H.T. Chugani & B. Dalla Bernardina, pp. 192–202. London: W.B. Saunders.

Curatolo, P. (1996): Tuberous sclerosis: relationships between clinical and EEG findings and magnetic resonance imaging. In: *Dysplasias of cerebral cortex and epilepsy*, eds. R. Guerrini, *et al.* New York: Lippincott-Raven.

Cusmai, R., Chiron, C., Curatolo, P., Dulac, O. & Tran Dinh, S. (1990): Topographic comparative study on MRI and EEG in 34 children with tuberous sclerosis. *Epilepsia* **31,** 745–755.

Di Chiro, G. & Lindgren, E. (1951): Radiographic findings in 14 cases of Sturge–Weber syndrome. *Acta Radiol.* **35,** 387–399.

Di Trapani, G., Di Rocco, C., Abbamondi, A.L., Caldarelli, M. & Pocchiari, M. (1982): Light microscopy and ultrastructural studies of Sturge–Weber disease. *Child's Brain* **9,** 23–36.

Dulac, O., Lemaitre, A. & Plouin, P. (1984): The Bourneville syndrome: clinical and EEG features of epilepsy in the first year of life. *Boll. Lega. Ital. Epil.* **45/46,** 39–42.

Elster, A.D. & Chen, M.Y. (1990): MR imaging of Sturge–Weber syndrome: Role of gadopentetate dimeglumine and gradient-echo techniques. *AJNR.* **11,** 685–689.

Falconer, M.A. & Rushworth, R.G. (1960): Treatment of encephalotrigeminal angiomatosis (Sturge–Weber disease) by hemispherectomy. *Arch. Dis. Child* **35,** 433–447.

Fryer, A.E., Chalmers, A.H., Connor, J.M. *et al.* (1987): Evidence that the gene for tuberous sclerosis is on chromosome 9. *Lancet* **i,** 659–661.

Garcia, J.C., Roach, E.S. & McLean, W.T. (1981): Recurrent thrombotic deterioration in the Sturge-Weber syndrome. *Child's Brain* **8,** 427–433.

Garwicz, S. & Mortensson, W. (1976): Intracranial calcification mimicking the Sturge–Weber syndrome: a consequence of cerebral folic acid deficiency? *Pediatr. Radiol.* **5,** 5–9.

Gilly, R., Lapras, C. & Tommas, M. (1977): Maladie de Sturge–Weber–Krabbe. Reflexions a partir de 21 cast, *Pediatrie* **32,** 45–64.

Gobbi, G., Bouquet, F., Greco, L., Lambertini, A., Tassinari, CA, Venture, A. & Zaniboni, M.G. (1992): Coeliac disease, epilepsy and cerebral calcifications. *Lancet* **340,** 439–443.

Gobbi, G., Sorrenti, G., Santucci, M., Giovanardi Rossi, P., Ambrosetto, P., Michelucci, R. & Tassinari, C.A. (1988): Epilepsy with bilateral occipital calcifications: a benign onset with progressive severity. *Neurology* **38,** 913–920.

Gomez, M.R. & Bebin, E.M. (1987): Sturge–Weber syndrome. In: *Neurocutaneous diseases: a practical approach*, ed. M. Gomez, pp. 356–367. London: Butterworths.

Gomez, M.R. (Ed) (1988): *Tuberous sclerosis*, 2nd edn. New York: Raven Press.

Hoffman, H.J., Hendrick, E.B., Dennis, M. & Armstrong, D. (1979): Hemispherectomy for Sturge-Weber syndrome. *Child's Brain* **5,** 233–248.

Hunt, A. & Dennis, J. (1987): Psychiatric disorders among children with tuberous sclerosis. *Dev. Med. Child Neurol.* **29,** 190–198.

Huttenlocher, P.R. & Wollmann, R.L. (1980): The fine structure of cerebral cortex in tuberous sclerosis: a Golgi study. *Ann. Neurol.* **8,** 223.

Huttenlocher, P.R. (1984): Tuberous sclerosis. In: *Recent advances in clinical neurology*, eds. W.B. Matthews & G.H. Glaser, pp. 281–298. London: Churchill Livingstone.

Italian Working Group on coeliac disease and epilepsy (1993): Coeliac disease, epilepsy and cerebral calcifications: a multicentric study. In: *Occipital seizures and epilepsies in children*, eds. F. Andermann, A. Beaumanoir, L. Mira, J. Roger, C.A. Tassinari, pp. 189–196. London: John Libbey.

Ito, M., Sato, K., Ohnuki, A. & Uto, A. (1990): Sturge–Weber disease: operative indications and surgical results. *Brain Dev.* **12,** 473–7.

Kandt, R.S., Haines, L., Smith, S., *et al.* (1992): Linkage of an important gene locus for tuberous sclerosis to a chromosome 16 marker for polycystic kidney disease. *Nature Genet.* **2,** 37–41.

Kingsley, D., Kendall, B. & Fitz, C. (1986): Tuberous sclerosis: a clinicoradiological evaluation of 110 cases with particular reference to atypical presentation. *Neuroradiology* **28,** 171–190.

Kuzniecky, R.I. & Jackson, G.D. (1995): *Magnetic resonunce in epilepsy*, pp. 222–225. New York: Raven Press.

Lipski, S., Brunelle, F., Aicardi, J., Hirsch, J.F. & Lallemand, D. (1990): Gd-DOTAenhanced MR imaging in two cases of Sturge–Weber syndrome. *AJNR.* **11,** 690–692.

Martin, N., de Brouker, T., Cambier, J., Marsault, C. & Nahum, H. (1987): MRI evaluation of tuberous sclerosis. *Neuroradiology* **29,** 437–443.

McCaughan, B., Ouvrier, R.A., DeSilva, K. & MgLaughlin, A. (1975): The value of the brain scan and cerebral arteriogram in the Sturge–Weber syndrome. *Proc. Aust. Ass. Neurol.* **12,** 185–190.

Nakamura, Y., & Becker, L.E. (1983): Subependymal giant cell tumor: astrocytic or neuronal? *Acta Neuropathol.* **60,** 271-277.

Norman, M.G. & Schoenee, W.C. (1977): Ultrastructure of Sturge–Weber disease. *Acta Neuropathol.* **37,** 199–205.

Oakes, W.J. (1992): The natural history of patients with the Sturge–Weber syndrome. *Pediatr. Neurosurg.* **18,** 287–290.

Ogunmekan, A.O., Hwang, P.A. & Hoffman, H.J. (1989): Sturge–Weber–Dimitri disease: role of hemispherectomy in prognosis. *Can. J. Neurol. Sci.* **16,** 78–80.

Poser, C.M. & Taveras, J.M. (1957): Cerebral angiography in encephalotrigeminal angiomatosis. *Radiology,* **68,** 327–36.

Rappaport, Z.H. (1988): Corpus callosum section in the treatment of intractable seizures in the Sturge-Weber syndrome. *Child's Nerv. Syst.* **4,** 231–232.

Rasmussen, Th., Mathieson, G. & Le Blanc, F. (1972): Surgical therapy of typical and a forme fruste variety of the Sturge–Weber Syndrome. *Arch Suisses de Neurol. Neurochir. Psych.* **111,** 393–409.

Revol, M., Gilly, R., Challamel, M.J. Isnard, H. & Lapras, C. (1984): Epilepsie et maladie de Sturge–Weber. *Boll. Lega. It. Epil.* **45/46,** 51–58.

Roach, E.S., Riela, A.R., Chugani, H.T., Shinnar, S., Bodensteiner, J.B. & Freeman, J. (1994): Sturge–Weber syndrome: Recommendations for surgery. *J. Child Neurol.* **9,** 190–192.

Roach, E.S., Smith, M., Huttenlocher, P., *et al.* (1992): Report of the diagnostic criteria committee of the National Tuberous Sclerosis Association. *J. Child Neurol.* **7,** 221–224.

Rosen, I., Salford, L. & Starck, L (1984): Sturge–Weber disease. Neurophysiological evaluation of a case with secondary epileptogenesis, successfully treated with lobectomy. *Neuropediatrics* **15,** 95–98.

Sammaritano, M., Andermann, F. Melanson, D., Guberman, A. *et al.* (1988): The syndrome of intractable epilepsy, bilateral occipital calcifications and folic deficiency. *Neurology* **37,** 1063–1064.

Schweitzer, J.S. & Spencer, D.D. (1996): Surgery of congenital, traumatic and infectious lesions and those of uncertain aetiologies. In: *The treatment of epilepsy,* eds. S. Shorvon, F. Dreifuss, D. Fish & D. Thomas, pp. 669–688. Oxford: Blackwell Science.

Stephan, M.J., Hall, B.D., Smith, D.W. & Cohen, M.M. (1975): Macrocephaly in association with unusual cutaneous angiomatosis *J. Pediatrics* **87,** 353–359.

Taly, A.B., Nagaraja, D., Das, S. *et al.* (1987): Sturge–Weber–Dimitri disease without facial nevus. *Neurology* **37,** 1063–1064.

Tiacci, C., D'Alessandro, P., Cantisani, T.A. *et al.* (1993): Epilepsy with bilateral occipital calcifications: Sturge–Weber variant or a different encephalopathy. *Epilepsia* **34,** 528–539.

Wohlwili, F.J., & Yakovlev, P.I. (1957): Histopathology of meningo-facial angiomatosis (Sturge-Weber disease). Report of four cases. *J. Neuropath. Exper. Neurol.,* **16,** 341–364.

Yamamoto, N., Watanabe, K., Negoro, T. *et al.* (1987): Long- term prognosis of tuberous sclerosis with epilepsy in children. *Brain Dev.* **9,** 292–295.

Epilepsy and other neurological disorders in coeliac disease, edited by G. Gobbi *et al.*
© 1997 John Libbey & Company Ltd, pp. 171–179.

Chapter 23

Clinical and pathological findings in Sturge–Weber syndrome without nevus flammeus

Masanori Ito* and Kiyoshi Sato**

Department of Neurosurgery, East Tokyo Metropolitan Hospital and Juntendo University School of Medicine**,
Tokyo, Japan*

Introduction

In recent years, an association between coeliac disease, epilepsy, and intracranial calcification has been reported especially in Italy and Argentina (Fois *et al.*, 1977). An increasing number of patients with epilepsy and bilateral occipital corticosubcortical calcifications without any sign of facial nevus have also been described (Gobbi *et al.*, 1988). However, these conditions have not been reported in Asia, including Japan, presumably because the staple food there is rice. We reviewed 14 patients with Sturge–Weber syndrome including three cases with an atypical form of the syndrome without facial nevus flammeus (Ito *et al.*, 1989; 1990). No patients were found with associated digestive disorders including coeliac disease. We highlighted one case without facial nevus who underwent surgical treatment with special reference to pathological findings and favourable surgical results, and another case with facial nevus with bilateral occipital calcification.

Patients and methods

The neurological and radiological findings, and management of 14 patients with Sturge–Weber syndrome with or without facial nevus are listed in Table 1. Neurosurgical intervention was not indicated for those in whom the convulsive seizures were being medically controlled, psychomotor development was not retarded, and no progression of calcified lesion on CT and/or ischaemic damage on MRI and SPECT. We carried out surgery on seven patients who had medically intractable seizures and psychomotor retardation.

Results

The three cases without facial nevus had had no digestive disorders. Surgical treatment was apparently effective for the control of medically-intractable seizures in six cases. The seizures disappeared postoperatively in all patients, and anticonvulsant administration was not needed except in case 14. Psychomotor retardation following onset of seizures was dramatically reversed immediately after subtotal hemispherectomy concomitant with the disappearance of seizures in six cases. However, in patient 14, progression of mental retardation and loss of motor function of the right fingers and hand could not be prevented by surgical management, probably because the patient already had a right hemiparesis and cerebral atrophy at 4 months of age.

Table 1.

No.	Onset	Nevus	Calcification	EEG	Control	MR	Surgery
Cases without facial nevus							
1	3 m	none	bilateral PO	right & left polyspike	yes	no	no
2	36 m	none	right TPO	right spike & wave	no	no	effective
3	3 m	none	left O	hypsarrhythmia	no	no	effective
Cases with facial nevus							
4	7 m	left	left O	left spike	yes	no	no
5	10 m	right	bilateral O	right spike	yes	no	no
6	14 m	right	bilateral O	right PO slow	yes	no	no
7	5 m	left	left FO	left slow	yes	no	no
8	14 m	left	left FPO	left slow	yes	yes	no
9	3 m	right	right FT	right FT slow	no	no	no
Cases with facial nevus treated by surgery							
10	8 m	right	right TPO	right PO slow	no	no	effective
11	12 m	right	right O	right PO slow	no	no	effective
12	5 m	right	right FP	right spike	no	no	effective
13	3 m	left	right FTPO	right slow	no	yes	effective
14	2 m	right	right F	hypsarrhythmia	no	yes	ineffective

F, frontal; m, month(s); MR, mental retardation; O, occipital; P, parietal; T, temporal.

Representative case reports

Case 2

A 3-year-old boy had shown completely normal psychomotor development until the onset of convulsive seizures at 3 years. The patient had had no episodes of diarrhoea. By age 4, the seizures had become increasingly intractable in spite of exhaustive anticonvulsive regimens. He had no facial nevus (Fig. 1). The patient was suffering convulsive attacks several times a day by 5 years of age, and during a one year period had become unable to sing, run, or count. Precontrast CT at 3 years of age revealed a typical finding of Sturge–Weber disease (serpentine calcified lesion) in the right occipital lobe (Fig. 2). The lesion was not enhanced by contrast medium. Since the patient did not have facial angioma, he was diagnosed as having Sturge–Weber syndrome without facial nevus (Ambrosetto *et al.*, 1983) or a form fruste of the syndrome. Precontrast CT at 4 years of age demonstrated extension of the calcified lesion into the temporal and parietal lobes concomitant with enlargement of the trigone and inferior horn of the right lateral ventricle (Fig. 2). T2-weighted MRI revealed marked dilatation of the trigone and inferior horn of the right lateral ventricle, while the T-2 weighted image showed an area of high signal intensity in the right temporoparietooccipital lobe, suggesting ischaemic change in the region (Fig. 3). Right carotid angiography revealed an

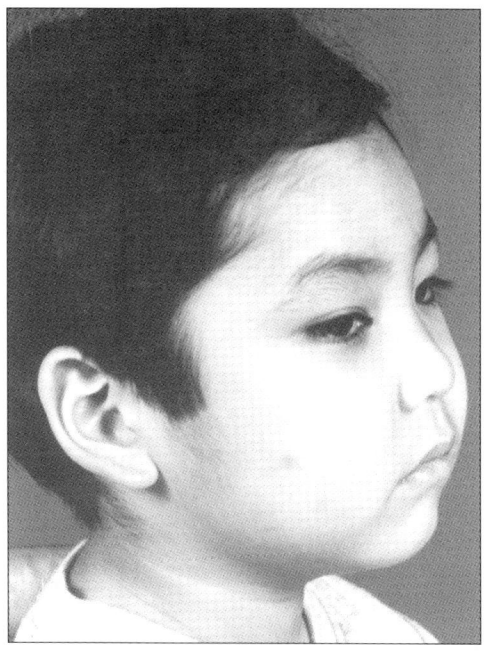

Fig. 1. Photograph of patient showing no facial nevus.

avascular area and a lack of cortical vein visualization in the right temporoparietooccipital region. There was no visualisation of deep veins such as the internal cerebral vein, basal vein and vein of Galen. N-isopropyl-p-^{123}I-iodoamphetamine (^{123}I-IMP)–SPECT revealed a marked reduction in blood flow in the right temporoparietooccipital lobes, corresponding to the area of high signal intensity on the T-2 weighted MRI image (Fig. 3). Right temporal-parietal-occipital lobectomy was performed preserving thalamus, and basal ganglia (Fig. 4). After the dura was opened, the leptomeningeal angiomatosis was observed in the atrophic right frontoparietal cortex. The postoperative course was uneventful. The patient has been free of seizures without the administration of anticonvulsants. Three months after the operation, the patient was able to sing, count, and run, and started going to kindergarten. At school he gets good marks, he loves music, and he won third place in the 100 m race in an athletic meeting. Histological findings of the case are shown in Fig. 5. There was extensive leptomeningeal angiomatosis and calcification within the brain paranchyma, both in the cortex and white matter. Neuronal atrophy, neuronal loss and gliosis were also found.

Case 5

This case is an example of a patient in whom we witheld surgical intervention. This 8-month-old

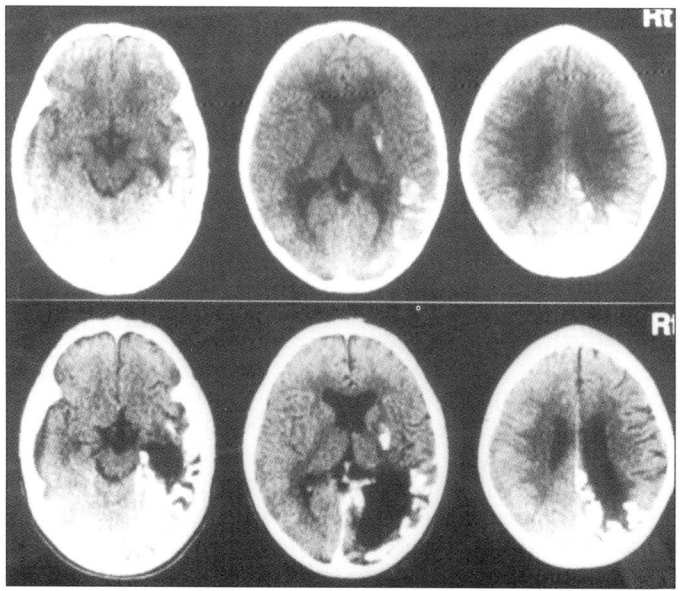

Fig. 2. Precontrast CT of Case 2 at 3 years of age revealing typical findings of Sturge–Weber syndrome (serpentine calcified lesion) in the right occipital lobe (upper). Precontrast CT at 4 years of age demonstrating extension of the calcified lesion into the temporal and parietal lobes concomitant with enlargement of the trigone and inferior horn of the right lateral ventricle (lower).

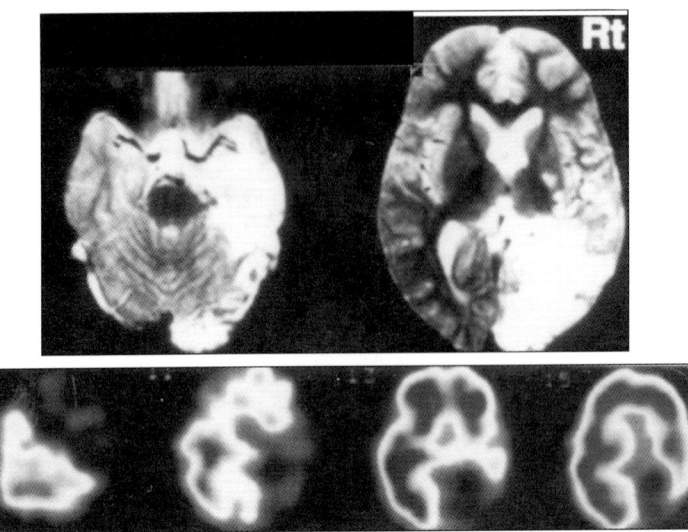

Fig. 3. T-2-weighted MRI (Case 2) revealing marked dilatation of the trigone and inferior horn of the right lateral ventricle, while the T-2 weighted image shows an area of high signal intensity in the right temporoparietooccipital lobe, suggesting ischaemic change (upper). ^{123}I-IMP – SPECT revealing marked reduction in blood flow in the right temporoparietooccipital lobes, corresponding to the area of high intensity signal on the T-2 weighted MRI image (lower).

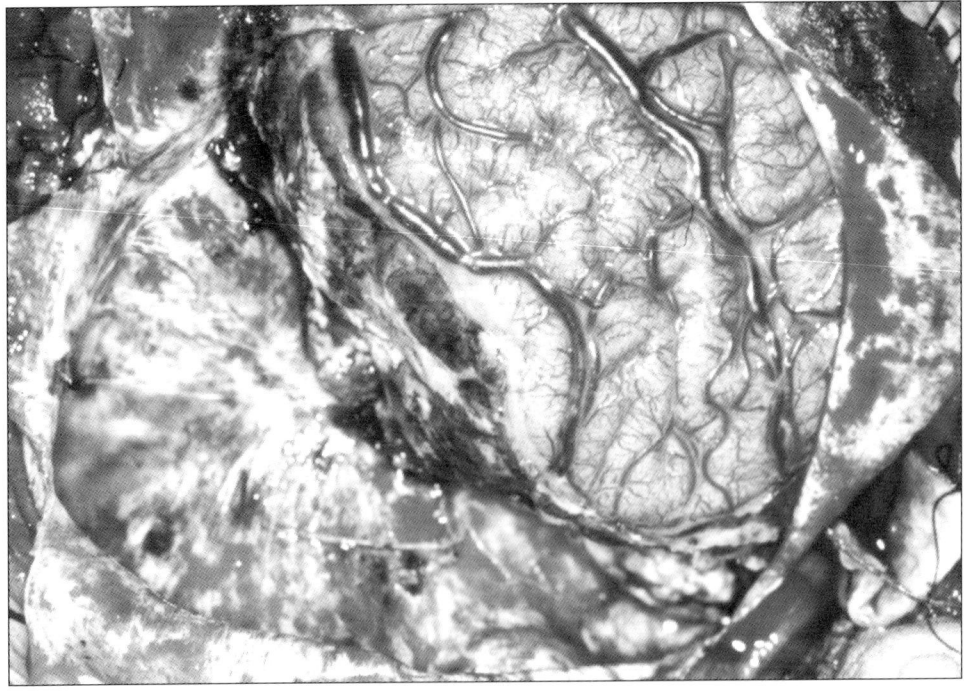

Fig. 4. The operative findings of Case 2: right temporal-parietal-occipital lobectomy subtotal hemispherectomy, preserving the thalamus and basal ganglia.

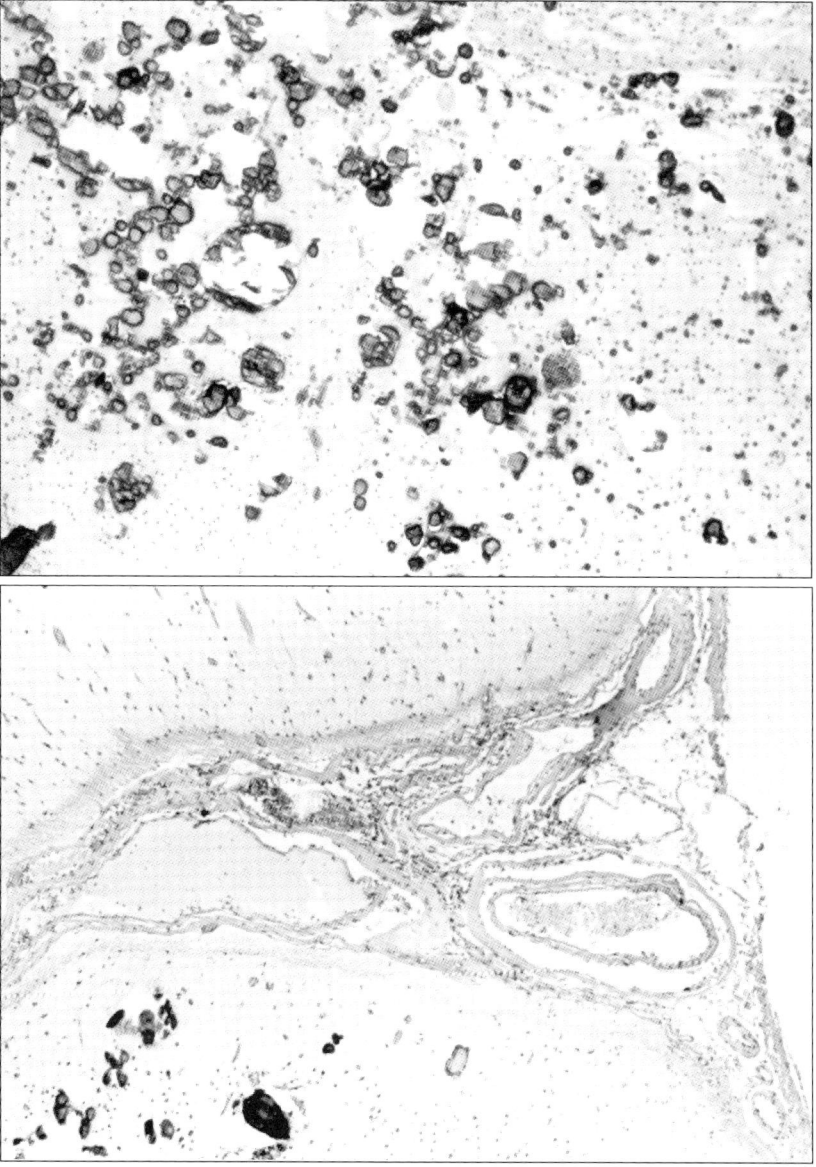

Fig. 5. The histological findings of case 2. There was extensive leptomeningeal angiomatosis and calcification within the brain parenchyma, both in the cortex and white matter. Neuronal atrophy, neuronal loss and gliosis were also found.

boy had a facial nervus on the left side. CT calcifications were present in both occipital lobes (Fig. 6, left). In the MRI, ischaemic lesion was present in the left side (Fig. 6, right). This boy had had right hemiconvulsive seizures several times in the first year of life. We considered surgical intervention when we first saw this patient. Figure 6 shows CBF study with $C^{15}O_2$ positron emission tomography (PET) at age 1 (left) and age 3 (right). There was no progression in the focal decrease in CBF during 2 years. Moreover, his seizures were gradually controlled by medical therapy, and at follow-up, his development was nearly normal. Therefore, we have treated him conservatively.

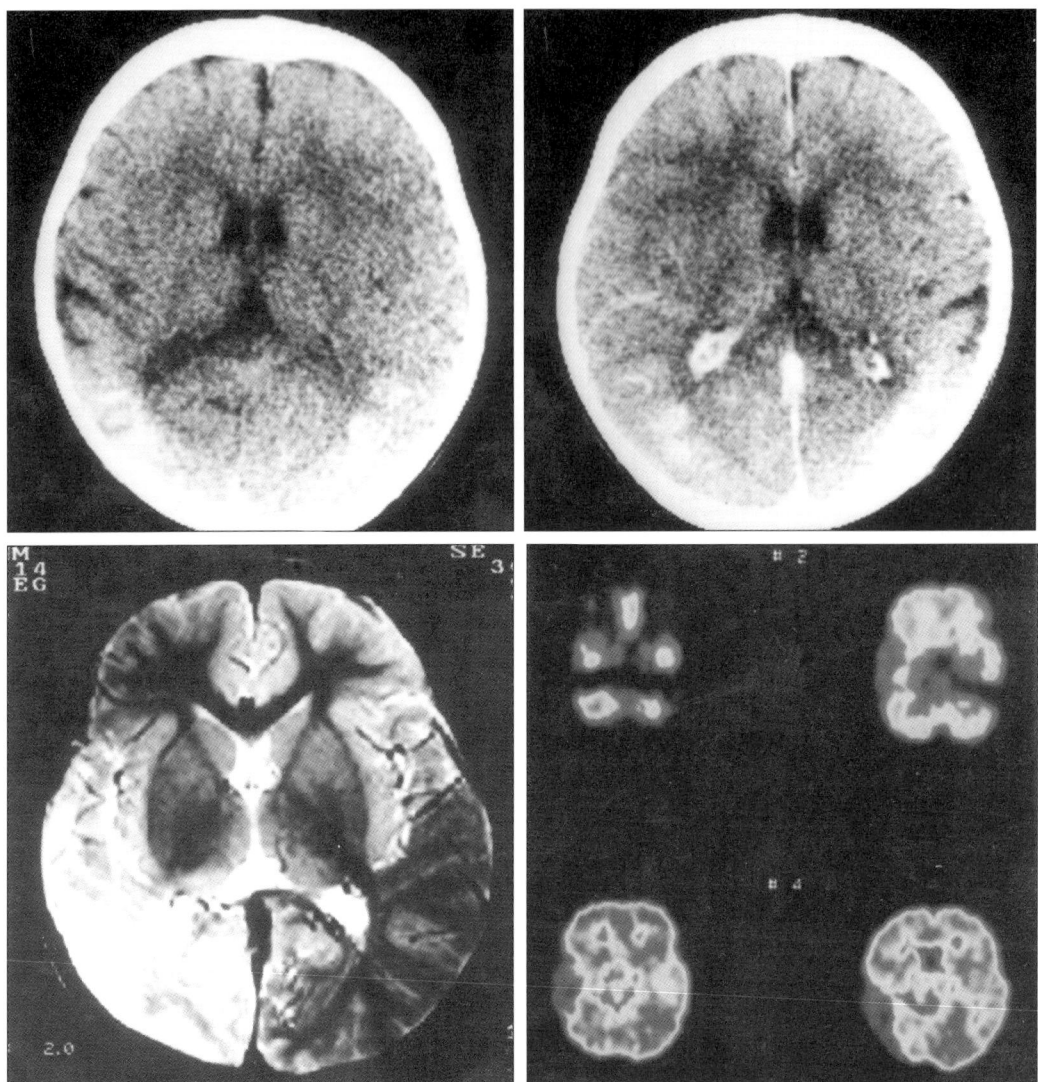

Fig. 6. Case 5: calcification was present in both occipital lobes in precontrast CT (upper left) and choroid plexus was enhanced bilaterally (upper right). An ischaemic lesion was noted in the left temporooccipital area in T-2 weighted image in MRI (lower right). Cerebral blood flow (CBF) study with with $C^{15}O_2$ positron emission tomography (PET) at age 1 (lower left) and at age 3 (lower right).

Discussion

We report clinical and pathological findings of 14 cases with Sturge–Weber syndrome with (typical form: 11 cases) and without facial nevus (atypical form: three cases). Case 2 described in this paper is defined as having an atypical form of Sturge–Weber syndrome without facial nevus flammeus. This patient had no digestive difficulties. After subtotal hemispherectomy, the patient became free of intractable seizures and regained normal psychomotor development. The pathological findings of leptomeningeal angiomatosis and in cerebral parenchyma were identical to those of typical Sturge–Weber syndrome. Case 5 had an epileptic disorder with bilateral occipital calcification, but he had facial nevus, indicating Sturge–Weber syndrome. For this patient we withheld surgical intervention because of good seizure control.

The natural history of Sturge–Weber syndrome remains unknown. Long-term follow-up studies reported from the Mayo Clinic (Peterman *et al.,* 1958) and the Hospital for Sick Children in Toronto (Tsuchida *et al.,* 1980) indicated that 30–40 per cent of patients had moderate to severe neurological deficits and epilepsy, and did poorly at home or were confined to institutions. Oakes (1992) reviewed the natural history of patients with Sturge–Weber syndrome. Of the 30 patient reviewed, 33 per cent had significant extremity weakness and 4 of the 30 died from their disease within the period of follow-up (a minimum of 10 years). Seizures in these patients were uncontrollable or poorly controlled in 83 per cent. All patients in whom seizures started within the first year of life had difficult-to-control seizures regardless of drug therapy. More significantly, no patients in the group developing seizures under age of 1 was living independently. Nevertheless, variability in natural course of the syndrome has been reported such as delayed onset of neurological signs (Gilly *et al.,* 1977). Our case 2 underwent surgical therapy at age 4 years, became free of intractable seizures and regained normal psychomotor development.

The clinical, radiological and histopathological features of our cases with Sturge–Weber syndrome without facial nevus are identical to those of patients with the typical Sturge–Weber syndrome with facial nevus (Oakes, 1992). Progressive vasculopathy occurs in the subependymal and deep medullary veins beneath the leptomeningeal angiomatosis, and the venous stasis that results leads to progressive cortical injury and subsequent calcifications over time (Oakes, 1992). The repeated convulsive seizures, which implicate abnormal excitation of the neural cells and relatively poor blood supply and pathologically enhanced energy metabolism, may result in neuronal damage similar or identical to ischaemic brain damage (Auer & Siejo, 1988; Tada *et al.,* 1993). Serial CT has been reported to demonstrate evolution of calcified parietooccipital lesions (Maki & Semba, 1979). Progressive enlargement of the calcified lesions was clearly demonstrated on CT scanning in three of our 14 cases and all of them presented with medically intractable seizures. In contrast, the calcified lesions remained unchanged during at least one to two years of follow-up in the seven patients in whom seizures were medically controlled. Recently, Marti-Bonmati *et al.* (1993) clarified the correlation between clinical status, CT and MRI findings. The extent of angiomatosis, degree of atrophy and white matter alterations were related to control of the seizures and the degree of hemiparesis and psychomotor development. However, there was no correlation with alterations in the grey matter signal intensity, the prominence of the choroid plexus, parenchymal venous anomalies, or the degree of cortical calcification. Serial PET (Chugani *et al.,* 1989) or SPECT (Chiron *et al.,* 1989) can be used to assess the progression of functional cerebral impairment.

If extensive areas of the hemisphere are involved in a child with Sturge–Weber syndrome who presents with a seizure disorder during the first year or two of life, early hemispherectomy may be considered (Oakes, 1992). Our algorithm for surgery on intractable epilepsy is as follows. (1) If a structural lesion is identified in a patient with intractable epilepsy, we first intend to remove this lesion by tumour surgery or AVM surgery, and then observe the patient. (2) If no structural lesions are found or if seizures are still uncontrolled after removal of structural lesions, we do functional imaging studies, video EEG monitoring, invasive EEG monitoring, or MEG studies. In cases with Sturge-Weber syndrome, we do lobectomy, subtotal or total hemispherectomy depending on the extent of involvement by the angiomatosis. Therefore, in case 2, we skipped video and invasive EEG monitoring, and carried out subtotal hemispherectomy. The area to be removed was determined by neuroimaging, i.e. a calcified lesion on CT, an area of reduced blood flow on SPECT or PET, and a high intensity area on T-2 weighted image, and by the intraoperative findings under the surgical microscope.

According to Falconer *et al.* (1960), Balder pioneered surgical intervention for cerebral angioma in this syndrome, and electrocoagulation of angiomatosis is reported to reduce the frequency of seizures. Peterman *et al.* (1958) reported that one of their four surgically treated patients showed an apparent increase in intelligence quotients after surgical excision, and seizures and behavioural problems decreased. Falconer & Rushworth (1960) reported the results of five hemispherectomies and concluded that surgery helped abolish seizures. Hoffman *et al.* reported 12 surgically-treated patients with Sturge–Weber syndrome (Hoffman & Raffel (1989). Eleven patients underwent hemispherectomy at 1 year of age or younger, of whom seven have a normal IQ (greater than 80). Two have moderate developmental delay and two patients are markedly retarded. Eight of the patients are seizure-free on no anticonvulsant medication, and two patients are having occasional seizures. Two patients continue to have seizures and are severely retarded. Three of the patients required shunting procedures, but none of the patients have had late deterioration during a follow-up from 3 to 22 years. Their results indicate that seizure control can be obtained with hemispherectomy and that if the surgery is performed before 1 year of age, a normal IQ can result. One patient who had had uncontrolled seizures since the age of 9 months had his operation at age 7 years. He had a marked hemiparesis and an IQ of 58. Postoperatively, he has remained seizure-free for 15 years; his intelligence has remained unchanged (Hoffman & Raffel, 1989). This case illustrates that even older patients can have a chance to be ameliorated by the surgery.

References

Ambrosetto, P., Ambrosetto, G., Michelucci, R. & Bacci, A. (1983): Sturge–Weber syndrome without portwine nevus. Report of 2 cases studied by CT. *Child's Brain* **10,** 387–392.

Auer, R.N. & Siejo, B.K. (1988): Biological differences between ischemia and hypoglycemia, and epilepsy. *Ann. Neurol.* **24,** 699–707.

Chiron, C., Raynaud, C., Tzourio, N., Diebler, C., Dulac, O., Zilbovicius, M. & Syrota, A. (1989): Regional cerebral blood flow by SPECT imaging in Sturge–Weber disease: an aid for diagnosis. *J. Neurol. Neurosurg. Psych.* **52,** 1402–1409.

Chugani, H.T., Mazziotta, J.C. & Phelps, M.E. (1989): Sturge–Weber syndrome: a study of cerebral glucose utilization with positron emission tomography. *J. Pediatr.* **114,** 244–253.

DiTrapani, G., DiRocco, C., Abbamondi, A.L., Caldarelli, M. & Pocchiari, M. (1989): Light microscopy and ultrastructural studies of Sturge–Weber disease (1982) **9,** 2326.

Falconer, M.A. & Rushworth, R.G. (1960): Treatment of encephalotrigeminal angiomatosis (Sturge–Weber disease) by hemispherectomy. *Arch. Dis. Child* **35,** 443–447.

Fois, A., Vascotto, M., Di Bartolo, R.M. & Di Marco, V. (1977): Celiac disease and epilepsy in pediatric patients. *Child's Nerv. Syst.* **10,** 450–454.

Gilly, R., Lapras, C., Tommasi, M., Revol, M., Challamel, M.J., Clavel, D. & Mamelle, J.C. (1977): Maladie de Sturge–Weber–Krabbe. *Pediatrie* **1,** 45–64.

Gobbi, G., Sorrenti, G., Santucci, M., Giovanardi Rossi, P., Ambrosetto, P., Michelucci, R. & Tassinari, C.A. (1988): Epilepsy with bilateral occipital calcifications: A benign onset with progressive severity. *Neurology* **38,** 913–920.

Hoffman, H.J. & Raffel, C. (1989): Hemispherectomy for intractable epilepsy. In: *Pediatric neurosurgery, surgery for the developing nervous system,* 2nd edn, eds. R. McLaurin, J.L. Venes, L. Schut & F. Epstein, pp. 549–555. Philadelphia: W.B. Saunders.

Ito, M., Sato, K., Maruki, C., Nitta, T., Ohnuki, A. & Ishii, S. (1989): Surgical treatment of Sturge–Weber syndrome–case report. *Neurol. Med. Chir.* (Tokyo) **29,** 60–64.

Ito, M., Sato, K., Ohnuki, A. & Uto, A. (1990): Sturge–Weber disease: operative indications and surgical results. *Brain Dev.* **12,** 473–477.

Maki, Y. & Semba, A. (1979): Computed tomography of Sturge–Weber disease. *Child's Brain* **5,** 51–61.

Marti-Bonmati, L., Menor, F. & Mulas, F. (1993): The Sturge–Weber syndrome: correlation between the clinical status and radiological CT and MRI findings. *Child's Nerv. Syst.* **9,** 107–109.

Oakes, W.J. (1992): The natural history of patients with the Sturge–Weber syndrome. **18,** 287–290.

Peterman, A.F., Hayles, A.B., Dockerty, M.B. & Love, J.G.A (1958): Encephalotrigeminal angiomatosis (Sturge–Weber disease). *JAMA* **167,** 2169–2176.

Tada, H., Ito, M. & Sato, K. (1993): Experimental study of calcified lesions in immature rat brains induced by ischemia and convulsive seizures. *Nerv. Syst. in Child* **18,** 307–314.

Tsuchida, T., Hoffman, H.J., Hendrick, E.B. & Thompson, H. (1980): Sturge–Weber syndrome. A clinical study of 41 cases of 153 facial angiomas. *No to Shinkei (Tokyo)* **32,** 949–956 (in Japanese).

Epilepsy and other neurological disorders in coeliac disease, edited by G. Gobbi *et al.*
© 1997 John Libbey & Company Ltd, pp. 181–184.

Chapter 24

Pathological findings of coeliac disease, epilepsy and cerebral calcifications

Paolo Tinuper

Neurological Institute, University of Bologna, Via Ugo Foscolo 7, 40123 Bologna, Italy

Introduction

The syndrome of coeliac disease (CD), epilepsy and cerebral calcifications has recently been described (Sammaritano *et al.*, 1985, 1988; Gobbi *et al.*, 1992; Magaudda *et al.*, 1993; Tiacci *et al.*, 1993). Since the first reports, investigators have questioned the nature of the cerebral calcified lesions, comparing them to those reported in Sturge–Weber syndrome (SWS).

Only two cases of CD, epilepsy and occipital calcifications, who underwent neurosurgery for intractable epilepsy, had a complete histopathological study on brain tissue removed during the operation.

The first case was described by Bye *et al.* in 1993. A young girl, with intractable occipital seizures and increasing bilateral occipital calcifications, underwent surgery with extensive resection of her right occipital cortex. Because of mild anaemia, folate and iron deficiency and delayed growth she had a complete gastrointestinal assessment. Antigliadin antibodies were elevated and small-bowel biopsy disclosed villous atrophy, hyperplastic crypts and plasma cell infiltrates, leading to a diagnosis of CD.

Anatomopathological study, performed on brain specimens removed during surgery, showed few foci of pial angiomatosis, separated by portions of normal leptomeninges and cortical small veins with calcified walls and intimal fibrosis almost completely occluding the lumen. Calcifications were large and coalescent and blurred the cortical lamination, destroying the normal parietoccipital cortex. Immunocytochemical analysis failed to disclose significant reactive gliosis.

The second case of occipital calcification, epilepsy and CD was reported by Plazzi *et al.* in 1994. A 28 year old Italian woman, with a long-lasting unrecognized history of gastrointestinal disturbances, developed simple occipital seizures at the age of 9 years. CT-scanning revealed a right occipital calcification; right carotid angiography did not show any vascular abnormality. Because of the coexistence of a clear-cut right occipital epileptic focus on EEG and her resistance to all antiepileptic drug trials she underwent neurosurgical treatment at the age of 17 years. However surgery did not modify the seizure frequency and the patient was examined eight years later for her

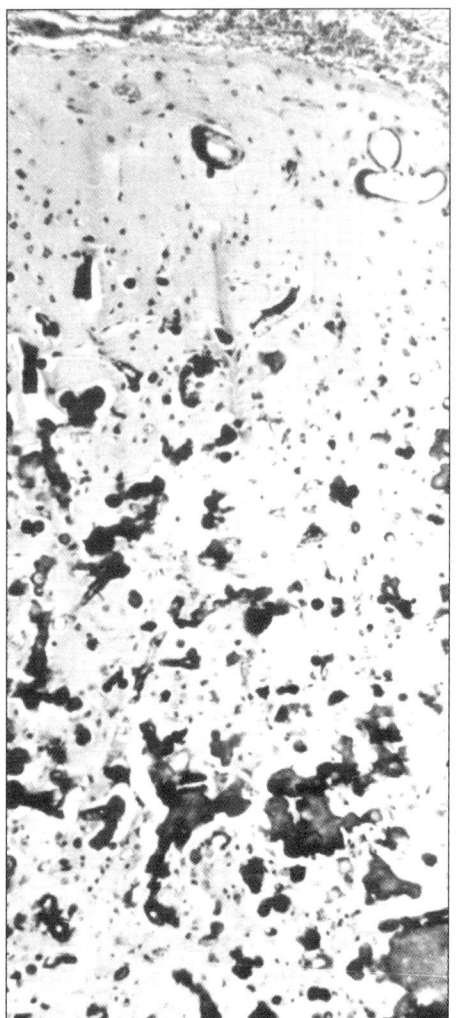

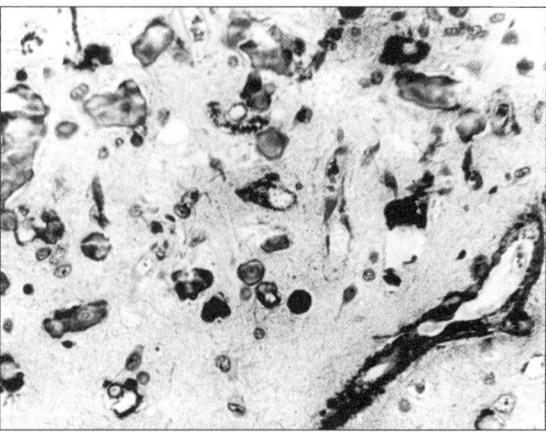

Fig. 2. Coralliform calcifications arising from the walls of cortical vessels of small and medium calibre. Absence of neurons in the calcified zone. HE × 200.

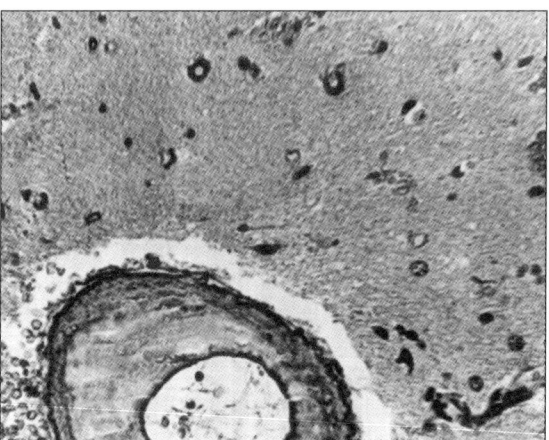

Fig. 1. Multiple cortical calcifications predominant in deeper layers, sparing the molecular layer. HE × 82.

Fig. 3 Thickened and calcified walls of cortical vessels. HE × 200.

drug-resistant seizures. The neurosurgical report was obtained from neurosurgical archives and anatomopathological specimens removed eight years before review (Fig. 1–5).

Histopathological examination revealed many cortical microcalcifications. Calcifications were often confluent and predominated in the deep cortical layers sparing the molecular layer. Small pearly calcifications were in contact with the endothelium of intracortical capillary vessels. Most cortical small veins appeared calcified, with stenosed or completely occluded lumina. There were few foci of pial angiomatosis. Cortical lamination appeared blurred. There was a diffuse neuronal loss but a moderate reactive gliosis in the neuropil close to the calcifications. These findings are identical to those described by Bye *et al.* in 1993.

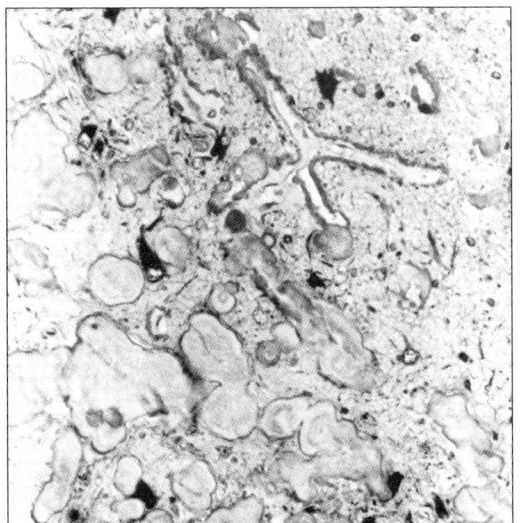

Fig. 4 Moderate reactive astrogliosis near the calcifications. GFPA × 200.

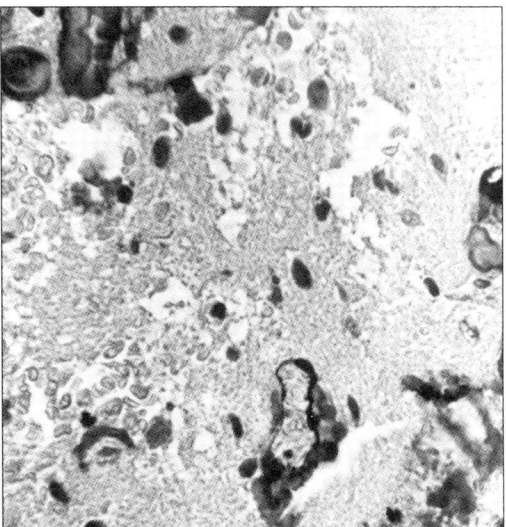

Fig. 5. Small pearly calcifications in contact with the endothelium and at the periphery of intracortical capillary vessels. Immunohistochemistry ULEX × 320.

Discussion

Two studies detailing the anatomopathological aspects of occipital calcifications in proven CD with epileptic seizures are not sufficient to establish the range of the anatomopathological picture of this syndrome. Some findings, however, are consistent and can differentiate this condition from the better known picture of SWS (Norman *et al.*, 1963). Microscopic examination in SWS shows subintimal calcification of meningeal arteries; angiomatous vessels rarely penetrate the brain. Calcium concretions of various sizes are small spherules that in the early stage are confined to the walls of the smaller vessels. In more advanced stages confluent concretions replace the molecular and outer pyramidal layers. Laminar cortical necrosis with calcium deposits is also present. Thus, the most distinctive anatomopathological features that differentiate occipital calcifications in CD from SWS are that, in SWS, cortical architecture is better preserved, and calcifications maintain a laminar distribution, at least in the early stages of disease (Taly *et al.*, 1987; Ito *et al.*, 1990).

Acknowledgement

We are grateful to Professor J.F. Pellissier, from the Department of Neuropathology, University of Aix-Marseille, Marseille, France, who reviewed surgical specimens of the Italian patient.

References

Bye, A.M.E., Andermann, F., Robitaille, Y., Oliver, M., Bohane, T. & Andermann E. (1993): Cortical vascular abnormalities in the syndrome of celiac disease, epilepsy, bilateral calcifications, and folate deficiency. *Ann. Neurol.* **34,** 399–403.

Gobbi, G., Bouquet, F., Greco, L., Lambertini, A., Tassinari, C.A., Ventura, A. & Zaniboni, M.G. (1992): Coeliac disease, epilepsy, and cerebral calcifications. *Lancet* **340,** 439–443.

Ito, M., Sako, K., Ohnuki, A. & Uto, A. (1990): Sturge–Weber disease: operative indications and surgical results. *Brain. Dev.* **12,** 473–477.

Magaudda, A., Dalla Bernardina, B., De Marco, P., Sfaello, Z., Longo, M., Colamaria, V., Daniele, O, Tortorella G, Tata MA, Di Perri R, & Meduri M. (1993): Bilateral occipital calcification, epilepsy and coeliac disease: clinical and neuroimaging features of a new syndrome. *J. Neurol. Neurosurg. Psychiatry* **56,** 885–889.

Norman, R.M. (1963): Malformations of the nervous system, birth injury and diseases of early life. In: *Greenfield's neuropathology*, 2nd edn., eds. W. Blackwood, W.H. McMenemey, A. Mayer, *et al.* pp. 324–440. Baltimore: Williams & Wilkins.

Plazzi, G., Tinuper, P., Provini, F., Cerullo, A., Marini, C., Gambardelli, D. & Pellissier, J.F. (1994): Epilepsy, occipital calcification, and celiac disease: anatomopathological findings and response to gluten-free diet. *Epilepsia* **35,** 81–82.

Sammaritano, M., Andermann, F., Melanson, D., Guberman, A., Tinuper, P. & Gastaut, H. (1985): The syndrome of epilepsy and bilateral occipital calcifications. *Epilepsia* **26,** 532.

Sammaritano, M., Andermann, F., Melanson, D., Guberman, A., Tinuper, P. & Gastaut, H. (1988): The syndrome of intractable epilepsy, bilateral occipital calcifications, and folic deficiency. *Neurology* **38,** (suppl 1), 239.

Taly, A.B., Nagaraja, D., Das, S., Shankar, S.K. & Pratibha, N.G. (1987): Sturge–Weber–Dimitri disease without facial nevus. *Neurology* **37,** 1063–1064.

Tiacci, C., D'Alessandro, P., Cantisani, T.A., Piccirilli, M., Signorini, E., Pelli, M.A., Cavalletti, M.L., Castellucci, G., Palmeri, S., Battisti, C. & Federico, A. (1993): Epilepsy with bilateral occipital calcifications: Sturge–Weber variant or a different encephalopathy? *Epilepsia* **34,** 528–539.

Part VII

Neuroradiological findings

Epilepsy and other neurological disorders in coeliac disease, edited by G. Gobbi *et al.*
© 1997 John Libbey & Company Ltd, pp. 187–194.

Chapter 25

Neuroradiological findings in coeliac disease, epilepsy and cerebral calcifications

F. Triulzi

Department of Neuroradiology, Scientific Institute H S. Raffaele, Milan, Italy

Introduction

Evidence of bilateral occipital calcifications on computerized tomography (CT) is one of the main features of the syndrome of coeliac disease, epilepsy and bilateral occipital calcifications (CEC). For a long time these calcifications were erroneously interpreted as part of the 'atypical Sturge–Weber syndrome' without facial port-wine angioma. Only recently it has been established that CEC syndrome and Sturge–Weber syndrome (SWS) are actually two separate entities.

In this report we will review the different neuroradiological findings of these two syndromes, the clinico-neuroradiological correlation in CEC and the possible future role of modern neuroradiological techniques in the diagnosis and clinical assessment of patients with CEC syndrome.

CEC syndrome is not an atypical SWS

SWS is a congenital disorder of the vasculature of the face, the meninges and the brain. The hallmark of this syndrome is the vascular lesion that involves the territory of the fifth cranial nerve plus the ipsilateral brain and meninges (Smirniotopoulos & Murphy, 1992). SWS has a number of neuroradiological features (Barkovich, 1995) that can be summarized as follow:

(1) The earliest neuroradiological sign of SWS is the *enhancement of the pial angioma* that can be detected on both CT (Fig. 1a, b) and Magnetic Resonance Imaging (MRI) (Fig. 1c, d). Angiography may reveal the pial angioma as well, even though contrast-enhanced MRI was reported as the most sensitive technique in depicting the pial vascular malformation (Sperner *et al.*, 1990; Benedikt *et al.*, 1993). In only less than 20 per cent of SWS patients is the angioma bilateral (Bolthauser *et al.*, 1976). The occipital lobe is most frequently involved, but all the hemisphere can be affected as well (Gardeur *et al.*, 1983).

(2) Due to poor venous drainage, the cerebral circulation in the affected areas becomes metabolically insufficient over time. This causes slow progressive neuronal death accompanied by *calcium deposition.* The calcium deposits begin in the subcortical white matter, the

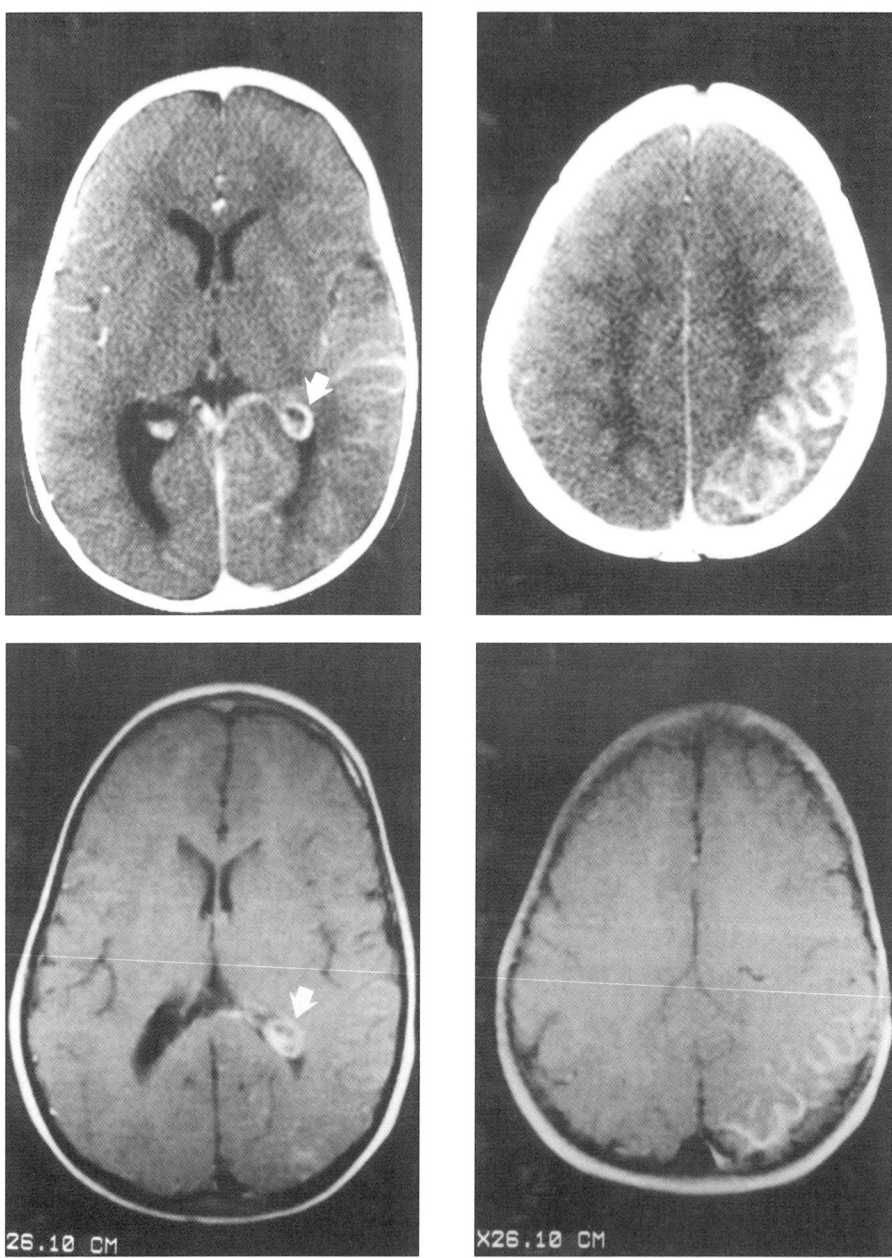

Fig. 1. Two-year-old patient with Sturge–Weber syndrome. Post-contrast CT (a, top left), (b, top right) and post-contrast T1-weighted MRI (c, bottom left), (d, bottom right). On both CT and MRI a parieto-occipital leptomeningeal enhancement is clearly visible on the left hemisphere (right on figure). No focal atrophy is detectable. Ipsilateral choroid plexus enlargement is also easily visible (arrows in a and c) (Courtesy Dr P. Tortori Donati, 'Gaslini' Institute and Children Hospital, Genoa).

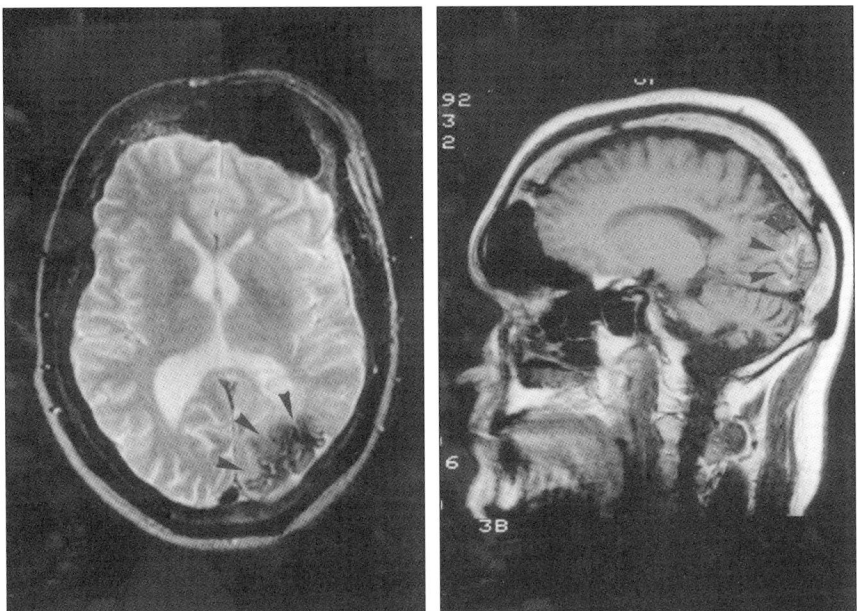

Fig. 2. Long-standing Sturge-Weber syndrome. MRI study, axial T2-weighted (right) and sagittal T1-weighted (left) images. Left hemisphere (right on fig.) atrophy is clearly evident together with ipsilateral skull thickening and enlargement of the frontal sinus. Ipsilateral occipital calcifications are visible as gyriform lesions, hypointense on T2- weighted image and hyperintense on T1-weighted image (arrowheads).

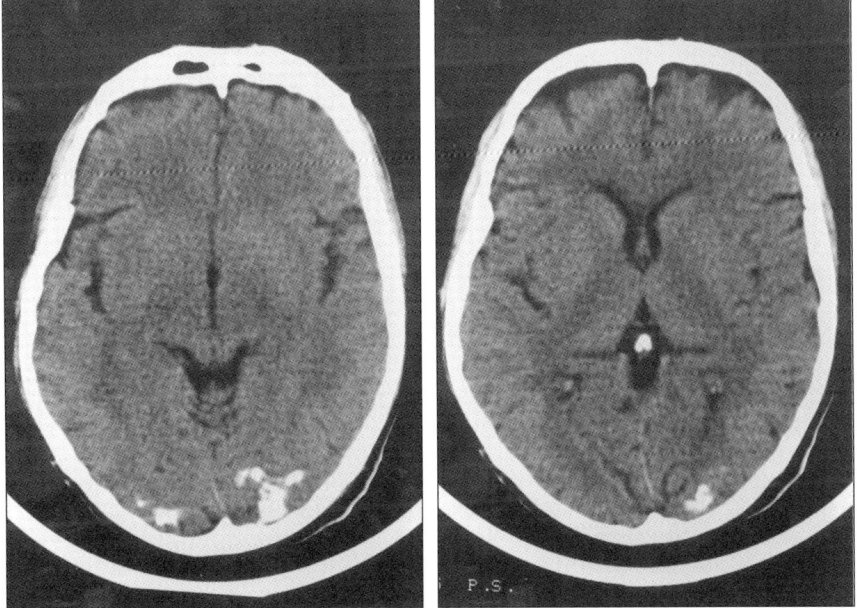

Fig. 3. Thirty-five-year-old patient with CEC syndrome with benign clinical course. Basal CT. Asymmetrical cortico-subcortical occipital calcifications, without focal atrophy.

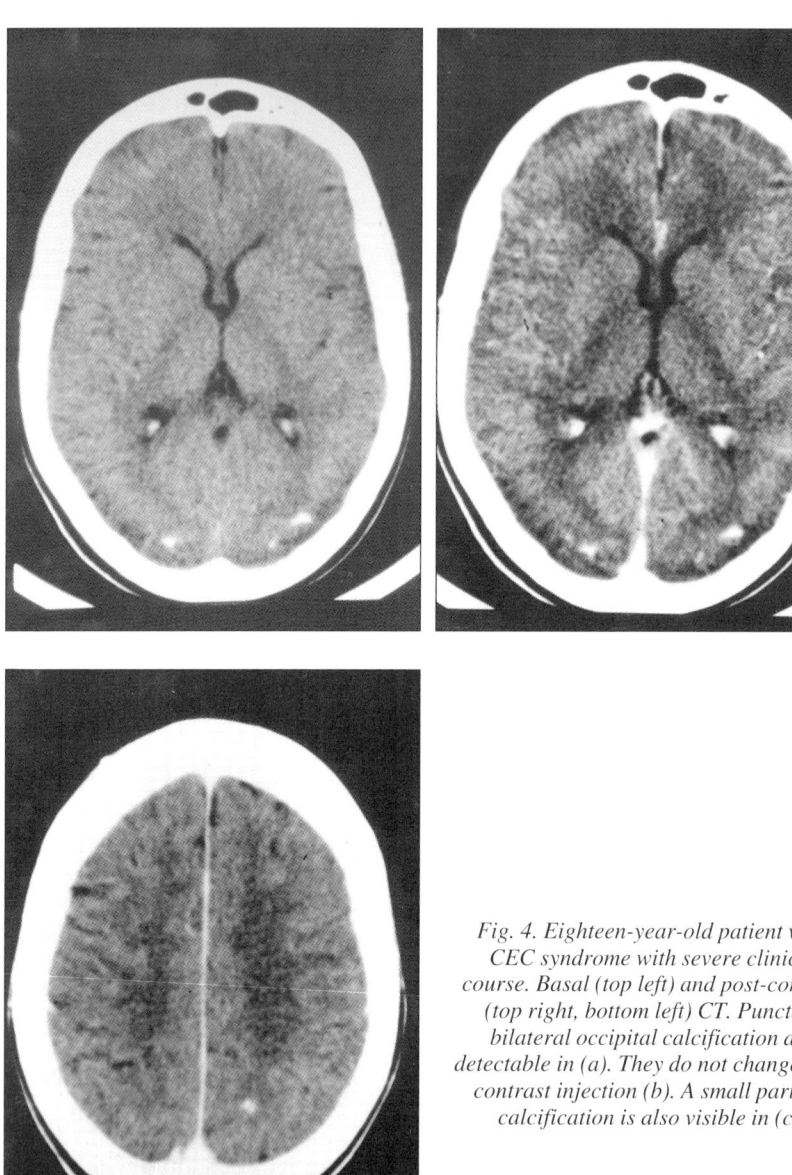

Fig. 4. Eighteen-year-old patient with CEC syndrome with severe clinical course. Basal (top left) and post-contrast (top right, bottom left) CT. Punctate bilateral occipital calcification are detectable in (a). They do not change after contrast injection (b). A small parietal calcification is also visible in (c).

middle layers of the cerebral cortex, and the walls of small intracerebral vessels (Smirniotopoulos & Murphy, 1992). Sometimes even before one year of age, CT easily demonstrated the cortico-subcortical calcifications, limited to the site of the enhancing angioma. Calcium deposits are normally well demonstrable also on T2-weighted MRI as linear hypointense signals within the cortex (Barkovich, 1995) (Fig. 2 right).

(3) *Progressive atrophy* occurs with the advent of calcifications. Cranial asymmetry frequently ensues from brain hemiatrophy, and the lack of cerebral growth on the affected side causes

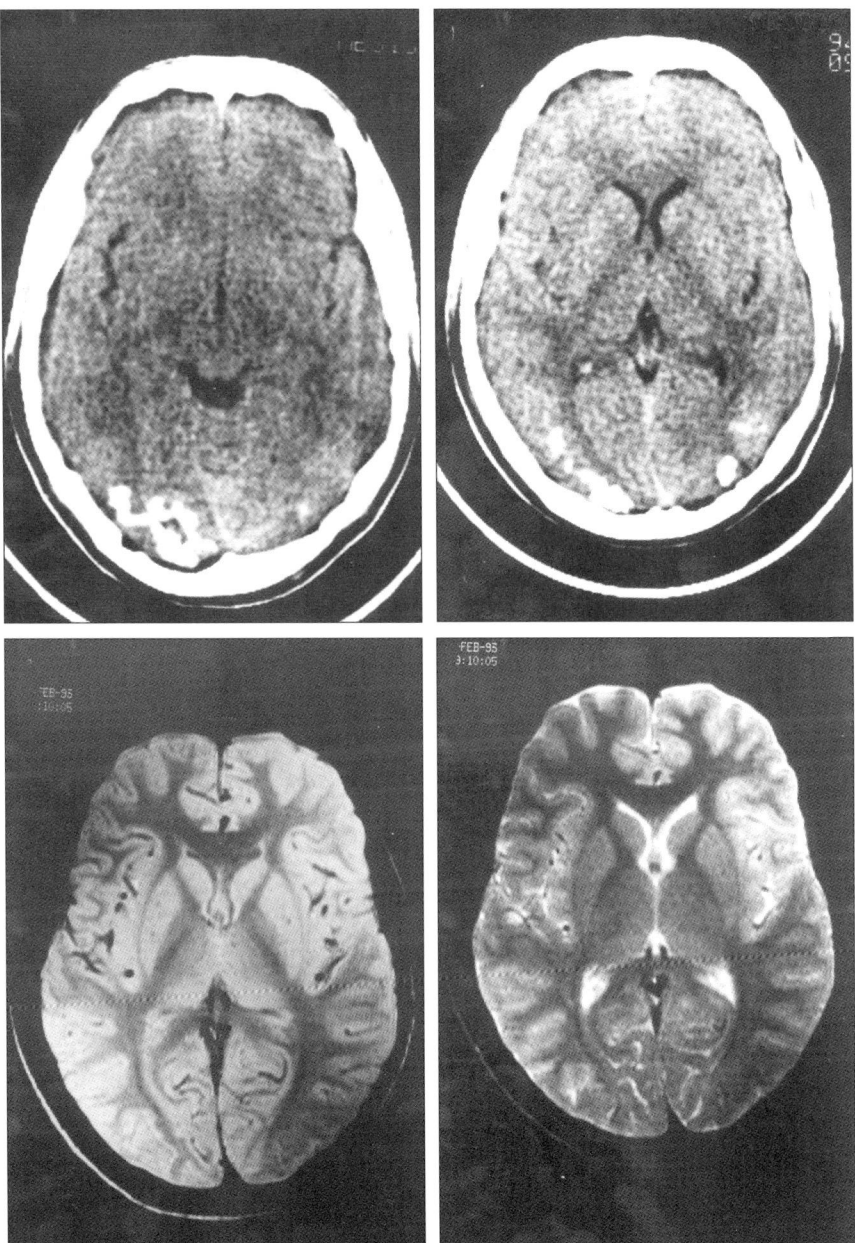

Fig. 5. Twenty-one-years-old patient with CEC syndrome and benign clinical course. Basal CT (a, top left) (b, top right) and basal, PD- (c, bottom left) and T2- (d, bottom right) weighted image, and post-contrast (e, top left, next page) MR. Large occipital calcifications are detectable on basal CT, whereas no significative changes are visible on both basal and post-contrast MR.

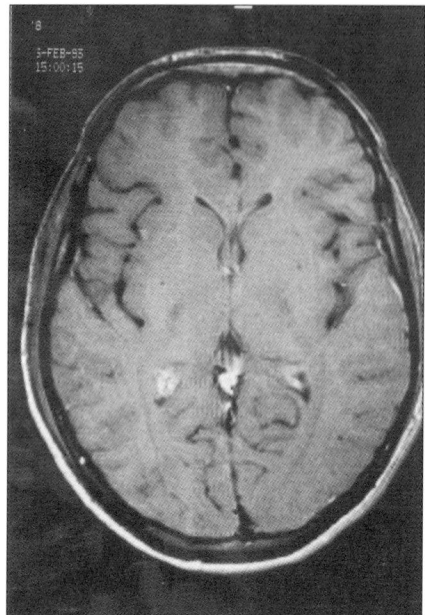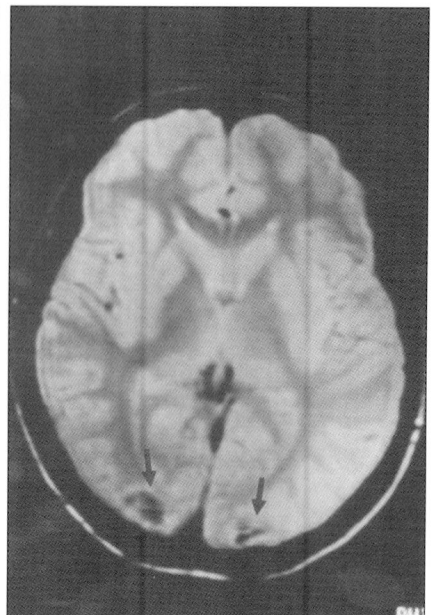

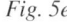

Fig. 5e.	*Fig. 6. Patient with CEC syndrome, PD-weighted MRI. Despite the low quality of the image bilateral hypointense occipital calcifications are visible (arrows).*

ipsilateral thickening of the calvarium with enlargement of the ipsilateral paranasal sinuses (Fig. 2).

(4) Sometimes *enlarged subependymal and periventricular vessels* and *an enlarged choroid plexus* are seen on both CT and MRI ipsilateral to the lesion (Stimac *et al.*, 1986) (Fig. 1a,c).

Apart from the presence of calcifications on CT, neuroradiological features of CEC syndrome greatly differ from SWS:

(1) In no series of CEC patients was leptomeningeal enhancement reported after contrast administration on both CT (Fig. 4b) and MRI (Fig. 5e) (Magaudda *et al.*, 1993; Gobbi *et al.*, 1988; Tiacci *et al.*, 1993). The reported angiographic studies (Magaudda *et al.*, 1993; Molteni *et al.*, 1988) were invariably normal.

(2) Calcifications are located only in the cortex and in the subcortical white matter, are not tram like and occur almost always bilaterally. They are rarely visible on MRI (Magaudda *et al.*, 1993; *et al.*, 1993)(Fig. 5c, d).

(3) Atrophy does not occur in the cerebral areas harbouring calcifications, and no modifications of skull thickening and size of paranasal sinuses are reported (Gobbi *et al.*, 1992; Ventura *et al.*, 1991).

(4) No enlarged subependymal – periventricular vessels or enlarged ipsilateral choroid plexus are reported.

CT and MR in CEC syndrome and clinical correlation

Typical CT features of CEC syndrome are:

  – bilateral subcortical, roughly symmetrical or asymmetrical, occipital calcifications;

  – absence of contrast enhancement;

  – absence of brain atrophy.

In some case additional calcifications may be encountered in frontal region, and scattered cases of unilateral occipital calcifications are reported (Gobbi *et al.*, 1992) (Figs. 3, 4).

Calcifications are extremely variable in size and at present no definite correlation between the extension of the calcifications and the severity of the disease has been demonstrated. Small or punctate calcifications may be sometimes associated with frequent and drug-resistant seizures and/or with progressive intellectual impairment (Fig. 4); or, on the contrary, large calcification may be detected in patients with a benign clinical course (Fig. 5).

The majority of CEC patients did not show a significant change in the size of calcification on follow-up studies. However, in some cases a significant extension of calcifications with time was reported (Magaudda *et al.*, 1993).

Only a small series of CEC patients was investigated with MRI which usually failed to reveal brain calcifications and it was normal even after contrast administration (Magaudda *et al.*, 1993; Tiacci *et al.*, 1993) (Fig. 5). In some cases however calcifications may be detected also on MRI as T2/PD hypointense lesions (Fig. 6).

Neuroradiology and CEC syndrome: future studies

Even though calcifications are an essential part of CEC syndrome, large and complete (both basal and contrast-enhanced CT and MRI) neuroradiological prospective studies are lacking. From the neuroradiological point of view the natural history of CEC syndrome is not well known and too much attention is probably still paid to the end-stage of an unknown phenomenon (calcifications).

Very little is also know about the pathological changes in CEC syndrome; however, in one of the reported cases (Bye *et al.*, 1993) a 'moderate degree of reactive gliosis, mostly localized to the edge of the microcalcification' was reported. Gliosis is usually well recognizable on T2/PD MRI, thus large MRI series of CEC patients studied with heavily T2-weighted sequences should clarify the real extent of gliosis in these patients. Furthermore, new MRI techniques could be used in CEC syndrome patients in order to achieve a better *in vivo* structural insight of CEC syndrome brains: with FLAIR technique the contrast between white matter lesions, such as gliosis or demyelination, and normal brain is maximized. White matter abnormality can also be quantitatively assessed by the magnetization transfer ratio technique or – using echo-planar techniques with very powerful gradients – by diffusion techniques. The presence of calcifications could, on the contrary, limit the use of MR spectroscopy techniques.

In conclusion apart from the classic CT evidence of bilateral occipital calcifications, neuroradiology and new MR techniques could play a significant role in the future clinical assessment of CEC syndrome.

References

Barkovich, A.J. (1995): *Pediatric neuroimaging*, 2nd edn., pp. 304–309. New York: Raven Press.

Benedikt, R.A., Brown, D.C., Walker, R., Ghaed, V., Metchell, M. & Geyer, C.A. (1993): Sturge–Weber syndrome: cranial MR imaging with Gd-DTPA. *Am. J. Neuroradiol.* **14,** 409–415.

Boltshauser, E., Wilson, J. & Hoare, R.D. (1976): Sturge–Weber syndrome with bilateral intracranial calcifications. *J. Neurol. Neurosurg. Psychiatry* **39,** 429–435.

Bye, A.M.E., Andermann, F., Robitaille, Y., Oliver, M., Bohane, T. & Andermann, E. (1993): Cortical vascular anomalies in the syndrome of celiac disease, epilepsy, bilateral occipital calcifications, and folate deficiency. *Ann. Neurol.* **34,** 399–403.

Gardeur, D., Palmieri, A. & Mashaly, R. (1983): Cranial computed tomography in the phakomatoses. *Neuroradiology* **25,** 293–304.

Gobbi, G., Sorrenti, G., Santucci, M., Giovanardi Rossi, P., Ambrosetto, P., Michelucci, R. & Tassinari, C.A. (1988): Epilepsy with bilateral occipital calcifications: a benign onset with progressive severity. *Neurology* **38,** 913–920.

Gobbi, G., Bouquet, F., Greco, I.L., Lambertini, A., Tassinari, C.A., Ventura, A. & Zaniboni, M.G. (1992): Coeliac disease, epilepsy, and cerebral calcifications. *Lancet* **340,** 439–443.

Magaudda, A., Dalla Bernardina, B., De Marco, P. *et al.* (1993): Bilateral occipital calcifications, epilepsy and coeliac disease: clinical and neuroimaging features of a new syndrome. *J. Neurol. Neurosurg. Psychiatry* **56,** 885–889.

Molteni, N., Bardella, M.T., Baldassarri, A.R. & Bianchi, P.A. (1988): Celiac disease associated with epilepsy and intracranial calcifications: report of two patients. *Am. J. Gastroenterol.* **83,** 992–994.

Smirniotopoulos, J.G. & Murphy, F.M. (1992): The phakomatoses. *Am. J. Neuroradiol.* **13,** 725–746.

Sperner, J., Schmauser, I., Bittner, R. *et al.* (1990): MR imaging findings in children with Sturge–Weber syndrome. *Neuropediatrics* **21,** 146–152.

Stimac, G.K., Solomon, M.A. & Newton, T.H. (1986): CT and MR of angiomatous malformations of the choroid plexus in patients with Sturge-Weber disease. *Am. J. Neuroradiol.* **7,** 623–627.

Tiacci, C., D'Alessandro, P. & Cantisani, T.A. *et al.* (1993): Epilepsy with bilateral occipital calcifications: Sturge–Weber variant or different encephalopathy? *Epilepsia* **34,** 528–539.

Ventura, A., Bouquet, F., Sartorelli, C., Barbi, E., Torre, G. & Tommasini, G. (1991): Coeliac disease, folic acid deficiency and epilepsy with cerebral calcifications. *Acta Paediatr. Scand.* **80,** 559–562.

Epilepsy and other neurological disorders in coeliac disease, edited by G. Gobbi *et al.*
© 1997 John Libbey & Company Ltd, pp. 195–199.

Chapter 26

Cerebral blood flow in patients with coeliac disease, epilepsy and cerebral calcifications: a SPECT study

Cristina Messa, Andrea d'Amico, Giovanni Lucignani and Ferruccio Fazio

INB – CNR, San Raffaele Institute, University of Milano, Italy

Introduction

The association of epilepsy, coeliac disease and cerebral calcification has been recently found in a series of 43 patients, and it is suspected to have an higher incidence than expected (Gobbi *et al.*, 1992a). The physiopathological mechanism underlying this syndrome has been poorly understood. The type of epilepsy in these patients is usually partial and more often it starts from the occipital lobes, where the cerebral calcifications are usually located. The severity of such epilepsy varies among different patients and, in a minority of cases, seizures are only partially controlled by medical therapy (Gobbi *et al.*, 1992a, b). Mental impairment can also be present (Gobbi *et al.*, 1992b). Although the type of epilepsy is in agreement with the location of the cerebral calcifications, there is not a correlation between the severity of disease and the size and extension of calcifications. The evaluation of regional cerebral blood flow (rCBF) by single photon emission computer tomography (SPECT) has emerged as a useful tool in patients with epilepsy, being able to demonstrate the site of the epileptogenic area. The sensitivity and specificity of this method varies greatly depending on the origin of seizures and time of injection (if it is during the seizure or not), being more accurate when the seizure is temporal and the study is perfomed during the ictal phase (up to 90–100 per cent) (Spencer *et al.*, 1994; Wieser *et al.*, 1994). Several studies have shown that there are particular patterns of perfusion and metabolism in patients with Sturge–Weber syndrome (Chiron *et al.*, 1989), a disorder which shows histopathological findings similar to those of CEC (Bye *et al.*, 1993).

Until now there have been no studies of functional imaging in these patients. We evaluated rCBF using SPECT and [99mTc]HM-PAO in patients with CEC in order to: (1) detect functional abnormalities and evaluate their relationship with epilepsy and other neurological disturbances and (2) combine the functional with the anatomical findings and particularly evaluate the effect of the calcification on brain function.

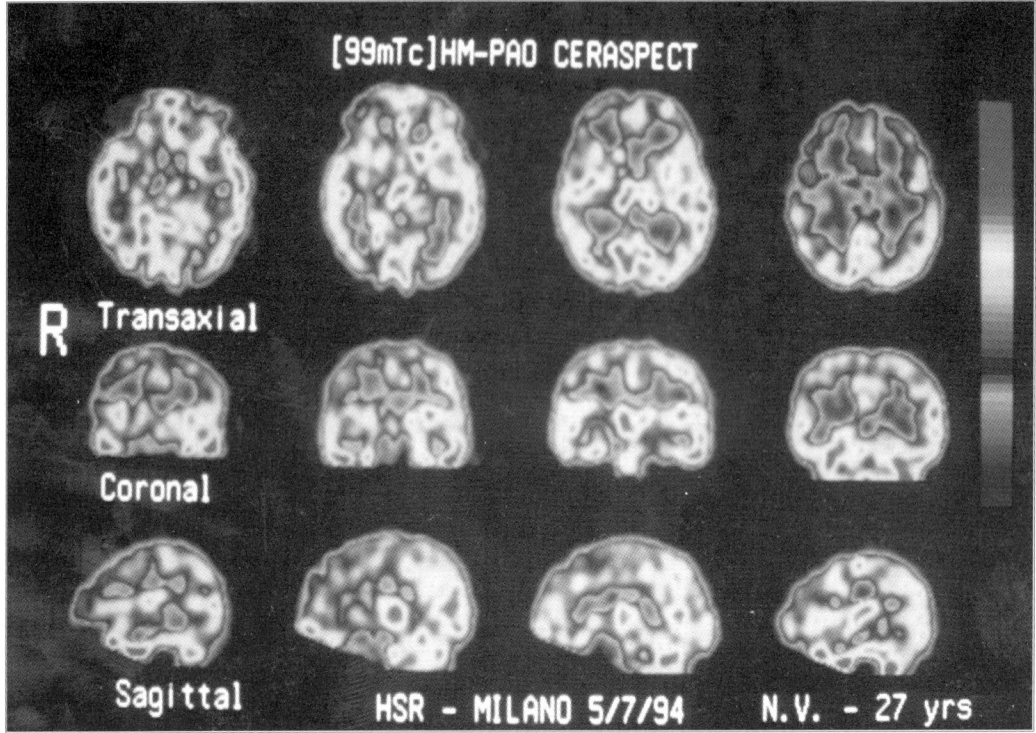

Fig. 1. Transaxial, coronal and sagittal images of cerebral blood flow of patient NV. The patient had a long history of epilepsy and, although she did not show cognitive impairment, she was depressed. Note the marked reduction of perfusion in the frontal cortex (evident on the sagittal planes) which corresponds to the depressive symptoms. Also small but evident areas of hypoperfusion are present bilaterally in the lateral occipital cortex (see transaxial images).

Materials and methods

Patients

Cerebral blood flow using SPECT was evaluated in eight patients (six males and two females, age range 16–28). Clinical characteristics of these patients are reported in Table 1. Seizures onset varied between 1 and 16 years and the type of seizures at onset were all occipital except for one patient in whom it was temporal. At the time of examination all patients had seizures only partially controlled by therapy. Electrical abnormalities were evident in all patients in the occipital cortex bilaterally, except for patient LF whose seizures were temporal. In 6/7 patients with occipital seizures, abnormalities were also spreading anteriorly to the temporal lobes. Mental impairment was present in 4/8 patients.

Calcifications were detected by cranial CT in the occipital cortex of all patients with different size and extension, being large in four patients and small in the remaining ones. All these lesions were present bilaterally with exception of patient CD (right hemisphere).

SPECT studies

SPECT imaging was performed with an annular SPECT system (CERASPECT – Digital Scintigraphic Inc., MA, 29), with a spatial resolution equal to 8.4 mm FWHM in the centre of the axial plane.

Table 1. Patient clinical characteristics

Patients	Sex	Age (years)	Age at seizure onset	EEG at SPECT examination	Mental impairment	X-ray CT calcification
LF	M	28	16	T	No	large
BE	M	24	14	O	No	large
NV	F	27	6	O (+)	No (Dep)	medium
CD	M	24	9	O (+)	Mild	small r
PM	M	24	2	O (+)	Sev.	small
CT	M	16	4	O (+)	Sev.	small
MC	F	20	3	O (+)	Mild	large
SM	M	16	1	O (+)	No	small

T, temporal; O, occipital; O (+), extending beyond the occipital area; Dep, depression; Sev., severe; r, right.

Images parallel to the orbito-meatal line were acquired beginning 15 min after intravenous injection of approximately 740–800 MBq of [99mTc]HM- PAO. The reconstructed images were corrected for attenuation with Chang's 1st order method (attenuation coefficient = 0.1 cm^{-1}). Four consecutive transaxial slices were added to obtain a slice thickness of 6.64 mm. Coronal and sagittal images were also reconstructed. None of the patients showed any seizures on the day of the SPECT study. Since the time elapsing between the latest seizures and SPECT examination was more than 94 h and none of the SPECT studies showed any increased activity, perfusion studies were considered to represent the interictal phase.

Images were qualitatively analysed by three expert observers unaware of the patients' symptoms, but provided with the latest CT of the patient. Observers were asked to describe the location and severity (mild or severe) of the hypoperfused area.

Table 2. SPECT findings

Patient	Area	Degree of hypoperfusion
LF	r TO	mild
BE	b O	mild
NV	b O	mild
	r TP	mild
	b F	severe
CD	r TO	severe
	b F	severe
PM	b F	mild
CT	r TPO	severe
	b F mesial	mild
MC	b O	mild
SM	b PO	mild

T, temporal; O, occipital; F, frontal; P, parietal; r, right; b, bilateral.

Results

Observer agreement was reached for all studies except for patients CT and SM, for whom 2/3 observers agreed. Perfusion abnormalities were present in all patients in various areas of the brain. Table 2 summarizes the results.

Occipital hypoperfusion was present in all patients except PM. The extension of the occipital hypoperfusion corresponded to the size of the calcification area, being more evident when corresponding to a larger calcified area. Hypoperfusion was not restricted to the occipital lobes but extended to temporo-parietal areas in all patients except for patients BE, PM and MC. In four patients an asymmetry of perfusion was observed which corresponded to the side electrically more involved.

Frontal hypoperfusion was present in three patients (CD, PM, CT) with mild to severe mental impairment and in one patient with depression (NV).

All perfusion defects in the occipital cortex were considered mild by all observers, while severe defects were found in the frontal cortex (NV and CD) and in the right temporo-parietal cortex (CD, CT).

Discussion

Our data show that in patients with coeliac disease, epilepsy and cerebral calcification, regional cerebral perfusion abnormalities are also present. This is to our knowledge the first study of functional imaging in such patients. Since 7/8 patients were showing signs and symptoms of epilepsy of the occipital lobes, these perfusion data can be interpreted as the functional correlate of occipital lobes epilepsy (Sveinbjornsdottir & Duncan, 1993). In fact all patients except for patient PM were showing occipital hypoperfusion in areas which corresponded to the calcification. The sparing of the occipital cortex in patient PM could be related to both the small size of the cerebral calcifications and to possible global impairment of perfusion in this particular case, who had a long history of epilepsy and was severely mentally impaired.

Interictal perfusion studies have shown a sensitivity of approximately 60 per cent in detecting the epileptogenic area in seizures of the temporal lobes and even less in other focal seizures, including those from the frontal lobes (Spencer, 1994). The fact that we quite consistently found hypoperfusion in the occipital cortex is probably related to the fact that there is also an anatomical abnormality in the same area. The only patient where hypoperfusion was not evident was the one with the smallest calcification.

The finding that perfusion was only mildly reduced in the occipital lobes can be explained by the relatively small size of the associative occipital cortex in comparison with the cortical areas, and consequently the poor visualization in emission imaging of such structures.

What appears more interesting is that in 6/8 patients functional abnormalities were extending either to the temporo-parietal or to frontal cortices or both. Frontal impairment was present in three patients with mild to severe mental impairment (CD, PM and CT). This is consistent with the well known importance of frontal lobes in cognitive functions. Furthermore, frontal hypoperfusion was present in a patient with normal mental functions but severe depression (NV), in agreement with previous findings of a correlation between depressed mood and psychomotor retardation with hypoperfusion of the left prefrontal cortex (Bench et al., 1993).

Finally, with exception of patient BE, who showed a purely occipital epilepsy, and MC, the area of hypoperfusion extended over the temporal and/or parietal cortex, in agreement with the clinical and EEG findings.

In conclusion the present data show that:

(1) in patients with CEC, focal CBF abnormalities are present in the occipital cortex, according to the type of epilepsy and the site of calcification areas;

(2) the functional defect can be larger than the anatomical defect, and its size and location usually correlate better with the clinical findings.

References

Bench, C.J., Friston, K.J., Brown, R.G., Frackowiak, R.S.J. & Dolan, R.J. (1993): Regional cerebral blood flow in depression measured by positron emission tomography: the relationship with clinical dimensions. *Psychol. Med.* **23,** 579–590.

Bye, A.M.E., Andermann, F., Robitaille, Y., Oliver, M., Bohane, T. & Andermann, E. (1993): Cortical vascular abnormalities in the syndrome of celiac disease, epilepsy, bilateral occipital calcifications and folate deficiency. *Ann. Neurol.* **34,** 399–403.

Chiron, C., Raynaud, C., Tzourio, N. *et al.* (1989): Regional cerebral blood flow by SPECT imaging in Sturge–Weber disease: an aid for diagnosis. *J. Neurol. Neuros. Psych.* **52,** 1402–1409.

Gobbi, G., Bouquet, F., Greco, L., Lambertini, A., Tassinari, C.A., Ventura, A. & Zaniboni, M.G. (1992a): Coeliac disease, epilepsy, and cerebral calcifications. *Lancet* **340,** 439–443.

Gobbi, G., Ambrosetto, P., Zaniboni, M.G., Lambertini, A., Ambrosioni, G. & Tassinari, C.A. (1992b): Celiac disease, posterior cerebral calcifications and epilepsy. *Brain Dev.* **14,** 23–29.

Spencer, S.S. (1994): The relative contributions of MRI, SPECT and PET imaging in epilepsy. *Epilepsia* **35,** S72–89.

Sveinbjornsdottir, S. & Duncan J.S. (1993): Parietal and occipital lobe epilepsy: A review. *Epilepsia* **34,** 493–521.

Wieser, H.G. (1994): PET and SPECT in epilepsy. *Eur. Neurol.* **34** Suppl 1:58–62.

Epilepsy and other neurological disorders in coeliac disease, edited by G. Gobbi *et al.*
© 1997 John Libbey & Company Ltd, pp. 201–207.

Chapter 27

Cerebral metabolic imaging in Sturge–Weber syndrome

Gregory J. Moore[*] and Harry T. Chugani[**]

[*]*Departments of Psychiatry and Behavioral Neurosciences and Radiology, Wayne State University School of Medicine, Children's Hospital of Michigan, Detroit, Michigan;* [**]*Departments of Neurology, Pediatrics, and Radiology, Wayne State University School of Medicine, Children's Hospital of Michigan, Detroit, Michigan, USA*

Introduction

Prior to the demonstration by Gobbi and colleagues (1992) that coeliac disease may be associated with occipital calcification, a number of such patients were described and reported as a forme fruste of the Sturge–Weber syndrome, since they lacked the typical port-wine stain. In the United States, where coeliac disease is not widely recognized, and the neurological complications even less, misdiagnosis continues to be a problem.

Sturge–Weber syndrome (SWS) classically manifests with facial and scalp port-wine stain (capillary hemangioma) in the divisions of the fifth cranial nerve and ipsilateral leptomeningeal angiomatosis (Enjolras *et al.*, 1985). The cerebral vascular malformations in SWS often lead to a number of neurologic abnormalities including epilepsy, intracerebral calcification, hemiparesis, hemiatrophy, and hemianopia. Other clinical features common in SWS are glaucoma (unilateral or bilateral) and mental retardation. Children with the highest risk for cerebral involvement are those with bilateral port-wine stain, or unilateral involvement of all three divisions of the trigeminal nerve, or involving the eyelid (Tallman, 1991). The term SWS should be reserved for only those patients with clear neurological symptoms. The reader can find a more comprehensive description of SWS in publications by Sujansky & Conradi (1995), Enjolras *et al.* (1985), Peterman *et al.* (1958), Alexander & Norman (1960), and Alexander (1972). The focus of this chapter is metabolic imaging of SWS, however we must briefly review anatomic imaging developments in SWS to properly set the stage for our discussion. The development of new high-resolution neuroimaging modalities in the past 10 years has had a significant impact on the diagnosis and management of SWS. Anatomical images obtained with X-ray computed tomography (CT) and magnetic resonance imaging (MRI) can readily detect gross anatomical abnormalities in the child with SWS. CT has played an important diagnostic role because of its sensitivity in the detection of early calcification in the brain (Maki & Semba, 1979). In infants younger than about 1–2 years of age, CT scanning may show the affected hemisphere to be enlarged, with small arachnoid spaces and lateral ventricles. Following the administration of contrast medium, CT may reveal opacification of the angioma and adjacent regions of the hemisphere. The choroid plexus on the involved side is typically enlarged. In some cases, contrast infusion may reveal enhancement of the affected cerebral convolutions. Calcifications may also be seen within the angioma. As the disease progresses and the angioma is progressively excluded from the circulation, large areas of calcification in the brain parenchyma may be seen on CT. This is accompanied by focal or generalized cerebral atrophy, presumably secondary to chronic ischemia. In general, MRI of patients with SWS has shown findings similar to CT. Although CT demonstrates better the calcifications in SWS, MRI is far superior to CT in demonstrating the vascular channels of the angioma. Gadolinium-enhanced MRI is extremely useful in accurately delineating the extent of the angiomatosis (Sperner et al., 1990; Lipski et al., 1990), even before the emergence of neurologic abnormalities (Pascual-Castroviejo et al., 1993). Jacoby et al. (1987) demonstrated accelerated myelination of the affected cerebral hemisphere in two infants (age 3 and 9 months) with SWS. These investigators suggested that this seemingly paradoxic finding of a hypermyelinative state may be due to ischemia of brain tissue underlying the leptomeningeal angioma, and in that way, may be analogous to the myelin-rich lesions (status marmoratus) seen in neonatal hypoxic-ischaemic insults.

Cerebral metabolic imaging

Since SWS causes large functional disturbances of the brain, cerebral metabolic neuroimaging modalities, such as positron emission tomography (PET) and magnetic resonance spectroscopy (MRS) can provide important information necessary for the early characterization, diagnosis, intervention and management of patients with SWS. In addition, the extent and progression of SWS can be monitored with these metabolic imaging techniques. Furthermore, new PET probes for metabolic imaging of SWS are being developed at a rapid pace, and this combined with the access to new metabolic windows recently made available by MRS technology will provide important insights into the biochemistry and pathophysiology of SWS.

Positron emission tomography (PET)

PET is a non-invasive imaging method which can be used to measure local metabolic functions in various body organs. The application of PET in the evaluation of patients with SWS has had a significant impact on management, particularly when there is progressive cerebral involvement and/or the associated epilepsy is refractory to pharmacotherapy and surgical intervention is being considered. PET provides a useful guide as to the type of resection to be performed (hemispherectomy vs. focal). Furthermore, PET can provide an assessment of the functional integrity of brain regions outside the regions with gross anatomical involvement and/or epileptogenic involvement.

Basic concepts of PET methodology

The PET technique employs a camera consisting of multiple pairs of oppositely-situated detectors which are used to record the paired high energy (511 KeV) photons traveling in opposite directions as a result of positron decay (Hoffman & Phelps, 1986). Tracer kinetic models which mathematically describe physiological or biochemical reaction sequences of compounds labeled with positron-emitting isotopes permit a characterization of the kinetics and the mathematical expression for calculating actual rates of the biological process being studied (Huang & Phelps, 1986). Because of the short half-life (minutes to hours) of the isotopes commonly used in PET, it is essential that the cyclotron used to generate these isotopes be situated either on-site or within one to two hours driving distance from the PET scanning facility. The clinical and research applications of PET methodology have been steadily increasing, and many substrates and drugs labeled with positron-emitters are now available for the study of various biological functions in vivo. In the brain, PET has been applied in the study of local glucose and oxygen utilization, blood flow, protein synthesis, and neurotransmitter uptake and binding (Wagner et al., 1995).

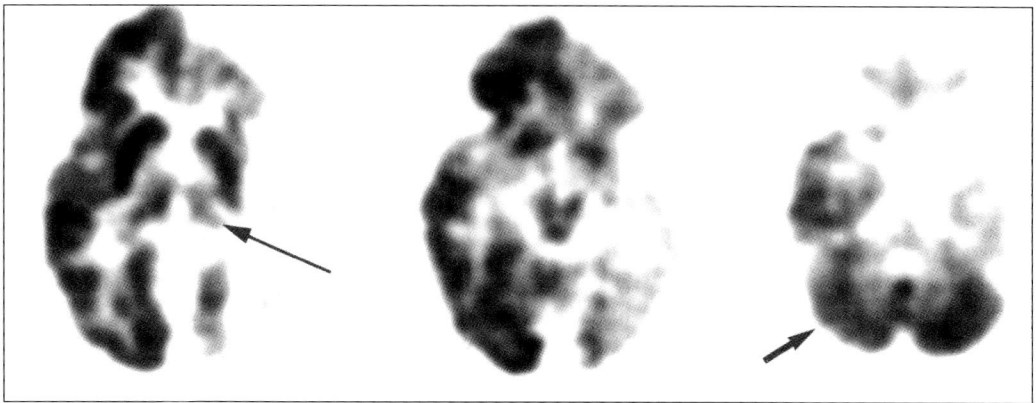

Fig. 1. Glucose metabolism PET images of an 11-year-old boy with Sturge–Weber syndrome. The port-wine stain was on the left side and he had a right hemiparesis. CT scan showed extensive left hemispheric calcification. The PET images show diffuse left cortical hypometabolism. Hypometabolism in the left thalamus (thin arrow) and right cerebellum (thick arrow) are probably due to diaschisis.

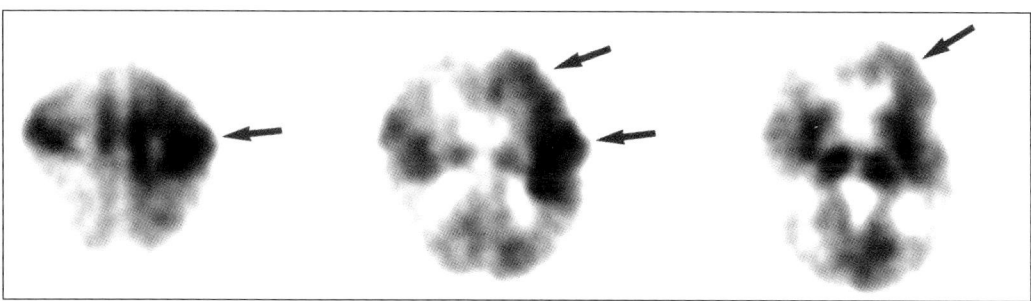

Fig. 2. Interictal glucose metabolism PET scan of a 2-month-old infant with seizures and Sturge–Weber syndrome. The left facial port-wine stain, left-sided epileptogenicity on the EEG, right hemiparesis, and subsequent development of left cerebral calcifications were all consistent with an abnormal left cerebral hemisphere. However, note the increased interictal glucose metabolism in left frontal, parietal and superior temporal cortex (arrows) compared to the right hemisphere which shows a normal pattern of glucose metabolism for a 2-month-old infant.

PET Findings in Sturge–Weber syndrome

PET with the tracer 2-deoxy-2[^{18}F]fluoro-D-glucose (FDG) has been used to image the regional cerebral glucose metabolism in recently diagnosed infants with SWS and in patients with more advanced disease (Chugani *et al.*, 1989). In children and adults with advanced SWS, FDG PET typically reveals a severe diffuse unilateral hypometabolism ipsilateral to the facial nevus in a distribution that extends well beyond the anatomic abnormalities depicted on CT or MRI (Fig. 1). This finding is of great importance in those SWS patients with intractable seizures for whom surgical intervention is contemplated. A paradoxical FDG PET finding in small infants (< 1 year of age) with SWS and recent seizure onset has shown a pattern of increased glucose utilization in the cerebral cortex of the anatomically affected hemisphere interictally. An example of this finding is shown in Fig. 2. As the disease progresses, repeat PET studies show diffuse cerebral glucose hypometabolism ipsilateral to the facial nevus, consistent with our findings in advanced cases of SWS. A number of possible explanations have been proposed for these findings (Chugani & Dietrich, 1992), however the exact mechanism remains unclear.

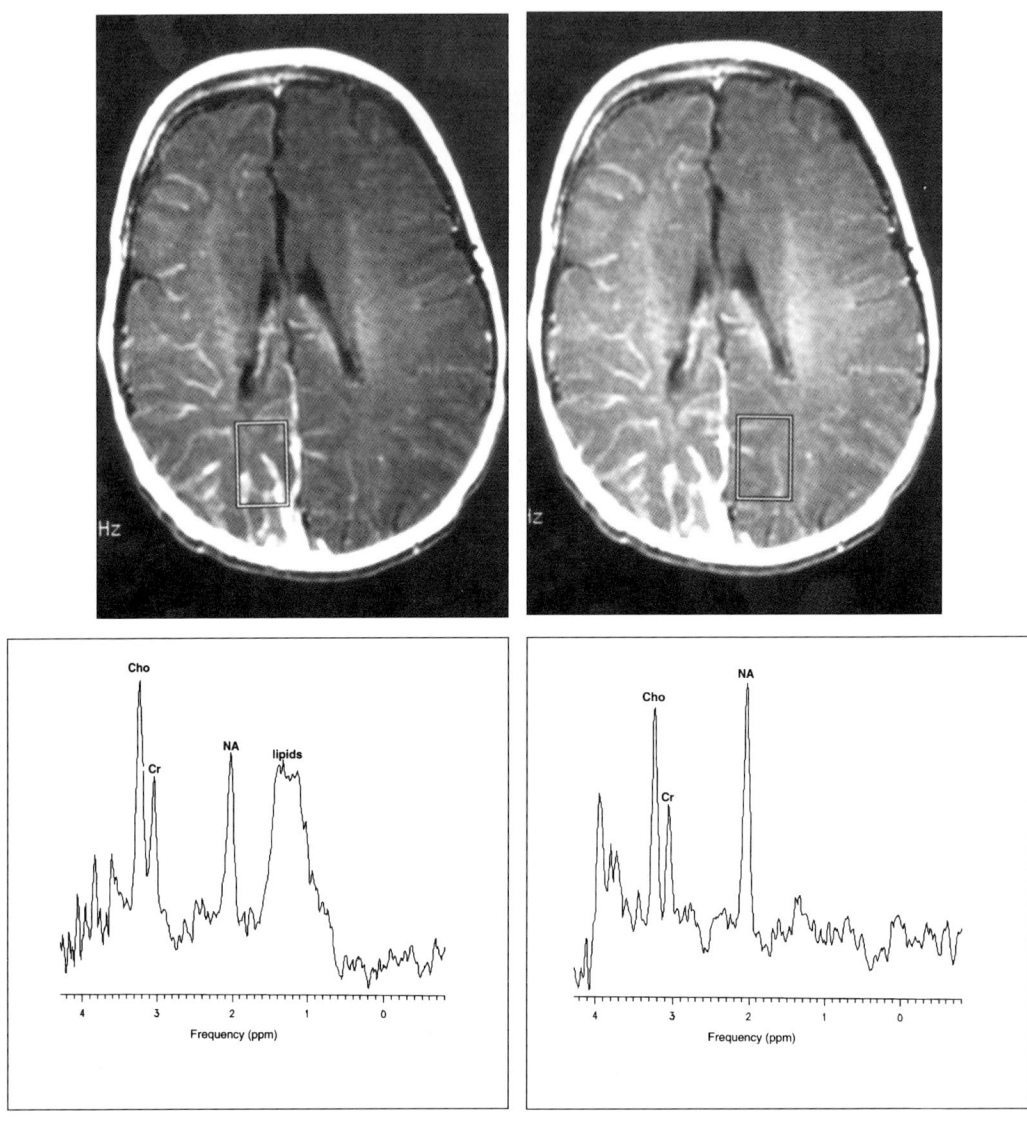

Fig. 3. Proton MRI/MRS study of a young female infant (4 months) with Sturge–Weber syndrome. (a) T1 weighted gadolinium enhanced axial MRI showing enhancement in the right parietal-occipital region. The box indicates the volume of interest for the 1-H MRS exam in (c). (b) Same MRI as in (a). The box represents the volume of interest for the l -H MRS exam in (c) which is an 1-H MRS profile from the affected region defined in (a). Acquisition parameters included an echo time 272 msec, repetition time 2000 ms, 128 averages, acquisition time 5.5 min. Refer to the text for abbreviations. (d) 1-H MRS profile from the unaffected contralateral region defined in (b). Acquisition parameters are identical to (c).

Magnetic resonance spectroscopy (MRS)

In vivo MRS is a tool which has recently been developed to study non-invasively cerebral metabolites (for an excellent review article, see Cousins, 1995). MRS uses the same basic instrument as a conventional MRI system, but differs in that it uses special pulse sequences (combinations of radiofrequency and gradient pulses) to acquire either localized metabolic profiles or spectroscopic images of the brain. Clinical research studies using MRS technology to investigate its potential utility in seizure disorders have focused primarily on proton (1-H) and phosphorus (31-P) containing brain metabolites. *In vivo* 1-H MRS technology can provide non-invasive concentration measures of choline (Cho), creatine (Cr), N-acetyl compounds, primarily N-acetyl-aspartate (NAA), lactate, myo-inositol, glutamine, glutamate, and lipids in the human brain. The NAA resonance has been the subject of considerable recent investigation and has been demonstrated to be a putative specific neuronal marker not found in mature glial cells (Birken & Oldendorf, 1989). *In vivo* 31-P MRS of the brain provides concentration measures of phosphocreatine (PCr), adenosine triphosphate, inorganic phosphate (Pi), phosphomonoesters (PME), and phosphodiesters. In addition, 31-P MRS also provides a non-invasive measure of the intracellular pH by determining the chemical shift of the Pi resonance referenced to PCr.

MRS methodology

We have recently used 1-H MRS to investigate the cerebral metabolic profile of children with SWS (Moore *et al.*, 1996). Young infants and older children with clinical and MRI evidence of SWS were examined. Single voxel 1-H MRS was performed using a clinical 1.5T scanner (GE Signa 5.4) following an MRI examination which included injection of a gadolinium contrast agent (Omniscan). Approximately 8 cc volumes of interest (VOI) were chosen in the enhancing region seen on MRI and in a comparable region in the contralateral hemisphere for each of the patients studied. A double spin-echo PRESS pulse sequence (Bottomley, 1987) technique was used to acquire a metabolic profile from each VOI. The area under each peak in the profile is proportional to the concentration of that compound within the chosen VOI. Essentially this technique allows the investigator to perform a non-invasive biopsy of the brain.

MRS findings in Sturge–Weber syndrome

The N-acetyl-aspartate (NAA)/Creatine (Cr) ratio was markedly reduced in all patients in the gadolinium-enhancing VOI as compared to the contralateral VOI. In addition, metabolic profiles obtained from the gadolinium-enhancing VOI revealed a large resonance in the lipid region of the spectrum in all but one of the patients studied. Only the oldest patient studied (15 years) showed no evidence of a lipid peak in the gadolinium-enhancing VOI. A 1-H MRS study from a 4 month old female diagnosed with SWS is shown in Fig. 3. The gadolinium-enhancing region showing the area of involvement is clearly visualized on the MRI scan in the right parietal-occipital region of the brain. The 1-H MRS profile from the affected region (Fig. 3c) shows a dramatically decreased NAA/Cr ratio and a large lipid peak in comparison to the profile from the contralateral unaffected region (Fig. 3d). A metabolic profile (not shown) acquired to determine if lactate was a major component of the peak in the lipid region indicated that lactate was not a significant contributor to this resonance.

Our 1-H MRS finding of decreased NAA/Cr in the gadolinium enhancing regions is consistent with neuronal loss and is presumably a consequence of the leptomeningeal angiomatosis and the associated cerebral ischemia which characterize this syndrome. The observation of a lipid signal in the gadolinium-enhancing regions may represent an intermediate metabolic step prior to intracranial calcification. Calcification is rarely present at birth, but is present in 90 per cent of these patients by adult age (Nellhaus *et al.*, 1967). These findings yield new information which may be helpful for understanding the pathophysiology and planning possible intervention in this syndrome. In addition, these findings may help in the differential diagnosis of SWS at an early age and/or in atypical cases. We conclude that 1-H MRS is a sensitive tool for the early characterization of SWS in a paediatric population.

Discussion

Cerebral metabolic imaging has given us valuable information useful for the presurgical evaluation of SWS patients with early-onset intractable epilepsy (Chugani *et al.*, 1988, Chugani *et al.*, 1990). In this subset of SWS patients, cerebral hemispherectomy or focal resection performed early in the course of the disease can prevent progressive clinical deterioration (Rosen *et al.*, 1984, Hoffman *et al.*, 1979). Hemispherectomy performed after one year of age in SWS patients generally has a less favorable outcome both in terms of intellectual development and motor impairment (Hoffman *et al.*, 1979). In the presurgical evaluation process, the role of FDG PET and 1-H MRS is complementary to that of the anatomic neuroimaging techniques. CT and/or MRI provide evidence of gross anatomic involvement, whereas the metabolic imaging techniques give sensitive information regarding the extent and severity of functional impairment as well as pathophysiological information regarding the process of epileptogenesis. It is the authors' experience that it is crucial to have both structural and functional information when surgical intervention is considered in SWS as well as in other seizure disorders.

Another area where cerebral metabolic imaging has proven useful is in the monitoring of disease progression in SWS (Chugani & Dietrich, 1992). The pattern of cerebral glucose metabolism seen on FDG PET undergoes dramatic changes as the disease progresses. Our preliminary findings with 1-H MRS (Moore *et al.*, 1996) also seem to indicate changes related to disease progression, although this finding will have to wait to be confirmed until the results of a longitudinal study are available.

These FDG PET and 1-H MRS findings give us new insight and raise novel questions regarding the pathophysiology of epileptogenesis and neuronal death in SWS. In a disease whose underlying etiology remains to be determined, we believe that cerebral metabolic imaging techniques will play an important role in the development of new management strategies, possible pharmacological interventions, and in the eventual determination of the pathophysiology of the disorder and its progression.

References

Alexander, G.L. & Norman. R.M. (1960): *The Sturge–Weber syndrome.* Bristol: Wright.

Alexander, G.L. (1972): The Sturge–Weber syndrome. In: *Handbook of clinical neurology*, vol. 14, eds. P.J. Vinken & G.W. Bruyn, pp. 223–240. Amsterdam: North-Holland.

Birken, D.L. & Oldendorf, W.H. (1989): N-acetylaspartic acid: a literature review of a compound prominent in 1-H NMR spectroscopic studies of brain. *Neurosci. Behav. Rev.* **13**, 23–31.

Bottomley, P.A. (1987): Spatial localization in NMR spectroscopy *in vivo*. *Ann. NY. Acad. Sci.* **508**, 333–348.

Chugani, H.T., Shewmon, D.A., Peacock, W.J., Shields, W.D., Mazziotta, J.C. & Phelps, M.E. (1988): Surgical treatment of intractable neonatal-onset seizures: the role of positron emission tomography. *Neurology* **38**, 1178–1188.

Chugani, H.T., Mazziotta, J.C. & Phelps, M.E. (1989): Sturge–Weber syndrome: a study of cerebral glucose utilisation with positron emission tomography. *J. Pediatr.* **114**, 244–253.

Chugani, H.T., Shields, W.D., Shewmon, D.A., Olson, D.M. & Phelps, M.E. (1990): Infantile spasms: I. PET identifies focal cortical dysgenesis in cryptogenic cases for surgical treatment. *Ann. Neurol.* **27**, 406–413.

Chugani, H.T. & Dietrich, R.B. (1992): Sturge-Weber syndrome: recent developments in neuroimaging and surgical considerations, In: *Fetal and perinatal neurology*, eds. Y. Fukuyama, Y. Suzuki, S. Kamoshita. & P. Casaer, pp. 187–196. Basel: S. Karger.

Cousins, J.P. (1995): Clinical MR spectroscopy: fundamentals, current applications, and future potential. *AJR* **164**, 1337–1347.

Enjolras, O., Riche, M.C. & Merland, J.J. (1985): Facial port-wine stains and Sturge–Weber syndrome. *Pediatrics* **76**, 48–51.

Gobbi, G., Bouquet, F., Greco L., Lambertini, A., Tassinari, C.A., Ventura, A. & Zaniboni, M.G. (1992): Coeliac disease, epilepsy, and cerebral calcifications. The Italian Working Group on Coeliac Disease and Epilepsy. *Lancet* **340**, 439–443.

Hoffman, E.J. & Phelps, M.E. (1986): Positron emission tomography: principles and quantitation. In: *Positron emission tomography and autoradiography: principles and applications for the brain and heart*, eds. M.E. Phelps, J.C. Mazziotta & H.R. Schelbert, pp. 237–286. New York: Raven Press.

Hoffman, H.J., Hendrick, E.B., Dennis, M. & Armstrong, D. (1979): Hemispherectomy for Sturge–Weber syndrome. *Child's Brain* **5**, 233–248.

Huang, S.C. & Phelps, M.E. (1986): Principles of tracer kinetic modeling in positron emission tomography and autoradiography. In: *Positron emission tomography and autoradiography: principles and applications for the brain and heart*, eds. M.E. Phelps, J.C. Mazziotta & H.R. Schelbert, pp. 287–346. New York: Raven Press.

Jacoby, C.G., Yuh, W.T.C., Afifi, A.K., Bell, W.E., Schelper, R.L. & Sato, Y. (1987): Accelerated myelination in early Sturge–Weber Syndrome demonstrated by MR imaging. *J. Comput. Assist. Tomogr.* **11**, 226–231.

Lipski, S., Brunelle, F., Aicardi, J., Hirsch, J.F. & Lallemand, D. (1990): Gd-DOTA-enhanced MR imaging in two cases of Sturge–Weber syndrome. *AJNR* **11**, 69–692.

Maki, Y. & Semba, A. (1979): Computed tomography of Sturge–Weber disease. *Child's Nerv. Syst.* **5**, 51–61.

Moore, G.J., Slovis, T.L. & Chugani, H.T. (1996): Proton magnetic resonance spectroscopy of Sturge–Weber syndrome in children. *Proceedings of the International Society of Magnetic Resources in Medicine: 968.*

Nellhaus, G., Haberland, C. & Hill, B.J. (1967): Sturge–Weber disease with bilateral intracranial calcification at birth and unusual pathologic findings. *Acta Neurol. Scand.* **43**, 314.

Pascual-Castroviejo, I., Diaz-Gonzalez, C., Garcia-Melian, R.M., Gonzalez-Casado, I. & Munoz-Hiraldo, E. (1993): Sturge–Weber syndrome: study of 40 patients. *Pediatr. Neurol.* **9**, 283–288.

Peterman, A.F., Hagles, A.B., Dockerty, M.B. & Love, J.G. (1958): Encephalotrigeminal angiomatosis (Sturge–Weber disease): Clinical Study of thirty-five cases. *JAMA* **167**, 2169–2176.

Rosen, I., Salford L. & Starck, L. (1984): Sturge–Weber disease: neurophysiological evaluation of a case with secondary epileptogenesis sucessfully treated with lobectomy. *Neuropediatrics* **15**, 95–98.

Sperner, J., Schmauser, I., Bittner, R., Henkes, H., Bassir, C., Sprung, C., Scheffner, D. & Felix, R. (1990): MR-imaging findings in children with Sturge–Weber syndrome. *Neuropediatrics* **21**, 146–152.

Sujansky, E. & Conradi, S. (1995): Sturge–Weber syndrome: Age of onset of seizures and glaucoma and the prognosis for affected children. *J. Child Neurol.* **10**, 49–58.

Tallman, B., Tan, O.T. & Morelli, J.G. (1991): Location of port-wine stains and the likelihood of opthalmic and/or central nervous system complications. *Pediatrics* **87**, 323.

Wagner, H.N., Zsolt, S. & Buchanan, J.W. (1995): *Principles of nuclear medicine*, 2nd edn., pp. 483-594. Philadelphia: W.B. Saunders.

Part VIII
Psychiatric disorders in coeliac disease

Epilepsy and other neurological disorders in coeliac disease, edited by G. Gobbi *et al.*
© 1997 John Libbey & Company Ltd, pp. 211–217.

Chapter 28

Depression in coeliac disease

Claes Hallert

Coeliac Centre, Linköping University, Sweden

C oeliac disease may be regarded as basically a disorder of the small intestinal mucosa caused by gluten peptides in the diet, with changes in the villous structure impairing nutrient absorption and leading to various degrees of malabsorption. One might, hence, expect coeliac patients to be generally aware of their gluten intolerance or at least show signs of overt malabsorption at presentation.

Unfortunately for all involved, this is seldom the case. Gastrointestinal symptoms may be frequent at presentation but constitutional symptoms are no less common. Indeed, in most series lassitude ranks with diarrhoea in frequency, making many adult coeliacs likely to present at almost any hospital department for related illnesses and remarkably unaware of their basic gluten intolerance.

Screening adult populations for coeliac disease and taking jejunal biopsy on wider indications have revealed a new concept of coeliac disease over the past decades with evidence accumulating to suggest that psychiatric morbidity may be a significant and neglected cause of disability among adult coeliacs.

In this chapter, current knowledge of the psychic features of adult coeliac disease is reviewed, highlighting the depressive signs and possible links to lack of essential nutrients.

'Bread and tears'

Mental symptoms have been known for many years to be a distinct feature of coeliac disease of all ages. In 1932 the Danish physician Hess Thaysen wrote in his classic study on non-tropical sprue: 'One of the chief complaints in non-tropical sprue is tiredness. This is probably in part of psychic origin, as the fatigue is often persisting long after a bad period has improved, and keeps on even when the patients have been gaining weight' making reference to observations by others of depression as a common finding in these patients (Thaysen, 1932).

However, his comments failed to attract general attention until things changed dramatically in 1950 at the time of Dicke's discovery of the noxious properties of gluten in coeliac disease, making it a treatable disorder. It was not long until reports were published on a striking and almost immediate improvement in mood taking place in children starting a gluten-free diet. Daynes (1956) was able to recognize a syndrome in over 40 coeliac children aged between 1 and 5 years characterized by naughtiness, irritablity, negativism and even fits, responding dramatically within two or three days to a gluten-free diet.

Daynes extended his observations to adult coeliac patients showing what he called a 'headache insomnia depression syndrome'. The immediate response in mood to the gluten-free diet reported by Daynes soon proved inconsistent as experience grew wider and the interest in exploring the mental features of the disorder waned. Instead, anecdotal observations came to dominate the literature, describing adult coeliacs as mentally peculiar, excessively nervous and unstable, depressive, or even schizophrenic (Paulley, 1959; Dohan, 1966).

For instance, the Dohan hypothesis suggesting a link between coeliac disease and schizophrenia was originally based on an observation of a strong association between hospital admissions for schizophrenia in three Scandinavian countries during World War II and the domestic cereal consumption. Although it was stated to be supported by 'numerous clinical observations', many gastroenterologists failed to feel convinced, and a need for studies on the coeliac personality emerged.

The psychic features of adult coeliac disease

Goldberg (1970) was the first to carry out a standardized psychiatric assessment of a series of 46 adult coeliacs. His patients, already diagnosed to be coeliac and taking a gluten-free diet, showed a high incidence of depressive traits with no obvious relationships to bowel symptoms or the nutritional state as assessed by serum folate recordings. Goldberg was seeing most of the patients on repeated occasions during the survey year and found that those remaining ill more often had a family history of psychiatric illness than those who felt well. He arrived at the conclusion that signs of depression are a common finding among adult coeliacs, possibly related to genetic factors. Interestingly, with respect to the Dohan hypothesis, no schizophrenics were recognized in his series.

Adopting a similar approach, Vaitl & Stouthamer-Geisel (1992) recently assessed the psychological complaints among adult coeliacs by mailing the Hopkins Symptom Check List (SCL-90-R) to 182 members (mean age 45 years) of the German Coeliac Society. Half of the series reported an experience that symptoms present prior to the diagnosis had been taken as psychologically determined, leading to drug treatment in 32 per cent and to psychotherapy in 14 per cent of cases. Summarizing the psychological complaints, the authors concluded that coeliacs are apt to show a distinct "psychovegetative" state of exhaustion featuring a depressive component. They found that patients who had gone unrecognized as coeliacs for many years, or were unable to keep a strict gluten-free diet after the diagnosis, were particularly at risk of showing symptoms of mental ill-health and to report more pronounced psychological complaints.

The observation by Vaitl & Stouthamer-Geisel of a past history of psychiatric illness among many adult coeliacs is in good agreement with Goldberg's figure of 40 per cent in his series. Hallert & Derefeldt (1982) had made similar observations in an area of Sweden with a high prevalence of coeliac disease, reporting that 21 per cent of their coeliac patients had attended a psychiatric department during a 10-year period before the diagnosis of coeliac disease. In their patients, depression proved the most common diagnosis and, on the whole, psychiatric illness was found to be the most frequent reason for granting disability pension to adults coeliacs.

Evidence of signs of genuine depression

So far, the only psychological study of newly detected and still untreated adult coeliacs was carried out by Hallert and Åström (1982), testing a series of 12 patients (mean age 47 years) by means of the Minnesota Multiphasic Personality Inventory (MMPI). They found high scores achieved on scale 2 (Depression) alone, which was the only significant difference from matched surgical controls awaiting cholecystectomy (Fig. 1). This MMPI profile would suggest a distinct depressive mood in coeliacs which is separate from that seen in other medical patient groups, e.g. colitis patients, who generally show high scores on scales 1–3 ('the neurotic triad') (Table 1), and further investigation into the depressive symptoms using the Harris subscales showed scores indicative of

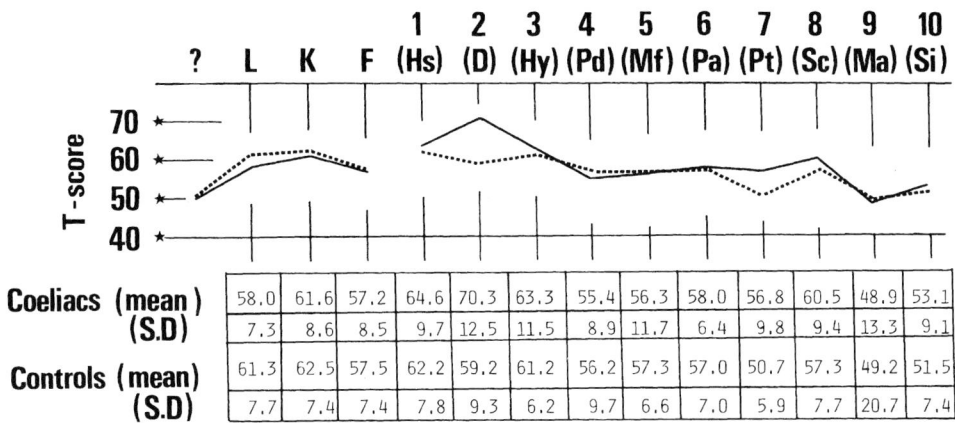

	?	L	K	F	1 (Hs)	2 (D)	3 (Hy)	4 (Pd)	5 (Mf)	6 (Pa)	7 (Pt)	8 (Sc)	9 (Ma)	10 (Si)
Coeliacs (mean)	58.0	61.6	57.2	64.6	70.3	63.3	55.4	56.3	58.0	56.8	60.5	48.9	53.1
(S.D)	7.3	8.6	8.5	9.7	12.5	11.5	8.9	11.7	6.4	9.8	9.4	13.3	9.1
Controls (mean)	61.3	62.5	57.5	62.2	59.2	61.2	56.2	57.3	57.0	50.7	57.3	49.2	51.5
(S.D)	7.7	7.4	7.4	7.8	9.3	6.2	9.7	6.6	7.0	5.9	7.7	20.7	7.4

Fig. 1. The mean MMPI profile of 12 coeliac patients (unbroken line) and of 12 matched surgical controls (broken line). ?, L, K, F denote validity scales, and 1–10 (Hs-Si) denote clinical scales explained in Table 1. The corresponding T-scores ± SD appear in the boxes. Reprinted from: Psychic disturbances in adult coeliac disease by Hallert & Åström, from Scand. J. Gastroenterol. 1982, 17, 21–24, by permission of Scandinavian University Press.

predominant subjective depression and psychomotor retardation. Again, as shown in Fig. 1, coeliacs did not to produce evidence of schizophrenia when undergoing a clinical test.

Further support for the presence of a genuine depression state afflicting adult coeliacs arrived with the demonstration of low cerebrospinal fluid (CSF) levels of major metabolites of the biogenic amines serotonin, dopamine, and norepinephrine (Hallert *et al.*, 1982a), i.e. recordings in a range displayed by depressed patients seeking psychiatric advice (Fig. 2).

No signs of dementia

Investigating the possibility of an organic brain syndrome underlying the monoamine abnormalities of coeliac disease, Hallert & Åström (1983) extended their original observations (Hallert & Åström, 1982) and examined the intellectual capacity of a series of 19 consecutive adults (mean age 48 years) at the time of the diagnosis, eight of whom reported a history of overt coeliac disease in childhood, mostly periods of unexplained diarrhoea accounting for treatment in hospital in three. Using a comprehensive test battery, they found no consistent signs of cognitive impairment and concluded that lifelong intestinal malabsorption as encountered in coeliac disease is not associated with apparent signs of dementia at least in middle-aged adults. Thus, the signs of reduced central monoamine metabolism displayed by untreated adult coeliacs are more likely to be accounted for by mechanisms other than cell degeneration in brain tissues.

Table 1. Number and name of the clinical scales of the MMPI

1. Hypochondriasis (Hs)
2. Depression (D)
3. Hysteria (Hy)
4. Psychopathic deviate (Pd)
5. Masculinity-femininity (Mf)
6. Paranoia (Pa)
7. Psychasthenia (Pt)
8. Schizophrenia (Sc)
9. Hypomania (Ma)
10. Social introversion (Si)

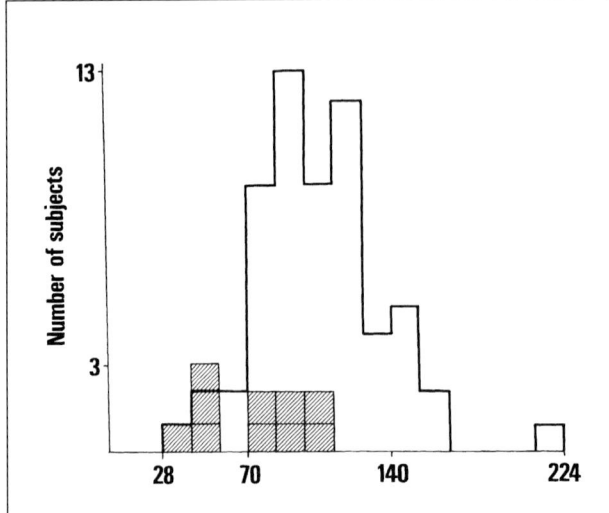

Fig. 2. The distribution of the serotonin metabolite 5-HIAA in CSF of 10 coeliac patients. Reference range, 70–140 pmol/ml. Hatched area denotes distribution in healthy controls. Reprinted from: Psychic disturbances in adult coeliac disease by Hallert, Åström & Sedvall, from Scand. J. Gastroenterol. 1982, 17, 25–28, by permission of Scandinavian University Press.

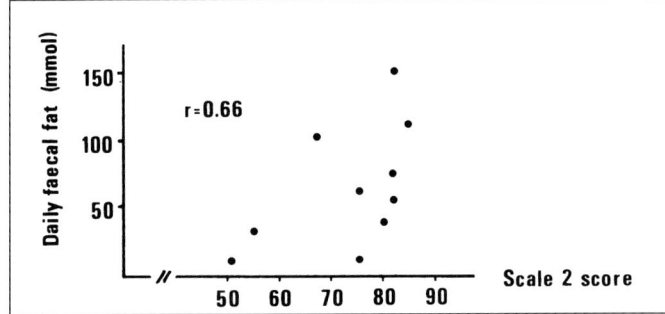

Fig. 3. A significant relationship between daily fat excretion on a 100-g fat diet and the score on scale 2 (Depression) in the MMPI (no. 10). Reprinted from: Psychic disturbances in adult coeliac disease by Hallert & Åström, from Scand. J. Gastroenterol. 1982, 17, 21–24, by permission of Scandinavian University Press.

Nutritional aspects of depression in adult coeliac disease

The association of a medical disorder and its emotional complications may be complex, and this may be particularly true for coeliac disease (Hallert, 1987). Disturbances in the early mother–child relationship and the tendency for retarded growth development to cause later feelings of inferiority and vulnerability in unrecognized patients may all have bearing on the personality of adult coeliacs. Yet, most current interest in the coeliac depression extends from the works of Wurtman (1979) and his colleagues, demonstrating that dietary control over monoamine production in brain operates also under physiological conditions.

The nutritional approach in elucidating mechanisms underlying the coeliac depression emerged from findings of a significant correlation between the degree of depression as assessed by the MMPI and the amount of steatorrhoea in untreated coeliacs (Fig. 3). It was further encouraged by the observation of improvement in central monoamine metabolism following the return of the villous structure in the jejunal mucosa when gluten was withdrawn from the diet (Hallert & Sedvall, 1983).

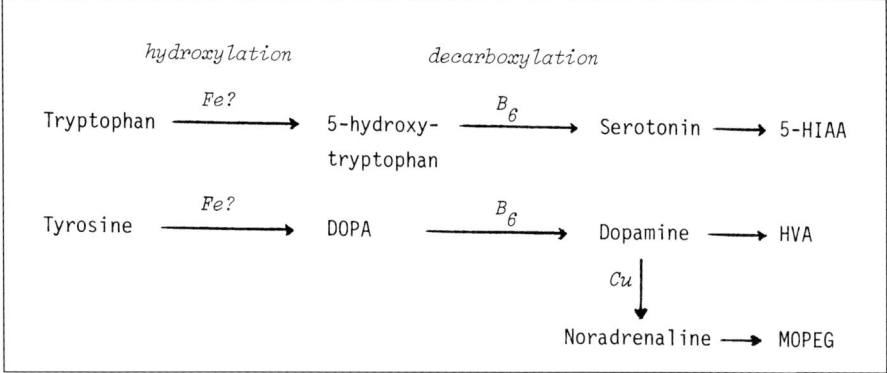

Fig. 4. Diagram showing the participation of essential dietary constituents in monoamine synthesis in the central nervous system.

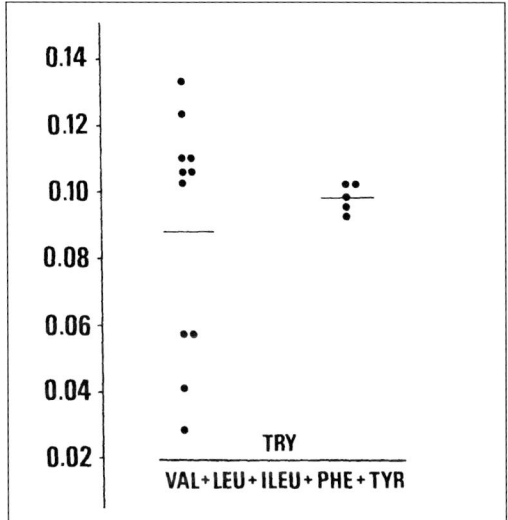

Fig. 5. Plasma tryptophan ratios in 11 adult coeliac patients (left), 0.09 ± 0.037, and in 5 healthy controls (right), 0.10 ± 0.011 (n.s.). Abbreviations: TRY=tryptophan; VAL=valine; LEU=leucine; ILEU=isoleucine; PHE=phenylalanine; TYR=tyrosine. Reprinted from: Brain availability of monoamine precursors in adult coeliac disease by Hallert, Mårtensson & Allgén, from Scand. J. Gastroenterol. 1982, 17, 87–89, by permission of Scandinavian University Press.

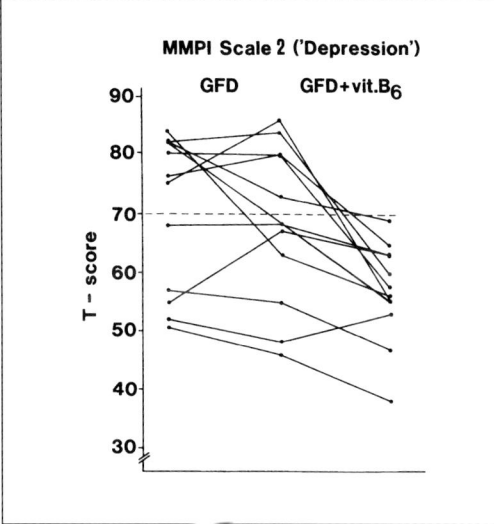

Fig.6. The MMPI scale 2 (Depression) as scored by 12 adult coeliac patients on three occasions: before starting the gluten-free diet (GFD), after one year on the GFD, and after three years on the diet + 6 months of pyridoxine (B6). Reprinted from: Reversal of psychopathology in adult coeliac disease with the aid of pyridoxine (vitamin B6), from Hallert, Åström & Walan, from Scand. J. Gastroenterol. 1983, 18, 299–304, by permission of Scandinavian University Press.

The synthesis of monoamines in the brain (Fig. 4) is carefully regulated by mechanisms, of which at least two are believed to be operating under environmental influence: the brain supply of dietary precursor substances, i.e. tryptophan and tyrosine, and the functional state of the coenzymes, respectively.

It is known that many untreated coeliacs have low levels of plasma tryptophan, for various reasons, but according to Wurtman (1979), it may rather be the ratio of plasma tryptophan to the sum of amino acids competing for entry to the brain that determines the availability of tryptophan to the brain and its role in regulating serotonin production in the brain. Adopting this approach, Hallert *et al.* (1982b) were able to show that most coeliacs show evidence of normal entry to the brain of the monoamine precursors tyrosine and tryptophan (Fig. 5). This is corroborated by the finding of normal CSF tryptophan concentrations in these people (Hallert & Sedvall, 1983). They concluded that reduced precursor supply to the brain fails to account for the generally reduced monoamine synthesis in the brain of coeliacs.

Vitamin B6 in the treatment of depression of adult coeliacs

As depicted in Fig. 4, a number of dietary factors are involved in the regulation of monoamine synthesis as coenzymes at different levels. Of these compounds, vitamin B6, generally malabsorbed by coeliac patients (Reiken & Zieglauer, 1978), may be the only one of physiological significance, prompting Hallert *et al.* (1983) to examine whether the depressive features of coeliac disease are amenable to treatment by dietary means.

They administered the MMPI to 12 adult patients while untreated and the patients were re-tested one year later when showing signs of remission in the small bowel mucosa. On this second occasion, only some minimal change in the MMPI profile was recorded, probably reflecting improvement on items associated with physical complaints, whereas more interestingly, the score on scale 2 (Depression) remained unchanged despite improvement in bowel functions and routine prescription of folate supplementation.

Considering the potential of vitamin B6, all in the series received pyridoxine 80 mg daily over a 6-month period and were retested by the MMPI carefully avoiding seasonal bias on the emotional items. As shown in Fig. 6, they showed substantial improvement in their MMPI profile, unlike coeliacs continuing on a gluten-free diet alone, with all abnormalites reverting to normal, including the signs of depression.

Conclusion

Depression should be regarded as a serious feature of coeliac disease which left unrecognized may complicate the clinical course and contribute to persistent feeling of ill-health despite adherence to a gluten-free diet. Evidence is presented to suggest that the depressed mood in adult coeliacs may in part be nutritional in origin and responsive to vitamin B6 supplementation.

It is recommended that adults seeking care for depression who give a history of unexplained nutritional deficiences should be routinely screened for coeliac diease.

References

Daynes, G. (1956): Bread and tears – naughtiness, depression and fits due to wheat sensitivity. *Proc. Royal Soc. Med.* **49**, 391–394.

Dohan, F.C. (1966): Cereals and schizophrenia: data and hypothesis. *Acta Psychiatr. Scand.*, **42**, 125–132.

Goldberg, D. (1970): A psychiatric study of patients with diseases of the small intestine. *Gut* **11**, 459–465.

Hallert, C. & Åström, J. (1982): Psychic disturbances in adult coeliac disease. II. Psychological findings. *Scand. J. Gastroenterol.* **17**, 21–24.

Hallert, C., Åström, J. & Sedvall, G. (1982a): Psychic disturbances in adult coeliac disease. III. Reduced central monoamine metabolism and signs of depression. *Scand. J. Gastroenterol.* **17**, 25–28.

Hallert, C. & Åström, J. (1983): Intellectual ability of adults after lifelong intestinal malabsorption due to coeliac disease. *J. Neurol. Neurosurg. Psych.* **46**, 87–89.

Hallert, C. & Derefeldt, T. (1982): Psychic disturbances in adult coeliac disease. I. Clinical observations. *Scand. J. Gastroenterol.* **17**, 17–19.

Hallert, C., Mårtensson, J. & Allgén, L-G. (1982b): Brain availability of monoamine precursors in adult coeliac disease. *Scand. J. Gastroenterol.* **17,** 87–89.

Hallert, C., Åström, J. & Walan A. (1983): Reversal of psychopathology in adult coeliac disease with aid of pyridoxine (vitamin B6). *Scand. J. Gastroenterol.* **18,** 299–304.

Hallert, C. & Sedvall, G. (1983): Improvement in central monoamine metabolism in adult coeliac patients starting a gluten-free diet. *Psychol. Med.* **13,** 267–271.

Hallert, C. (1987): Nutritional deficiencies and psychological problems in adult celiac disease. In: *Nutrition in gastrointestinal disease*, eds. L. Barbara, G. Bianchi Porro, R. Cheli & M. Lipkin, pp. 127–134. New York: Raven Press.

Hess Thaysen, H.E. (1932): *Non-tropical Sprue*. Munksgaard, Copenhagen.

Paulley, J.W. (1959): Emotion and personality in the etiology of steatorrhea. *Am. J. Dig. Dis.* **4,** 352–360.

Reinken, L. & Zieglauer, H. (1978): Vitamin B6 absorption in children with acute celiac disease and in control subjects. *J. Nutr.* **108,** 1562–1565.

Vaitl, D. & Stouthamer-Geisel, F. (1992): Die Zöliakie – eine psychosomatisch fehleingeschätzte Störung. *Münch. Med. Wschr.* **134,** 370–375.

Wurtman, R. J. (1979): When and why should nutritional state control neurotransmitter synthesis? *J. Neural. Transm.* Suppl. **15,** 69–79.

Epilepsy and other neurological disorders in coeliac disease, edited by G. Gobbi *et al.*
© 1997 John Libbey & Company Ltd, pp. 219–221.

Chapter 29

Autism and coeliac disease

Mary Coleman

Georgetown University School of Medicine Washington DC, USA

Introduction

Autism is a major behaviour syndrome of very young children that can be caused by many different injuries to the infant brain (Gillberg & Coleman, 1992). These children appear to lack interest in other people; they are alone, autistic. Their social/emotional behaviour is immature and often inappropriate. Often there is little or only fleeting eye contact. They have major problems in comprehension of human speech, gesture and mime so that social imitation usually is missing. Speech is delayed or, in up to half of the children, totally missing. Many children develop rituals, such as hand flapping, either when they are excited or apparently just to pass time. Another major disability in these children is their level of cognitive functioning; the majority appear mentally retarded. Even the approximately 15 per cent who do not test as retarded retain the immature and inappropriate social behaviour.

With regard to age of onset, the majority of clinicians and researchers agree that the behavioural disorder – or some major indication of abnormal development – must be apparent before 30–36 months of age (Gillberg & Coleman, 1992). Other investigators would require an earlier date of onset while a couple of clinicians accept cases that begin as late as 5 years (Wing & Gould, 1979) or even 7 years of age (Bohman *et al.*, 1983)

The discussion of the age of onset is relevant to the possibility of the symptoms of autism being caused by the intake of foods. Certainly the greatest number of young children that present at a clinician's office with autism have symptoms prior to 18 months of age. This gives a limited amount of time for the infant to have ingested gluten-containing foods. However it may be noted in passing that the protein in milk (casein), which is somewhat similar to gluten, has been ingested since birth.

In cases that present as late as 30 months or 36 months (or possibly even later), there may have been significant exposure to gluten-containing foods. A question of possible coeliac disease has been raised in some of these children with both autism and gastrointestinal symptoms. Is coeliac disease one of the subgroups underlying the symptoms of autism?

A review of the literature

Coeliac disease was first reported by Asperger in 1961 in patients with his syndrome (Asperger, 1961). Asperger's syndrome is considered as the upper cognitive end of the autistic spectrum disorders. Regarding autism as described by Kanner, the first report was in 1969 by Goodwin &

Goodwin. A 6-year-old boy with autism had an improvement in both his behavior and his physical condition when placed on treatment with a gluten-free diet (Goodwin & Goodwin 1969). A normal diet, ordered in error, produced a brief relapse with exacerbation of autistic symptoms; reinstitution of the gluten-free diet restored his previous course (Goodwin *et al.*, 1971). Since that publication, a number of other case reports have been published of children diagnosed by their pediatricians as having both autism and coeliac disease (Rimland, 1972; Reichelt *et al.*, 1986; Shattock, 1988; Braffet 1994).

Two research studies have been conducted trying to sort out the possibility of coeliac disease in some children with autism. The first was by John Walker-Smith in 1973. This study of 18 children with autism assessed the general physical health of the children, the frequency of gastrointestinal symptoms, sought evidence of malabsorption and determined the presence or absence of coeliac disease (Walker-Smith, 1973). In seven of the children, a history of gastrointestinal symptoms was identified. However, all children were well nourished and on physical examination there were no findings to suggest coeliac disease. Laboratory studies failed to demonstrate steatorrhea and/or the presence of dietary antibodies including antibodies to gliadin. For the three children on whom small intestinal biopsies were possible, the results were negative. In fact, laboratory studies were generally unimpressive except that for 11 of the children, α-1 globulin levels were noted to be low and in seven of the children the level of α-1 antitrypsin fell into the reported heterozygous range for α-1 antitrypsin deficiency.

The other research study performed by McCarthy & Coleman studied eight autistic children selected because of steatorrhea greater than 6 g of fat/day in the stool, documented hypocalciuria and a parental report of behavioral improvement on gluten-free diets. The patients ingested 20 grams of gluten powder per day added to their food for 4 weeks prior to the procedure. As in the Walker-Smith study, the struggle to obtain a jejunal biopsy on each child was a battle royal. Nevertheless, each child had a jejunal biopsy and all eight revealed entirely normal intestinal villus structure (McCarthy & Coleman, 1979).

Discussion

Detection of coeliac disease by jejunal biopsy in a child with autism has been most difficult in the past because these children are so tactilely defensive. They often shrink to a simple human touch, so the confinement involved in the invasive procedure of a jejunal biopsy is a frightening, overwhelming experience to them. Although case histories have been suggestive of coeliac disease, systematic research studies in groups of patients have not been able to verify coeliac disease in the patients receiving jejunal biopsy so far. However, current techniques of diagnosing coeliac disease by blood testing for antiendomysial antibodies, antigliadin antibodies and HLA allele testing should allow the question of coeliac disease in autism to be settled. With testing limited to blood samples, large number of patients could be examined and more definitive information obtained.

References

Asperger, H. (1961): Die psychopathologie des coeliakiekranken Kindes. *Ann. Paediatr.* **197**, 146–151.

Bohman, M., Bohman, I.L., Bjorck, P.O. & Sjoholm, E. (1983): Childhood psychosis in a northern Swedish county: some preliminary findings from an epidemiological survey. In: *Epidemlological approaches in child psychiatry* 11, eds. M.H. Schmidt & H. Remschmidt, pp. 164–173. Stuttgart: Thieme.

Braffet, C. (1994): No milk; no bread please. *Autism Society of Indiana Quarterly Update* **1**, 7–9.

Gillberg, C. & Coleman, M. (1992): *The Biology of the autistic syndromes* – 2nd edition. London: MacKeith Press.

Goodwin, M.S. & Goodwin, T.C. (1969): In a dark mirror. *Mental Hygiene* **53**, 550.

Goodwin, M.S., Cowen, M.A. & Goodwin, T.C. *et al.* (1971): Malabsorption and cerebral dysfunction: a multivariate and comparative study of autistic children. *J. Autism Child. Schizophr.* **1**, 48.

Mc Carthy, D.M. & Coleman, M. (1979): Response of intestinal mucosa to gluten challenge in autistic subjects. *Lancet* **ii,** 877–878.

Reichelt, K.L., Saelid, G., Lindback, T., Boler, J.B. *et al.* (1986): Childhood autism: a complex disorder. *Biol. Psych.* **21,** 1 279–1 290.

Rimland, B. (1972): *Progress in Research.* Proceedings of the Fourth Annual Meeting of the National Society for Autistic Children. Washington, DC.

Shattock, P. (1988): Autism: Possible clues to the underlying pathology. A parent's view. In: *Aspects of autism*, ed. L. Wing, pp. 11–18. London: Gaskell.

Walker-Smith, J. (1973): Gastrointestinal disease and autism – the results of a survey. Symposium on Autism. Abbott Laboratories, Sydney, Australia,

Wing, L. & Gould, J. (1979): Severe impairments of social interaction and associated abnormalities in children: epidemiology and classification. *J. Autism Dev. Dis.* **9,** 11–29.

Epilepsy and other neurological disorders in coeliac disease, edited by G. Gobbi *et al.*
© 1997 John Libbey & Company Ltd, pp. 223–226.

Chapter 30

Neurotransmitters in autistic children

Giovanni Lanzi, Carlo Alberto Zambrino, Umberto Balottin, Emma Bettaglio and Paolo Manfredi

Child Neuropsychiatry Division, C. Mondino Foundation, IRCCS, University of Pavia, 27100 Pavia, Italy

Introduction

The possible involvement of central monoaminergic systems in the pathogenesis of autism, or of some of its symptoms at least, is a frequently debated hypothesis in the literature, even though the results differ widely.

It has been hypothesized that a possible dysfunction of the catecholaminergic systems (dopamine (DA) and norepinephrine/plus epinephrine (NE/E)) may be involved in producing certain symptoms of autism, such as hyperactivity, stereotypes, self-stimulation, and abnormal reactions to environmental stimuli. On the one hand, this thesis would appear to be supported by clinical and pharmacological observations: dopaminergic receptor antagonists efficaciously control certain behavioural symptoms of autism, while some partial dopaminergic agonists, such as dextro- and levamphetamine lead to a worsening of the autistic symptomatology. On the other hand, experimental data exist in relation to the role played by the dopaminergic systems of the accumbens and striatum in modulating the capacity of the motor cortex and the limbic lobe to activate complex behaviours in response to various kinds of stimuli, and on the role played by these systems in motivational processes. Similarly, behavioural disorders such as hyperactivity, high levels of anxiety, and the regulation of arousal and attention are attributed to a dysfunction of the central norepinephrinergic systems. The results of neurochemical studies aimed at investigating levels of monoamines and of their metabolites in the biological fluids of autistic subjects are often at variance with one another.

We recall the valuable contribution made by Martineau *et al.* (1992, 1994). Investigations on a wide population revealed an increase in urinary homovanillic acid (HVA) and 3-methoxy tyramine (3-MT) levels, as opposed to a slight drop in DA levels, as well as high blood levels of DA and E. A further, and particularly interesting finding was the slower decrease of HVA over time in autistic subjects, indicating a possible maturational defect of the catecholaminergic system. No significant results emerged from the link with the genetic study of the locations containing the genes for enzymes involved in the biosynthesis of the monoamines, even though experimental evidence exists suggesting a linkage between the D4 and D2 receptors (one of which is situated on the short arm and the other on the long arm of chromosome 11) which could prove an interesting area for future research. Another major problem concerns the difficulties in defining sub-groups within the context of the whole syndrome of autism. This must be done by refining the clinical criteria so as to be able to identify homogeneous groups of subjects who are often characterized by polymorphic behaviour.

As long ago as 1973, Coleman hypothesized the involvement of serotoninergic systems on the basis of the modulatory effects these circuits have on psychophysiologic processes often affected in autism: an alteration of these pathways at brainstem level occurring in an early period of CNS maturation could lead to peripheral and central sensory defects, as well as dysfunction of the midbrain locomotion region and of electrophysiological sleep patterns. The detection of hyperserotonaemia is not entirely specific to autism as it has also been found in sub-groups of mentally retarded subjects. The fact that the mechanisms underlying the hyperserotonaemia are also difficult to explain is probably due to changes in the number and characteristics of the platelets or to the presence of serotoninergic antireceptor-antibodies in the blood and in the CSF. More recent studies have revealed an imbalance, in platelets, between the serotonin and some amino acids, which supports the theory that the platelets represent a peripheral model of what is occurring on a neuronal level, even though there is no experimental evidence to suggest that high blood serotonin levels correspond to high serotonin levels in the CNS.

In short, the different findings emerging from studies of neurotransmission do not allow conclusions to be reached regarding a specific pathogenetic role of the system in autism; likewise, due to the absence of specificity, researchers are not drawn to consider neurotransmitters as possible diagnostic markers. Furthermore, the peripheral alterations found may constitute, rather than primary dysfunctions, the epiphenomena of alterations of other systems which interact with and regulate the activity of the monoaminergic circuits. The capacity of peptides to influence the release of dopamine through interaction with D2 receptors is, indeed, well known, and there is also the model proposed by Chamberlain & Herman (1990), in which hyperserotonaemia would appear to represent a response to increased melatonin secretion.

It is, finally, important to bear in mind the strictly technical difficulties linked to biological fluid sampling methods and the capacity of extrinsic factors, such as stress (which affects NE and E in particular) and diet, to affect the levels of monoamines and monoamine metabolites.

Materials and methods

In the present study we examined a group of 30 children (24 male and six female) referred to the Division of Child Neuropsychiatry of Pavia between 1990 and 1994 and who were diagnosed as having Pervasive Development Disorder (PDD) according to DSM-III-R criteria. Of these patients, 24 could be classified as belonging to the autistic disorder sub-type, while the other six fell into the category of pervasive developmental disorder – Not Otherwise Specified (NOS). Diagnosis was made on the basis of an anamnestic investigation, a neuropsychiatric examination, compilation of the BSE scale, determination of the development quotient and on a series of laboratory and instrumental tests (karyotype, EEG, evoked potentials, CT-scan or MRI).

On the basis of the data thus obtained, six of the 24 patients diagnosed as having the autistic disorder presented with a psychosis with signs of CNS damage. The control group was made up of 35 children (28 male and seven female) recruited from the Paediatric Surgery Division of the 'Policlinico S. Matteo', in Pavia, where they had undergone surgery for the following disorders: inguinal hernia, epithelioma, cysts, phimosis, varicocele, hypospadias or cystoscopy. No child had a history of neuropsychiatric disorders and all had a normal neurological examination. The patients and the control group were age- and sex-matched (Table 1).

Table 1. Patients studied

	PDD[*]	Controls	Total
Males	24	28	52
Females	6	7	13
Total patients	30	35	65

[*]Diagnosis performed using DSM-III-R criteria 24 pts subgroup 'autistic disorder' 6 pts sub-group 'pervasive developmental disorder nos'.

After two days in which a tryptophan-free and tyrosine-free diet was followed, a blood sample was taken from each child, while under anaesthetic. Narcosis was induced in order to perform surgery, or, in the case of the autistic children, using halothane in order to carry out neuroradiological investigations. A sample of approximately 5 ml of blood was taken through venopuncture without using a turniquet, by drops. The first urine passed on the day of surgical operation, or of the neuroradiological examination, was also collected at approximately the same time in each case (8.00 a.m.–9.00 a.m.).

We were able to measure the blood plasma level of NE and E in 45 subjects, and of DA in 43 subjects, as well as the urinary levels of NE, E, DA in 46, of vanilmandelic acid (VMA) in 38, of 5-HT in 28, of HVA in 34, and of 5-hydroxy indolacetic acid (5-HIAA) in 36 subjects. High Performance Liquid Chromatography (HPLC) was used to separate and determine the concentration of all the neurotransmitters and their metabolites. Statistical analysis was performed using one way ANOVA.

Results

While the results relating to blood NE and E levels were statistically diverse, no significant differences emerged between the group of autistic children and the group of non-autistic children. The same was true of the results of blood DA level analysis.

Processing of data relating to urinary values revealed no statistically significant differences between the two groups as far as NE, E, DA, VMA, 5-HT, and 5-HIAA were concerned, unlike HVA which was found to be significantly higher in autistic than in normal subjects ($P < 0.05$) (Table 2).

No statistically significant difference emerged between male and female subjects in relation to any of the substances being studied.

Conclusions

Even taking into account, as described in the introduction, the limits imposed by the considerable variation in results reported in the literature, the hypothesis of a possible correlation between an alteration in catecholamines and dopamine and certain behavioural disorders present in autism seems tenable. This thesis appears to be supported by experimental evidence (Salamone, 1992) and has been strengthened by the results of studies carried out by Martineau & Herault who found higher levels of HVA, 3-MT, and 5-HT and lover levels of DA in the urine of autistic children, in comparison with the results obtained from a control group made up of normal and mentally retarded children.

In our study, we paid particular attention to the methods used to collect the biological fluids, striving to achieve a condition in which the influence of extrinsic factors (i.e. diet and stress brought on by the blood sampling procedure) was reduced to a minimum.

Table 2. Results of determinations

	Patients (No.)	F	P
Plasma			
NE	45	3.76	0.06
E	45	0.31	0.58
DA	43	0.45	0.50
Urine			
NE	46	0.06	0.79
E	46	1.77	0.19
DA	46	3.19	0.08
VMA	38	0.22	0.64
5HT	28	1.2	0.28
HVA	34	4.89	*0.034
5HIAA	36	0.42	0.83

$^{*}P < 0.05$; one way analysis of variance between PDD patients and controls.

The results we obtained, while based on a small population (which nevertheless reflects the low incidence of autism and the complexity of the methods used), did allow us to draw several conclusions which can be compared with information contained in the literature.

Our results indicate that, as far as blood plasma levels of DA, NE, and E are concerned, there are no significant differences between autistic subjects and controls. These results are, for example, in conflict with the findings of other studies. The results we obtained in relation to urinary levels of NE, E and VMA also failed to demonstrate significant differences, indicating normal noradrenergic and adrenergic functioning. Our findings appear to be in agreement with the results of recent data reported by Martineau *et al.* (1992) who cast doubt over the pathogenetic role of noradrenergic systems. The only altered urinary value found was that of HVA was significantly increased in autistic subjects. Many investigators have reported similar results. Furthermore, the increase of HVA in the urine correlates with the values found in the CSF. While realizing that urinary HVA values cannot be taken as a direct indication of central dopamine metabolism, the studies of Maas *et al.* (1979) demonstrate that at least 33 per cent of HVA in the urine derives from the catabolism of dopamine in the CNS.

It has been hypothesized, on the basis of results obtained, that the increase of urinary HVA reflects a disorder of dopamine metabolism. Given that, in our sample, there was no alteration of the levels of dopamine in the blood plasma or in the urine, one can suppose that the increase of HVA is to be ascribed to an accelerated turnover of the dopamine itself.

References

Chamberlain, R.S. & Herman, B.H. (1990): A novel biochemical model linking dysfunction in brain melatonin, proopiomelanocortin peptides, and serotonin in autism. *Biol. Psych.* **28**, 773–793.

Maas, J.W., Hattox, S.E., Martin, D.M. & Landis, D.H. (1979): A direct method for determining dopamine synthesis and output of dopamine metabolites from brain in awake animals. *J. Neurochem.* **32**, 839–843.

Martineau, J., Barthélémy, C., Jouve, J., Muh, J.P. & Lelord, G. (1992): Monoamines (serotonin and catecholamines) and their derivatives in infantile autism: age-related changes and drug effects. *Dev. Med. Child Neurol.* **34**, 593–603.

Martineau, J., Hérault, J., Petit, E., Guérin, P., Hameury, L., Perrot, A., Mallet, J., Sauvage, D., Lelord, G. & Muh, J.P. (1994): Catecholaminergic metabolism and autism. *Dev. Med. Child Neurol.* **36**, 688–697.

Salamone, J.D. (1992): Complex motor and sensimotor functions of striatal and accumbens dopamine: involvement in instrumental behaviour processes. *Psychopharmacology* **107**, 160–174.

Epilepsy and other neurological disorders in coeliac disease, edited by G. Gobbi *et al.*
© 1997 John Libbey & Company Ltd, pp. 227–237.

Chapter 31

The possible role of peptides derived from food proteins in diseases of the nervous system

W.H. Reichelt and K.L. Reichelt

Institute of Paediatric Research, University of Oslo, Rikshospitalet, N-0027 Oslo, Norway

Introduction

A role of gluten and possibly casein in schizophrenia was proposed by Dohan (1980). He found a correlation of gluten consumed to the incidence of schizophrenia of 0.96. In cultures where gluten was sparse or absent so was schizophrenia (Dohan *et al.*, 1984).

Dietary acculturation led to a sharp increase in the incidence of schizophrenia (Lorenz, 1977). We found a large increase in peptides in the urines of schizophrenics (Reichelt *et al.*, 1981; Reichelt *et al.*, 1985). These peptides showed bioactivities relevant to schizophrenia (Hole *et al.*, 1979; Reichelt *et al.*, 1985). The opioid activity found in urine is also found in serum as part of a general hyperpeptidaemia (Drysdale *et al.*, 1982; Idet *et al.*, 1982; Lindstrøm *et al.*, 1986). Increased opioid receptor binding peptides were also found in the CSF (Lindstrøm *et al.*, 1986).

Hyperpeptiduria has also been found in autism (Reichelt *et al.*, 1981; Reichelt *et al.*, 1986; Israngkun *et al.*, 1986; Shattock *et al.*, 1990). Bovine casomorphin 1–8 was found in both urine and dialysis fluid of DSM III diagnosed autistic patients (Reichelt *et al.*, 1991). Increased serum opioid activity has likewise been found in this syndrome (Gillberg *et al.*, 1985; LeBoyer *et al.*, 1994). In general hyperpeptidaemia is accompanied by hyperpeptiduria.

Methods

Demonstration of hyperpeptiduria

To counteract possible diurnal variations in peptide secretion, 24 h complete urines were used. Creatinine was measured twice for each urine by the Department of Clinical Chemistry, Rikshospitalet, Oslo. 0.5 ml urine was applied to Costar spin-X centrifugal cellulose acetate filters 0.22 μm and centrifuged at $2315 \times g$ for 10 min at 4 °C.

Urine equivalent to 250 nmol of creatinine was then applied to C18 reverse phase columns on the HPLC system Gold for analysis. The fractionation is based on Guillemin's method to separate peptides from amino acids and salts (Bøhlen, 1980). The column was Vydac C18 250×4.6 mm with

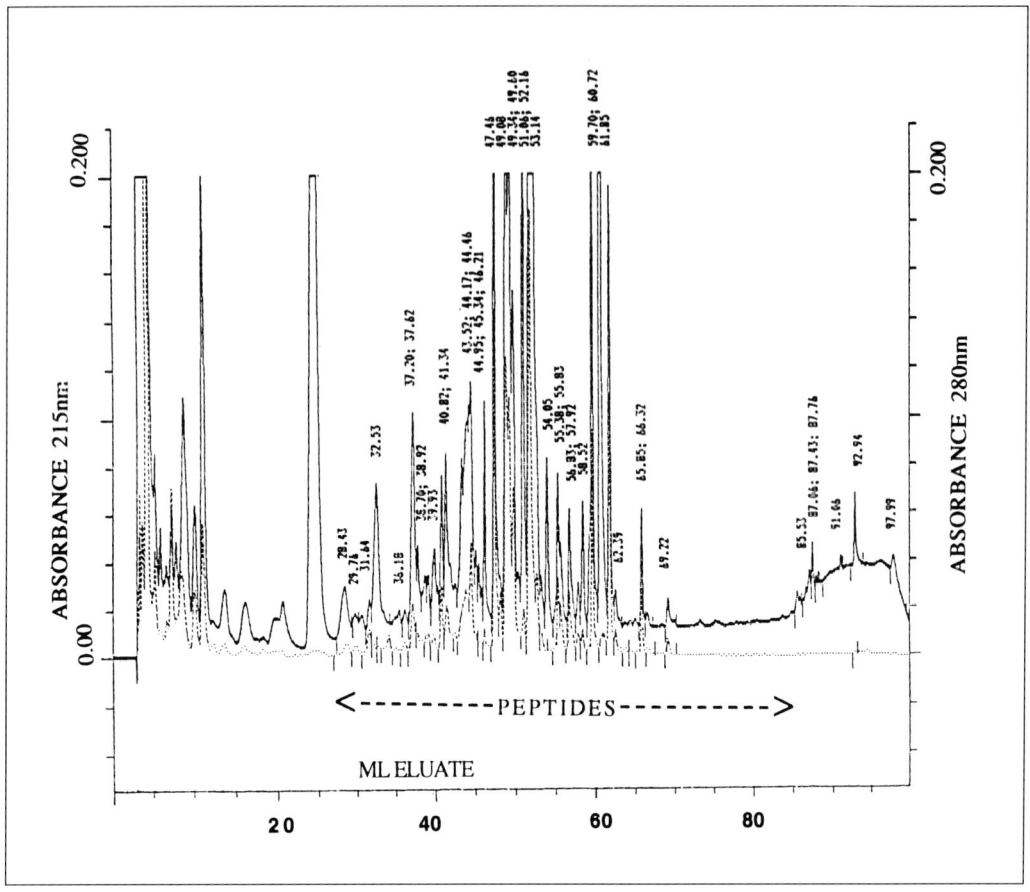

Fig. 1. The peptide pattern of a 27 year old male schizophrenic (DSM III 295.9) after HPLC analysis (see text).

the same pre-column and a column heater (BioRad Code no 1250 426) kept at 35 °C (Shattock *et al.*, 1990). Flow rate was 1 ml/min with detection at 215 and 280 nm and sensitivity 0.2. Buffer A was 0.1 per cent trifluoroacetic acid (TFA) and buffer B: 0.1 per cent TFA in 94.9 per cent acetonitrile and 5 per cent water. The elution was performed with: Step 1, using buffer A with 1 per cent B for 15 min to wash out most amino acids, urea, and salts; Step 2, a gradient from 1–40 per cent B was run for 60 min linearly (15–75 min); Step 3, from 75–80 min with B from 40–60 per cent; Step 4, from 80–89 min isocratically at 60 per cent buffer B; Step 5, return to 1 per cent B from 89–94 min; Step 6, re-equilibration at 1 per cent B from 89–115 min.

An automatic sample applicator (Waters 717 Autosampler from Millipore) was used, and the computer integrated the area under the curve over the peptide area on the column at 215 and 280 nm. The thymol peak eluting at 85 ml was subtracted.

Purification of peptides

(1) Batch isolation of peptides was done on complete 24 h urines filtered through Whatman 3MM filter after adjusting the pH to 3 and then passed through a C-18 preparative column of dimension 2.6 × 50 cm at pH 3. After washing with 100 ml 10 mM TFA the peptides were eluted in 80 per cent methanol/water by volume and rotavapored (Bøhlen *et al.*, 1980).

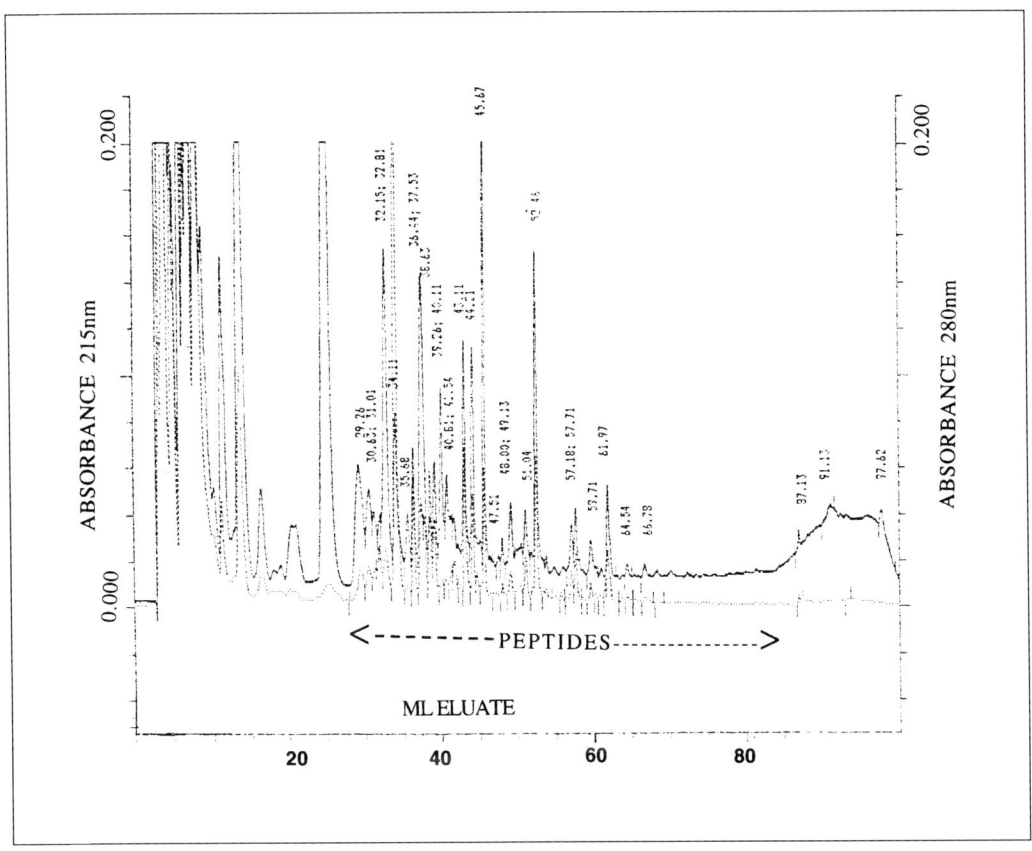

Fig. 2. Another HPLC pattern of a schizophrenic (DSM III 295.9) male of the same age as in Fig. 1

(2) First fractionation was a gel filtration on P 2 gels 1.6 × 90 cm in 0.5 M acetic acid with elution rate 24 ml/h and fractions of 4 ml. The application volume was 10 ml 0.5 M acetic acid at room temperature (acetic acid is a protease inhibitor). Off-line ninhydrin colour was developed after alkaline hydrolysis (Reichelt *et al.*, 1981).

(3) The stepwise further purification has been extensively described for tissue specific mitosis inhibitors (Reichelt *et al.*, 1990). Briefly the following purification sequence was used: (a) Cation exchange to separate protonable from nonprotonable mainly N-substituted peptides, (b) Anion exchange to separate out the strong anions, (c) Gel filtration on Fractogel MG 2000 from Merck in 1 M acetic and 20 mM HCl to determine size, (d) C-18 reverse phase gradient chromatography in TFA with n-propanol, methanol and acetonitrile gradients, (e) C-8 reverse phase in TFA acetonitrile gradients.

Characterization of the peptides

The complete amino acid composition was ensured by 6 M HCl hydrolysis in closed vials, evaporation of acid over KOH and P_2O_5 in vacuum and amino acid analysis on the α-plus (Pharmacia) amino acid analyser using ninhydrin technique. Sequencing was performed by manual Edman degradation (Reichelt *et al.*, 1990).

Cochromatography with synthetic peptide in two different buffer systems and gradients on the HPLC was also taken as proof of identity.

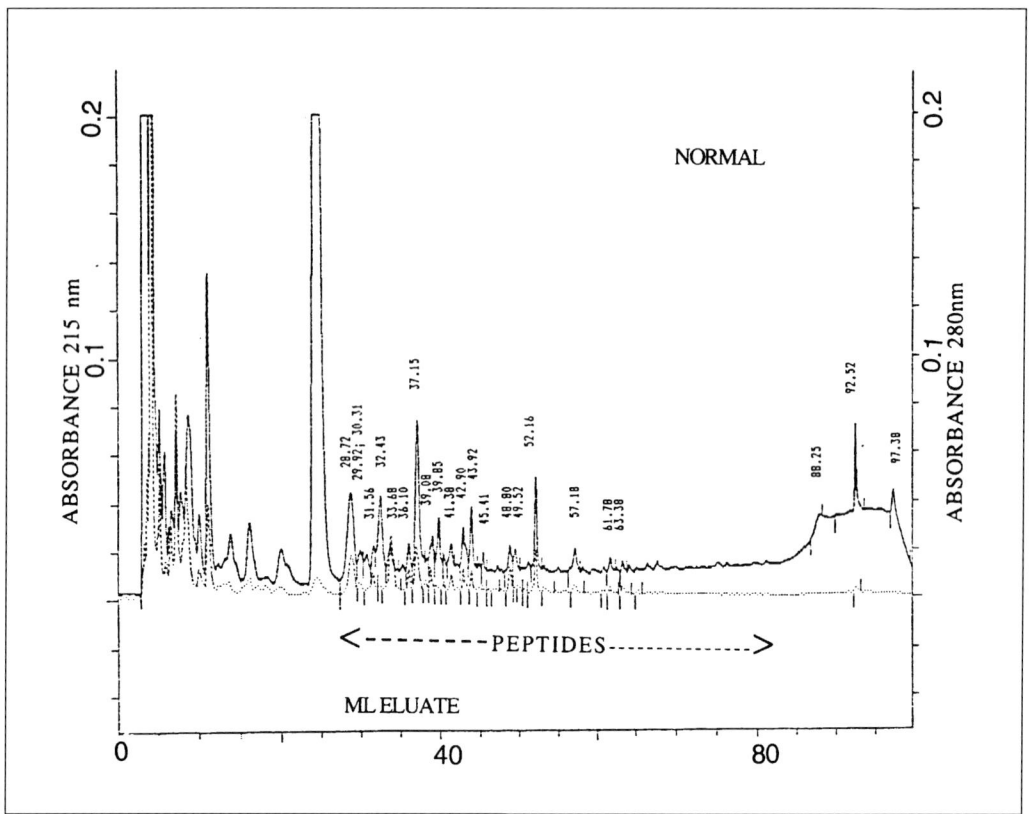

Fig. 3. A normal male of the same age as in Figs. 1 and 2.

Receptor assay of opioids

The opioid receptor displacement by material from the different peaks after C-18 peptide separation was carried out as described (Terenius & Wahlstrom, 1975) using synaptic plasma membranes. The first assays were performed by Terenius who is thanked for this help.

Immunoassay

Demonstration of binding to antibodies against bovine casomorphin was first carried out by Prof. Teschemacher in Giessen (Koch et al., 1988). He generously donated antibody and also gave training sessions to several members of our group. Cross reactivity with human casomorphins was below 0.01 per cent (Koch et al., 1988).

Table 1. Quantitative data on schizophrenia and autism

	N	Schizophrenics	N	Autistic individuals
Average	10	1250	57	913.5
95% C.I.		401–2099		704.5–1122.5

All patients were without medication. The autistic patients were obtained from seven countries. The schizophrenic patients are all Norwegian collected over three years. DSM III diagnoses were used. C.I. is Confidence Interval.

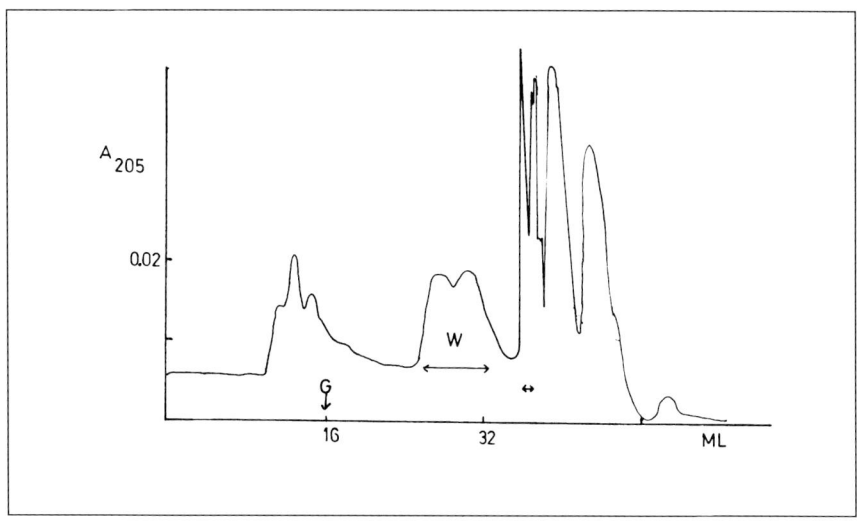

Fig. 4. C-18 semipreparative HPLC as described of the batch isolated peptide fraction from one patient. Gradient starts at point G. (10 nM TFA 0.1 per cent n-propanol to 10 nM TFA and 60 per cent n-propanol over 30 min). Opioid receptor and immune reactive peaks are marked with arrows. Absorbance read at 205 nm.

Results

Schizophrenia

Figure 1 and 2 compared to Fig. 3 illustrates: (a) The large increase in peptides in the peptide region compared to normal; (b) the enormous heterogeneity of the patterns obtained in spite of the same diagnosis and rating (not shown). This confirms our earlier data with a different method (Reichelt *et al.*, 1985). In Table 1 the quantitative data are given for untreated schizophrenics and autistic patients. Figure 4 shows the gradient HPLC on semipreparative C-18 reverse phase columns (Partisil M9 10/25 ODS) of the peptide peaks from the batch isolation of peptides (Bøhlen *et al.*, 1980). The peaks that showed opioid receptor binding and effects are marked (Hole *et al.*, 1979). In Table 2 the effect of diluting the test sample in the receptor assay for opioids is shown. This is quite common for peptides.

Table 2. Opioid receptor binding

Purification step	Specific activity undiluted	Specific activity diluted (×10)
6	0.78	4.27
7	1.8	64.0

Specific activity = displacement of labelled dehydromorphine measured in picomoles opioid / micromole hydrolysis released amino acids in the peptide peak.

Immunoreactivity against antibodies to bovine casomorphin 1–8 is shown in Table 3 for fractions obtained from peak W in Fig. 4. The rechromatography can be seen in Fig. 5. This immunoreactivity could be diluted away and severely reduced by preincubation with cold casomorphin.

After several chromatographic steps the peptide E showed cochromatography with synthetic bovine casomorphin 1–8 (Fig. 6). In addition to immunoreactivity it showed receptor binding to opioid

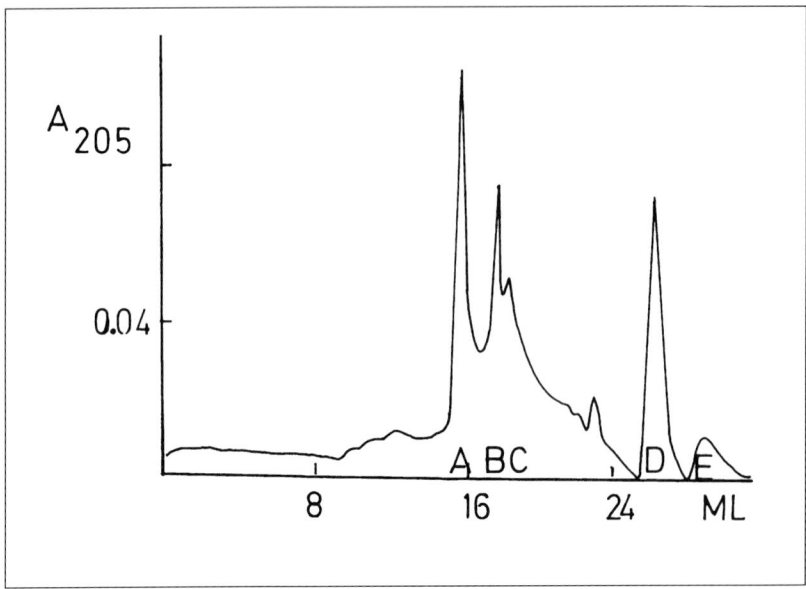

Fig. 5. Gradient elution on semipreparative HPLC of the peak W seen in Fig. 4. Gradient from 6–60 per cent n-propanol over 30 min and Abs. at 205 nm. Immuno- and receptor-active peaks labelled A–E.

receptors. Amino acid analysis showed the same composition as the synthetic compound obtained from Novabiochem, UK. (Y 0.9; P 3.8 ; F 1; G 1; I 0.95). Y-P-F was the N-terminal sequence. The other immunoreactive peaks were not analysed.

Autism

The quantitative aspects can be seen in Table 1. Fig. 6 demonstrates the gel filtration of a peak containing an opioid binding peptide from autistic subjects (Reichelt *et al.*, 1991). The immunore-activity can be seen in Table 3. This peptide showed cochromatography with synthetic bovine casomorphin 1–8 (Reichelt *et al.*, 1991) and the correct amino acid composition after hydrolysis.

Table 3. Bovine casomorphin 1–8 immunoreactive peaks in schizophrenics (Fig. 4)

Peak	Dilution	F-Moles/peak
A	1:100	2001
	1:10000	17
B	1:100	1330
C	1:100	1526
D	1:100	1280
E	1:100	1040
Controls	1:1	0.17
	1:100	0.05
Autistic subjects (Fig. 7)	1:1	1162.04
	1:10	187.07

1/30 of each peak was tested. For autistic subjects only the peak where immunoreactivity was found is shown. Only a few examples of dilution included.

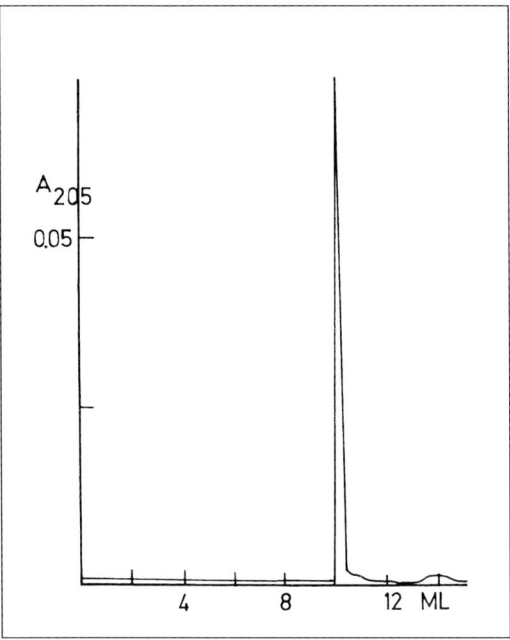

Fig. 6. Cochromatography of purified peak E and
equal amounts of bovine casomorphin 1–8 on HPLC
with 9–60 per cent n-propanol gradient as described.

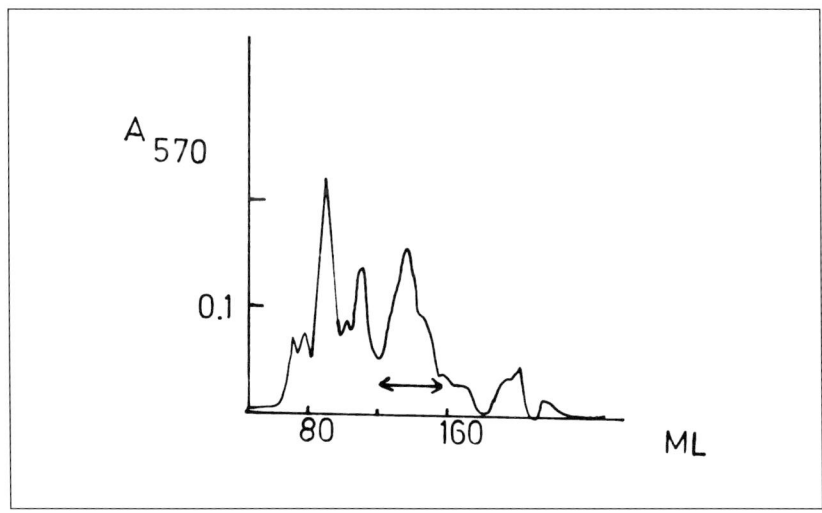

Fig. 7. Fractogel MG 2000 gel filtration of the opioid active fraction from autistic
children run in 1 M acetic acid 20 mM HCl. Off-line ninhydrin on a 5 per cent aliquot
after alkaline hydrolysis read at 570 nm.

Previously published findings

We found increases over the upper normal limit in IgA antibodies against gliadin, β-lactoglobulin
and casein (Reichelt & Landmark, 1995). The stable epitopes were the exorphin sequences. The

behavioural effects induced by partly purified peptide fractions from schizophrenics clearly demonstrated opioid activity (Hole *et al.*, 1979; Drysdale *et al.*, 1982; Idet *et al.*, 1982). Also GABA and Glutamate releasing peptides were found (Reichelt *et al.*, 1981, 1985).

Discussion

The presence of casomorphin antibody reactive peptides in autistic subjects (Reichelt *et al.*, 1991) and in schizophrenics described support Dohans (1980) hypothesis. Dohan thought that schizophrenia was caused by gluten and possibly casein overloading a genetic defect in their breakdown. Schizophrenia is rare in cultures without gluten (Dohan *et al.*, 1984; Lorenz, 1990). This view is reinforced by the immune data (Sugarman, 1982). Serum from schizophrenics inhibits the chemotactic movement of lymphocytes (Ashkenazi *et al.*, 1979), and the gliadin peptide that causes this effect contains the gliadinomorphin sequence (Graf *et al.*, 1987) and binds to opiate receptors. In male schizophrenics statistically significant increase in IgA antibodies against gliadin, β-lactoglobulin and casein were found (Reichelt & Landmark, 1995). In autistic subjects an increased frequency of higher than normal IgA values against casein and gliadin and gluten was also found (Reichelt *et al.*, 1991)

The following can be deduced from the autistic and schizophrenic patterns (Figs. 1 and 2) : (a) There is an enormous quantitative spread in the level of peptides secreted in the urine (Reichelt *et al.*, 1985). (b) There are large variations in the pattern of peptide peaks obtained. This must mean that autism and schizophrenia are syndromes caused by different enzymes in different patients ending up with peptides of different chain lengths but the same bioactivity. The multiple peaks immunoreactive to casomorphin (bovine) 1–8 antibodies (Fig. 4; Table 3) confirm that opioids of different chain lengths are present as with most bioactive peptides. (c)The opioid activity found shows bell-shaped dose–response curves (increasing receptor binding on dilution). This may explain the contradictory data on opioids in schizophrenia and autism. Very concentrated opioid solutions do not bind to the receptor (Table 2). It is therefore not suprising that the effect of naloxone and naltrexone varies too (Gunne *et al.*, 1977; Janowsky *et al.*, 1977). Peptides very frequently show bell-shaped dose–response curves (Moon, 1988; Pincus *et al.*, 1990; Reichelt *et al.*, 1990). It is therefore quite important to test out isolated peptide factors over a very wide range of concentrations.

Because peptiduria is caused by defects in peptide metabolism (Abassi *et al.*, 1992; Watanabe *et al.*, 1993), it is reasonable to expect that different peptidases in different families may be the cause. Because peptidases are regulated by and often inhibited by hormones (Griffiths, 1975) like testosterone and cortisone, the relationship of disease to puberty and stress in schizophrenia is understandable.

Increased uptake from the gut of exorphins can furthermore be caused by peptidase defects or inhibition (Mahe *et al.*, 1989) but also by transulphation defects (Waring & Ngung, 1993). Uptake of intact and bioactive proteins (Husby *et al.*, 1986; Jakobsson *et al.*, 1986) may be the cause of multiple sequences of opioids present in one molecule of protein (Fukudome & Yoshikawa, 1991), causing large peptide increases if poorly broken down. Uptake of intact proteins is confirmed by finding intact and dietary proteins in mother's milk (Stuart *et al.*, 1984; Troncone *et al.*, 1987). Botulinum toxin is a case of such small but tragic uptake.

Sufficiently prolonged treatment with gluten-free diet has therapeutic effects in at least some schizophrenics (Dohan & Grasberger, 1973; Singh & Kay, 1976; Reichelt *et al.*, 1990b), and in autistic individuals (Reichelt *et al.*, 1991; Knivsberg *et al.*, 1995). Because the improvements progressed over four years in autistic children (Knivsberg *et al.*, 1995) this probably excludes placebo effects. Those that quit the diet showed regression (Reichelt *et al.*, 1991, Knivsberg *et al.*, 1995).

Finally the long term effect of neuroleptics supports a peptidase involvement, because they induce peptidases (Traficante & Turnbull, 1982; Koning *et al.*, 1990; Konkoy *et al.*, 1993). Neuroleptics cause decrease in peptides found in the urine (Reichelt & Teigland-Gjerstad, 1995). Furthermore Lithium in therapeutic doses directly stimulates pyroglutamyl aminopeptidase (DeGandaries *et al.*, 1994). Because about half the peptides in the urine are pyroglupeptides (Reichelt *et al.*, 1985), this direct enzyme activation may also be important.

Consequences of opioid accumulation

Opioid increases would inhibit the normal maturation of the CNS. (Zagon & McLaughlin, 1987). Inhibited maturation is found in schizophrenia (Crow, 1994; Roberts & Bruton, 1990). Opioids may well also interfere with the important maturational pruning process (Feinberg, 1982/83) and thus cause progressive dysfunction. Casomorphins are known to be the mediators of the dramatic state of post-partum psychosis (Lindstrøm *et al.*, 1984).

Opioids furthermore inhibit socialization and inhibit separation distress calls in chicken, puppies and kittens (Panksepp *et al.*, 1978; Panksepp, 1978). It is therefore possible that opioids may be the mediators of the social isolation typical of both schizophrenia and autism. This has been proposed (Panksepp *et al.*, 1980).

Conclusions

Immune data and the high levels of peptides indicate a dietary source of hyperpeptidaemia and hyperpeptiduria. The effect of diet and the isolation of probable exorphins from the urine and dialysis fluid all support Dohan's hypothesis (Dohan, 1980).

Because opioids can enter the cerebrospinal fluid, the inhibition of maturation of the CNS may be ascribed to such compounds. Opioids furthermore may cause social isolation of significance to both autism and schizophrenia.

References

Abassi, Z., Golomb, E. & Keiser, H.R. (1992): Neutral endo-peptidase inhibition increases urinary excretion and plasma level of Endothelin. *Metabolism* **41**, 683–685.

Ashkenazi, A., Krasilowsky, D., Levin ,S., Idar, D., Kalian, M., Hyala, O., Ginat, Y. & Halperin, B. (1979): Immunological reaction of psychotic patients for fractions of gluten. *Am. J. Psychiat.* **136**, 1306–1309.

Bhlen, P., Castillo, F., Ling, R. & Guillemin, R. (1980): An efficient procedure for the separation of peptides from amino acids and salts. *Int. J. Peptide Prot. Res.* **16**, 306–310.

Crow, T.J. (1994): Aetiology of schizophrenia. *Curr. Opin. Psychiat.* **7**, 39–42.

DeGandaries, J.M., Irazusta, J., Gil, J., Fernandez, D. & Casis, L. (1994): Effects of acute Lithium administration on pyroglutamyl-aminopeptidase I activity in several brain areas of the rat. *Arzneimittel. Forsch.*. **44**, 119–121.

Dohan, F.C. & Grasberger, J.C. (1973): Relapsed schizophrenics: Earlier discharge from hospital after a cereal-free, milk-free diet. *Am. J. Psychiat.* **130**, 685–688.

Dohan, F.C. (1980): Hypothesis: genes and neuroactive peptides from food as cause of schizophrenia. In: *Neuronal peptides and neuronal communication*, eds. E. Costa & M. Trabucchi. pp. 535–548. New York: Raven Press.

Dohan, F.C., Harper, E.H., Clark, M.H., Rodrigue, R.B. & Zigas, V. (1984): Is schizophrenia rare if grain is rare? *J. Biol. Psychiat.* **19**, 385–399.

Drysdale, A., Deacon, R., Lewis, P., Olly, S., Electricwala, A. & Sherwood, R. (1982): A peptide containing fraction of plasma of schizophrenic patients which binds to opiate receptors and induces hyperactivity in rats. *Neuroscience.*, **7**, 1567–1574.

Feinberg, I. (1982/83): Schizophrenia: caused by a fault in programmed synaptic elimination during adolescence? *J. Psychiat. Res.* **17**, 319–334.

Fukudome, S.-I. & Yoshikawa, M. (1991): Opioid peptides derived from wheat gluten: their isolation and characterization. *FEBS Lett.* **296**, 107–111.

Gardner, M.L.G. (1994): Absorption of intact proteins and peptides. In: *Physiology of the gastrointestinal tract,* 3rd edn., ed. L.R. Johnson, pp. 1795–1820. New York: Raven Press.

Gardner, M.L.G. (1995): A review of current knowledge of gastrointestinal absorption of intact proteins including medicinal preparations of proteolytic enzymes In: *Absorption of orally administered enzymes.* eds. M.L.G. Gardner & K.-J. Steffens. pp. 1–8. Berlin: Springer Verlag.

Gillberg, C., Terenius, L. & Lønnerholm, G. (1985): Endorphin activity in childhood psychosis. *Arch. Gen. Psychiat.* **42,** 780–783.

Graf, L., Horvath, K., Walcz, E., Berzetei, I. & Burnier, J. (1987): Effect of two synthetic α-gliadin peptides on lymphocytes in celiac disease: identification of a novel class of opioid receptors. *Neuropeptides* **9,** 113–122.

Griffiths, E.C. (1975): Peptidase inactivation of hypothalamic releasing hormones. *Hormone. Res.* **7,** 179–191.

Gunne, L.-M., Lindstrøm L.H. & Terenius L. (1977): Naloxone-induced reversal of schizophrenic hallucinations. *J. Neural Transmiss.* **40,** 13–19.

Hole, K., Bergslien, A.A., Jørgensen, H., Berge, O.-G., Reichelt K.L. & Trygstad, O.E. (1979): A peptide containing fraction in the urine of schizophrenia patients which stimulates opiate receptors and inhibits dopamine uptake. *Neuroscience* **4,** 1139–1147.

Husby, S., Jensenius, J.C. & Svehag, S.E. (1985): Passage of undegraded dietary antigen into the blood of healthy adults. *Scand. J. Immunol.* **22,** 83–92.

Idet, M., Grof, J., Menyhart, J. & Pajor, A. (1982): Elevated opioid activity in sera of chronic schizophrenics. *Acta. Physiol. Hung.* **60,** 121–127.

Israngkun, P., Newman, H.A., Patel, S.T., Duruibe, V.A. & Abou-Issa, H. (1986): Potential biochemical markers for infantile autism. *Neurochem. Pathol.* **5,** 51–70.

Jakobsson, I., Lindberg, G.T., Lothe, L., Nilsson, I. & Benediktsson, B. (1986): Human β-lactoglobulin as a marker of macromolecular absorption. *Gut* **27,** 1029–1034.

Janowsky, D.S., Segal, D.S., Abrams, A., Bloom, F. & Guillemin, R. (1977): Negative naloxone effects in schizophrenic patients. *Psychopharmacology* **53,** 295–297.

Knivsberg, A-M., Reichelt, K.L., Nødland, M. & Høien, T. (1995): Autistic syndromes and diet. A four year follow-up study of 15 subjects. *Scand. J. Educat. Res.* **39,** 223–236.

Koch, G., Wiedemann, E, Drebes E., Zimmermann, W., Link, G. & Teschemacher, H. (1988): Human β-casomoprhin-8 immunoreactive material in the plasma of women during pregnancy and after delivery. *Regul. Pept.* **20,** 107–117.

Koning, P.N., Colling-Berglund, A. & Davis, T.P. (1990): Chronic haloperidol and chlorpromazine treatment alters *in vitro* β-endorphin metabolism in rat brain. *Eur. J. Pharmacol.* **97,** 15–28.

Konkoy, C.S., Oakes, M.G. & Davis, T.P. (1993): Chronic treatment with neuroleptics alters neutral endopeptidase 24.11 activity in rat brain regions. *Peptides* **14,** 1017–1020.

Lindstrøm, L.H., Besev, G., Gunne, L.-M. & Terenius, L. (1986): CSF levels of receptor-active endorphins in schizophrenic patients: correlation with symptomatology and monoamine metabolites. *Psychiat. Res.* **19,** 93–100.

Lindstrøm, L.H., Nyberg, F., Terenius, L., Bauer, K., Besev, G., Gunne, L.M., Lyrenås, S., Willdeck-Lund, G.J. & Lundberg, B. (1984): CSF and plasma beta-casomorphin-like opioid peptides in post-partum psychosis. *Am. J. Psychiat.* **141,** 1059–1066.

LeBoyer, M., Bouard, M.P., Recasens, C., Philippe, A., Guillod-Bataille, M., Bondeux, D., Tabuteau, F, Fugas, M., Panksepp, J. & Launoy, J.-M. (1994): Difference between plasma N- and C-terminally directed β-endorphin immunoreactivity in infantile autism. *Am. J. Psychiat.* **151,** 1797–1801.

Lorenz, K. (1990): Cereals and schizophrenia. *Adv. Cereal Science and Technol.* **X,** 435–469.

Mahe, S., Tome, D., Dumontier, A.M. & Deseux, J.J. (1989): Absorption of intact morphiceptin by diisopropyl-fluorophosphate-treated rabbit ileum. *Peptides* **10,** 45–52.

Moon, T.D. (1988): The effct of opiates upon prostatic carcinoma cell growth. *Biochem. Biophys. Res. Comm.* **153,** 722–727.

Panksepp, J. (1978): A neurochemical theory of autism. *Trends Neurosci.* **2,** 174–177.

Panksepp, J., Normansell, L., Sively, S., Rossi, J. & Zolovick, A.J. (1978): Casomorphins reduce separation distress in chickens. *Peptides* **5,** 829–831.

Panksepp, J., Herman, B.H., Vilberg, T., Bishop, P. & DeEskinazi, F.G. (1980): Endogenous opioids and social behavior. *Neurosci. Biobehav. Rev.* **4,** 473–487.

Pincus, D.W., DiCicco-Bloom, E.M. & Black, I.B. (1990): Vasoactive intestinal peptide regulates mitosis, differentiation and survival of cultured sympathetic neuroblasts. *Nature* **343,** 564–567.

Reichelt, K.L., Hole, K., Hamberger, A., Sælid, G., Edminson, P.D., Bræstrup, C., Lingjærde, O., Ledaal, P. & Ørbeck, H. (1981): Biologically active peptide-containing fractions in schizo-phrenia and childhood autism. *Adv. Biochem. Psycho-pharmacol.* **28,** 627–643.

Reichelt, K.L., Edminson, P.D. & Toft, G. (1985): Urinary peptides in schizophrenia and depression. *Stress Med.* **1,** 169–181.

Reichelt, K.L., Sælid, G., Lindback, T. & Bøler, J.B. (1986): Childhood autism: a complex disorder. *Biol. Psychiat.* **21,** 1279–1290.

Reichelt, K.L., Paulsen, J.-E., & Elgjo, K. (1990a): Isolation of a growth and mitosis inhibitory peptide from mouse liver. *Virchows Arch. B.* **59,** 137–142.

Reichelt, K.L., Sagedal, E., Landmark, J., Tschumi-Sandvik, B., Eggen, O. & Scott H. (1990b): The effect of gluten free diet on glycoprotein attached urinary peptide excretion and behaviour in schizophrenia. *J. Ortomol. Med.* **5,** 223–239.

Reichelt, K.L, Knivsberg, A.-M., Lind, G. & Ndland, M. (1991): Probable etiology and possible treatment of childhood autism. *Brain Dysfunct.* **4,** 308–319.

Reichelt, K.L. & Landmark, J. (1995): Specific IgA antibody increases in schizophrenia. *J. Biol. Psychiat.* **37,** 410–413.

Reichelt, K.L. & Teigland-Gjerstad, B. (1995): Decreased urinary peptide excretion in schizophrenic patients after neuroleptic treatment. *Psychiat. Res.* **58,** 171-176.

Roberts, G.W. & Bruton, C.J. (1990): Annotation. Notes from the graveyard: neuropathology and schizophrenia. *Neuropathol. Appl. Neurobiol.* **16,** 3–16.

Shattock, P., Kennedy, A., Rowell F. & Berney, T. (1990): Role of neuropeptides in autism and their relationships with classical neurotransmitteres. *Brain Dysfunct.* **3,** 328–345.

Singh, M.M. & Kay, S.R. (1976): Wheat gluten as a pathogenic factor in schizophrenia. *Science* **191,** 401–402.

Stuart, C.A., Twiselton, R., Nicholas, M. & Hide, D.W. (1984): Passage of cows milk protein in breast milk. *Clin. Allergy* **14,** 533–535.

Sugarman, A.A, Southern, D.L. & Curran, J.F.U. (1982): A study of antibody levels in alcoholic, depressive and schizophrenic patients. *Ann. Allergy* **48,** 166–171.

Terenius, L. & Wahlstrom, A. (1975): Morphine-like ligand for opiate receptor in human CSF. *Life Sci.* **16,** 1759–1764.

Traficante, L.S. & Turnbull, B. (1982): Neuropeptide degrading enzyme(s) in plasma and brain: Effect of *in vivo* neuroleptic administration. *Pharm. Res. Comm.* **14,** 341–348.

Troncone, R., Scarcella, A., Donatiello, A., Cannataro, P., Tarabuso, A. & Auricchio, S. (1987): Passage of gliadin into human breast milk. *Acta Paed. Scand.* **76,** 453–456.

Waring, R.M. & Ngong, J.M. (1993): Sulphate metabolism in allergy-induced autism: relevance to the disease etiology. In: *Biological perspectives in autism,* ed. The autism Research Unit, Sunderland Univ. pp. 25–33. UK: Sunderland Univ.

Watanabe, Y., Kojima-Komatsu, T., Iwaki-Egura, S. & Fujimoto, Y. (1990): Increased excretion of proline-containing peptides in dipeptidyl peptidase IV deficient rats. *Res. Comm. Clin. Pathol. Pharmacol.* **81,** 323–330.

Zagon, I.S. & McLaughlin, P.J. (1987): Endogenous opioid systems regulate cell proliferation in the developing rat brain. *Brain Res.* **412,** 68–72.

Epilepsy and other neurological disorders in coeliac disease, edited by G. Gobbi *et al.*
© 1997 John Libbey & Company Ltd, pp. 239–243.

Chapter 32

Coeliac disease and schizophrenia

Chiara Marson, Rossella Michetti and Vittorio Volterra

Institute of Psychiatry, University of Bologna, Italy

One of the first reports on the relationship between schizophrenia and cereal consumption was made by Lauretta Bender (1953), who noted that schizophrenic children were often affected by coeliac disease (CD). She recorded 20 cases among over 2000 schizophrenic children.

Graff & Handford (1961) published data reporting that, over a period of one year, four out of 37 hospitalized male adult schizophrenics had suffered from CD in infancy.

Dohan *et al.* (1969), starting from the assumption that both CD and schizophrenia were characterized by the existence of a polygenic susceptibility, advanced the hypothesis that the presence of one of these diseases could favour the development of the other.

The hypothesis that CD could constitute a research model for the aetiology of schizophrenia was based on the results of studies by gastroenterologists and psychiatrists from Philadelphia, New York and Baltimore, carried out on schizophrenic patients affected by CD (Table 1) and from case histories of CD in infancy in schizophrenic patients. This combination of the two diseases seemed to derive from genetic factors. Mc Guffin (1979), supporting this hypothesis, suggested an association between nuclear forms of schizophrenia and haplotype HLA-B8, and that the distribution of the titers of anti-gluten antibodies was related to the presence or absence of haplotype HLA-B8 in groups of schizophrenic patients.

Since 1960, the principal external agents responsible for CD in patients with a susceptible genotype have been identified in some types of cereal. From this starting point, Dohan (1983) hypothesised that these cereals could be a possible cause of schizophrenia, again on the basis of a genetic predisposition.

Dohan listed a series of results to support this hypothesis:

1. The discovery by Zioudrou *et al.* (1979) of peptides similar to endorphins (exorphins) in the enzymatic digestion of various cereals;

2. The discovery by Mycroft *et al.* (1982) that a fraction of the gliadin in wheat gluten contains the Pro-Leu-Gly sequence of the Migration Inhibition Factor (MIF), a neural peptide that increases dopaminergic activity;

3. The abnormal behaviour of rats following intracerebral injection of gluten peptides (Dohan *et al.*, 1969);

4. The demonstration by Ashkenazi *et al.* (1979) that the lymphocytes of 50 per cent of schizophrenic patients react to some gluten peptides in a similar way to the lymphocytes of CD patients;

5. A statistically significant correlation between the pattern of amino acids in the blood serum of schizophrenic and CD patients (Manowitz, 1978);

6. A strong link between the first hospitalization for schizophrenia and cereal consumption (Dohan, 1980);

7. An inverse relationship between schizophrenia and a gluten-free diet (Dohan *et al.* 1982);

8. A significant percentage of relapses or improvements in the symptoms of schizophrenia according to the presence or absence of gluten in the diet (Dohan & Grasberger, 1973; Singh & Kay, 1976).

As far as the relationship between gluten enteropathy and schizophrenia is concerned, Dohan *et al.* (1982), starting from the observation that during the Second World War food reserves were scarce and cereal consumption fell, studied the number of hospitalized schizophrenic patients in psychiatric units in Canada, Europe and the United States. He found a decrease in numbers, even though hospitalization for other forms of psychosis increased over the same period. In the same paper, Dohan pointed out the low prevalence of schizophrenia reported in previous studies made on populations in remote regions of the world (Papua New Guinea, Malaysia, the Solomon Islands, Yap, Micronesia), where the consumption of wheat was unusual or practically non-existent. The prevalence of schizophrenia reached European levels only when their diet was transformed as a result of westernization.

Double-blind research based on the introduction of a cereal and milk-free diet in schizophrenic patients on admission to hospital, demonstrated a considerable and rapid improvement in their condition within one week (Dohan *et al.*, 1969). When gluten was secretly added to this diet no improvement was noted. The same result did not occur with non-schizophrenic patients. These results support the hypothesis that cereal consumption can prove to be a pathogenic factor in subjects with a genetic predisposition to schizophrenia.

In 1973, Baker advanced the hypothesis that a diet of gluten and milk could contain an inhibiting factor for phenothiazines, thus competing with their pharmacological action. Dohan (1973) responded that there was no relationship between the positive results obtained in schizophrenic patients and treatment with phenothiazines. Singh & Kay (1976) had arrived at the same conclusions from a study of schizophrenic patients treated with neuroleptics and a cereal-free and milk-free diet. In these patients, symptoms had been aggravated by the addition of gluten to the diet in a double-blind trial, which was not affected by a change in the dosage of neuroleptics.

Research has been carried out to verify the role of antibodies to gliadin, discovered both in some schizophrenic patients and in some patients affected by coeliac disease. In fact, Dohan & Grasberger (1973) revealed that although the frequency of gliadin Abs in hospitalized schizophrenic patients increased considerably, it also increased in non-schizophrenic hospitalized psychiatric patients. The frequency (20.3 per cent) in all psychiatric patients (presumably the most highly stressed group of patients in the study) was six times greater than in the control sample (3.15 per cent, $P < 0.005$), and it was even more significant when compared with the group of hospitalized non- psychiatric patients, probably less stressed (13.7 per cent, $P < 0.005$). According to Dohan, this would presuppose the development of anti-gliadin antibodies provoked by prolonged stress factors (hospitalization, psychiatric illness). The increased number of antibodies to gliadin would determine a change in the function of the intestinal mucosa with an additional increase in the absorption of gliadin peptides, some of which could be harmful to patients genetically susceptible to schizophrenia or to coeliac disease. Abnormal intestinal absorption has been identified as an aetiologic factor in schizophrenia. In fact, Wood *et al.* (1987), showed in a study of a group of schizophrenic patients, that a remarkable percentage of these had abnormal intestinal permeability that could not be attributed to gastrointestinal illness. The alteration of the intestinal functions resulted in an increased absorption of molecules similar to endorphins, responsible for behavioural disorders.

Table 1. Association: coeliac disease (CD) and schizophrenia (SC). Observations made before 1965 in or near Philadelphia

By gastroenterologists/internists	Coeliacs with SC[*]	Total
J. Cerda. C. Dohan	1	12
M. Sleisenger	3	32
T. Bayless	1	36
G. Barbero	1	35

By psychiatrists/psychologists	Schizophrenics with CD[**]	Total
H. Graff	4	37
C. Pfeiffer	4	300
L. Bender	4	100
B. Fish	3	300
M. Gittleman	4	96

[*]All had diagnosis of CD confirmed by gut biopsy. [**]By history (adults) or concurrent symptoms (children); CD symptoms occurred before general use of intestinal biopsy.
From Dohan F.C. *et al.* (1969): Relapsed schizophrenics: more rapid improvement on a milk and cereal free diet. *Br. J. Psychiat.* **115,** 595–596.

Manowitz (1978) reported a positive relationship between amino acid levels in the plasma of both treated and untreated schizophrenics and CD patients. Simpson (1982), reconsidering the same data, criticized the results as not being statistically reliable. He also highlighted some limitations of this research: the limited size of the sample of patients with coeliac disease; the lack of information about the diagnostic criteria for schizophrenia; the absence of data on the co-variance of individual levels of amino acids.

The production of a factor inhibiting the migration of leucocytes from the lymphocytes in the peripheral blood (MIF) of schizophrenics and other psychotics in response to an antigenic stimulus with fractions of gluten was also studied and compared with that of normal subjects and adolescents with coeliac disease (Ashkenazi *et al.,* 1979). Two groups of psychotics were identified, of which one group responded with the production of MIF, as did the CD patients, and the other responded in the same way as the normal control group. On the basis of these results, the authors hypothesized that gluten could interfere with the biological processes of the brain. In fact, Klee *et al.* (1978) reported the presence in gluten of polypeptides, similar to endorphins and the antagonists of opioids. After intestinal absorption, these polypeptides could be responsible for the production of psychotic symptoms in susceptible individuals.

In 1981, Rudin (1981) considered eight different epidemiological studies and reported on the high statistical coincidence between schizophrenia, coeliac disease and herpetiform dermatitis, suggesting the existence of a gluten-dependent syndrome. According to Rudin, the data supporting this hypothesis are:

(1) the presence of the B8 and Dw3 genes of chromosome 6, both in coeliac disease and in herpetiform dermatitis and the positive correlation between Ag HLA and Cw4 in paranoid schizophrenia;

(2) the presence of a gluten-dependent enteropathy in the majority of subjects affected by this syndrome, even though some patients may be asymptomatic;

(3) the fact that the incidence of gluten-dependent syndrome in the population could decrease with a drastic reduction in cereal consumption;

(4) the fact that a gluten-free diet could be more effective than phenothiazines for the treatment of schizophrenia.

(5) the fact that the use of haemodialysis to remove gluten-derived peptides would induce an improvement in schizophrenic symptomatology. In 1982, Hallert (1982)questioned the hypothesis, mainly sustained by Dohan, of coeliac disease as a model for schizophrenia. He underlined the need for clear clinical evidence of an increase in the development of schizophrenia in CD patients. In fact, Stevens *et al.* (1977) discovered no sufferers from CD among 380 schizophrenic patients. In a retrospective psychiatric study of adult CD patients in an area of Sweden where CD sufferers represent 1: 1000, Hallert (1982) found that psychiatric illness in this population was due to problems of depression. No cases of schizophrenia were recorded. Other criticisms of this model came from Singh (1976), who pointed out the impossibility of evaluating the pathogenetic effect of gluten, since the continuing presence of this factor could be a sign of chronic illness and there was therefore no reason to presume that its increase would aggravate the symptoms. Singh criticized the method of conducting research, since he should have started with the exclusion of gluten from the diet and then assessed the changes after adding it once again. Another criticism concerned the inclusion in the study of patients with chronic symptomatology, including symptoms that presumably were therefore irreversible.

Considering these reports in the literature, we decided to undertake a prospective study in order to establish whether there is any real association between CD and schizophrenia. In order to do this we looked for Ab-anti-gliadin (AGA) and anti-endomysium (EMA) antibodies in the blood serum of 101 schizophrenic patients (65 male and 36 female).

The IgG and IgG class of Ab-anti-gliadin were methodically calculated using ELISA. The results were expressed in Arbitrary ELISA Units, choosing as a cut-off the result obtained from the average plus two standard deviations of the values obtained from a large number of healthy volunteers.

The IgA class Ab-anti-endomysium were calculated in indirect immunofluorescence using commercial sections of monkey oesophagus as a substratum. The specific pattern of antibodies was identified from the presence of fluorescence in the endomysium around the myofibrils of smooth oesophageal muscle tissue. Blood serum samples with values equal to or greater than 1:5 were considered positive.

According to our results, AGA and EMA have a sensitivity and specificity respectively of 92 and 90 per cent for AGA and of 99 and 100 per cent for EMA, previously checked in a wide range of patients.

None of the tested blood serums were positive, so that our research, although still preliminary, does not confirm the association between the two conditions.

References

Ashkenazi, A. *et al.* (1979): Immunologic reaction of psyhcotic patients to fractions of gluten. *Am. J. Psychiat.* **136**, 1306–1309.

Baker, A.G. (1973): Effects of nutrition on schizophrenia. *Am. J. Psych.* **130**, 1400.

Bender, L. (1953): Childhood schizophrenia. *Psych. Quart.* **27**, 3–81

Dohan, F.C. *et al.* (1969): Relapsed schizophrenics: more rapid improvement on a milk and cereal free diet. *Br. J. Psychiat.* **115**, 595–596.

Dohan, F.C. (1983): More on celiac disease as model for schizophrenia. *Biol. Psych.* **18**, (5) 561–564.

Dohan, F.C. (1980): Hypothesis: genes and neuroactive peptides from food as cause of schizophrenia. In: *Neural peptides and neuronal communication*, eds. E. Costa & M. Trabucchi, pp. 535–548. New York: Raven Press.

Dohan, F.C. (1973): Relapsed schizophrenics: earlier discharge from hospital after cereal-free, milk-free diet. *Am. J. Psychiat.* **130,** 685–688.

Dohan, F.C. *et al.* (1982): Is schizophrenia rare if grain is rare? *Biol. Psych.* **19,** 385–399.

Dohan, F.C. (1973): Dohan Replies. *Am. J. Psych.* **130,** 1400–1401.

Graff, H. & Hanford, A. (1961): Celiac syndrome in the case history of five schizophrenics. *Psych. Quart.* **35,** 306–313.

Hallert, C. (1982): Psychiatric illness, gluten, and celiac disease. *Biol. Psych.* **17,** 959–961.

Klee, W.A. *et al.* (1978): Exorphins, peptides with opioid activity isolated from wheat gluten, and their possible role in the etiology of schizophrenia. In: *Endorphins in mental health research*, ed. E. Usdin. New York: Macmillan

Manowitz, P. (1978): Amino acid levels in schizophrenia: a clue to etiology. *Biol. Psychiat.* **13,** 489–491.

Mc Guffin, P. (1979): Is schizophrenia an HLA-associated disease? *Psychol. Med.* **9,** 721–728

Mycroft , F.J. *et al.* (1982): MIF-like sequences in milk and wheat proteins. *N. Engl. J. Med.* **307,** 895.

Rudin, D. (1981): The choroid plexus and system disease in mental illness. III.The exogenous peptide hypothesis of mental illness. *Biol.Psych.* **16, (5)**, 489–512.

Simpson, J. (1982): Amino acid levels in schizophrenia and celiac disease: another look. *Biol. Psych.* **17,** 1353–1357.

Singh, M. & Kay, S.R. (1976): Wheat gluten as a pathogenic factor in schizophrenia. *Science* **191,** 401–402.

Singh, M. (1976): Letter to the editor. *Am. J. Psych.* **136,** 733.

Stevens F M. *et al.* (1977): Schizophrenia and celiac disease, the nature of relationship. *Psychol. Med.* **7,** 259–263.

Wood *et al.* (1987): Abnormal intestinal permeability. *Br. J. Psych.* **150,** 853–856.

Zioudrou, C. *et al.* (1979): Opioid peptides derived from food proteins. The exorphins. *J. Biol. Chem.* **254,** 2446–2449.

Epilepsy and other neurological disorders in coeliac disease, edited by G. Gobbi *et al.*
© 1997 John Libbey & Company Ltd, pp. 245–248.

Chapter 33

Coeliac disease and schizophrenia: hypotheses of a possible association

G. Bersani*, F. De Palma*, G. Sandri** and M. Mazzetti di Pietralata**

*Department of Psychiatry, University of Rome 'La Sapienza', Viale dell'Università 30, 00185 Rome, Italy;
**I Medical Division, S. Eugenio Hospital, Piazzale dell'Umanesimo 10, 00144 Rome, Italy*

Introduction

The hypothesis of a possible association between coeliac disease and schizophrenic spectrum disorders has been formulated on the basis of evidence accumulated during the last 30 years (Graff & Hanford, 1961; Dohan, 1976; Singh & Kay, 1976; McGuffin *et al.*, 1981; Pfeiffer, 1984).

The clinical observation of increased incidence of coeliac disease in schizophrenic populations with respect to expected incidence of coeliac disease in the general population (about 3 ‰) prompted several investigators to test such observation; however, studies carried out on this subject yielded inconsistent results (Dohan, 1983). Furthermore, family studies also showed an increased incidence of coeliac disease or schizophrenia in various members of the same family (Table 1) (Perisic *et al.*, 1990).

Data that apparently support such a hypothesis of clinical association between the two diseases refer to the finding of an abnormal intestinal permeability (Wood, 1987; Lambert, 1989) and of altered amino acid plasma levels in subgroups of schizophrenic patients (Manowitz, 1983; Waziri, 1985; Macciardi *et al.*, 1990); further, it has been reported that, in some samples of psychiatric patients, diets appear to affect psychotic symptomatology (Dohan, 1979; Storms, 1982). Moreover, several studies reported increased levels of food antibodies in subgroups of psychotic patients (McGuffin *et al.*, 1981).

Table 1. Family studies on the association between schizophrenia and coeliac disease

Authors	No. families investigated	No. families with both diseases
Goodwin (1969)	65	5
Dohan (1970)	–	6
Goldberg (1970)	46	12
Peresic *et al.*, (1990)	554	3

On the other hand, the possibility of brain neurochemical abnormalities in untreated coeliac patients (Hallert *et al.*, 1982) and the occasional presence of neurological and neuromorphological correlates (Cooke, 1978, Finelli *et al.*, 1980, Kinney *et al.*, 1982; Ventura *et al.*, 1991) provides a theoretical bridge with the biological bases underlying schizophrenic disorders (Pancheri *et al.*, 1992).

In the present study we investigated whether antibodies to gluten are present in a sample of psychiatric patients. Our objective was to seek possible relations between antibody to gluten, a food-substance involved in the pathogenesis of coeliac disease, and schizophrenia. We studied a sample of psychiatric patients composed of schizophrenics and patients affected by mood disorders, the latter serving as a control, in order to avoid non-specific findings.

Methods

Eighty-eight adult, male, hospitalized psychiatric patients were included in the study. The sample was split into two subgroups on the basis of diagnosis (DSM-III-R). The first subgroup included 56 patients with schizophrenic spectrum disorders (schizophrenia catatonic, disorganized, paranoid, undifferentiated and residual type, delusional disorder and schizophreniform disorder). The second group used as a control, was composed of 32 patients with affective disorders (bipolar disorder, manic and depressed, major depression, dysthymia). Patients with somatic disease, both acute and chronic, were excluded.

Blood samples were drawn from each patient independently of disease stage and evaluated by ELISA for anti-gliadin IgA and IgG antibodies. Coeliac disease family history was investigated.

Results and discussion

Positivity for anti-gluten IgG antibodies was found in two patients with a diagnosis of schizophrenia (3.6 per cent). One of them was found to have coeliac disease at jejunal biopsy, that was carried out due to the presence of clear intestinal symptoms. Familial coeliac disease was found in another two patients, both schizophrenic and negative for anti-gluten antibodies, one of whom had a sibling who was both schizophrenic and coeliac.

These results are in agreement with the reported trend of increased association of the two disorders, and do not exclude the hypothesis of a relationship between schizophrenia and coeliac disease. The main hypotheses related to this association concerns the role of genetic factors and neurotransmitter–biochemical factors (De Palma & Bersani, 1995).

It was suggested that the two disorders share particular major histocompatibility loci (HLA) inherited through *linkage disequilibrium* (Ivanyi *et al.*, 1978; McGuffin & Sturt, 1986; Metzer *et al.*, 1988). The immunoregolatory role of these genetic sequences matches the finding of an abnormal immune reactivity in subgroups of schizophrenic patients. Table 2 shows the results of some of these studies.

The neurotransmitter–biochemical hypotheses suggest an abnormal regulation of peptidergic systems consequent to intestinal malabsorption with the possibility of early alterations of neurodevelopment, followed by abnormal neuromodulatory activity. The exorphin properties of gliadin have been implicated in the determination of psychotic symptoms (Dohan, 1976; Singh & Kay, 1976; Huebner *et al.*, 1984). The physiopathological effects of gluten exorphin derivatives may include an alterated modulation of central neurotransmission processes. Figure 1 shows the possible role of gliadin in the opioid-imbalance hypothesis of schizophrenia. Alternatively, increased levels of plasma amino acids, such as glutamate, glycine and serine, could alter their modulation of N-methyl-D-aspartate (NMDA) receptors (Manowitz, 1983; Waziri, 1985; Macciardi *et al.*, 1990; Baruah 1991).

These results should be considered as preliminary, due to small sample size. Further studies are needed to clarify the relationships between schizophrenia and coeliac disease.

Table 2. Studies on the association between schizophrenia and HLA loci

Authors	No. schizophrenics	HLA Ag
Cazzullo *et al.* (1974)	144	A10, A11, B27
Eberhard *et al.* (1975)	47	A9, A11, B5
Smeraldi *et al.* (1976)	"	Bw15, Bw35
McGuffin *et al.* (1978)	80	A29, Bw27, Bw17
Ivanyi *et al.* (1978)	200	A28, B18, Bw16, Cw4
Crowe *et al.* (1979)	45	non-significant
Luchins *et al.* (1980)	92	A2
Asaka *et al.* (1981)	136	A9, A10
Frangos *et al.* (1982)	56	Bw35
Rudduck *et al.* (1984)	116	A1–3, A11, B8, B17
Miyanaga *et al.* (1984)	77	A1, B12, Dr1, Dr8
Chadda *et al.* (1986)	16	Non-significant
Bersani *et al.* (1989)	91	Non-significant
Alexander (1990)	55	Non-significant
Campion *et al.* (1992)	33 (families)	Non-significant
Sasaki *et al.* (1994)	47	DR1

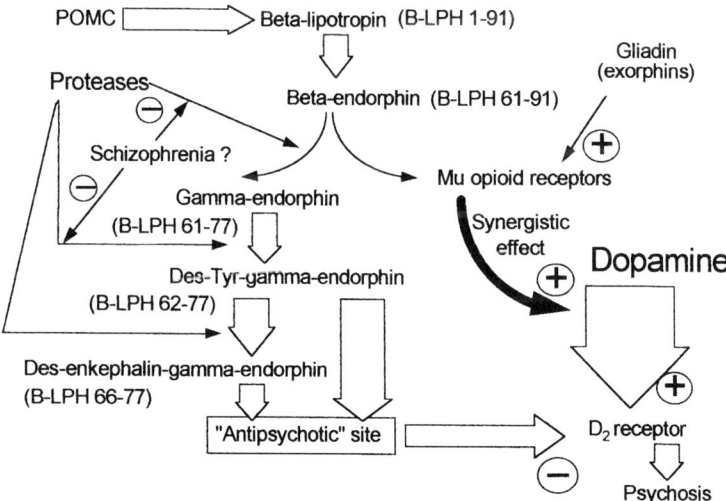

Fig. 1. Possible influence of exorphins in the opioid-imbalance hypothesis of schizophrenia.

References

American Psychiatric Association: *Diagnostic and Statistical Manual of Mental Disorders,* 3rd ed. revised (DSM-III-R). American Psychiatric Press, Washington, 1987.

Baruah, S., Waziri, R., Hegwood, T.S. & Mallis, L.M. (1991): Plasma serine in schizophrenics and controls measured by gas chromatography-mass spectrometry. *Psych. Res.* **37,** 261–270.

Cooke, W.T. (1978): The neurological manifestations of malabsorption. *Postgrad. Med. J.* **54,** 760–762.

De Palma, F. & Bersani, G. (1995): Malattia celiaca e schizofrenia: ipotesi di una possibile associazione. *Rivista di Psichiatria,*

Dohan, F.C. (1979): Celiac-type diets in schizophrenia. *Am. J. Psych.* **136,** 732–733.

Dohan, F.C. (1983): More on celiac disease as a model for schizophrenia. *Biol. Psych.* **18,** 561–564.

Dohan, F.C. (1976): The possible pathogenic effect of cereal grains in schizophrenia. *Acta Neurol.* **31,** 195–205.

Finelli, P.F., McEntee, W.J., Ambler, M. & Kestenbaum, D. (1980): Adult coeliac disease presenting as cerebellar syndrome. *Neurology* **30,** 245–249.

Graff, H. & Hanford, A. (1961): Celiac syndrome in the case history of five schizophrenics. *Psychiat. Quart.* **35,** 306–313.

Hallert, C., Åström, J. & Sedvall, G. (1982): Psychic disturbances in adult coeliac disease III. Reduced central monoamine metabolism and signs of depression. *Scand. J. Gastroenterol.* **17,** 25–28.

Huebner, F.R., Lieberman, K.W., Rubino, R.P. & Wall, J.S. (1984): Demonstration of high opioid-like activity in isolated peptides from wheat gluten hydrolysates. *Peptides* **5,** 1139–1147.

Ivanyi, D., Zemek, P. & Ivanyi, P. (1978): HLA antigens as possible markers of heterogeneity in schizophrenia. *J. Immunogenet.* **5,** 165–172.

Kinney, H.C., Burger, P.C., Hurwitz, B.J., Humans, J.C. & Grant, J.P. (1982): Degeneration of the central nervous system associated with coeliac disease. *J. Neurol. Sci.* **53,** 9–22.

Lambert, M.T., Bjarnason, I., Connelly, J., Crow *et al.* (1989). Small intestine permeability in schizophrenia. *Br. J. Psychiatry* **155,** 619–622.

Macciardi, F., Lucca, A., Catalano, M., Marino, C., Zanardi, R. & Smeraldi, E. (1990): Amino acid patterns in schizophrenia: some new findings. *Psychiatry Res.* **32,** 63–70.

Manowitz, P. (1983): Schizophrenia, amino acids, and celiac disease. *Biol. Psychi.* **18,** 942–943.

McGuffin, P. & Sturt, E. (1986): Genetic markers in schizophrenia. *Human Heredity* **36,** 65–88.

McGuffin P., Gardiner P. & Swinburne, L.M. (1981): Schizophrenia. celiac disease, and antibodies to food. *Biol. Psych.* **16,** 281–285.

Metzer, W.S., Newton, J.E.O., Steele, R., Claybrook, M., McMillan, D.E. & Hays, S. (1988): HLA antigens and haplotypes in schizophrenia. Neuropsychiat. *Neuropsychol. Behav. Neurol.* **1,** 39–46.

Pancheri, P., Macciardi, F., Bersani, G. & Martini, G. (1992): Etiopatogenesi (Disturbi schizofrenici). In: *Trattato Italiano di Psichiatria,* eds. P.Pancheri. & G.B. Cassano, vol. 2, pp. 1337–1434. Milano: Masson.

Perisic, V.N., Lopicic, Z. & Kokai, G. (1990): Celiac disease and schizophrenia: family occurrence. *J. Pediatr. Gastroenterol. Nutr.* **11,** 279.

Pfeiffer, C.C. (1984): Schizophrenia and wheat gluten enteropathy. *Biol. Psych.* **19,** 279–280.

Singh, M.M. & Kay, S.R. (1976): Wheat gluten as a pathogenic factor in schizophrenia. *Science* **191,** 401–402.

Storms, L.H., Clopton, J.M. & Wright, C. (1982): Effects of gluten on schizophrenics. *Arch. Gen. Psych.* **39,** 323–327.

Ventura, A., Bouquet, F., Sartorelli, C., Barbi, E., Torre, G. & Tommasini G. (1991): Coeliac disease, folic acid deficiency and epilepsy with cerebral calcifications. *Acta Paediatr. Scand.* **80,** 559–562.

Waziri, R. (1985): Serine metabolism, psychosis, and coeliac disease. *Biol. Psych.* **20,** 120–122.

Wood, N.C. (1987): Abnormal intestinal permeability: an aetiological factor in chronic psychiatric disorders? *Br. J. Psychiatry* **150,** 853–856.

Part IX
Neurological disorders in coeliac disease

Epilepsy and other neurological disorders in coeliac disease, edited by G. Gobbi *et al.*
© 1997 John Libbey & Company Ltd, pp. 251–264.

Chapter 34

Neurological and psychiatric complications in coeliac disease

G.K.T. Holmes

Department of Medicine, Derbyshire Royal Infirmary, London Road, Derby DE1 2QY, United Kingdom

Historical perspectives

The early literature contains descriptions of neuropathy complicating sprue, a term used at that time to cover tropical and non-tropical sprue (Cooke & Holmes, 1984). These reports are difficult to evaluate and many of the abnormalities would now be attributed to the effects of fluid and electrolyte imbalance (Woltman & Heck, 1937). Evidence continued to accumulate however, that non-tropical sprue was complicated by a disorder of the nervous system resembling subacute combined degeneration of the cord, already associated with pernicious anaemia (Richmond & Davidson, 1958). The importance of a report from New York was recognition for the first time that 'although most of the neurological manifestations in the malabsorption syndrome are minor and related to anaemia, a progressive crippling myeloradiculoneuropathy (a pseudotabes) can ensue which is refractory to all known medications' (Sencer, 1957). Clinical and pathological studies have further delineated this progressive disorder and other neurological and psychiatric complications of coeliac disease, but there is still much that remains unknown (Cooke & Smith, 1966; Cooke, Johnson & Wolff, 1966; Kinney *et al.*, 1982; Muller *et al*, 1996). The prevalence is not known for certain and it is not clear which, if any, of the conditions are specific for coeliac disease. Whether the disorders arise as a result of deficiencies due to malabsorption or because of an underlying mechanism inherent in coeliac disease, possibly related to gluten, is also unknown. Other than perhaps some cases of peripheral neuropathy and epilepsy there are no satisfactory treatments for these complications. These issues are considered in this chapter.

Prevalence

Prevalence data for neurological and psychiatric complications are difficult to obtain for a number of reasons. Firstly, information from referral centres is often unreliable because patients do not come from an unselected group. Secondly, different authors have included different conditions under the term neuropathy and in some instances what has been included is not clearly stated (Cooke, 1976). For example, some have included myopathy (Banerji & Hurwitz, 1971), and epilepsy and mental illness (Morris *et al.*, 1970) in the total figures but others have not (Cooke *et al.*, 1963). These considerations have given rise to widely differing estimates for prevalence. In New York, Sencer (1957) reported that appoximately half of patients with sprue had symptoms and signs of neurological involvement, most of which were minor and reversible. Of 49 patients regarded as having neurological abnormalities, 21 had paraesthesiae, 16 tetany and eight tetany with other neurological symptoms. One had syphilis and another symptoms due to osteoporosis. Thus only two (2 per cent) of 94 cases had severe neurological impairment which could be attributed to the malabsorption syndrome. An early study of 100 coeliac patients from Birmingham, UK, revealed that only two had minor neurological signs that disappeared with improvement in the general condition (Cooke *et al.*, 1953).

Table 1. Psychiatric disturbances among 388 patients with adult coeliac disease

Disorder	Number of cases	Percentage
Depression	39	10.1
Anxiety	9	2.3
Self-poisoning	8	2.1
Schizophrenia	2	0.5
Hysteria	1	0.3
Psycho-sexual problem	1	0.3
Schizoid personality	1	0.3

Table 2. Neurological disturbances among 388 patients with adult coeliac disease

Disorder	Number of cases	Percentage
Epilepsy	14	3.6
Migraine	12	3.1
Carpal tunnel syndrome	8	2.1
Stroke	6	1.5
Myopathy	5	1.3
Parkinsonism	3	0.8
Learning difficulties	2	0.5
Meningitis	2	0.5
Peripheral neuropathy	2	0.5
Sensori-neural deafness	2	0.5
Sydenham's chorea	2	0.5
Ant. spinal artery thrombosis	1	0.3
Benign essential tremor	1	0.3
Brain abscess	1	0.3
Cerebral metastases	1	0.3
CSF leak	1	0.3
Dementia	1	0.3
Friederich's ataxia	1	0.3
Ischaemic optic atrophy	1	0.3
Migrainous neuralgia	1	0.3
Sciatica	1	0.3
Spinocerebellar disease	1	0.3
Subdural haematoma	1	0.3
Transverse myelitis	1	0.3

Of the 388 patients with adult coeliac disease attending my own clinic at the Derbyshire Royal Infirmary, 102 (26 per cent) have developed 132 neurological or psychiatric disturbances (several patients had more than one disturbance) (Tables 1 and 2). Since patients were unselected and drawn from the local area served by the hospital, these data are likely to reflect the numbers and types of neuro-psychiatric disorder that occur among coeliac patients in the community. Many of the conditions were only encountered as single cases but several such as depression, epilepsy and migraine were well represented. Depression occurred in 10 per cent of the group and in some cases was severe. It is still not clear whether depression is more common or more severe among coeliacs than in the general population but there is no doubt that it is an important feature in some patients. Only two cases of schizophrenia were found. Epilepsy occurred in 14 (3.6 per cent) patients. Chapman *et al.* (1978) recorded a prevalence of epilepsy in coeliac disease of 5.5 per cent and accepted a figure of 0.5 per cent for the community, indicating that epilepsy may be more common among coeliacs than in the general population (Sander & Shorvon, 1987). Migraine does not appear to be any more common in coeliac disease than in the community (Waters & O'Connor, 1975). Myopathy was always a result of osteomalacia and responded to treatment with vitamin D and a gluten-free diet. Two patients had peripheral neuropathy which in one led to the diagnosis of coeliac disease. Only one patient who developed ataxia had evidence of spinocerebellar disease. In this case deficiencies of folate, B_{12} or vitamin E were not found although supplements were given. The condition has very slowly progressed. It may well be that with the earlier diagnosis of coeliac disease and the wider use of the gluten-free diet, the prevalence of severe neuropathy is decreasing, as appears to be the case for malignant complications (Holmes *et al.*, 1989).

In one investigation, the frequency of antigliadin antibodies and coeliac disease were looked for in neurological patients (Hadjivassiliou *et al.*, 1996). In this study, of 53 patients with neurological dysfunction of unknown cause of whom 25 had ataxia and 20 peripheral neuropathy, 30 were antigliadin antibody positive. Duodenal biopsies were performed in 26 of these antibody positive patients and nine (35%) were found to have coeliac disease which in the majority was clinically silent. These data indicate that a search for coeliac disease should be undertaken in patients with unexplained neurological disturbances.

Clinical presentations

In most cases intestinal symptoms precede the onset of neuropathy and patients may already be established on a gluten-free diet. Occasionally neuropathy appears first (Cooke & Smith, 1966; Binder *et al.*, 1967; Telerman-Toppet *et al.*, 1969; Finelli *et al.*, 1980). Presenting features will depend on which part of the nervous system is affected but patients usually come to medical attention because of symptoms affecting the legs which include numbness, tingling, pain, weakness and unsteadiness. Rapidly developing sensory ataxia is the most prominent feature in the majority of cases. Symptoms may affect the arms but are less common and milder. Epilepsy is an important presentation. Dysarthria, dysphonia, diplopia (Cooke & Smith, 1966; Telerman-Toppet *et al.*, 1969) and palatal myoclonus (Finelli *et al.*, 1980) may occur. The muscles are usually weak and incoordination is invariably present. The ankle jerks are diminished early and more markedly than the knee jerks but brisk reflexes may be encountered. Extensor planter responses are only occasionally found. Sensory impairment of glove and stocking type is frequently found. Coeliac patients with malignancy may rarely exhibit neurological disturbance (Camillieri *et al.*, 1993).

Neurological disorders encountered

Spinocerebellar degeneration and cerebellar disease

Spinocerebellar degeneration is a common presentation (Cooke & Smith, 1966; Finelli *et al.*, 1980; Kinney *et al.*, 1982). The cerebellar syndrome may occur without evidence of spinal cord disease (Kristoferitsch & Pointer, 1987; Hermaszewski *et al.*, 1991; Mauro *et al.*, 1991; Dick *et al.*, 1995). Cord involvement may be minimal (Finelli *et al.*, 1980. If cerebellar signs are marked these may mask dorsal column lesions. Two patients with the Ramsey-Hunt syndrome who exhibited a progressive cerebellar ataxia, mild seizures and severe myoclonus are reported (Lu *et al.*, 1986) and other cases have since been described (Tison *et al.*, 1989; Bhatia *et al.*, 1995; Mumford *et al.*, 1996).

There are no satisfactory treatments for these conditions but one patient appeared to improve on vitamin E supplements (Mauro *et al.*, 1991).

Myelopathy

Cord abnormalities are common and a lesion resembling subacute combined degeneration of the cord can occur (Cooke & Smith, 1966). No treatment is available.

Peripheral neuropathy

A patient with coeliac disease and peripheral neuropathy improved following the institution of a gluten-free diet (Farmer & Richards, 1964). Kaplan *et al.* (1988) described one patient and reviewed 11 others with peripheral neuropathy and coeliac disease and identified a consistent clinical pattern. Most patients were middle-aged men who developed intense paraesthesiae, numbness, hyporeflexia and sensory ataxia with varying degrees of weakness. None had central nervous system signs. A distal axonopathy was evident in 83 per cent of cases. Improvement may follow a gluten free diet and vitamin supplements (Cooke & Smith, 1966).

Epilepsy

Recent observations have highlighted the association between coeliac disease, epilepsy and intra-cranial calcifications although why these disorders should occur together is not clear. Garwicz & Mortensson (1976) reported two children with epilepsy and intracranial calcifications; one of whom had coeliac disease. Gobbi *et al.* (1988) described four patients with epilepsy and bilateral occipital calcifications, all had coeliac disease (Zaniboni *et al.*, 1989). The clinical course was similar in all patients and evolved from a benign onset to severe encephalopathy with progressive mental impair-ment. Whether this represents an atypical form of the Sturge–Weber syndrome was thought unlikely by these authors and others (Molteni *et al.*, 1988; Sammaritano *et al.*, 1988; Tiacci *et al.*, 1993). Since then several more reports of coeliac disease, epilepsy and cerebral calcifications have ap-peared (Ventura *et al.*, 1991; Crosato and Senter, 1991; Gobbi *et al.*, 1992a, b; Fois *et al.*, 1992; Ambrosetto *et al.*, 1992; Fois *et al.*, 1993; Magaudda *et al.*, 1993; Bye *et al.*, 1993; Piattella *et al.*, 1993; Fois *et al.*, 1994; Cernibori and Gobbi, 1994; Lea *et al.*, 1995). In the largest study to date, of 31 patients with epilepsy and cerebral calcifications, 24 had coeliac disease and conversely, of 12 with coeliac disease and epilepsy, five had calcifications (Gobbi *et al.*, 1992b). At the time of presentation with these features, the majority of patients were asymptomatic with regard to coeliac disease but most had a past history of malabsorption. In 27 of the 29 patients with epilepsy, calcifications and coeliac disease, the calcifications were localized to the parieto-occipital region. At the time of the biopsy, seizures were resistant to antiepileptic drugs in 25 cases. Of 20 patients who were given a gluten-free diet for longer than six months, seizures were reduced by 50 per cent in four, stopped in six, worsened in one and were unchanged in nine. Patients whose seizures stopped were younger and their epilepsy was of shorter duration at the start of the gluten-free diet. Bardella *et al.* (1994) also found a gluten-free diet to be of benefit in coeliac patients with epilepsy. Of 81 patients on a strict diet or only taking gluten occasionally, none had epilepsy, compared with five of 47 on an unrestricted diet. The geographical distribution of patients with these abnormalities is puzzling because, to date, the vast majority have been reported from Italy. It is likely that cases will be identified in other locations with greater awareness of the syndrome.

The aetiology of the calcifications is not understood but several unconvincing possibilities have been considered. These include folate deficiency, the use of anticoagulant drugs, vasculitis in the cerebral blood vessels and genetic factors (Gobbi *et al.*, 1992a, b).

Dementia

This is uncommon in established coeliac disease (Smith & Cooke, 1966; Kinney *et al.*, 1982).

Collin *et al.* (1991) reported five patients with dementia who were later found to have coeliac disease. The gastrointestinal symptoms were mild. There was no convincing evidence that vitamin B_{12}, folic acid or pyridoxine deficiencies were the cause although deficiencies were found. A gluten-free diet did not improve the mental state. The mental state of a man with coeliac disease, ataxia and confusion improved on gluten free diet and vitamin E (Beversdorf *et al.*, 1996).

Myopathy

This is included as a neurological disorder in some reports although it is invariably due to to osteomalacia and responds to vitamin D supplements (Hardoff *et al.*, 1980; Rossi, 1982). A 12 year old girl with coeliac disease presented with an isolated ocular myopathy which was reversed by a gluten-free diet and vitamins (Sandyk & Brennan, 1983).

Basilar impression

Of 22 patients with coeliac disease investigated for basilar impression or platybasia, seven fulfilled the criteria. Two of these had neurological features with posterior column and pyramidal tract lesions. (Hurwitz & Banerji, 1972). It was argued that basilar impression of the skull had occurred secondary to bone softening due to malabsorption in early life.

Miscellaneous conditions

Other neurological disorders are encountered in coeliac disease but the significance of the associations is not clear. These include, acute quadriparesis (Coers *et al.*, 1972), progressive multifocal leukoencephalopathy (Kepes *et al.*, 1975), chronic inflammatory neuromuscular disorders (Bernier *et al.*, 1978) amyotrophic lateral sclerosis, syringomyelia, Guillain-Barré syndrome (Cooke & Holmes, 1984), encephalitis (Brucke *et al.,* 1988), neuropathic joint disease (Cooke & Holmes, 1984), disseminated intravascular coagulation with cerebral involvement (Ryan *et al.*, 1977), and cerebral thrombosis (Florholmen *et al.,* 1980). The Floating-Harbor syndrome which comprises speech impediment, developmental delay and facial anomalies occurs in association with coeliac disease (Chudley & Moroz, 1991). Patients with multiple sclerosis and coeliac disease have have been reported by some (Lange & Shiner, 1976; Cook *et al.*, 1978; Fantelli *et al.*, 1978) but not others (Gupta *et al.*, 1977; Bateson *et al.*, 1979). It is almost certain that this is only a chance association. Optic atrophy has been recorded (Bundey, 1967; Banerji & Hurwitz, 1971), and macular degeneration (Mitchell & Robinson, 1996).

Mental disturbance

It has long been recognized that psychiatric disturbances accompany coeliac disease (Daynes, 1956; Paulley, 1959). In a study of neuropathy in coeliac disease it was noted that three of 30 patients had severe depression (Morris *et al.,* 1970). Hallert & Derefeldt (1982) found five of 42 patients to be depressed. It has been claimed that depression among coeliac patients can be treated successfully by giving supplements of pyridoxine (Hallert *et al.*, 1983). Psychiatric assessment carried out on 80 patients with small intestinal disorders, the largest group of whom were coeliacs, found a high prevalence of various psychiatric abnormalities, but no differences emerged between the different disorders (Goldberg, 1970). There is no evidence that autism is associated with coeliac disease and such children should not be put on a gluten-free diet (Walker-Smith & Andrews, 1972; McCarthy & Coleman, 1979).

Dohan (1966) called attention to a possible association between schizophrenia and coeliac disease and provided some evidence in support of this view (Dohan, 1970). Studies from Ireland however, have not upheld the proposition (Dean *et al.*, 1975; Stevens *et al.*, 1977). No cases of schizophrenia were discovered by Hallert & Derefeldt (1982) in their series. Correlation of the frequency of schizophrenia with consumption of wheat and rye was proposed (Dohan, 1966) but this assertion were criticized because the data quoted in support were not unselected (Lancet, 1983). Cereal-free, milk-free diets have appeared to benefit schizophrenic patients (Dohan *et al.*, 1969; Dohan & Grasberger, 1973; Singh & Kay, 1976) but these studies have been criticized on methodological grounds (Lancet, 1983).

Aetiology

The aetiology of these neurological complications of coeliac disease is unknown but heredity, infection, absorption of toxic substances, autoimmune mechanisms, vasculitis and vitamin deficiencies have to be considered. Whether gluten is of any importance also requires attention.

Heredity

Some spinocerebellar ataxias are linked to HLA loci (Haines *et al.*, 1984). Although it is possible that a subgroup of coeliac patients is more likely to develop neurological disorders because of the presence of a particular HLA profile there is no evidence for this assertion at present.

Infection

There are defects in the immunological status of coeliac patients which may cause them to react abnormally to particular infections. It has been suggested that a basic protein as a by-product of viral synthesis may become a myelinotoxic antigen by triggering an immune response of lymphocytes (Kepes *et al.*, 1975).

Toxins

The small intestinal mucosa in coeliac disease is more permeable than normal and could allow through substances that are toxic to neural tissue.

Autoimmunity

Many immunological disturbances can be identified in coeliac disease and autoimmune mechanisms may be of importance in the causation of neurological disorders. Immunosuppressants were effective in preventing deterioration in one case (Cordonnier *et al.*, 1983). In a patient with cerebellar ataxia antibodies against Purkinje cells were not detected (Dick *et al.*, 1995).

Vasculitis

Two patients with seizures had vasculitis (Holdstock & Oleesky, 1970; Rush *et al.*, 1986). Vasculitis might play a part in the development of other neurological disturbances.

Deficiencies

Folic acid

Neurological syndromes are associated with folic acid deficiency (Hansen *et al.*, 1964; Grant *et al.*, 1965; Horwitz *et al.*, 1968; Ahmed, 1972; Manzoor & Runcie, 1976; Botez, 1976; Parry, 1990) and dementia has also been reported (Strachan & Henderson, 1966). Patients exhibit peripheral neuropathy with or without myelopathy which may be indistinguishable from subacute combined degeneration of the cord (Grant *et al.*, 1965; Manzoor & Runcie, 1976; Parry, 1990). In some instances improvement has occurred following the administration of folic acid supplements (Grant *et al.*, 1965; Strachan & Henderson, 1966; Ahmed, 1972; Manzoor & Runcie, 1976).

In some patients a flat jejunal mucosa has been demonstrated (Fehling *et al.*, 1974; Pallis & Lewis, 1974; Botez, 1976). Folic acid deficiency in coeliac disease is common but neurological disorder is uncommon. If folic acid deficiency is of importance in producing neurological complications it could be argued that these should occur much more commonly than is the case.

Vitamin B₁₂

Vitamin B_{12} deficiency develops by two main mechanisms – by malabsorption as in coeliac disease or due to lack of intrinsic factor. The mechanism by which vitamin B_{12} may cause neurological damage has emerged from the observation that exposure to nitrous oxide produces megaloblastic changes in the bone marrow, myelopathy closely resembling subacute combined degeneration of the cord and peripheral neuropathy. Nitrous oxide selectively inhibits a B_{12}-dependent enzyme, methionine synthetase. This leads to a failure to synthesize methionine from homocysteine and a deficiency of S-adenosylmethionine ensues which is involved in myelin synthesis.

Among 145 patients with coeliac disease, 20 or 14 per cent had low levels of vitamin B_{12} in the serum (Cooke & Holmes, 1984). Others have found a higher incidence, 37 per cent of 52 patients (Stewart *et al.,* 1967) and 53 per cent of 30 patients, reverting to normal with a gluten-free diet (Fausa, 1974). Low levels have been found in 27 (21 per cent) of 129 patients with dermatitis herpetiformis (Kastrup *et al.,* 1986). Concentrations are usually marginally below normal but can be very reduced (Stene-Larson *et al.,* 1988; Kastrup *et al.,* 1986). Pernicious anaemia is rare in coeliac disease (Jarvinen & Lapvalahti, 1958; Shiner, 1963; Ellis *et al.,* 1966; Quigley *et al.,* 1986; Stene-Larson *et al.,* 1988).

Is vitamin B_{12} implicated in coeliac neuropathy? A patient with idiopathic steatorrhoea and impairment of vitamin B_{12} absorption was considered to have subacute combined degeneration of the cord (Richmond & Davidson 1958). As far as these authors were aware this had not previously been described in coeliac disease. A similar case was reported by Banerji & Hurwitz (1972). A patient with pernicious anaemia and a flat small intestinal biopsy developed posterolateral spinal cord disease which progressed during treatment with vitamin B_{12} therapy (Ellis *et al.,* 1966). There is little evidence to suggest that vitamin B_{12} is concerned with the neurological complications of coeliac disease (Cooke & Smith, 1966).

Vitamin E

Vitamin E is fat-soluble and found particularly in vegetable oils. Bile is essential for absorption of vitamin E which is found in the blood in the low density lipoproteins. Its active form is D-α-tocopherol which functions as an anti-oxidant and may help to stabilize biological membranes by protecting unsaturated lipids from oxidation. Evidence has accumulated which indicates that vitamin E has an important role in maintaining the integrity of neurological tissues. Support for this assertion comes from observations made in abetalipoproteinaemia and other chronic disorders of fat malabsorption (Muller, 1986). In abetalipoproteinaemia vitamin E is undetectable in the plasma from birth. Towards the end of the first decade of life an ataxic neuropathy and retinal lesions develop, and by the age of 20 years virtually all patients are affected. Spontaneous improvement does not occur. Muller *et al.* (1983) treated eight cases with supplements of vitamin E and the results were impressive: the manifestations of the disease either did not appear in those who were treated early or were arrested or reversed in those treated later. In the group with other chronic disorders of fat absorption the majority are children with cholestatic liver disease who have low concentrations of vitamin E in the serum and develop neurological disorders of the cerebellum, posterior columns and peripheral nerves. These features are similar to those found in abetalipoproteinaemia (Rosenblum *et al.,* 1981; Elias *et al.,* 1981; Frydman *et al.,* 1981; Guggenheim *et al.,* 1982, 1983). Neurological disturbances have also been found in adults with vitamin E deficiency associated with pseudointestinal obstruction and ileal resection for Crohn's disease (Harding *et al.,* 1982), and in cystic fibrosis (Elias *et al.,* 1981; Bye *et al.,* 1985; Willison *et al.,* 1985). The clinical features include dysarthria, cerebellar ataxia, severe proprioceptive loss and depressed or absent reflexes. Improvement may occur following supplementation with vitamin E (Tomasi, 1979; Elias *et al.,* 1981; Harding *et al.,* 1982; Guggenheim *et al.,* 1982; Howard *et al.,* 1982).

Frydman *et al.* (1981) drew attention to the similarities between the neurological abnormalities in their cases and those reported in adult coeliac disease by Cooke & Smith (1966). So the question arises whether lack of vitamin E is of importance in the development of the neurological compli-cations of coeliac disease. Binder *et al.* (1967) reported four patients with malabsorption and neurological disease, two of whom with severe peripheral neuropathy, had low serum concentra-tions of vitamin E. A progressive and fatal neurological disorder occurred in a man with coeliac disease who showed no response to intravenous nutrition including vitamin E administration for six months (Kinney *et al.*, 1982). Vitamin E deficiency was found in two patients with coeliac disease, one of whom with cerebellar syndrome, improved on vitamin E therapy (Ackerman *et al.*, 1989; Mauro *et al.*, 1991). Two patients with coeliac disease and the Ramsay Hunt syndrome had low serum vitamin E levels but supplements given to one of these did not result in any benefit (Lu *et al.*, 1986). When vitamin E was given to a coeliac patient with myoclonus who had mild deficiency there was no improvement (Tison *et al.*, 1989). A patient with brown bowel syndrome and coeliac disease had peripheral neuropathy and low serum vitamin E levels but supplements were unhelpful (Connolly *et al.*, 1994). Low concentration was found in a coeliac patients who died of encephalitis (Brucke *et al.*, 1988). Peripheral neuropathy (Kaplan *et al.*, 1988), spinocerebellar degeneration (Ward *et al.*, 1985) and cerebellar ataxia (Dick *et al.*, 1995) can arise in coeliac patients who have normal levels of vitamin E.

Pyridoxine

Pyridoxine is important in many enzyme reactions. It is, for example, a cofactor in the conversion of 5-hydroxytryptophan to 5-hydroxytryptamine (serotonin) and acts at other points in the metabo-lism of tryptophan. Interest in serotonin metabolism in coeliac disease began with the observation that the urinary excretion of 5-hydroxyindoleacetic acid (5HIAA) was increased in adults (Kow-lessar *et al.*, 1958; Haverback *et al.*, 1960) and in children (Challacombe & Wheeler, 1987) and an augmented shunt of serotonin to 5HIAA was suggested as a cause (Kowlessar *et al.*, 1964). Those with coeliac disease metabolize a tryptophan load abnormally and in a similar way to patients with pyridoxine deficiency (Kowlessar *et al.*, 1964). Low levels of pyridoxine have been found in half of an unselected series of coeliac patients but low values did not correlate with neurological problems or with delay in nerve conduction (Morris *et al.*, 1970). Cooke & Smith (1966) reported improvement in five patients with peripheral neuropathy who were treated with large parenteral doses of vitamins including pyridoxine. Mood changes experienced by patients with coeliac disease could be related to disturbances of tryptophan metabolism in adults (Hallert *et al.*, 1982a, b) and in children (Challacombe & Wheeler, 1987; Hernanz & Polanco, 1991). It has been shown that supplements of pyridoxine may reverse depression suffered by some patients (Hallert *et al.*, 1983).

Biopterin compounds

There is increasing appreciation of the role of biopterin compounds in human metabolism and in particular, in the synthesis of neurotransmitters. If this system is disturbed, neurological disorder may ensue (Smith *et al.*, 1975). Significantly low levels of crithidia factor have been found in senile dementia, schizophrenia, and untreated coeliac disease (Leeming & Blair, 1980; Leeming *et al.*, 1976).

The metabolisms of folates, vitamin B₁₂, pyridoxine, biopterins and amines are closely related although the mechanism and functions are poorly understood (Smith *et al.*, 1975; Smith *et al.*, 1986: Scott, 1992).

Gluten

There is no evidence that gluten directly damages neural tissues. Several patients of Cooke & Smith (1966) developed neurological disorders whilst taking a gluten free diet, although it is not clear how strictly they were adhering to this. A gluten-free diet, however, benefits patients with epilepsy (Gobbi *et al.*, 1992b; Bardella *et al.*, 1994). It has been suggested that gluten peptides might be important in the aetiology of psychiatric disturbances. Lymphocytes from about half of patients with schizophrenia and other psychoses reacted to subfractions of gluten in the migration inhibition test (Ashkenazi *et al.*, 1979). None of the patients showed evidence of malabsorption but it was speculated that there might be a link between the absorption of cereal peptides and mental illness in some patients. Peptides with opioid activity are found in pepsin hydrolysates of wheat and α-casein (Zioudrou, 1979) and in rats, peptide material from gliadin can be found in the brain (Hemmings, 1978). It has been speculated that antigliadin antibodies may be directly or indirectly neurotoxic (Hadjivassiliou *et al.*, 1996).

Pathology

Some of the pathological lesions are reminiscent of certain deficiency states. Thus, loss of Nissl granules in the pyramidal cells of the cerebral cortex, especially the Betz cells and in the neurons of the basal ganglia and the brain stem, are similar to changes described in pellagra. Systematized demyelination in the posterior and lateral tracts of the spinal cord are also found in pellegra and in malnourished prisoners of war. Changes in the hypothalamus are similar to those that occur in Wernicke's encephalopathy. Astrocytic hypertrophy is also found in liver coma. Changes in the spinal cord (patchy non-systematized, spongiform demyelination of the posterior and posterolateral columns) resemble subacute combined degeneration of the cord. There is great variation in the character and distribution of the lesions within the nervous system (Cooke *et al.*, 1996; Cooke & Smith, 1966; Finelli *et al.*, 1980; Kepes *et al.*, 1985). Cortical or cerebellar atrophy may be sufficiently marked to be recognized macroscopically. Atrophy and focal loss of neurones are common findings. Astrocytic hypertrophy is sometimes associated with neuronal degeneration. In the spinal cord, the lesions tend to be patchy and non-systematized, with spongy demyelination of the posterior and posterolateral columns associated with varying degrees of axonal degeneration. In the peripheral nerves the most striking features are globular swellings of the terminal axons and fusion of the terminal axonic expansions.

Treatment

Comments about treatments for the neurological complications have already been made in the section on the various disorders encountered in clinical practice. As indicated, some patients with peripheral neuropathy or epilepsy may improve when given a gluten-free diet and vitamin supplements. In general, however, no satisfactory treatments are available, certainly not for the severe neuropathy of coeliac disease which affects the central nervous system. A gluten-free diet should always be given for it improves general health and well-being and may prevent neurological complications by reconstituting the integrity of the small intestinal mucosa and so prevent absorption of potential neuro-toxic substances, or damp-down immune responses that might originate in the mucosa and be damaging to neural tissues. A mucosa that has been normalized will absorb more efficiently and so make up deficiencies of nutrients, lack of which may cause neural damage. It is the impression that neurological complications are less common than they were which might reflect the earlier diagnosis of coeliac disease before severe nutritional deficiencies occur and the more widespread use of the gluten-free diet. If vitamin and iron deficiencies are present, supplements should be given. Neurological disturbance may not be affected but the general condition, anaemia and myopathy should improve. There is no conclusive beneficial role for steroids although it is likely that these will be tried in a rapidly progressing neuropathy. Immunosuppressants may be given but there is no evidence that these are effective.

References

Ackerman, Z., Eliashiv, S., Reches, A. & Zimmerman, J. (1989): Neurological manifestations in coeliac disease and vitamin E deficiency. *J. Clin. Gastroenterol.* **11**, 603–605.

Ahmed, M. (1972): Neurological disease and folate deficiency. *BMJ* **1**, 181.

Ambrosetto, G., Antonini, L. & Tassinari, A. (1992): Occipital lobe seizures related to clinically asymptomatic coeliac disease in adulthood. *Epilepsia* **33,** 476–481.

Ashkenazi, A., Krasilowsky, D., Levin, S., Idar, D., Kalian, M., Or, A., Ginat, Y. & Halperin, B. (1979): Immunologic reaction of psychotic patients to fractions of gluten. *Am. J. Psych.* **136,** 1306–1309.

Banerji, N.K. & Hurwitz, L.J. (1971): Neurological manifestations in adult steatorrhoea (probable gluten enteropathy). *J. Neurol. Science* **14,** 125–141.

Bardella, M.T., Molteni, N., Prampolini, I., Giunta, A.M., Baldassarri, A.R., Morganti, D. & Bianchi, P.A. (1994): Need for follow up in coeliac disease. *Arch. Dis. Child* **70,** 211–213

Bateson, M.C., Hopwood, D. & MacGillivray, J.B. (1979): Jejunal morphology in multiple sclerosis. *Lancet* **i** 1108–1110

Bemier, J.J., Buge, A., Rambaud, J.C., Rancurel, G., Hauw, J.J., L'Hirondel, C. & Denvil, D. (1978): Chronic inflammatory neuromuscular disorders associated with treated coeliac disease. In: *Perspectives in coeliac disease*, eds. B. McNichol, C.F. McCarthy & P.F. Fottrell, pp. 495–497. Lancaster: MTP press.

Beversdorf, D., Moses, P., Reeves, A. & Dunn, J. (1996): A man with weight loss, ataxia, and confusion for 3 months. *Lancet* **i,** 446

Bhatia, K.P., Brown, P., Gregory, R., Lennox, G.G., Manji, H., Thompson, P.D., Ellison, D.W. & Marsden, C.D. (1995): Progressive myoclonic ataxia associated with coeliac disease. *Brian* **118,** 1087–1093

Binder, H.J., Solitaire, G.B. & Spiro, H.M. (1967): Neuromuscular disease in patients with steatorrhoea. *Gut* **8,** 605–611.

Botez, M.I. (1976): Folate deficiency and coeliac disease. *BMJ* **ii,** 699–700

Brucke, T., Kollegger, H., Schmidbauer, M., Muller, C., Podreka, I. & Deecke, L. (1988): Adult coeliac disease and brainstem encephalitis. *J. Neurol. Neurosurg. Psych.* **51** 456–457.

Bundey, S. (1967): Adult coeliac disease and neuropathy. *Lancet* **i,** 851–852 (letter).

Bye, A.M.E., Andermann, F., Robitaille, Y., Bohane, T., Oliver, M., & Andermann, E. (1993): Cortical vascular abnormalities in the syndrome of coeliac disease, bilateral occipital calcifications and folate deficiency. *Ann. Neurol.* **34,** 399–403.

Bye, A.M.E., Muller, D.P.R., Wilson, J., Wright, V.M. & Mearns, M.B. (1985): Symptomatic vitamin E deficiency in cystic fibrosis. *Arch. Dis. Child* **60,** 162–164.

Camillieri, M., Krausz, T., Lewis, P.D., Hodgson, H.J.F., Pallis, C.A. & Chadwick, V.S. (1983): Malignant histiocytosis and encephalomyeloradiculopathy complicating coeliac disease. *Gut* **24,** 441–447.

Cerniborni, A. & Gobbi, G. (1995): Partial seizures, cerebral calcifications and coeliac disease. *Ital J Neurol Sci.* **16,** 187–191

Challacombe, D.N. & Wheeler, E.E. (1987): Are the changes of mood in children with coeliac disease due to abnormal serotonin metabolism? *Nutr. Health* **5,** 145–152.

Chapman, R.W.G., Laidlow, J.M., Colin-Jones, D., Eade, O.E. & Smith, C.L. (1978): Increased prevalence of epilepsy in coeliac disease. *BMJ* **ii,** 250–251.

Chudley, A.E. & Moroz, S.P. (1991): Floating-Harbor syndrome and coeliac disease. *Am. J. Med. Genet.* **38,** 562–564.

Coers, C., Telerman-Toppet, N. & Cremer, M. (1972): Acute quadriparesis with muscle spasms related to electrolyte disturbances in steatorrhoea. *Am. J. Med.* **52,** 849–856.

Collin, P., Pirttila, T., Nurmikko, T., Somer, H., Erila, T. & Keyrilainen, O. (1991): Coeliac disease, brain atrophy, and dementia. *Neurology* **41,** 372–375.

Connolly, C.E., Kennedy, M., Stevens, F.M. & McCarthy, C.F. (1994): Brown bowel syndrome occurring in coeliac disease in the West of Ireland. *Scand. J. Gastroenterol.* **29,** 91–94.

Cook, A.W., Gupta, J.K., Pertschuk, L.P. & Nidzgorski, F. (1978): Multiple sclerosis and malabsorption. *Lancet* **i,** 1366.

Cooke, W.T. (1976): Neurologic manifestations of malabsorption. *Handbook of Clinical Neurology* **28,** 225–241.

Cooke, W.T., Fone, D.J., Cox, E.V., Meynell, M.J. & Gaddie, R. (1963): Adult coeliac disease. *Gut* **4,** 279–291.

Cooke, W.T. & Holmes, G.K.T. (1984): *Coeliac Disease*. Edinburgh: Churchill-Livingstone.

Cooke, W.T., Johnson, A.G. & Woolf, A.L. (1966): Vital staining and electron microscopy of the intramuscular nerve endings in the neuropathy of adult coeliac disease. *Brain* **89,** 663–682.

Cooke, W.T., Peeney, A.L.P. & Hawkins, C.F. (1953): Symptoms, signs and diagnostic features of idiopathic steatorrhoea. *Quart. J. Med.* **22,,** 59–77.

Cooke, W.T. & Smith, W.T. (1966): Neurological disorders associated with adult coeliac disease. *Brain* **89,** 683–722.

Cordonnier, M., Robin, M. & Cornette, M. (1983): Neuro-myeloencephalopathy in coeliac disease. *Act. Gastroenterol. Belg.* **46,** 47–54.

Crosato, F., Senter, S. (1991): Cerebral occipital calcifications in coeliac disease. *Neuropediatrics* **23,** 214–217

Dalgleish, A.G. (1996): Adult coeliac disease. *Lancet* **i,** 908

Daynes, G. (1956): Bread and tears – naughtiness, depression and fits due to wheat sensitivity. *Proc. R. Soc. Med.* **49,** 391–394.

Dean, G., Hanniffy, L., Stevens, F.M., Temperley, I., O'Broin, J.D., Scott, J. & Cahalane, S.F. (1975): Schizophrenia and coeliac disease. *J. Irish. Med. Assoc.* **68,** 545–546.

Dick, D.J., Abraham, D., Falkous, G. & Hishon, S. (1995): Cerebellar ataxia in coeliac disease – no evidence of humoral aetiology. *Postgrad. Med. J.* **71,** 186 (letter).

Dohan, F.C. (1966): Cereals and schizophrenia: data and hypothesis. *Acta Psychiatr. Scand.* **42,** 125–152.

Dohan, F.C. (1970): Coeliac disease and schizophrenia. *Lancet* **i,** 897–898.

Dohan, F.C. & Grasberger, J.C. (1973): Relapsed schizophrenics: earlier discharge from the hospital after cereal-free milk-free diet. *Am. J. Psych.* **130,** 685–688.

Dohan, F.C., Grasberger, J.C., Lowell, F.M., Johnston, H.T. & Arbegast, A. W. (1969): Relapsed schizophrenics: more rapid improvement on a milk- and cereal-free diet. *Brit. J. Psychiat.* **115,** 595–596.

Elias, E., Muller, D.P.R. & Scott, J. (1981): Association of spinocerebellar disorders with cystic fibrosis or chronic cholestasis and very low serum vitamin E. *Lancet* **ii,** 1319–1321.

Ellis, G.J., Breuer, R.I., Owen, E.E. & Laszlo, J. (1966): Pernicious anaemia and malabsorption, with spinal cord degeneration developing during vitamin B12 treatment. *Ann. Intern. Med.* **64,** 654–658.

Fantelli, F.J., Mitsumoto, H. & Sebek, B.A. (1978): Multiple sclerosis and malabsorption. *Lancet* **i,** 1039–1040.

Farmer, R.G. & Richards, N.G. (1964): Malabsorption syndrome and peripheral neuropathy. Report of two cases. *Cleve. Clin. Q.* **31,** 163–168.

Fausa, O. (1974): Vitamin B$_{12}$ absorption in intestinal diseases. *Scand. J. Gastroent.* 9, supplement **29,** 75–79.

Fehling, C., Jagerstad, M., Lindstrand, K. & Elmqvist, D. (1974): Folate deficiency and neurological disease. *Arch. Neurol.* **30,** 263–265.

Finelli, P.F., McEntee, W.J., Ambler, M. & Kestenbaum, D. (1980): Adult coeliac disease presenting as cerebellar syndrome. *Neurology* **30,** 245–249.

Florholmen, J., Waldum, H. & Nordoy, A. (1980): Cerebral thrombosis in two patients with malabsorption syndrome treated with vitamin K. *BMJ* **ii,** 541.

Fois, A., Balestri, P., Vascotto, M., Farnetani, M.A., Di Bartolo, R.M. & Di Marco, V. (1992): Epilepsy, progressive cerebral calcifications, and coeliac disease. *Lancet* **ii,** 1095.

Fois, A., Balestri, P., Vascotto, M., Farnetani, A., Rosanna, M., Di Bartolo, R.M., Di Marco, V. & Vindigni, C. (1993): Progressive cerebral calcifications, epilepsy, and coeliac disease. *Brain Dev.* **15,** 79–82.

Fois, A., Vascotto, M., Di Bartolo, R.M. & Di Marco, V. (1994): Coeliac disease and epilepsy in paediatric patients. *Child's Nerv. Syst.* **10,** 450–454.

Frydman, M., Rotter, J.I., Kazimiroff, P. & Phelps, D.L. (1981): Neurological syndrome in liver disease. *N. Engl. J. Med.* **305,** 108.

Garwicz, A. & Mortensson, W. (1976): Intracranial calcification mimicking the Sturge–Weber syndrome. *Paediat. Radiol.* **5,** 5–9.

Gobbi, G., Ambrosetto, P., Zaniboni, M.G., Lambertini, A., Ambrosioni, G. & Tassinari, C.A. (1992a): Coeliac disease, posterior cerebral calcifications and epilepsy. *Brain Dev.* **14,** 23–29.

Gobbi, G., Bouquet, F., Greco, L., Lambertini, A., Tassinari, C.A., Ventura, A. & Zaniboni, M.G. (1992b): Coeliac disease, epilepsy, and cerebral calcifications. *Lancet* **ii,** 439–443.

Gobbi, G., Sorrenti, G., Santucci, M., Giovanardi Rossi, P., Ambrosetto, P., Michelucci, R. & Tassinari, C.A. (1988): Epilepsy with bilateral occipital calcifications: A benign onset with progressive severity. *Neurology* **38,** 913–920.

Goldberg, D. (1970): A psychiatric study of patients with diseases of the small intestine. *Gut* **11,** 459–465.

Grant, H., Hoffbrand, A.V. & Wells, D.G. (1965): Folate deficiency and neurological disease. *Lancet* **ii,** 763–767.

Guggenheim, M.A., Jackson, V., Lilly, J. & Silverman, A. (1983): Vitamin E deficiency and neurologic disease in children with cholestasis: A prospective study. *J. Paediatr.* **102**, 577–579.

Guggenheim, M.A., Ringel, S.P., Silverman, A. & Grabert, B.E. (1982): Progressive neuromuscular disease in children with chronic cholestasis and vitamin E deficiency: Diagnosis and treatment with alpha tocopherol. *J. Paediatr.* **100**, 51–58.

Gupta, J.K., Ingogno, A.P., Cook, A.W. & Pertschuk, L.P. (1977): Multiple sclerosis and malabsorption. *Am. J. Gastroenterol.* **68**, 560–565.

Hadjivassiliou, M., Gibson, A., Davies-Jones, G.A.B., Lobo, A.J., Stephensen, T.J., Milford-Ward, A. (1996): Does cryptic gluten sensitivity play a part in neurological illness? *Lancet* **i**, 369–377

Haines, J.L., Schut, L.J., Weitkamp, L.R., Thayer, M. & Anderson, V.E. (1984): Spinocerebellar ataxia, in a large kindred: age at onset, reproduction, and genetic linkage studies. *Neurology* **34**, 1542–1548.

Hallert, C., Astrom, J. & Sedvall, G. (1982a): Psychic disturbances in adult coeliac disease III. Reduced central monoamine metabolism and signs of depression. *Scand. J. Gastroenterol.* **17**, 25–28.

Hallert, C., Astrom, J. & Walan, A. (1983): Reversal of psychopathology in adult coeliac disease with the aid of pyridoxine (vitamin B6). *Scand. J. Gastroenterol.* **18**, 299–304.

Hallert, C. & Derefeldt, T. (1982): Psychic disturbances in adult coeliac disease I. Clinical observations. *Scand. J. Gastroenterol.* **17**, 17–19.

Hallert, C., Martensson, J. & Allgen, L.G. (1982b): Brain availability of monoamine precursors in adult coeliac disease. *Scand. J. Gastroenterol.* **17**, 87–89.

Hansen, H.A., Nordqvist, P. & Sourander, P. (1964): Megaloblastic anaemia and neurologic disturbances combined with folic acid deficiency. *Acta Med. Scand.* **176**, 243–251.

Harding, A.E., Muller, D.P.R., Thomas, P.K. & Willison, H.J. (1982): Spinocerebellar degeneration secondary to chronic intestinal malabsorption; a vitamin E deficiency syndrome. *Ann. Neurol.* **12**, 419–424.

Hardoff, D., Sharf, B. & Berger, A. (1980): Myopathy as a presentation of coeliac disease. *Dev. Med. Child Neurol.* **22**, 781–783.

Haverback, B.J., Dyce, B., Heriberto, V. & Thomas, M.S. (1960): Indole metabolism in the malabsorption syndrome. *N. Eng. J. Med.* **262**, 754–757.

Hemmings, W.A. (1978): The entry into the brain of large molecules derived from dietary proteins. *Proc. R. Soc. Med.* (B) **200**, 175–192.

Hermaszewski, R.A., Rigby, S. & Dalgleish, A.G. (1991): Coeliac disease presenting with cerebellar degeneration. *Postgrad. Med. J.* **67** 1023–1024.

Hernanz, A, Polanco (1991): Plasma precursor amino acids of central nervous system monoamines in children with coeliac disease. *Gut* **32**, 1478–1481.

Holdstock, D.J. & Oleesky, S. (1970): Vasculitis in coeliac disease. *BMJ* **2**, 369.

Horwitz, S.J., Klipstein, F.A. & Lovelace, R.E. (1968): Relation of abnormal folate metabolism to neuropathy developing during anticonvulsant drug therapy. *Lancet* **i**, 563–565.

Howard, L., Ovesen, L., Satya-Murti, S. & Chu, R. (1982): Reversible neurological symptoms caused by vitamin E deficiency in a patient with short bowel syndrome. *Am. J. Clin. Nutr.* **36**, 1234.

Hurwitz, L.J. & Banerji, N.K. (1972): Basilar impression of the skull in patients with adult coeliac disease and after gastric surgery. *J. Neurol. Neurosurg. Psych.* **35**, 92–96.

Jarvinen, K.A.J. & Lapvalahti, J. (1958): Some observations on non-tropical sprue. A case with hypocalcaemia, intrinsic factor deficiency and diabetes mellitus. *Ann. Clin. Res.* **47**, 39–46.

Kaplan, J.G., Pack, D., Horoupian, D., De Souza, T., Brin, M. & Schaumburg, H. (1988): Distal axonopathy associated with chronic gluten enteropathy: A treatable disorder. *Neurology* **38**, 642–645.

Kastrup, W., Mobacken, H., Stockbrugger, R., Swolin, B. & Westin, J. (1986): Malabsorption of vitamin B_{12} in dermatitis herpetiformis and its association with pernicious anaemia. *Acta Med. Scand.* **220**, 261–268.

Kepes, J.J., Chou, S. & Price, L.W. (1975): Progressive multifocal leukoencephalopathy with a 10-year survival in a patient with nontropical sprue. *Neurology* **25**, 1006–1012.

Kinney, H.C., Burger, P.C., Hurwitz, B.J., Hijmans, J.C. & Grant J.P. (1982): Degeneration of the central nervous system associated with coeliac disease. *J. Neurol. Sci.* **53**, 9–22.

Kowlessar, O.D., Williams, R.C., Law, D.H. & Sleisenger, M.H. (1958): Urinary excretion of 5-hydroxyindoleacetic acid in diarrhoeal states, with special reference to nontropical sprue. *N. Eng. J. Med.* **259**, 340–341.

Kowlessar, O.D., Haeffner, L.J. & Benson, G.D. (1964): Abnormal tryptophan metabolism in patients with adult coeliac disease, with evidence for deficiency of vitamin B$_6$ *J. Clin. Invest.* **43,** 894–903.

Kristoferitsch, W. & Pointner, H. (1987): Progressive cerebellar syndrome in adult coeliac disease. *J. Neurol.* **234,** 116–118.

Lancet (Leading Article) (1983): Gluten in schizophrenia. *Lancet* **i,** 744–745.

Lange, L.S. & Shiner, M. (1979): Jejunal morphology in multiple sclerosis. *Lancet* **i,** 1300–1301.

Lea, M.E., Harbord, M, Sage, M.R. (1995): Bilateral occipital calcification associated with coeliac disease, folate deficiency, and epilepsy. *Am. J. Neuroradiol.* **16**, 1498–1500.

Leeming, R.J. & Blair, J.A. (1980): Serum Crithidia levels in disease. *Biochem. Med.* **22,** 122–125.

Leeming, R.J., Blair, J.A., Melikian, V. & O'Gorman, D.J. (1976): Biopterin derivatives in human body fluids and tissues. *J. Clin. Path.* **29,** 444–451.

Lu, C.S., Thompson, P.D., Quinn, N.P., Parkes, J.D. & Marsden, C.D. (1986): Ramsay Hunt Syndrome and coeliac disease: A new association? *Mov. Dis.* **1** 209–219.

Magaudda, A., dalla Bernardina, B., De Marco, P., Sfaello, Z., Colamaria, V., Daniele, O., Tortorella, G., Tata, M.A., Di Perri, R. & Meduri, M. (1993): Bilateral occipital calcification, epilepsy and coeliac disease: clinical and neuroimaging features of a new syndrome. *J. Neurol. Neurosurg. Psych.* **56,** 885–889.

Manzoor, M. & Runcie, J. (1976): Folate-responsive neuropathy: report of 10 cases. *BMJ* **1,** 1176–1178.

Mauro, A., Orsi, L., Mortara, P., Costa, P. & Schiffer, D. (1991): Cerebellar syndrome in adult coeliac disease with vitamin E deficiency. *Acta Neurol. Scand.* **84** 167–170.

McCarthy, D.M. & Coleman, M. (1979): Response of intestinal mucosa to gluten challenge in autistic children. *Lancet* **ii,** 877–878.

Mitchell, M., Robinson, T.J. (1996): Gluten sensitivety and neurological dysfunction. *Lancet* **i,** 904.

Molteni, N., Bardella, M.T., Baldassarri, A.R. & Bianchi, P.A. (1988): Coeliac disease associated with epilepsy and intracranial calcifications: report of two patients. *Am. J. Gastroenterol.* **83,** 992–994.

Morris, J.S., Ajdukiewicz, A.B. & Read, A.E. (1970): Neurological disorders and adult coeliac disease. *Gut* **11,** 549–554.

Muller, A.F., Donnelly, M.T., Smith., C.M.L. Grundman, M.J., Holmes, G.K.T., Toghill, P.J. (1996). Neurological complications of coeliac disease: a rare but continuing problem. *Am. J. Gastroenterol.* **91,** 1430–1435.

Muller, D.P.R. (1986): Vitamin E its role in neurological function. *Postgrad. Med. J.* **62,** 107–112.

Muller, D.P.R., Lloyd, J.K. & Wolff, O.H. (1983): Vitamin E and neurological dysfunction. *Lancet* **i,** 225–228.

Mumford, C.J., Fletcher, N.A., Ironside, J.W., Warlow, C.P. (1996) Progressive ataxia, focal seizures, and malabsorption syndrome in a 41 year old woman. *J. Neurol. Neurosurg. Psych.* **60**, 225–230.

Pallis, C.A. & Lewis, C.D. (1974): Neurology of gastrointestinal disease. London: Saunders.

Parry, T. E. (1990) Folate deficiency neuropathy. *Acta Haematol.* **84,** 108.

Paulley, J.W. (1959): Emotion and personality aetiology of steatorrhoea. *Am. J. Dig. Dis.* **4,** 352–360.

Piattella, L., Zamponi, N., Cardinali, C., Porfiri, L. & Tavoni, M.A. (1993): Endocranial calcifications, infantile coeliac disease, and epilepsy. *Child's Nerv. Syst.* **9,** 172–175.

Quigley, E.M.M., Carmichael, A. & Watkinson, G. (1986): Adult coeliac disease (coeliac sprue), pemicious anaemia and IgA deficiency. *J. Clin. Gastroenterol.* **8,** 277–281.

Richmond, J. & Davidson, S. (1958): Subacute combined degeneration of the spinal cord in non-Addisonian megaloblastic anaemia. *Quart. J. Med.* **27,** 517–531.

Rosenblum, J.L., Keating, J.P., Prensky, A.L. & Nelson, J.S. (1981): A progressive neurologic syndrome in children with chronic liver disease. *N. Eng. J. Med.* **304,** 503–508.

Rossi, E. (1982): Monosymptomatic forms of coeliac disease. *Eur. J. Paediatr.* **138,** 4–5.

Rush, P.J., Inman. R., Bernstein, M., Carlen, P. & Resch, L. (1986): Isolated vasculitis of the central nervous system in a patient with coeliac disease. *Am. J. Med.* **81,** 1092–1094.

Ryan, F.P., Timperley, W.R., Preston, F.E. & Holdsworth, C.D. (1977): Cerebral involvement with disseminated intravascular coagulation in intestinal disease. *J. Clin. Path.* **30,** 551–555.

Sammaritano, M., Andermann, F., Melanson, D., Guberman, A., Tinuper, P. & Gastaut, H. (1988): The syndrome of intractable epilepsy, bilateral occipital calcifications, and folic acid deficiency. *Neurology* **38,** (Suppl. 1) 239.

Sander, J.W.A. & Shorvon, S.D. (1987); Incidence and prevalence studies in epilepsy and their methodological problems: a review. *J. Neurol. Neurosurg. Psych.* **50,** 829–839.

Sandyk, R. & Brennan M. J. W. (1983) Isolated ocular myopathy and coeliac disease in childhood. *Neurology* **33,** 792

Scott, J.M. (1992): Folate-vitamin B_{12} interrelationships in the central nervous system. *Proc. Nutr. Soc.* **51,** 219–224.

Sencer, W. (1957): Neurologic manifestations in the malabsorption syndrome. *J. Mt. Sinai. Hosp.* **24,** 331–345.

Shiner, M. (1963): Effect of gluten free diet in 17 patients with idiopathic steatorrhoea. *Am. J. Dig. Dis.* **8,** 969–983.

Singh, M.M. & Kay, S.R. (1976): Wheat gluten as a pathogenic factor in schizophrenia. *Science* **191,** 401–402.

Smith, I., Clayton, B.E. & Wolff, O.H. (1975): New variant of phenylketonuria with progressive neurological illness unresponsive to phenylalanine restriction. *Lancet* **i,** 1108–1111.

Smith, I., Howells, D.W. & Hyland, K. (1986): Pteridines and mono-amines: relevance to neurological damage. *Postgrad. Med. J.* **62,** 113–123.

Stene-Larsen, G., Mosvold, J. & Ly, B. (1988): Selective vitamin B_{12} malabsorption in adult coeliac disease. *Scand. J. Gastroenterol.* **23,** 1105–1108.

Stevens, F.M., Lloyd, R.S., Geraghty, S.M.J., Reynolds, M.T.G., Sarsfield, M.J., McNicholl, B., Fottrell, P.F., Wright, R. & McCarthy, C.F. (1977): Schizophrenia and coeliac disease–the nature of the relationship. *Psychol. Med.* **7,** 259–263.

Stewart, J.S., Pollock, D.J., Hoffbrand, A.V., Mollin, D.L. & Booth, C.C. (1967): A study of proximal and distal intestinal structure and absorptive function in idiopathic steatorrhoea. *Quart. J. Med.* **36,** 425–444.

Strachan, R.W. & Henderson, J.G. (1966): Dementia and folate deficiency. *Quart. J. Med.* **36,** 189–204.

Telerman-Toppet, N., Coers, C. & Desneux, J.J. (1969): Ophthalmoplegie externe progressive associee a une polyneuropathie sensitivomotrice chez un patient atteint de maladie coelique. *Revue Neurologique (Paris)* **121,** 57–70.

Tiacci, C., D'Alessandro, P., Cantisani, T.A., Piccirilli, M, Signorini, E., Pelli, M.A., Cavalletti, M.L., Castellucci, G., Palmeri, S., Battisti, C. & Federico, A. (1993): Epilepsy with bilateral occipital calcifications: Sturge–Weber variant or a different encephalopathy? *Epilepsia* **34,** 528–539.

Tison, F., Arne, P. & Henry, P. (1989): Myoclonus and adult coeliac disease. *J. Neurol.* **36,** 307–308.

Tomasi, L.G. (1979): Reversibility of human myopathy caused by vitamin E deficiency. *Neurology* **29,** 1182–1186.

Ventura, A., Bouquet, F., Sartorelli, C., Barbi, E., Torre, G. & Tommasini, G. (1991): Coeliac disease, folic acid deficiency and epilepsy with cerebral calcifications. *Acta Paediatr. Scand.* **80,** 559–562.

Walker-Smith, J.A. & Andrews, J. (1972): Alpha-l-antitrypsin, autism, and coeliac disease. *Lancet* **ii,** 883–884.

Ward, M.E., Murphy, J.T. & Greenberg, G.R. (1985): Coeliac disease and spinocerebellar degeneration with normal vitamin E status. *Neurology* **35,** 1199–1201.

Waters, W.E. & O'Connor, P.J. (1975): Prevalence of migraine. *J. Neurol. Neurosurg. Psych.* **38,** 613–616.

Woltman, H.W. & Heck F.J. (1937): Funicular degeneration of the spinal cord without pernicious anaemia. Neurological aspects of sprue, nontropical sprue and idiopathic steatorrhoea. *Arch. Int. Med.* **60,** 272–300.

Willison, H.J., Muller, D.P.R., Matthews, S., Jones, S., Kriss, A., Stead, R.J., Hodson, M.E. & Harding, A.E. (1985): A study of the relationship between neurological function and serum vitamin E concentrations in patients with cystic fibrosis. *J. Neurol. Neurosurg. Psych.* **48,** 1097–1102.

Zaniboni, M.G., Lambertini, A., Romeo, N., Conti, R., Ambrosioni, G., Gobbi, G., Ambrosetto, P., Santucci, M., Michelucci, R. & Tassinari, C.A. (1989): Coeliac disease and epilepsy with occipital calcification: an unusual association. In: *First Joint Meeting of the European Society of Paediatric Gastroenterology and Nutrition and Italian Society of Peadiatrics [Abstact book]* eds. G. Bianchini, S. Guandalini, G.L. De Angelis & J.A. Walker-Smith, September 21–23, 1989: 54, Parma.

Zioudrou, C., Streaty, R.A. & Klee, W.A. (1979): Opioid peptides derived from foods. *J. Biol. Chem.* **254,** 2446–2449.

Epilepsy and other neurological disorders in coeliac disease, edited by G. Gobbi *et al.*
© 1997 John Libbey & Company Ltd, pp. 265–270.

Chapter 35

Neurological disorders associated with adult coeliac disease: clinical and pathogenetic aspects

Antonio Federico, Carla Battisti and Maria Teresa Dotti

Neurometabolic Diseases Unit and Chair of Neurology (OPD), Institute of Neurological Sciences, Medical School, University of Siena, Viale Bracci – 53100 Siena, Italy

Introduction

Coeliac disease (non-tropical sprue) is a malabsorption syndrome characterized by loss of weight, steatorrhoea, diarrhoea, abdominal distension, flatulence, evidence of intestinal absorption, abnormal small bowel mucosa, and intolerance to gluten.

Neurologic complications in adult coeliac disease occur in about 10 per cent of patients and include peripheral neuropathy, myelopathy, encephalopathy, cerebellar encephalopathy, myopathy, leucoencephalopathy, myoclonus and seizures.

Here we review the different clinical presentations and discuss the pathogenetic mechanism which may be fundamental to this combination of disorders.

Adult coeliac disease and neurologic complications

Among 16 patients with neurologic disorders complicating coeliac disease (CD), Cooke & Smith (1966) noted that gastrointestinal manifestations preceded neurologic abnormalities in all but one, in whom gastrointestinal and neurologic symptoms coincided. A simultaneous onset of coeliac disease and neurologic symptoms was discovered in the cases reported by Finelli *et al.* (1980), Kinney *et al.* (1982), Tison *et al.* (1989), Ward *et al.* (1985), Lu *et al.* (1986), while a 15-year history of gluten enteropathy was reported in the case of Kaplan *et al.* (1988).

The gastrointestinal lesion is generally chronic and steatorrhoea is prominent when neurologic disturbancies start; the only patient in whom the neurologic signs predated the malabsorption syndrome had been on chronic steroid therapy, which was postulated to prevent the development of intestinal symptoms (Binder *et al.*, 1967).

Adult coeliac disease presenting as cerebellar syndrome and/or myoclonic ataxia

The main clinical neurologic findings in adults with coeliac disease consist of a cerebellar syndrome characterized by ataxia, marked speech impairement (associated in some cases with memory loss), myoclonus, fibrillation and hypoareflexia.

The most consistent neuropathologic changes are in the cerebellum, deep-grey and brain-stem nuclei, and spinal cord. There is a variable but generally severe depopulation of Purkinje cells with associated gliosis and loss of granule cells. In contrast to alcoholic cerebellar degeneration (Victor & Ferrendelli, 1970; Adams, 1976) the cortical atrophy involves all folia without regionalization. The neuronal loss and gliosis in the dentate nuclei and inferior olive also distinguishes this disorder from nutritional cerebellar degeneration. Focal neuronal loss and/or gliosis in deep-grey and brain-stem nuclei are evident, mainly involving thalamus, caudate nucleus, globus pallidus, putamen, amygdala, anterior hypothalamic nuclei, periaqueductal grey, corpora quadrigemina, substantia nigra, red nuclei, and motor and sensory cranial nerve nuclei. In the spinal cord, symmetrical demyelination of posterior columns, especially the fasciculus gracilis and lateral columns, is evident. In some patients neuronal changes and gliosis of anterior horns are present.

In the cerebral cortex, focal neuronal atrophy and/or loss, chromatolysis and gliosis are found.

Finelli *et al.* (1980) first reported myoclonus associated with adult coeliac disease–cerebellar syndrome: it was palatal myoclonus, combined with rhythmic tremor of the eyelids; chin-myoclonus has been described by Kinney *et al.* (1982).

Reviewing 14 consecutive patients with Ramsay-Hunt syndrome (a descriptive term indicating patients with progressive cerebellar ataxia, seizures and severe myoclonus), Lu *et al.* (1986) found two cases with coeliac disease. More recently, Tison *et al.* (1989) described a 56-year old woman with cortical and palatal myoclonus in combination with subcortical white matter changes on magnetic resonance and a moderate vitamin E deficiency.

Distal axonopathy associated with chronic gluten enteropathy

Peripheral neuropathy is rarely described and it is often overshadowed by cerebellar dysfunction, myelopathy or dementia. Isolated peripheral neuropathy was reported by Cooke & Smith (1966, five cases), by Bannerji & Hurwitz (1971, two cases), Binder *et al.* (1967, two cases), Farmer *et al.* (1964), Morris *et al.* (1970), and Kaplan *et al.* (1988). The disorder appears as an isolated peripheral neuropathy and is reversible when recognized and treated. None of the patients has signs of central nervous system (CNS) dysfunction. Neuropathy occurs later in the course of the disease, usually after moderate–severe steatorrhoea. Clinical signs are characterized by intense paresthesias, hyporeflexia, sensory ataxia, weakness. Nerve conduction velocities and biopsy studies show evidence of distal axonopathy in 83 per cent of cases. Neuropathy most frequently occurs without evidence of vitamin E or B deficiency and improves after gluten restriction.

Down's syndrome (DS) and coeliac disease

The association of Down's syndrome and coeliac disease has been described in several reports (Dias & Smith, 1990; Bentley, 1975; Howell *et al.*, 1983; Nowak *et al.*, 1983; Ruch *et al.*, 1985; Santer *et al.*, 1991; Simila & Kokkonen, 1990; Storm, 1990; Hilhorst *et al.*, 1993; Zubillaga *et al.*, 1993; Castro *et al.*, 1993).

Of 70 DS patients, Zubillaga *et al.* (1993) found positive IgA antigliadin antibodies in nine (13 per cent). Castro *et al.* (1993), examining 155 DS cases, found high IgA AGA levels in 26 per cent of DS patients, and total villous atrophy in seven of them (33 per cent), confirming the data about higher levels of IgA AGA in DS and the relatively high incidence of CD in this syndrome.

Coeliac disease and vitamin E

It is generally accepted that vitamin E deficiency causes a characteristic syndrome in children with cholestatic liver diseases. Low levels of serum vitamin E secondary to impaired fat absorption in the small intestine were also found in children with coeliac disease (Muller *et al.,* 1983). Weder *et al.* (1984) reported neurologic disorder and vitamin E deficiency in a 49-year old man with acquired intestinal malabsorption, in which neurologic symptoms appeared 15 years after the onset of a malabsorption syndrome.

In 1985, Ward *et al.* reported a 47-year-old man with spinocerebellar degeneration and malabsorption due to coeliac enteropathy: the serum vitamin E level was normal. However, a positive change of small bowel histology on a gluten-free diet and vitamin E therapy were described.

Tison *et al.* (1989) reported moderately low serum vitamin E levelin a patient with myoclonus and adult coeliac disease. Highly reduced serum level of vitamin E (10.5 – 8.4 µmoles/l n.v. 11–35) has been reported in two cases of Ramsay-Hunt syndrome and coeliac disease (Lu *et al.,* 1986).

Low levels of vitamin E have been reported in case 2 described by Binder *et al.* (1967) as a combination of coeliac disease and peripheral neuropathy.

Vitamin E deficiency has been implicated in the aetiology of neurologic disorders with chronic fat malabsorption in abetalipoproteinaemia (Muller & Lloyd, 1982), chronic cholestasis, cystic fibrosis (Sung *et al.,* 1980) and small bowel resection (Federico *et al.,* 1991). The neurological complications described in coeliac disease are similar. Coeliac patients lack the pigmentary retinal degeneration that is, on the other hand, a consistent feature of vitamin E-related forms of neurologic degeneration.

Case report

We describe an adult onset case of coeliac disease and severe vitamin E deficiency, neurologically characterized by cerebellar dysfunction and peripheral neuropathy (Battisti *et al.,* 1993). Significant clinical, neurophysiological and histological improvement with the recovery of normal serum levels of vitamin E have been obtained after prolonged vitamin E treatment and a gluten-free diet.

The patient was a 62-year-old architect with negative family and medical history. At the age of 56, he complained of abdominal symptoms with severe diarrhoea and steatorrhoea, associated with loss of weight (about 20 kg in 2 years). Six months later paresthesias of the fingers and toes, tremor of the hands and head gradually appeared in association with respiratory distress. Neurologic examination showed ataxic gait, diffuse muscle hypotrophy with slight hypotonia, hypopallestesia and hypoaestesia, weak deep tendon reflexes, dysmetria and positive Romberg sign.

Routine blood chemistry showed hypochromic anaemia, low cholesterol levels (118 mg/dl) and electrolyte deficiency (potassium 2.5 mEq/1, calcium 4 mEq/1, magnesium 0.89 mEq/1). Several aspecific indices of inflammation, such as C3, C4, VES, and C reactive protein were elevated. Folate (0.24 ng/ml, n.v. 3–17 ng/ml) and IgA (28 mg/dl, n.v. 90–450 mg/dl) levels, were low. FSH, LH, prolactin, GH, cortisol, calcitonin, vitamin D and vitamin B_{12}, T3, T4 and TSH were normal. No acanthocytes were evident and apoprotein assay revealed deficiency of Apo A1 (53.3 mg/100 ml, n.v. 102–215 mg/100 ml) and normal levels of Apo B (84 mg/100 ml). Antigliadin antibodies were within normal limits. Serum vitamin E was undetectable and an oral vitamin E loading test (2 g bolus) confirmed malabsorption.

At neurophysiological investigations sensory potentials could not be evoked in the right sural nerve and motor conduction velocity was slightly decreased (46.8 m/s) in the right deep peroneal nerve. Somatosensory evoked potentials (SEPs) in the lower limbs indicated bilateral cortical abnormalities (Cz') with increased central conduction time (CCT), suggesting medullary involvement. Motor evoked potentials (MEPs) were normal. Visual evoked potentials (VEPs) showed responses of extremely reduced amplitude to bilateral stimulation (suggesting foveal involvement). An electroretinogram (ERG) was severely impaired.

Brain NMR showed mild cortical atrophy mainly in frontal and parietal regions.

Ultrastructural examination of skin biopsy showed lipofuscin storage in cytoplasm of endothelial and glandular cells. Methylene blue-stained semithin cross sections of the sural nerve after biopsy showed reduction of large myelinated axons and single-fibre degeneration.

A jejunal biopsy showed chronic duodenal inflammation with almost total atrophy of the villi and hyperplasia of the crypts. Coeliac disease was diagnosed and the patient was put on a gluten-free diet.

Chronic vitamin E supplementation and gluten-free diet were able to improve the clinical signs and to normalize the serum vitamin E level. A second skin biopsy performed after 2 years was normal, in particular with the disappearance of lipofuscin material previously detected in dermal cells.

Pseudo-glutaric aciduria type II in a patient with coeliac disease

A possibility of misdiagnosis of a rare neurometabolic disorder in presence of coeliac disease has been reported by Largilliere *et al.* (1993). They described a 6-month-old boy, with vomiting, failure to thrive, hypotonia, hypotrophy and amyotrophy. Urinary examination of dicarboxylic acids (glutaric acid, adipic acid, suberic acid, dodecanoid acid, etilmalonic acid) showed a profile compatible with a diagnosis of glutaric aciduria type II.

To investigate the possibility of malabsorption, intestinal biopsy was performed which showed total villous atrophy suggestive of coeliac disease. Gluten-free diet (with carnitine and riboflavine) led to dramatic clinical improvement and progressive normalization of urinary organic acid excretion after 2 months. Primitive glutaric aciduria type II was excluded by measurement of myristate oxidation on skin fibroblasts.

Glutaric aciduria in this patient may be due to coeliac disease and the pathogenesis could be due to a subclinical deficiency of riboflavin, cofactor of acyl-CoA dehydrogenases, which is very sensitive to riboflavin deficiency.

Some digestive diseases with subclinical deficiency caused by malabsorption could be misdiagnosed as inherited mitochondrial fatty acid oxidation defects if enzymatic studies are not carried out.

Conclusions

It appears clear that a number of adults with coeliac disease may be at risk of superimposed neurological disorders of the central and/or peripheral nervous system whose pathogenesis is not known.

An underlying immunologic disorder involving both the small bowel and neural tissues has been proposed as a direct effect of gluten toxicity on the CNS (Dohan, 1983). Alteration in the CNS monoamine metabolism in untreated coeliac disease has also been described (Hallert & Sedvall, 1983). As reported by Kinney *et al.* (1982), the CNS degeneration may reflect a neuronal insult related to toxins accumulation in the intestinal tract or to deficiency of nutrient substances vital to the integrity of the central and peripheral nervous system. The finding of abnormal amounts of vitamin E in the serum in several neurologic patients with complicated CD, and some similarities with the clinical signs of primary vitamin E deficiency, may lead to speculation about a possible role of an abnormality in peroxidation and free radicals in the pathogenesis of the neuronal and myelin changes. Because only few patients with CD develop neurologic complications it is possible that these patients may have an inborn predisposition to develop such disease under appropriate environmental stress, as clearly indicated in the case of pseudoglutaric aciduria II (Fig. 1).

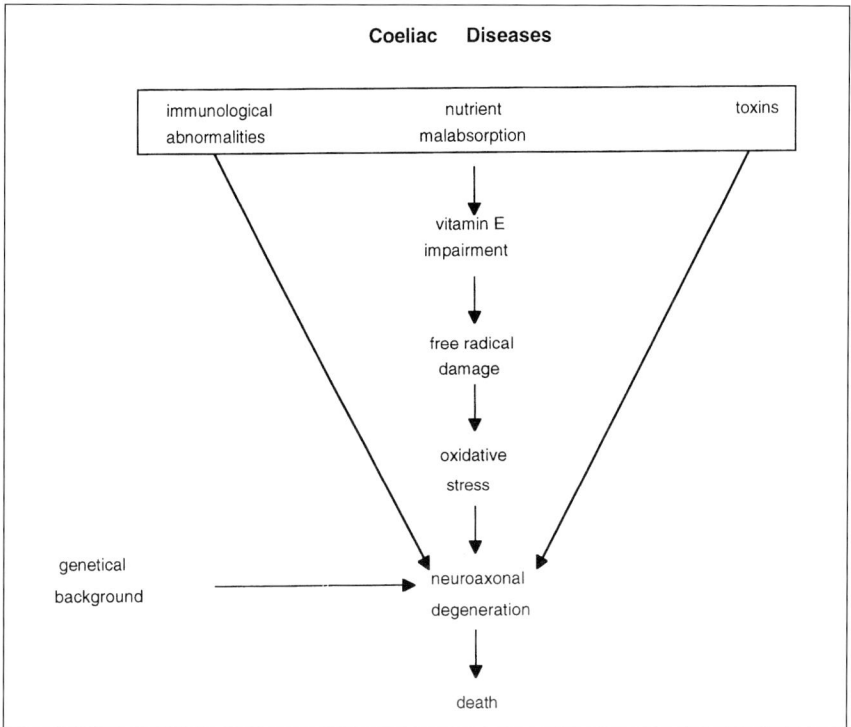

Fig. 1.

Acknowledgement

Research in part supported by a grant from Regione Toscana and MURST to AF.

References

Adams, R.D. (1976): Nutritional cerebellar degeneration. In: *Handbook of clinical neurology,* Vol. 28, (Metabolic and deficiency diseases of the nervous system Part II), eds. P.J. Vinken & G.W. Bruyn, pp. 271–283. Amsterdam: North Holland.

Amil Dias, J. & Walker-Smith, J. (1990): Down's syndrome and coeliac disease. *J. Pediatr. Gastroenterol. Nutr.* **10,** 41–43.

Bannerji, N.K. & Hurwitz, L.J. (1971): Neurological manifestations in adult steatorrhea (probably gluten enteropathy). *J. Neurol. Sci.* **14,** 125–141.

Battisti, C., Bonuccelli, U., Dotti, M.T., Maremmani, C., Muratorio, A., Malandrini, A. & Federico, A. (1993): Late onest multisystem disorder associated with coeliac disease and vitamin E deficiency (clinical, histopathological and biochemical study). *Ital. J. Neurol. Sci.* **14,** (Suppl.7), 113.

Bentley, D. (1975): A case of Down's syndrome complicated by retinoblastoma and coeliac disease. *Pediatrics* **56,** 131–133.

Binder, H.J., Solitare, C.B. & Spiro, H.M. (1967): Neuromuscular disease in patients with steatorrhea. *Gut* **8,** 605–611.

Castro, M., Crino, A., Papadatou, B., Purpura, M., Giannotti, A., Ferretti, F., Colistro, F., Mottola, L., Digilio, M.C., Lucidi, V. & Borrellli, P. (1993): Down's syndrome and coeliac disease: the prevalence of high IgA-antigliadin antibodies and HLA-DR and DQ antigens in trisomy 21. *J. Pediatr. Gastroenterol.* **16,** 265–268.

Cooke, W.T. & Smith, W.T. (1966): Neurological disorders associated with coeliac disease. *Brain* **89,** 683–722.

Dohan, F.C. (1983): More on coeliac disease as a model for schizophrenia. *Biol. Psychiat.* **18,** 561–564.

Farmer, R.G. & Richards, N.G. (1964): Malabsorption syndrome and peripheral neuropathy. *Cleve. Clin. Q.* **31**, 163–168.

Federico, A., Battisti, C., Eusebi, M.P., De Stefano, N., Malandrini, A., Mondelli, M. & Volpi, N. (1991): Vitamin E deficiency secondary to chronic intestinal malabsorption and effect of vitamin supplement: a case report. *Europ. Neurol.* **31**, 366–371.

Finelli, P.F., McEntee, W.J., Ambler, M. & Kestenbaum, D. (1980): Adult coeliac disease presenting as a cerebellar syndrome. *Neurology* **30**, 245–249.

Hallert, C. & Sedvall, G. (1983): Improvement in central monoamine metabolism in adult coeliac patients starting a gluten free diet. *Psychol. Med.* **13**, 267–271.

Hilhorst, M.I., Brink, M., Wauters, E.A.K. & Houwen, R.H.J. (1993): Down's syndrome and coeliac disease: five new cases with a review of the literature. *Eur. J. Pediat.* **152**, 884–887.

Howell, S.J.L., Foster, K.J. & Reckless, J. (1983): Protracted survival in patients with Down's syndrome. *BMJ* **287**, 1429–1430.

Kaplan, J.G., Pack D., Horoupian, D., Desouza, T., Brin, M. & Schaumburg, H. (1988): Distal axonopathy associated with chronic gluten enteropathy: a treatable disorder. *Neurology* **38**, 642–645.

Kinney, H.C., Burger, P.C., Hurwitz, B.J., Humans, J.C. & Grant, J.P. (1982): Degeneration of central nervous system associated with coeliac disease. *J. Neurol. Sci.* **53**, 9–22.

Largilliere, C., Fontaine, M., Marrakchi, S. & Voisin-Tabourreau, O. (1993): Pseudo-glutaric aciduria type II in a patient with coeliac disease. *J. Pediat.* **123**, 504.

Lu, C.S., Thompson, P.D., Quinn, N., Parkes, J.D. & Marsden, C.D. (1986): Ramsay Hunt syndrome and coeliac disease: a new association? *Mov. Dis.* **1**, 209–219.

Morris, J.S., Ajdukiewicz, A.B. & Read, A.E. (1970): Neurological disorders and adult coeliac disease. *Gut* **11**, 549–554.

Muller, D.P.R. & Lloyd, J.K. (1982): Effect of large oral dose of vitamin E on the neurological sequelae of patients with abetalipoproteinemia. *Ann. NY. Acad. Sci.* **393**, 133–144.

Muller, D.P.R. Lloyd, J.K. & Wolff, O.H. (1983): Vitamin E and neurological function. *Lancet* **i**, 225–227.

Nowak, T.V., Ghishan, F.K. & Schulze-Delrieu, K. (1983): Coeliac sprue in Down's syndrome: considerations on a pathogenetic link. *Am. J. Gastroenterol.* **78**, 280–283.

Ruch, W., Schurmann, K., Gordon, P., Burgin-Wolff, A. & Girard, J. (1985): Coexistent coeliac disease, Graves disease and diabetes mellitus type I in a patient with Down syndrome. *Eur. J. Pediatr.* **144**, 89–90.

Santer, R., Sievers, E. & Oldigs, H.D. (1991): Coeliac disease in Down's syndrome. *J. Pediatr. Gastroenterol. Nutr.* **13**, 121.

Simila, S. & Kokkonen, J. (1990): Coexistence of coeliac disease and Down's syndrome. *Am. J. Ment. Ret.* **95**, 120–122.

Storm, W. (1990): Prevalence and diagnostic significance of gliadin antibodies in children with Down syndrome. *Eur. J. Pediatr.* **149**, 833–834.

Sung, J.H., Park, S.H., Mastri, A.R. & Warwick, W.J. (1980): Axonal dystrophy in the gracile nucleus in congenital biliary atresia and cystic fibrosis (mucoviscidosis): beneficial effect of vitamin E therapy. *J. Neuropathol. Exp. Neurol.* **39**, 584–597.

Tison, F., Arne, P. & Henry, P. (1989): Myoclonus and adult coeliac disease. *J. Neurol.* **236**, 307–308.

Victor, M. & Ferrendelli, J.A. (1970): The nutritional and metabolic diseases of the cerebellum – clinical and pathological aspects. In: *The cerebellum in health and disease*, eds. W.S. Fields & W.D. Willis, pp. 412–449. St. Louis MO: Warren H Green Inc.

Ward, M.E., Murphy, J.T. & Greenberg, G.R. (1985): Coeliac disease and spinocerebellar degeneration with normal vitamin E status. *Neurology* **35**, 1199–1201.

Weder, B., Meinberg, O., Wildi, E. & Meier, C. (1984): Neurologic disorders of vitamin E deficiency in acquired intestinal malabsorption. *Neurology* **334**, 1561–1565.

Zubillaga, P., Vitoria, J. C., Arrieta, A., Echaniz, P. & Garci-Masdevall, M.D. (1993): Down's syndrome and coeliac disease. *J. Pediatr. Gastroenterol.* **16**, 168–171.

Epilepsy and other neurological disorders in coeliac disease, edited by G. Gobbi *et al.*
© 1997 John Libbey & Company Ltd, pp. 271–274.

Chapter 36

Progressive myoclonic ataxia associated with coeliac disease

Kailash P. Bhatia and C. David Marsden

University Department of Clinical Neurology, Institute of Neurology, Queen Square, London WC1N 3BG, UK

Introduction

Neurological disorders can occur in 10 per cent of patients with coeliac disease (Finelli *et al.*, 1980) and although seizures are commonly described, reports of a myoclonic syndrome in coeliac disease have been rare (Finelli *et al.*, 1980; Kinney *et al.*, 1982). In 1986, our group described two cases of progressive myoclonic ataxia (PMA) associated with coeliac disease (Lu *et al.*, 1986), but we wondered whether this was a chance association as coeliac diease is fairly common in the general population. Subsequently two other cases of myoclonic syndromes associated with coeliac disease were reported (Brucke *et al.*, 1988; Tison *et al.*, 1989). Brucke *et al.* (1988) described a 45-year-old man with coeliac disease with pathologically proven brainstem encephalitis who presented with tongue and palatal myoclonus, mild dysarthria and ataxia. Tison *et al.* (1989) reported a 56-year-old woman who developed stimulus-sensitive myoclonus of the upper limbs, neck, lower face and palate, one month after the diagnosis of coeliac disease at a time when the gastrointestinal symptoms were improving on a gluten-free diet. Electrophysiological studies suggested that the myoclonus was of cortical origin. Recently, we described four further patients with a progressive myoclonic ataxic syndrome associated with coeliac disease (Bhatia *et al.*, 1995) and these cases are summarized here.

Case summaries

Case 1 (AH). This 44-year-old man presented with a three year history of involuntary jerking of the limbs. The onset was in the fingers of the the left hand and then spread to the legs, causing many falls. There was no history of malabsorption. In the past he had developed dermatitis herpetiformis which was treated with dapsone for 7 years with resolution of symptoms. Examination revealed spontaneous and stimulus-sensitive myoclonus of all limbs, with mild gait ataxia. Eye movements and the rest of the neurological examination were normal. Psychometry revealed a verbal IQ of 114 and a performance IQ of 100. Investigations included normal haematological and biochemical screens, autoantibodies, anti-reticulin, anti-gliadin anti-Hu and anti-purkinje cell antibodies, white cell enzymes, spinal fluid analysis and serological tests for infection. There was no evidence of mitochondrial cytopathy on muscle biopsy blood DNA analysis. Endoscopic duodenal biopsy showed typical changes consistent with coeliac disease. The MRI brain scan showed mild cerebral

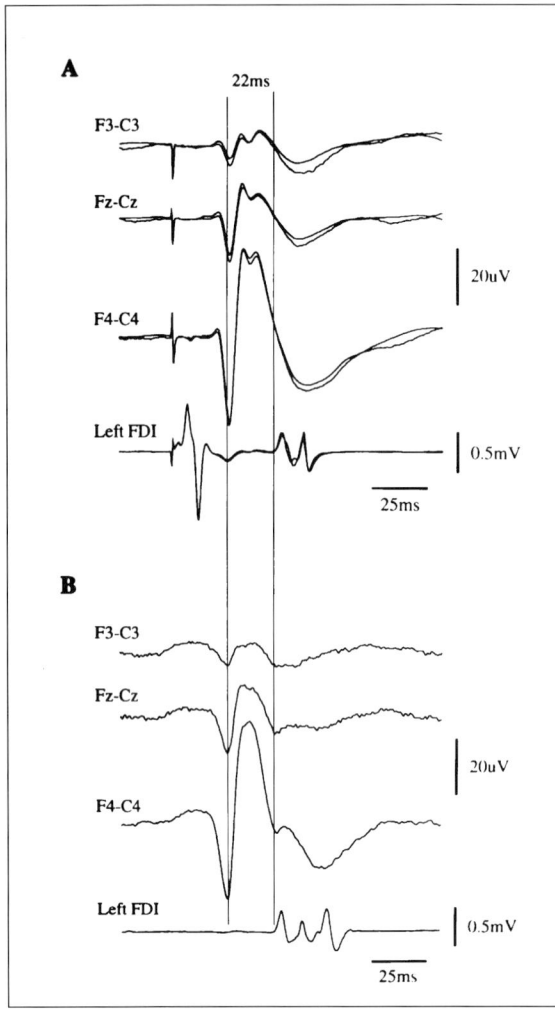

Fig. 1. (A) Cortical SEPs to electrical stimulation of the left ulnar nerve at the wrist and (B) back-averaged EEG activity preceding voluntary action jerks in case 1. (A). Two superimposed averages of 256 shocks. A giant P1N2 complex is clearly seen, largest contralateral to the stimulated limb (F4-C4). The P1 wave is followed 22 ms later by a C reflex in the left first dorsal interosseus (FDI0. A similar delay was recorded to this muscle with transcutaneous magnetic stimulation of the motor cortex. (B).Back-average of 30 jerks in the left FDI. A positive cortical wave precedes myoclonic activity by 22 ms. This EEG wave is maximal contralateral to the moved hand (F4-C4). Reprinted with permission of Oxford University Press.

and cerebellar atrophy. Electrophysiological studies confirmed the presence of both cortical action and reflex myoclonus (Fig. 1A, B). EEG showed frequent centro-parietal epileptiform discharges most marked on the right. Treatment with clonazepam, piracetam and subsequently sodium valproate improved control of the myoclonic jerks to some extent.

However his neurological condition gradually deteriorated despite plasma exchanges which were undertaken without sustained benefit. The patient comitted suicide. A limited post-mortem examination of the brain (1275 g) was possible which revealed no abnormality, except for histological changes in the cerebellar hemispheres which showed Purkinje cell loss and marked Bergmann astrocytosis. There was also astrocytosis of the dentate nucleus and the inferior olives which showed mild neuronal loss. No vasculitis was found.

Case 2 (BH). At age 60 years, this woman was diagnosed to have coeliac disease on duodenal biopsy when investigated for diarrhoea, weight loss, and anaemia. On a gluten-free diet and supplements she regained weight and her symptoms resolved, although two subsequent duodenal biopsies showed persistent pathological changes without histological improvement. Seven years later she developed spontaneous myoclonic jerks initially of the left leg and then the right leg causing many falls. On examination she had decreased visual acuity and colour vision due to previous retinal vein haemorrhage. Spontaneous and stimulus-sensitive myoclonus was evident in the left leg and to a lesser extent in the right leg, triggered by touch, pin-prick, and tendon taps. The rest of the examination was normal except for reduced touch and vibration sense in a glove and stocking distribution and mild dysdiadochokinesis of the upper limbs. Neuropsychological testing showed evidence of mild cognitive decline.

Haematological and biochemical screens, folate, vitamin B_{12} and calcium levels were normal. An auto-antibody screen including anti-endomysial, anti-gliadin and anti-GAD antibodies was negative. Nerve conduction studies revealed a mild sensory neuropathy. An EEG showed mildly abnormal theta activity in the right posterior temporal region but no definite epileptic activity. CT brain scan was normal. Electrophysiological studies confirmed that the myoclonus was of cortical origin.

Case 3 (NS). This 52-year-old left handed man developed anaemia and abdominal pain at age 25 and was subsequently found to have coeliac disease, with subtotal villous atrophy on duodenal biopsy. His symptoms improved on a gluten-free diet and supplements. At age 50 years, he developed an intermittent action tremor of the left hand and involuntary jerky movements of the right foot. That year he had one generalized tonic–clonic seizure which began with involuntary jerking of the right foot. The neurological examination was normal except for action myoclonus and dystonic posturing of the right foot and a mild action tremor of the left hand.

Haematological and biochemical investigations were normal. Auto-antibody screen was negative and antineuronal antibodies were not detected. Brain and spinal cord MRI were normal. Neuropsychological assessment found evidence of deficits in tests of abstraction and reasoning suggesting frontal lobe dysfunction. An electroencephalogram was normal and detailed electrophysiology revealed findings typical of cortical reflex myoclonus.

Drug therapy including sodium valproate and clonazepam were found to be of limited benefit. Plasma exchanges were undertaken but did not produce a sustained benefit, nor did subsequent treatment with cyclophosphamide.

Case 4 (MH). This woman developed malabsorption at age 48 years and a diagnosis of coeliac disease was confirmed on jejunal biopsy. Her symptoms responded to a gluten-free diet; 10 years later, she developed dysarthria and ataxia and involuntary jerks of her arms. Examination revealed an ataxic gait and myoclonus of the face and legs without evidence of a cognitive decline. At age 62 years, she had a repeat intestinal biopsy due to weight loss which showed partial villous atrophy suggestive of a partial response to diet. Her condition deteriorated and she developed generalized seizures. She received treatment with carbamazepine, phenytoin, prednisolone, azathioprine, imipramine, vitamin E and iron supplements, without benefit. Haematological and biochemical investigations, vitamin E, vitamin B_{12} levels, auto-antibody screens, and reticulin antibodies were all negative or normal. On one occasion the CSF contained 12 white cells (eight lymphocytes, four polymorphs) protein 4.2 g/l, and normal glucose. On another occasion the CSF contained six lymphocytes, and protein of 1.4 g/l. MRI brain scan showed multiple tiny high signal areas in the white matter of both hemispheres. A right carotid cerebral angiogram was normal. An EEG showed multifocalpolyspike and slow-wave paroxysmal activity with no photosensitivity. Her condition progressively worsened and terminally she became demented.

Discussion

The four cases described here are similar to the two reported previously by our group (Lu *et al.*, 1986) and to the case described by Tison *et al.* (1989), suggesting that there is a definite association between coeliac disease and the PMA syndrome seen in these patients. These seven cases had a characteristic phenotype dominated by action myoclonus (7/7) with prominent stimulus sensitivity in some (4/7); mild cerebellar ataxia (6/7); and infrequent seizures (4/7). Detailed electrophysiological assessment revealed a cortical origin for the myoclonus in five of these cases.

The other three reported cases of myoclonus associated with coeliac disease are somewhat different (Finelli *et al.*, 1980; Kinney *et al.*, 1982; Brucke *et al.*, 1988). Myoclonus was a minor and a late feature of clinical syndromes dominated by other signs, e.g. internuclear opthalmoplegia and pyramidal signs (Finelli *et al.*, 1980), and dementia (Kinney *et al.*, 1982). Two of these cases had palatal myoclonus and other prominent brain-stem signs (Finelli *et al.*, 1980; Brucke *et al.*, 1988), perhaps suggesting a brain-stem origin of their myoclonus. Interestingly, in the seven typical cases of PMA, the neurological syndrome appeared after the onset of the gastrointestinal manifestations of coeliac disease, often as the patients showed symptomatic (and in some cases histological) improvement of their gastrointestinal symptoms on a gluten-free diet. Furthermore, despite improvement of the gastrointestinal symptoms on a gluten-free diet, the neurological syndrome usually showed steady progression perhaps suggesting that the neurological symptoms were not due to the malabsorption itself. There has been speculation that the cause of neurological dysfunction in coeliac disease may be due to altered immune function (Cooper *et al.*, 1978; Perry *et al.*, 1986; Gobbi *et al.*, 1992). However, we did not detect antineuronal or other antibodies in our patients and plasmapheresis in two of these patients, one of whom subsequently was also treated with immunosuppressive drugs, did not improve their neurological condition.

In conclusion, it appears that PMA associated with coeliac disease is a definite entity which should be considered in the differential diagnosis of all patients presenting with this syndrome. The exact pathophysiological basis of this association is still unclear.

Acknowledgements

We thank Drs R. Gregory, G.G. Lennox, H. Manji for referring their patients to us. We also thank Dr P. Brown for providing the results of electrophysiological studies of the myoclonus in these patients and Dr D.W. Ellison for the neuropathology report on case 1. We would also like to thank Oxford University Press for giving us permission to use the data of the four cases cited here from the original publication in *Brain* (1995), **118**, 1087–1093.

References

Bhatia, K.P., Brown, P., Gregory, R., Lennox, G.G., Manji, H., Thompson, P.D., Ellison, D.W. & Marsden, C.D. (1995): Progressive myoclonic ataxia associated with coeliac disease. The myoclonus is of cortical origin, but the pathology is in the cerebellum. *Brain* **118**, 1087-1093.

Brucke, T., Kollegger, H., Schmidbauer, M., Muller, C., Podreka, I. & Deecke, L. (1988): Adult coeliac disease and brain stem encephalitis. *J. Neurol. Neurosurg. Psychiatry.* **51**, 456–457.

Cooper, B.T., Holmes, G.K.T. & Cooke, W.T. (1978): Coeliac disease and immunological disorders. *BMJ* **i**, 537–539.

Finelli, P.F., McEntee, W.J., Ambler, M. & Kestenbaum, D. (1980): Adult coeliac disease presenting as a cerebellar syndrome. *Neurology* **30**, 245–249.

Gobbi, G., Bouquet, F., Greco, L., Lambertini, A., Tassinari, C.A., Ventura, A. & Zaniboni, M.G. (1992): Coeliac disease, epilepsy and cerebral calcifications. *Lancet* **340**, 439–443.

Kinney, H.C., Burger, P.C., Hurwitz, B.J., Hijmans, J.C. & Grant, J.P. (1982): Degeneration of the central nervous system associated with coeliac disease. *J. Neurol. Sci.* **53**, 9–22.

Lu, C.S., Thompson, P.D., Quinn, N.P., Parkes, J.D. & Marsden, C.D. (1986): Ramsay Hunt syndrome and coeliac disease: a new association? *Mov. Dis.* **1**, 209–219.

Perry, R.J., Inman, R., Bernstein, M., Carlen, P. & Resch, L. (1989): Isolated vasculitis of the central nervous system in a patient with coeliac disease. *Am. J. Med.* **81**, 1092–1094.

Tison, F., Arne, P. & Henry, P. (1989): Myoclonus and adult coeliac disease. *J. Neurol.* **236**, 307–308.

Epilepsy and other neurological disorders in coeliac disease, edited by G. Gobbi *et al.*
© 1997 John Libbey & Company Ltd, pp. 275–284.

Chapter 37

Neurological complications associated with coeliac disease: a personal study

Luigi Piattella*, Nelia Zamponi*, Cesare Cardinali*, Giuseppe Caramia**,
Rolando Gagliardini** and Roberto Rossi***

*Children's Neuropsychiatry Division, **Paediatric Division, 'G. Salesi' Regional Paediatric Hospital, Via
Corridoni 12, Ancona; ***Radiology, I.N.R.C.A, Via della Montagnola, Ancona, Italy*

Introduction

Coeliac disease is a malabsorption syndrome characterized by chronic gluten intolerance. Although its aetiology is unknown, an immunologic mechanism seems to be prominent. Numerous neurological and psychiatric disorders can be related to coeliac disease ranging from 10 to 30 per cent of all cases, depending upon the various case histories. The more frequent complications are epilepsy, mental retardation, schizophrenia, organic dementia, cerebellar disorders, myopathy and peripheral neuropathy. Over the last ten years, numerous cases have been reported, mostly in Italy, of coeliac patients affected by epilepsy having biooccipital cerebral calcifications, to the extent that a specific syndrome (CEC) has been identified and its clinical, electroencephalographic and neuroradiological characteristics defined (Fois *et al.*, 1994; Gobbi *et al.*, 1992; Molteni *et al.*, 1988; Piattella *et al.*, 1986; Piattella *et al.*, 1987; Piattella *et al.*, 1987; Piattella *et al.* 1990; Piattella *et al.*, 1993; Sammaritano, 1985; Sammaritano *et al.*, 1988; Zaniboni *et al.*, 1989).

Materials and methods

Data are reported regarding the neurological complications observed during the course of coeliac disease in 58 patients (15 M, 43 F), mean age 12.5 years, admitted to the Pediatric Neuropsychiatry Division and to the Medicine Division of the Regional Paediatric Hospital of Ancona. The diagnosis of coeliac disease was defined according to the criteria of either ESPGAN or the Paediatric Gastroenterology Group (1987). Coeliac disease was subdivided according to initial symptoms and the results of laboratory investigation into three categories: typical, atypical or latent. At diagnosis, the age of the patients was less than 6 years in 35 cases, between 6 and 12 in 10, and over 12 years in the remaining 13. All patients underwent dietary therapy and were periodically checked both from a clinical standpoint as well as with biochemical tests (AGA, antiendomysial antibodies, nutritional indices, complete haematological profile, etc.). Furthermore, positive anamnaestic factors for headaches, convulsions, behavioural and psychic disorders and peripheral nervous system disorders specifically questionned. All patients underwent a neurological examination and EEG. In patients with neurological symptoms and/or altered EEG, the neurodiagnostic investigation was followed by neuroradiological (CT, MRI, SPECT), and neurophysiological (EP, EMG, MCV, SCV) examinations and psychodiagnostic evaluation.

Results

The more frequently observed neurological disorders were:

- Cerebral calcifications + epilepsy – 5
- Epilepsy without calcifications – 1
- Acute cerebral ischaemia – 1
- Migraine headaches – 4
- Cerebral neoplasia (with epilepsy) – 2
- Febrile convulsions – 3
- Isolated EEG alterations –3
- Psychiatric disorders– 2

Cerebral calcifications – epilepsy – coeliac disease

From 1983 onwards, there have been ever-increasing reports of Sturge–Weber-like bioccipital cerebral calcifications in patients affected by epilepsy and other neurological disorders; some of these patients were also shown to have coeliac disease.Therefore, an aetiopathogenic correlation has been suggested between the intestinal pathology and the cerebral parenchymal alterations found on neuroradiological examination. The pathogenesis of the calcified lesions and, more generally, of the neuropathological lesions found in patients with coeliac disease (gliosis, focal neuronal loss, chromatolysis, axonal damage, demyelination), is still unknown although various mechanisms have been invoked:

- folic acid deficiency with consequent mineralizing microangiopathy and alteration of the normal myelinization process (Bye *et al.*, 1993; Fois *et al.*, 1994; Garwicz & Mortennson, 1976; Piattella *et al.*, 1987; Piatella, 1990; Sammaritano *et al.*, 1988);

- vitamin and oligoelement deficiency, particularly selenium and vitamin E (Gregori *et al.*, 1988; Ward *et al.*, 1985);

- mechanisms of an immunological type causing repeated vasculitises with consequent damage to the surrounding cerebral parenchyma. The chronic hypoperfusion and successive calcium and, perhaps, silicon deposits would represent the eventual evolution of the disease (Fois *et al.*, 1994; Gobbi *et al.*, 1992). The anatomico–pathological alterations seen in those rare cases where biopsy of the calcific lesions has been carried out show vascular anomalies (intimal fibrosis, pial angiomatosis, microcalcifications) similar to, but not identical to, those found in Sturge–Weber disease (Bye *et al.*, 1993).

In recent years, five subjects of paediatric age affected by epilepsy, endocranial calcifications and coeliac disease were identified at the Pediatric Neuropsychiatry Division of the Regional Paediatric Hospital of Ancona; in particular, all cases had an atypical form of coeliac disease in that no intestinal symptoms were readily apparent, but rather the syndrome was manifested by low stature, constipation, pubertal retardation and anaemia.

The five patients (3 F, 2 M), ranging from 6 to 15 years of age, were admitted for observation due to epileptic syndromes of varying seriousness. In particular, two of the subjects had rare seizures at the outset, and these were partial and secondarily generalized, associated with slow EEG anomalies and centro-posterior foci; the evolution of the epileptic symptoms was favourable in both cases, entirely independent of dietary therapy.

The other three patients presented a clinical-EEG picture characteristic of the CEC syndrome recently identified and amply described in the literature (drug-resistant partial epilepsy with early onset polymorphous seizures evolving in phases, EEG alterations characterized by biooccipital focal anomalies suppressed by eye opening, psychointellectual regression). Its subsequent clinical evolution over a long-term follow-up (in some cases more than 10 years) has shown persistence of the drug-resistant epilepsy and psychic regression in two cases; in the third case, the seizures have disappeared, EEG has normalized, and psychointellectual capabilities have improved, and antiepileptic therapy could be discontinued. In this patient, the seizures were already under control by antiepileptic therapy at the time dietary therapy was initiated. The parenchymal structural alterations persisted without change over the entire period of observation. One year after therapy was suspended, the patient developed insulin-dependent diabetes.

The diagnostic investigations showed the following:

• Anti-gliadin antibodies (AGA) and jejunal biopsy compatible in all cases with the presence of coeliac disease;

• Low folate in four of the five cases;

• HLA: positive for haplotype DR3 and DQW2 in all patients;

• Constantly abnormal EEG with, in three cases occipital spike-waves of large amplitude reacting to opening of the eyes, with important secondary diffusion during sleep (Figs. 1–2);

• Cerebral CT with biooccipital multiple hemispheric intraparenchymal calcifications (Fig. 3);

• Cerebral MRI: negative in all cases but one, in which a void signal compatible with calcification was seen in biparietal-occipital areas (Fig. 4);

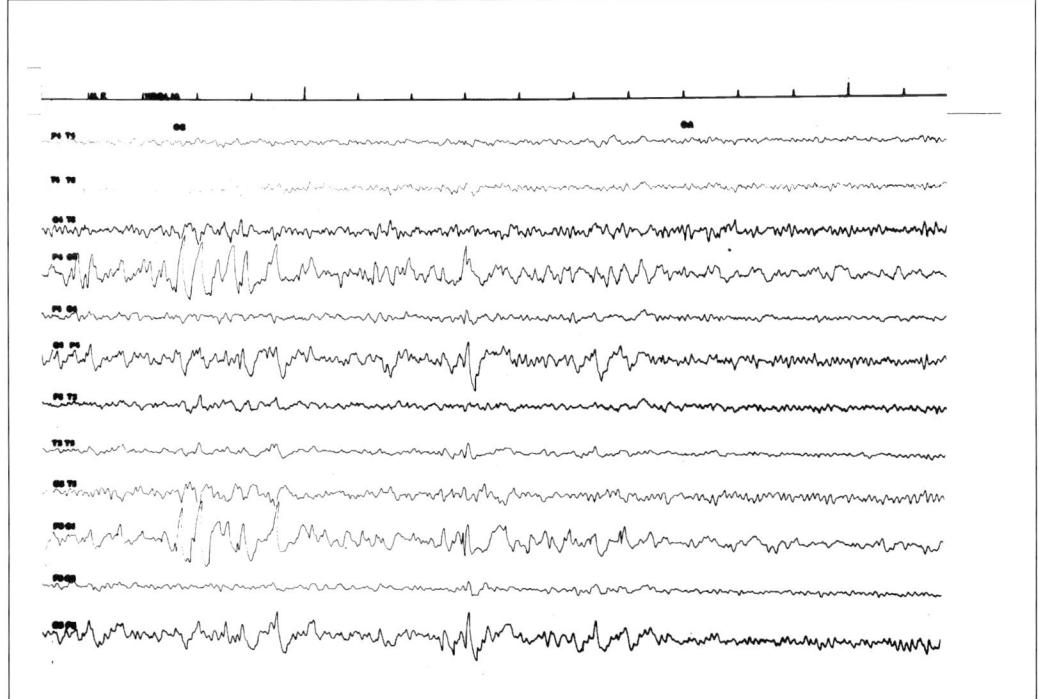

Fig. 1. EEG (wakefulness): Slow spike-waves over both occipital regions suppressed by eye opening.

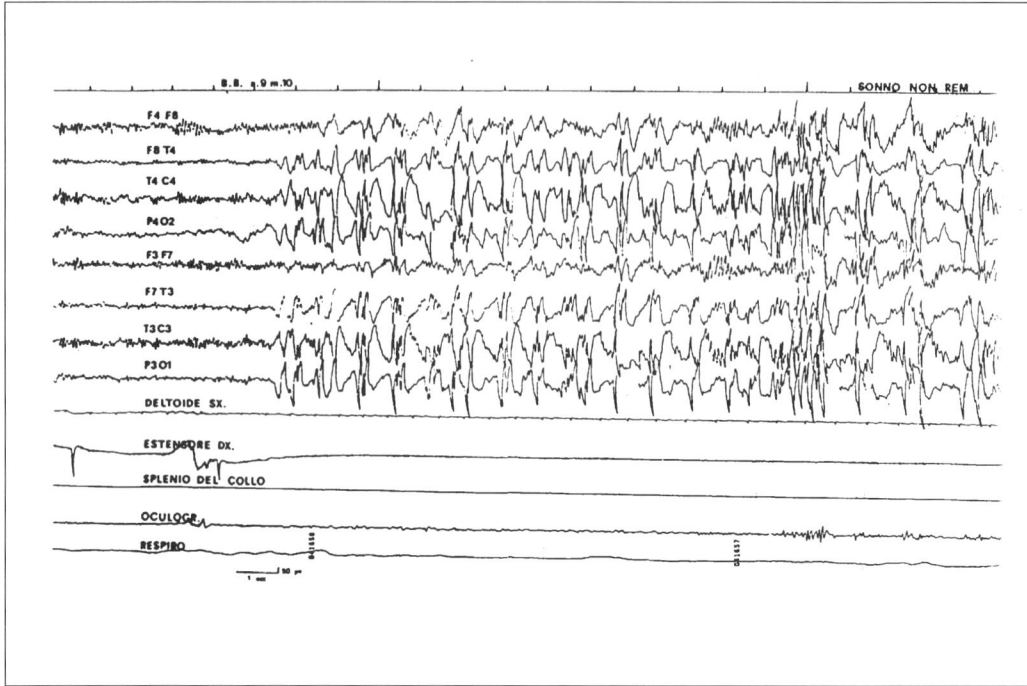

Fig. 2. EEG (nonREM sleep); Continuous spikes and spike-waves discharges in both parietal-occipital areas with a tendency to diffuse.

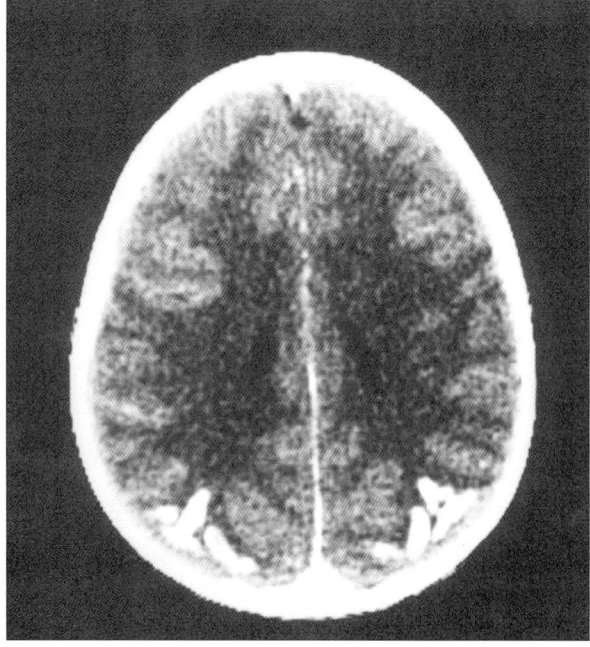

Fig 3. Cranial, CT; Bilateral cortical-subcortical occipital curvilinear symmetrical calcifications.

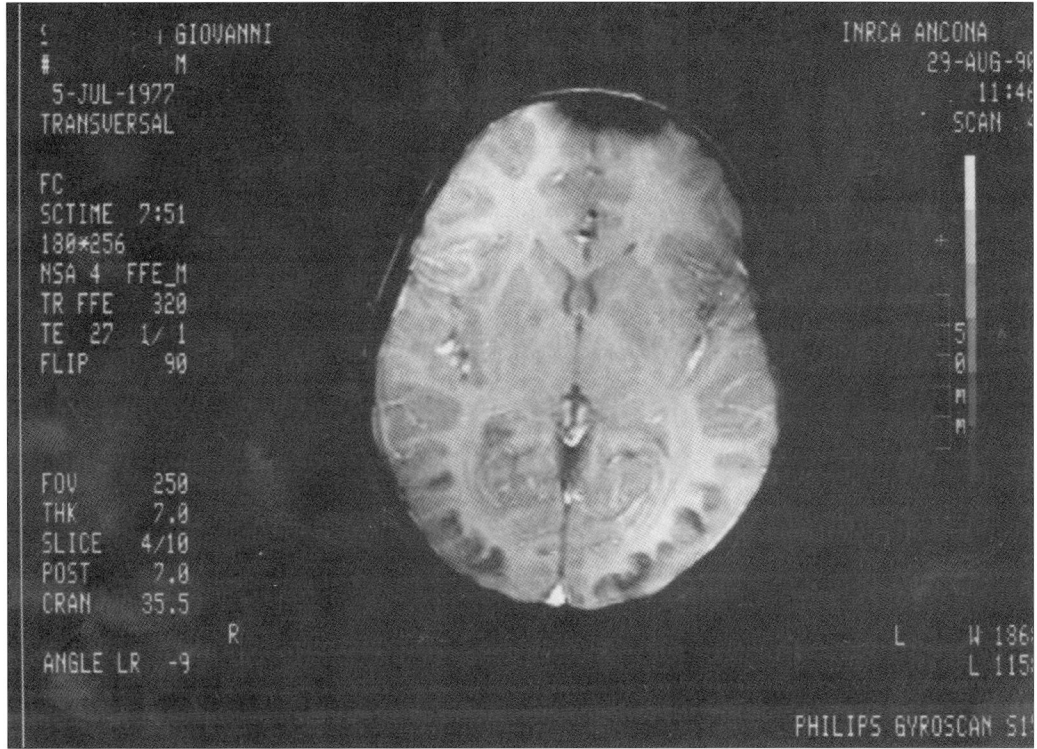

Fig. 4. Magnetic resonance imaging (FFE); Areas of reduced signal in the parietal occipital regions, compatible with a supposition of calcifications.

• SPECT: reduced radiotracer bilaterally in parieto-occipital areas in one patient;

• Evoked potentials (VEPs, SEPs, BAEPs): normal cortical responses in all subjects except one in whom pattern stimulation resulted in a lengthening of the P100 latency;

• EMG + MCV + SCV: normal in all.

These findings may lead to the following deductions:

• The cerebral calcification and epilepsy are almost certainly correlated aetiologically to coeliac disease even though the pathogenic mechanism is not entirely clear. The clinical manifestations may be heterogenous but in some cases one may speak of a syndromic entity, with its own EEG and clinical characteristics and course.

• The role of the cerebral calcification in the genesis and evolution of the epilepsy appears uncertain.

• The role of diet in seizure control and in the evolution of endocranial structural lesions cannot be evaluated; the control, whenever obtained, seems to be unrelated to dietary therapy and, moreover, neuroradiological findings were the same regardless of clinical course or compliance with dietary therapy.

• In the absence of positive anatomo-pathological results, even the more recent neuroradiological methods do not seem capable of furnishing definitive information with regard to the composition of the deposits shown by CT. In fact, in four of our five cases, MRI and SPECT showed that the cerebral parenchyma was structurally and functionally normal, even in those sites where the CT showed the presence of calcific hyperdensities; only in one case did the imaging and neurophysiological investigations show a pattern analogous to that of Sturge–Weber disease.

• The neurophysiological examinations (MCV, SCV, SEP) excluded early involvement of the peripheral nervous system.

Epilepsy

A greater incidence of epilepsy in coeliac disease is described in the literature even though definitive statistical data do not exist. Recent data lead us to believe that the incidence of epilepsy in coeliac disease is no different from that in the general population. Certain authors have signalled the possible occurrence of a peculiar form of occipital epilepsy in coeliac patients with no cerebral calcification, thus suggesting the need for medical tests (AGA, antiendomysial antibodies) for patients with complex partial seizures, particularly when these are originating in the occipital lobe (Ambrosetto et al., 1991; Fois et al., 1994).

In our case studies, epilepsy, although it represents one of the more frequent neurological disorders (8/58, or 13.8 per cent), is almost always associated with a parenchymal anatomical lesions (bioccipital or parieto occipital calcifications in five cases, cerebral neoplasia in two). Only one patient had complex partial seizures with their focus revealed by EEG in the right temporal lobe. There were no structural lesions on neuroradiological investigation; the seizures were completely controlled by antiepileptic therapy.

Acute cerebral ischaemia

Cortical vascular anomalies, with pial angiomatosis, venous fibrosis and microcalcifications have been recently described in a patient with CEC (Bye et al., 1993), but as early as 1986 the possibility was raised signalled the possibility of an acute ischaemic episode occurring in an adult with coeliac disease. Neuropathologic findings suggested a vasculitic phenomenon, probably of an immunologic nature similar to that already been seen in other sites (skin, kidneys) (Rush et al., 1986).

Toxic exogenous substances of bacterial or food origin could be absorbed by the damaged intestinal mucosa leading to the formation of circulating immunocomplexes which could be deposited in the smaller cerebral vessels and provoke vasculitic phenomena. Furthermore, local inflammatory phenomena could arise following activation of the alternate pathway of complement by the gliadin itself or by the in situ formation of IgA containing immunocomplexes (Gobbi et al., 1992; Rush et al., 1986; Ward et al., 1985).

At 30 years of age, our patient, diagnosed as a child but poorly compliant with dietary therapy, had an acute ischaemic episode which began with a headache that worsened over a period of a few days with dysarthria, and transient left brachio-crural hemiparesis.

On neurological examination (CT, MRI) the patient showed diffuse cerebral vasculopathy with ischaemic lesions localized in both frontal and parietal areas, more evident on the right at the level of the right internal capsule (Fig. 5).

The evolution was characterised by periods of well-being alternating with recurrences of transitory ischaemic disorders and headaches, which prompted further investigation.

MRI revealed a greater extension of the ischaemic lesions in the right hemisphere, while the focus in the homolateral internal capsule was less evident (Fig. 6).

The bilateral lesions, revealed by the neuroradiological investigations, and their further extension as seen during follow-up examinations, is compatible with the diagnostic hypothesis of vasculitis.

Headaches and migraine

Migraine, among the various neurological disorders manifested during the course of coeliac disease, is quite frequently reported in the literature, whether associated or not with bioccipital calcifications

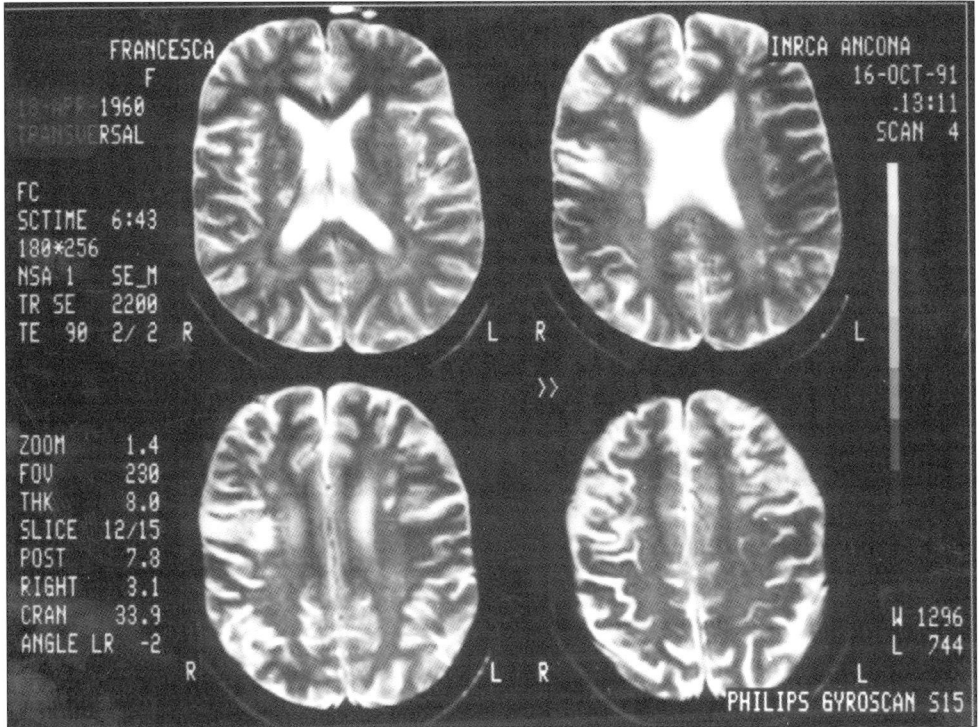

Fig. 5. Magnetic resonance imaging (Spin-Echo Axial images): Presence of hyperintense areas in the right parietal and frontal cortical and subcortical regions and other punctiform areas in the left frontal region compatible with ischemic foci.

and epilepsy. The interest in this is related to the fact that the occipital cerebral regions seem to be those more often involved, both in migraine syndromes and coeliac disease. The pathogenic mechanism is unknown, especially in cases without calcifications, although the presence of 'minor' vasculitic phenomena or, in any event, alteration in regional cerebral flow, could be suspected.

Our four cases presented the clinical manifestations of classic migraine (three cases) and common migraine (one case). The cephalgic episodes, even though in some cases intense and accompanied by visual symptoms and sensory disturbances, were never very frequent and responded well to therapy, never leading to a progressive disorder. Convulsive attacks never occurred during the course of the illness. On CT scan, structural anomalies, particularly those of a calcific nature, were absent in all. One migraine episode with flashing scotomas and dysmorphopsia corresponding to slow activity of the theta-delta frequency in posterior location was recorded by EEG.

Cerebral neoplasias

The predisposition to neoplasias in coeliac disease is well known, particularly with regard to lymphomas (50 per cent) and other gastrointestinal neoplasias (25 per cent), although other sites can be involved as well (25 per cent) (Swinson *et al.,* 1981). Deficiency of selenium, as found in coeliac disease and persisting even after dietary therapy, may represent a heightened risk factor in neoplastic pathology. Selenium would carry out its anticancerogenous activity by mechanisms in part still unknown, but these would include the ability to protect cell membranes, alter the metabolism of carcinogens and stimulate the immune system (Gregori *et al.,* 1988).

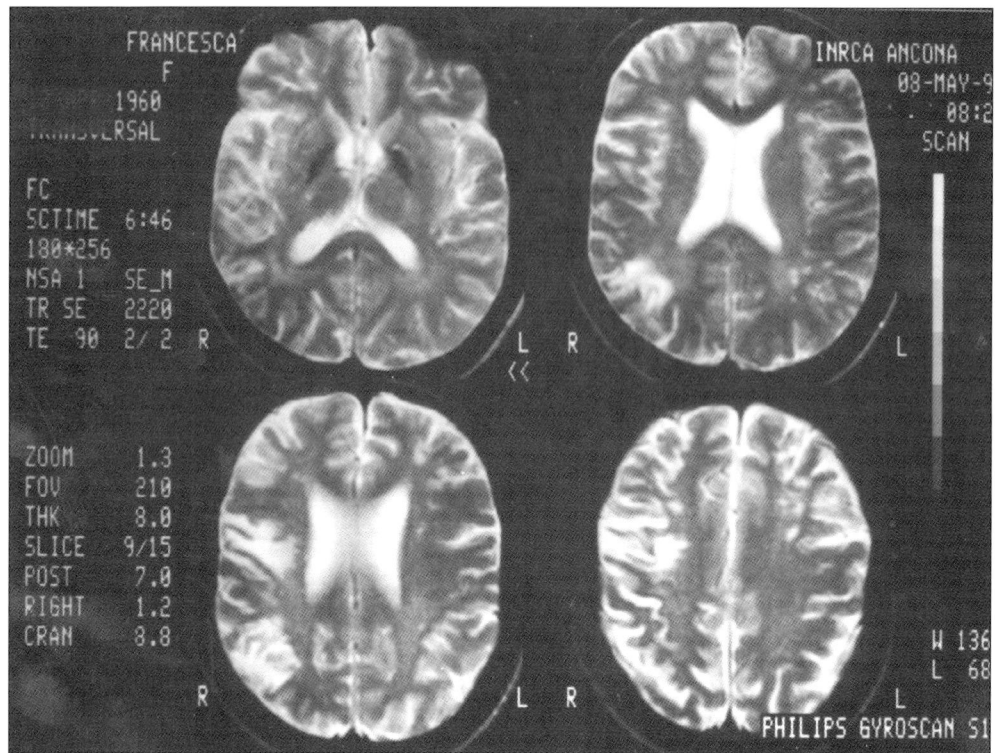

Fig. 6. Magnetic resonance imaging (Spin-echo Axial images): When compared with the previous examination, a greater extension of the ischaemic foci is observed in the right hemissphere.

We know of no cases of cerebral neoplasias associated with coeliac disease reported in the literature. Our cases included a subependymoma of the brain stem and one right frontal cortical astrocytoma. Both patients had been diagnosed as being affected by typical coeliac disease and had been received an adequate therapeutic diet early on. The neoplastic lesions occurred, respectively, at the ages of 7 and 12 years. Both patients had partial seizures not fully controllable by drug therapy. In particular, the patient with the frontal astrocytoma began having seizures at 2 years of age; the EEG revealed a slow focus in the right anterior head region while a CT scan carried out at 7 years of age gave negative results. The sudden appearance of signs and symptoms of increased intracranial pressure at the age of 12 years led to identification of the neoplastic lesion. The patient later died.

The dosage of selenium administered to the patient affected by low grade epeudymona of the brain-stem was equal to 40 µ/l (v.n. 107 ± 6.4 µ/l whole blood).

Other neurological disorders

Since coeliac disease is not a rare pathology, certain neurological disorders could have only a casual association with it; such is the case with febrile convulsions, which are quite frequent in paediatric age, and with isolated EEG anomalies, especially if localized in centro-temporal region. Even with regard to psychiatric disorders, so frequently described in the literature and concerning mainly depression and schizophrenia, recent studies have not shown a significant relationship with malabsorption syndrome.

In our study, one patient had learning disability and the other mental retardation with psychotic behaviour. Both children were affected by typical coeliac disease and both were following dietary therapy. Examinations and diagnostic investigations to determine the presence of other risk factors were all negative.

Conclusions

Coeliac disease is associated in a considerable number of cases with neurological pathology. Nonetheless, there are no statistical studies which define with certainty the real incidence of coeliac disease in the individual pathologies. The pathogenic mechanisms, which are the basis of these pathological associations, have also not been entirely explained.

Currently, the neurological disorder most frequently associated with coeliac disease is the cerebral calcifications–epilepsy syndrome, even though certain questions here remain unresolved: why the bioccipital localisation? What role do the calcifications play in the onset and evolution of the epileptic syndrome? What explanation can be given for the wide-ranging differences in the clinical manifestations of structural lesions which are identical?

Furthermore, nothing is currently known with certainty regarding the mechanism which causes the calcific lesions: the course of the clinico-neuroradiological aspects presented by our case with acute cerebral ischaemia seems to reinforce the hypothesis that vascular anomalies of an inflammatory nature can play a role in the onset of permanent parenchymal structural lesions.

We also find it worthy of note that in our study there are two instances of cerebral neoplasia associated with coeliac disease. Although the possibility that this association was fortuitous cannot be ruled out, we deem that it warrants further study in order to determine a possible aetiopathogenic correlation, with the aim of improving prognosis and finding possible preventive measures.

References

Ambrosetto, G., De Mara G. & Antonini, L. (1991): Crisi occipitali e celiachia in assenza di calcificazioni cortico-sottocorticali: presentazione di due casi. *Boll. Lega It. Epil.* **74,** 135–137.

Bye, A.M.E., Andermann, F., Robitaille, Y., Bohane, T., Oliver, M. & Andermann, E. (1993): Cortical vascular abnormalities in the syndrome of celiac disease, epilepsy, bilateral calcifications, and folate deficiency. *Ann. Neurol.* **34,** 3.

Fois, A., Vascott, M., Di Bartolo, R.M. & Di Marco, V. (1994): Celiac disease and epilepsy in pediatric patients. *Child's Nerv. Syst.* **10,** 450–454.

Garwicz, S. & Mortennson, W. (1976): Intracranial calcifications mimicking the Sturge–Weber syndrome (a consequence of cerebral folic acid deficiency?) *Pediatr. Radiol.* **5,** 5–9.

Gobbi, G., Bouquet, F. & Greco, L. (Italian Working Group on Coeliac Disease and Epilepsy) (1992): Coeliac disease, epilepsy and cerebral calcifications. *Lancet* **340,** 22, 439–443.

Gregori, G., Minoila, C., De Angelis, G.L. & Bianchini, G. (1988): Carenza di Selenio in corso di malattia celiaca: un problema potenziale. *Riv. Ital. Ped.* (IJP) **14,** 303–306.

Molteni, N., Bardella, M.T., Baldassarri, A.R. & Bianchi, P.A. (1988): Celiac disease associated with epilepsy and intracranial calcifications: report of two patients. *Am. J. Gastroenterol.* **83,** 992–994.

Piatella, L., Zamponi, N. & Cenci, L., (1986): Calcificazioni bioccipitali ed epilessia: Malattia di Sturge–Weber atipica o nuova sindrome? *Boll. Lega. It. Epil.* **54/55,** 139–142.

Piatella, L., Cardinali, C., Zamponi, N. *et al.* (1987): Encefalopatia epilettica tardiva con calcificazioni occipitali. In: *Atti del Convegno sulle Sindromi Epilettiche-Aspetti diagnostici, assistenziali e terapeutici*, pp. 21–24. **Ancona**

Piattella, L., Cardinali, C., Zamponi, N. & Tavoni, M.A. (1987): Sindrome di Sturge–Weber atipica e incompleta: Problemi di inquadramento diagnostico. *Acta Paediatrica. Latina.* **40,** 402–414.

Piatella, L., Zamponi, N. & Porfiri, L. (1990): Calcificazioni cerebrali multiple e celiachia. *Boll. Lega It. Epil.* **70/71,** 263–264.

Piattella, L., Zamponi, N., Cardinali, C., Porfiri, L. & Tavoni, M.A. (1993): Endocranial calcifications, infantile celiac disease, and epilepsy. *Child's Nerv. Syst.* **9,** 172–175.

Rush, P.J., Inman, R., Bernstein, M., Carlen, P. & Resch, L. (1986): Isolated vasculitis of the central nervous system in a patient with celiac disease. *Am. J. Med.* **6,** 1092–1094.

Sammaritano, M. (1985): The syndrome of epilepsy and bilateral occipital cortical calcifications. *Epilepsia* **26,** (5) 532.

Sammaritano, M., Andermann, F., Melanson, D., Guberman, A., Tinuper, P., & Gastaut, H (1988): The syndrome of intractable epilepsy, bilateral occipital calcifications and folic acid deficiency. *Neurology* **38,** (Suppl 1), 239.

Swinson, C.M., Slavin, G., Coles, E.C. & Booth, C. (1981): Coeliac disease and malignancy. *Gut* **22,** 872.

Ward, M.E., Murphy, J.T. & Greenberg, G.R. (1985): Celiac disease and spinocerebellar degenerations with normal vitamin E status. *Neurology* **35,** 1199–1201.

Zaniboni, M.G., Lambertini, A., Romeo, N., Conti, R., Ambrosioni, G., Gobbi G. *et al.* (1989): Coeliac disease and epilepsy with occipital calcifications: an uncasual association. In: *First Joint Meeting of the British Society of Paediatric Gastroenerology and Nutrition and Italian Society of Paediatrics* (abstract book), eds. Bianchini, G., Guandalini, S., De Angelis, G.L & Walker-Smith, J.A., p. 54. Parma.

Chapter 38

Dementia and coeliac disease

Pekka Collin[*,**], Anne Eerola[***] and Tuula Pirttilä[*,***]

[*]*Medical School, University of Tampere, PO Box 607, FIN-33101 Tampere, Finland;* [**]*Department of Medicine, Tampere University Hospital, PO Box 2000, FIN-33521, Tampere, Finland;* [***]*Department of Neurology, Tampere University Hospital, PO Box 2000, FIN-33521, Tampere, Finland*

The clinical pattern of coeliac disease has changed

Coeliac disease (CD) is characterized by a small bowel villous damage. Ingestion of gluten results in villous atrophy and crypt hyperplasia. The treatment consists of lifelong withdrawal of gluten-containing cereals. When untreated, the mucosal atrophy can lead to severe malabsorption of essential nutrients.

A wide range of neurological symptoms has been described as a complication of CD; of these, the symptoms of peripheral neuropathy are most frequent (Cooke & Holmes, 1984; Cooke & Smith, 1966; Morris *et al.*, 1970). Particularly in earlier series, many neurological symptoms have been the consequence of severe malabsorption. Banerji & Hurvitz (1971) reported neurological complications in as many as 37 per cent of their coeliac patients. Most of these complications were due to deficiency of vitamin D, hypocalcaemia, or hypokalaemia.

The clinical course of CD has changed from sprue and malabsorption syndrome towards milder forms (Logan *et al.*, 1983). The diagnostic delay can last for many years or even decades. The disease can present with atypical symptoms such as unspecific arthritis, or it can even be clinically silent, with no symptoms at all. Coeliac disease may also be latent: patients have initially normal small bowel mucosa but later develop typical villous atrophy (Ferguson *et al.*, 1993).

The changing pattern of CD will probably also alter our knowledge of the neurological complications. The complications of malabsorption will become rare, whereas new complications, not earlier connected with CD, will emerge. Dementia and brain atrophy may be previously unrecognized complications of CD. These neurological complications may sometimes be the main presentation, leading to the diagnosis of CD.

Mental deficiency and coeliac disease

Cognitive functions of CD patients have not been extensively studied and large cross-sectional studies are lacking. Thus, the extent of intellectual deterioration in patients with CD remains obscure, as well as the significance of gluten-free diet in its prevention. Hallert & Åström (1983) examined the intellectual impact on 19 untreated coeliac patients using a comprehensive test battery: no consistent signs of cognitive impairment were found.

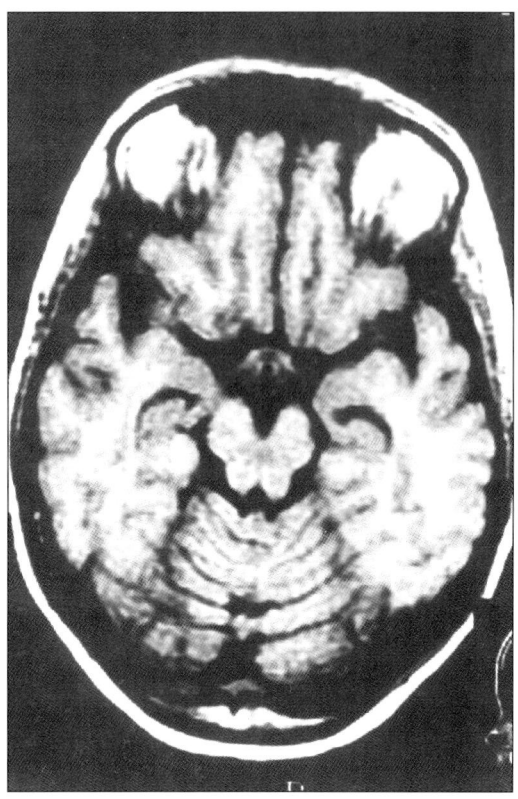

Fig. 1. A woman aged 27 with moderate to severe brain atrophy and coeliac disease (patient number 12 in Table 1).

Some other studies, however, have shown that CD patients might develop degenerative changes in the brain subsequently leading to dementia. Kinney *et al.* (1982) presented one case and quoted nine earlier cases with CD and brain damage. All 10 cases were fatal and an autopsy was carried out. Although the character and site of nervous involvements were variable, there was evidence of a specific neurological manifestation. The onset of neurological symptoms was insidious, and the progression was steady. Involvement was seen in the cerebellum, deep grey and brain stem nuclei, and spinal cord tracts. The most consistent neuropathological findings were neuronal loss and gliosis. Only two out of 10 patients suffered from dementia; the authors describe in detail a 57-year-old man with CD, progressive central nervous system disorder and dementia.

Cooke & Holmes (1984) described three patients with organic dementia. The first, reviewed by Kinney *et al.* (1982) was fatal. The autopsy revealed atrophy of frontal cortex with multiple small foci of neuronal loss. The condition of the second patient stabilized, and the third patient improved on a gluten-free diet.

Some coeliac patients can develop a progressive cerebellar disease. Finelli *et al.* (1980) described such a patient whose condition deteriorated despite the gluten-free diet. Kristoferitsch & Pointner (1987) described a coeliac patient having a cerebellar disease with a progressive course: the patient did not maintain the gluten-free diet.

In 1991 we reported five patients with CD, brain atrophy and dementia (Collin *et al.*, 1991). In four of them the diagnosis of CD was suspected on neurological examination, even though most patients also had unequivocal signs of malabsorption. Most of the patients had cerebellar, spinal and peripheral neurological symptoms. Intellectual deterioration ranged from moderate to severe. The neurological disease deteriorated despite treatment with the gluten-free diet.

Table 1. Cognitive impairment and brain atrophy in coeliac disease

Patient No.	Age and sex	Reference	Cognitive impairment	Brain atrophy[1]	Electroence-phalography	Malabsorption	Course of disease
1	59/M	(Cooke & Smith, 1966)	Severe	Cerebral	Multifocal spike activity	Many	Death
2	57/M	(Kinney *et al.,* 1982)	Progressive	None	Not available	Folic acid	Death
3	51/M	(Cooke & Holmes, 1984)	Progressive	Not known	Not available	Weight loss	Stable
4	56/M		Severe	Enlargement of the ventricles	Episodic low frequency activity	Megaloblastic anaemia	Improved
5	37/F	(Collin *et al.,* 1991)	Progressive	Cerebral	General slowing	Folic acid	Progressive
6	39/F		Progressive	Cerebral	General slowing	Vitamin B_{12}	Progressive
7	41/F		Progressive	Cerebral and cerebellar	Spike- and wave discharges	Folic acid	Progressive
8	58/F		Progressive	Cerebral	General slowing	Folic acid	Progressive
9	43/M		Mild	Cerebellar	General slowing	No	Stable
10	55/M	(Ferroir *et al.,* 1993)	Severe	No	Delta discharges	Asthenia	Death
11	53/M	Unpublished	Moderate	Cerebral and cerebellar	Normal	Vitamin B_{12}	Stable
12	27/F		No	Cerebral and cerebellar	Normal	No	Stable
13	55/F[2]		No	Cerebral	Normal	No	Stable
14	27/M[2]		Moderate	Cerebral and cerebellar	Not done	No	Progressive
15	57/M		No	Cerebral and cerebellar	Normal	Vitamin B_{12}, folic acid	Stable
16	55/F		Moderate	Cerebellar	Not done	Vitamin B_{12}	Follow-up time short
17	50/F		Moderate	Enlargement of the ventricles	General slowing	No	Improved

[1]By computer tomography, magnetic resonance imaging or autopsy;
[2]previously diagnosed insulin-dependent diabetes mellitus.

Table 1 summarizes CD patients with dementia or brain atrophy described in the literature, and additionally seven unpublished cases of our own. The magnetic resonance image of one patient is shown at Fig. 1. Only two of 17 patients showed clear improvement in cognitive functions while on gluten-free diet. However, it is possible that an earlier diagnosis of CD would have improved the outcome of neurological complications. One patient (patient number 14) suffered simulta-neously from insulin-dependent diabetes mellitus, dementia, and CD. Interestingly, his small bowel mucosa had been normal 12 years earlier, when he was examined due to positive reticulin anti-bodies. However, after developing dementia, a new biopsy specimen showed subtotal villous atrophy. The case raises the question whether even latent CD may be deleterious. On the other hand, it is possible that concomitant diabetes is a special risk factor for brain atrophy in patients with CD.

The aetiology of brain atrophy and dementia in coeliac disease

The impact of malabsorption of essential nutrients, due to damaged villous structure, cannot be excluded. Lindenbaum *et al.* (1988) showed that vitamin B_{12} (cobalamin) deficiency can lead to paraesthesiae, sensory loss, ataxia and memory loss. Low B_{12} levels are frequently detected in primary dementia (Karnaze & Carmel, 1987; Nijst *et al.*, 1990) , and the deficiency may contribute to defective brain function (Pirttilä *et al.*, 1993).

Neurological symptoms are frequently seen in patients with inborn errors of folic acid deficiency. In the study of Reynolds *et al.* (1973), a psycho-organic syndrome was common in patients with folic acid deficiency. Renvoize *et al.* (1985) reported a 45 per cent prevalence of folic acid deficiency in patients with dementia. On the other hand, Nijst *et al.* (1990) found no difference in serum and cerebrospinal fluid folic acid concentrations in patients with dementia. Folic acid deficiency alone cannot explain the occurrence of dementia in the patients described in Table 1, because the deficiency was found only in a minority of patients.

Vitamin E deficiency has been implicated in the aetiology of neurological disorders of CD patients (Ackerman *et al.*, 1989; Mauro *et al.*, 1991; Trabert *et al.*, 1992). The vitamin E deficiency does not, however, explain neurological complications in all cases (Kaplan *et al.*, 1988; Ward *et al.*, 1985).

Immune activation may contribute the pathogenesis of CD. Activated gliadin-specific T-cells have been cloned in CD patients (Gjertsen *et al.*, 1994), and an increase MCH II expression is seen in small bowel mucosa (Holm *et al.*, 1994). Wekerle *et al.* (1987) showed that activated T-cells cross the intact blood–brain barrier. In the pathogenesis of multiple sclerosis the presence of activated T-cells in the brain may be deleterious due to secretion of immune mediators, that induce the expression of MCH II molecules in astrocytes, microglial, and perivascular cells, or are toxic to myelin or myelin-producing cells (Raine, 1994). It is possible that immune activation may participate in the pathogenesis of neurological symptoms in CD. Gliosis, which has been detected in some CD patients with nervous involvement, may develop as the end-product of the inflammatory process.

We conclude that the aetiology of neurological complications in CD is probably multifactorial. In many patients described in Table 1, intellectual deterioration was associated with brain atrophy. Immunological mechanisms in brain can be vascular, antibody mediated, or parenchymal, T-cell mediated. Vitamin deficiency in connection with brain atrophy can worsen cognitive functions (Pirttilä *et al.*, 1993).

Future prospects

A cross-sectional study of the intellectual ability of new and earlier diagnosed CD patients is needed. The impact of the gluten-free diet on intellectual ability must be evaluated. The association of brain atrophy in CD must be examined in controlled longitudinal studies.

References

Ackerman, Z., Eliashiv, S., Reches, A. & Zimmerman, J. (1989): Neurological manifestations in celiac disease and vitamin E deficiency. *J. Clin Gastroenterol.* **11,** 603–605.

Banerji, N.K. & Hurwitz, L.J. (1971): Neurological manifestations in adult steatorrhoea. *J. Neurol. Sci.* **14,** 125–141.

Collin, P., Pirttilä, T., Nurmikko, T., Somer, H., Erilä, T. & Keyriläinen, O. (1991): Celiac disease, brain atrophy and dementia. *Neurology* **41,** 372–375.

Cooke, W. T. & Holmes, G. K. T. (1984): Neurological and psychiatric complications. In: *Coeliac disease*, eds. W.T. Cooke & G. K. T. Holmes, pp. 197–213. Edinburgh: Churchill Livingstone.

Cooke, W.T. & Smith, W.T. (1966): Neurological disorders associated with adult coeliac disease. *Brain* **89,** 683–722.

Ferguson, A., Arranz, E. & O'Mahony, S. (1993): Clinical and pathological spectrum of coeliac disease—active, silent, latent, potential. *Gut* **34,** 150–151.

Ferroir, J., Cosnes, J., Stankoff, B., Lequintrec, J.-L., Spelle, L., Guillard, A. & Lequintrec, Y. (1993): Maladie coeliaque et demence d'evolution rapidement mortelle. *Ann. Med. Interne. Paris* **144,** 499–500.

Finelli, P.F., McEntee, W.J., Ambler, M. & Kestenbaum, D. (1980): Adult celiac disease presenting as cerebellar syndrome. *Neurology* **30,** 245–249.

Gjertsen, H.A., Lundin, K.E., Sollid, L.M., Eriksen, J.A. & Thorsby, E. (1994): T cells recognize a peptide derived from alpha-gliadin presented by the celiac disease-associated HLA-DQ (α1*0501, β1*0201) heterodimer. *Hum. Immunol.* **39,** 243–252.

Hallert, C. & Åström, J. (1983): Intellectual ability of adults after lifelong intestinal malabsorption due to coeliac disease. *J. Neurol. Neurosurg. Psychiatry* **46,** 87–89.

Holm, K., Savilahti, E., Koskimies, S., Lipsanen, V. & Mäki, M. (1994): Immunohistochemical changes in the jejunum in first degree relatives of patients with coeliac disease and the coeliac disease marker DQ genes. HLA class II antigen expression, interleukin-2 receptor positive cells and dividing crypt cells. *Gut* **35,** 55–60.

Kaplan, J. G., Pack, D., Horoupian, D., DeSouza, T., Brin, M. & Schaumburg, H. (1988): Distal axonopathy associated with chronic gluten enteropathy: a treatable disorder. *Neurology* **38,** 642–645.

Karnaze, D.S. & Carmel, R. (1987): Low serum cobalamin levels in primary degenerative dementia. *Arch. Intern. Med.* **147,** 429–431.

Kinney, H.C., Burger, P.C., Hurwitz, B.J., Hijmans, J.C. & Grant, J.P. (1982): Degeneration of the central nervous system associated with celiac disease. *J. Neurol. Sci.* **53,** 9–22.

Kristoferitsch, W. & Pointner, H. (1987): Progressive cerebellar syndrome in adult coeliac disease. *J. Neurol.* **234,** 116–118.

Lindenbaum, J., Healton, E.B., Savage, D.G., Brust, J.C.M., Garret, T.J., Podell, E.R., Marcell, P.D., Stabler, S.P. & Allen, R.H. (1988): Neuropsychiatric disorders caused by cobalamin deficiency in the absence of anemia or macrocytosis. *N. Engl. J. Med.* **318,** 1720–1728.

Logan, R.F.A., Tucker, G., Rifkind, E.A., Heading, R.C. & Ferguson, A. (1983): Changes in clinical features of coeliac disease in adults in Edinburgh and the Lothians 1960–79. *BMJ* **286,** 95–97.

Mauro, A., Orsi, L., Mortara, P., Costa, P. & Schiffer, D. (1991): Cerebellar syndrome in adult celiac disease with vitamin E deficiency. *Acta Neurol. Scand.* **84,** 167–170.

Morris, J.S., Adjukiewicz, A.B. & Read, A.E. (1970): Neurological disorders and adult coeliac disease. *Gut* **11,** 549–554.

Nijst, T.Q., Wevers, R.A., Schoonderwaldt, H.C., Hommes, O.R. & de Haan, A.F.J. (1990): Vitamin B12 and folate concentrations in serum and cerebrospinal fluid of neurological patients with special reference to multiple sclerosis and dementia. *J. Neurol. Neurosurg. Psych.* **53,** 951–954.

Pirttilä, T., Salo, J., Laippala, P. & Frey, H. (1993): Effect of advanced brain atrophy and vitamin deficiency on cognitive functions in non-demented subjects. *Acta Neurol. Scand.* **87,** 161–166.

Raine, C.S. (1994): Multiple sclerosis: immune system molecule expression in the central nervous system. *J. Neuropathol. Exp. Neurol.* **53,** 328–337.

Renvoize, E.B., Gastkell, R.K. & Klar, H.M. (1985): Results of investigations in 150 demented patients consecutively admitted to a psychiatric hospital. *Br. J. Psychiatry* **147,** 204–205.

Reynolds, E.H., Rothfeld, P. & Pincus, J.H. (1973): Neurological disease associated with folate deficiency. *BMJ* 2, 398–400.

Trabert, W., Collin, P., Pirttilä, T., Nurmikko, T., Somer, H., Erilä, T. & Keyriläinen, O. (1992): Celiac disease and vitamin E deficiency. *Neurology* **42,** 1641–1642.

Ward, M.E., Murphy, J.T. & Greenberg, G.R. (1985): Celiac disease and spinocerebellar degeneration with normal vitamin E status. *Neurology* **35,** 1199–1201.

Wekerle, H., Sun, D., Oropeza-Wekerle, R.L. & Meyermann, R. (1987): Immune reactivity in the nervous system modulation of T-lymphocyte activation by glial cells. *J. Exp. Biol.* **132,** 43–57.

Epilepsy and other neurological disorders in coeliac disease, edited by G. Gobbi *et al.*
© 1997 John Libbey & Company Ltd, pp. 291–293.

Chapter 39

Cognitive disturbances in children with coeliac disease

L. Pavone, D. Mazzone, G. Incorpora, F. Drago[*] and G. Bottaro

Clinica Pediatrica, Università di Catania, [*]Istituto di Farmacologia, Università di Catantia, Italy

Introduction

The existence of a linkage between untreated coeliac disease (CD) and neurological manifestations is well known. Behavioural disorders such as irritability and apathy are frequently observed at the onset of first symptoms, while schizophrenia, depression and obsessional neurosis have been described in adults (Dohan, 1970; Hallert & Derefeldt, 1982; Hallert *et al.*, 1982) and also in children although with lower frequency (Sheldon, 1959; Cooke & Holmes, 1984).

We have evaluated the cognitive aspects in CD children followed-up at the Pediatric Clinic of Catania during the period 1989–94.

Patients and methods

120 patients, age 2.9 to 16 years, with a diagnosis of CD made according to ESPGAN criteria on the basis of clinical, immunological and bioptical features and of good response to diet, were investigated, after informed consent was obtained from their parents.

They were divided into two groups:

Group A : 69 children on a strict gluten-free diet, mean age 7 years (range 2.9 to 16) with IgA and IgG antigliadin antibodies lower than 12 per cent and 17 per cent respectively (assayed by Eurospital kit and expressed as percentage of the standard).

Group B : 51 children not completely compliant with the gluten-free diet, mean age 6.4 years (range 3.4 to 14) and IgA and IgG antigliadin antibodies lower than 32.3 per cent and 42.2 per cent respectively.

The investigation was extended to a control group of 20 age-matched children without clinical signs of gastrointestinal, nutritional or metabolic disease (Group C).

All children in this study, were studied with regard to motor and cognitive skills, language, sociability and school performance. Moreover, 29 of them were randomly chosen and submitted to IQ tests (WISC-R). Perceptive cognition was evaluated applying the RAVEN-PM test and visual discrimination ability in short term memory by the REY-Test. The results were compared to those obtained in the control group.

Results

The results of our investigation are summarized in Tables 1 to 4.

Motor skills, language, sociability, cognition and school performance evaluation showed no significant statistical differences between the two groups of patients and the controls (Table 1). In fact, none of the subjects showed impaired motor skills. A small percentage of patients, was found to have impairment of language, sociability, perceptive cognition and school performance, but again no statistically significant differences were encountered when compared to the control group.

The lowest IQ rates (65 and 70) were found in one patient from group A and one from group B (Table 2). Mental retardation, however did not appear to be correlated to CD since it was already present before the onset of gastrointestinal symptoms. Raven test for perceptive cognition gave values below the 25th centile in only three patients of group A (18 per cent) and one of group B (11 per cent), but without any statistical significance (Table 3).

Visual discrimination and short-term memory, tested by REY-test, were found to be impaired (lower than the 25th centile) in four patients of group A and seven of group B (Table 4). The data concerning group B, were statistically significant, mainly for memory ability ($P < 0.001$).

Discussion

Our results demonstrate that CD children on a strict gluten-free diet, or not completely compliant to the diet, failed to show neurological or psychiatric involvement. The only significant difference observed between the two groups of CD patients and the control group concerns visual discrimination abilities and short-term memory, with a slightly more significant occurrence of impairment of these abilities in patients not compliant with the diet. Hernanz & Polanco (1991) observed that untreated CD patients showing behavioural disturbances have tryptophan plasma concentrations lower that CD patients without behavioural signs. The impaired tryptophan availability could have played a role in determining the slight neuropsychological dysfunction observed in our group B patients. Conversely also, the inadequate nutritional supply and the psychological problems deriving from a strict diet might contribute to the onset of the behavioural and psychological problems.

Table 1.

	Group A 69 patients	Group B 51 patients	Group C 20 controls	P*
Disorders of Motor Skills	0	0	0	NS
Language	2 (2.8%)	2 (3.9%)	1 (5%)	NS
Sociability	1 (1.4%)	2 (2.9%)	1 (5%)	NS
Cognition	2 (2.8%)	1 (1.9%)	1 (5%)	NS
School Performance	1 (1.4%)	2 (3.9%)	0 (5%)	NS

* Comparison between group A, group B and controls was not significant: *P** A *vs* C, B *vs* C, A *vs* B.

Table 2.

WISC-R Test	Group A 16 patients	Group B 9 patients	Group C 20 controls	P*
I.Q. < 70	1 (6.2 %)	1 (11.1%)	0	NS

WISC-R Test (I.Q. < 70) in two groups of coeliac patients (A and B) and control group. A *vs.* C, B *vs.* C, A *vs.* B not significant

292

All children in this study were investigated regarding motor and cognitive skills, language, sociability and school performance. Moreover, 29 out of them were randomly chosen and submitted to IQ tests (WISC-R). Perceptive cognition was evaluated applying RAVEN-PM test and visual discrimination ability with short term memory by REY-Test. The results were compared to those obtained in the control group.

Table 3.

| Group A
16 patients | Group B
9 patients | Group C
20 controls | P* |
|---|---|---|---|
| 3 (18.7%) | 1 (11%) | 1 (5%) | NS |

Raven Test (< 25° centile) in two groups of coeliac patients (A and B) and control group was not significantly different

Table 4.

| | Group A
16 patients | Group B
9 patients | Control
subjects
n = 20 | P* |
|---|---|---|---|---|
| Copy | 2 (12.5%) | 3 (33.3%)* | 1 (5%) | |
| Memory | 2 (12.5%) | 4 (44.4%)** | 1 (5%) | |

Rey-test (copy and memory < 25° centile) in two groups of coeliac patients. (A and B) *vs.* control group. A *vs* B, A *vs* C. not significant. B *vs* C, P* 0.025 (copy); P** 0.001 (memory)

References

Cooke, W.T. & Holmes G.K.T. (1984): Neurological and psychiatric complications. In: Cooke, W.T. & Holmes, G.K.T. eds. Coeliac disease, pp. 197–213. Churchill-Livingstone, Edinburgh.

Dohan, F. C. (1970): Coeliac disease and schizophrenia. *Lancet* **i,** 897–898

Hallert, C., Derefeldt, T. (1982): Psychic disturbances in adult coeliac disease. Clinical observation. *Scand J Gastroenterol.* **17,** 17–19

Hallert, C., Astrom, J. & Sedwall, G. (1982): Psychic disturbances in adult coeliac disease. III: reduced central monoamine metabolism and signs of depression. *Scand J Gastroenterol.* **17,** 25–28

Hernanz, A. & Polanco, I. (1991): Plasma precursor aminoacids of central nervous system monoamines in children with coeliac disease. *Gut,* **32,** 1478–1481.

Sheldon, W. (1959):Coeliac disease. *Paediatrics* **23,** 132–145

Epilepsy and other neurological disorders in coeliac disease, edited by G. Gobbi *et al.*
© 1997 John Libbey & Company Ltd, pp. 295–300.

Chapter 40

Peripheral neuropathies associated with coeliac disease

P.A. Battistella[**], G. Guariso, A. Simonati[*], C. Nichetti and N. Rizzuto[*]

[*]*Department of Paediatrics, University of Padua, Italy; Department of Neurological and Visual Sciences, University of Verona, Italy;* [**]*Department of Paediatrics, University of Padova, Padova, Italy*

Introduction

Coeliac disease (CD), also named gluten-sensitive enteropathy, is a permanent intestinal intolerance to dietary wheat gliadin and related proteins that produces mucosal lesions in genetically susceptible individuals (Auricchio & Troncone, 1993). The most important clinical symptoms of CD are: chronic diarrhoea, abdominal distension, anorexia, short stature, muscle wasting, delayed puberty, unexplained nutritional deficiencies such as iron deficiency anaemia, folic acid deficiency, and rickets (Visakorpi, 1992).

A recent multicentric European survey of the frequency of identified cases of childhood CD reported rates ranged from 0.078 to 3.51 cases per 1000 (Greco *et al.*, 1992), while the estimated prevalence of CD in an Italian study seemed to be much higher, 3.87 per 1000 subjects (Catassi *et al.*, 1994). To date there is also an increasing number of atypical cases with symptoms such as isolated short stature, pubertal delay, recurrent abdominal pain, associated diseases, constipation, bulimia, diabetes, liver dysfunction, faecal blood loss and pseudo-obstruction (Greco *et al.*, 1992) and of subclinical or 'silent' forms, which lead to temporally delayed diagnosis (Visakorpi, 1992).

Many diseases have been found associated with CD, and many extensive reviews of these associations have been published (Muller *et al.*, 1974; Visakorpi, 1992).

Disorders associated with CD can be divided into three main groups: (a) firmly related and frequently reported diseases, such as dermatitis herpetiformis, insulin-dependent diabetes mellitus, selective IgA deficiency, lymphoma, small-intestinal cancer; (b) probably related conditions, such as autoimmune thyroid diseases, asthma and atopic diseases, epilepsy with cerebral calcification, Sjögren's syndrome, pharingeal and oesophageal cancer; (c) possibly associated ones, with single case reports: Addison disease, dementia, inflammatory bowel disease, sarcoidosis, primary biliary cirrhosis and other chronic liver disease, pancreatic insufficiency and connective tissue diseases (Collin & Maki, 1994).

Neurologic complications may occur in about 10 per cent of patients with CD and include encephalopathy, cerebellar ataxia, progressive multifocal leucoencephalopathy, seizures, myelopathy, myopathy, peripheral neuropathy and psychiatric disorders (Banerji & Hurwitz, 1971; Binder *et al.*,

1970; Chapman *et al.*, 1978; Collin *et al.*, 1991; Cooke, 1976; Cooke & Holmes, 1984; Cooke & Smith, 1966; Finelli *et al.*, 1980; Gobbi *et al.*, 1992; Hallert & Aström, 1982; Hallert & Darefeldt, 1982; Mulder & Tytgat, 1987; Pallis & Lewis, 1974; Ventura *et al.*, 1991).

A progressive cerebellar disease was reported in CD patients. In some cases the neurological condition worsened despite a gluten-free diet (Finelli *et al.*, 1980; Hermaszewski *et al.*, 1991), as it did in other patients who did not follow any specific dietary restriction (Kristoferitsch & Pointner, 1987). Moreover, signs and symptoms of spino-cerebellar involvement in CD patients were associated with normal serum vitamin E levels (Ward *et al.*, 1985), but also occurred in patients who had undetectable plasma levels of vitamin E (Mauro *et al.*, 1991).

Neuropathological features were reviewed by Cooke & Smith (1966): main findings are diffuse degeneration of the spinal cord – mainly the posterior roots – myelin loss of the nerve roots and spinal tracts, neuronal loss in the spinal sensory ganglia and anterior horns, cerebellar cortical atrophy, loss of neurons in the cerebral cortex, globus pallidus, thalamus, substantia nigra, astrocytic hypertrophy (Alzheimer type II astrocytes) in the basal ganglia, and in a few cases peculiar hypothalamic degeneration. Such changes occurred independently of the diet patients were taking. More recently, inflammatory cell infiltrates have been reported in the central nervous system (CNS): this has been considered as an abnormal immune response within the CNS, similar to that occuring in the diseased intestine (Finelli *et al.*, 1980; Marsh, 1992).

About one century ago Brown Carnegie (1908) reported two patients with 'sprue' who were also affected with 'peripheral neuritis localized to legs'. The association between CD and peripheral neuropathy is less frequent than CNS involvement: according to Cooke (1976): about 7 per cent of CD patients develop peripheral neuropathy, which affects lower limbs particularly. This condition was described by several authors (Cooke & Smith, 1966; Morris *et al.*, 1970; Pallis & Lewis, 1974).

The characteristic features of the CD-associated polyneuropathy were outlined by Kaplan *et al.* (1988): it shows a delayed onset, several years after gluten enteropathy and steatorrhea have started; there is no contemporary involvement of CNS; circulating levels of vitamins (vitamin B_1, B_6, B_{12}, E, folic acid) are normal; there is clinical improvement following gluten restriction, in contrast to the poorly responsive CNS symptoms. In a few reports, however, vitamin deficiencies have been shown. Vitamin E deficiency was postulated in two adults with severe peripheral neuropathy (Binder *et al.*, 1970; Connolly *et al.*, 1994), and folic acid deficiency was demonstrated in an adult patient, who improved following folic acid supplementation (Viader *et al.*, 1995).

Neurophysiological investigations show sensory action potentials to be decreased or even absent; both motor and sensory conduction velocities are also slowed. These findings are consistent with distal involvement of nerve trunks, particularly of the large myelinated axons and they are confirmed by morphological study of nerve biopsy. A moderate loss of myelinated fibres is observed, mainly affecting the larger ones; sporadic figures of wallerian-like degeneration are also reported. Intra-muscular nerve trunks show collateral branching and diffuse swelling of terminal axons, as shown in distal axonopathy (Cooke *et al.*, 1966). Clustered myelin fibres as well as hypertrophic Schwann cells, indicating repair changes, are also observed. Recently, demyelination has been reported on teased fibres, therefore suggesting a demyelinating neuropathy (Viader *et al.*, 1995). Myelin sheath abnormalities were also outlined by Bernier *et al.* (1976), who described the presence of inflammatory perivascular cuffing of the endoneurial vessels, which suggests an immune-mediated mechanism leading to the nerve pathology.

Peripheral nervous system (PNS) involvement is particularly rare in the early stages of CD, and therefore pediatric cases are rarely reported (Papadatou *et al.*, 1991). Clinical, neurophysiological and neuropathological findings are reported herein a child affected with CD and polyneuropathy, unassociated with vitamin deficiencies.

Case report

B.F. is an only child of non-consanguineous parents. Pregnancy and delivery were normal. Birth weight was 3.9 kg. During the first year the physical and neuropsychic mental were normal: he sat early, crawled at 5 months and walked at 13 months. After the 18th month, stools were abundant and frequent, resulting in decreased weight. At 24 months of age there was hypoproteinemia, sideropenic anaemia, he had an abnormal xylose test and antigliadin (AGA) was positive (IgG and IgA): CD was therefore suspected and later confirmed by a jejunal biopsy (mucosa subatrophy) and a gluten free diet was started. The HLA typing showed DQW_2, DR_3 and DR_7.

Notwithstanding the rapid weight recovery with normalization of blood chemistry indices at 30 months of age, he developed a clumsy gait, distal amyotrophy of the inferior limbs and a marked hyporeflexia of all limbs. A diagnosis of polyneuropathy was confirmed by neurophysiological examinations (motor nerve conduction velocity of left median nerve was 33 m/s, somatosensory evoked potentials from ulnar and median nerve were bilaterally absent). Serum vitamin E was always normal (30–45 µmol/l; n = 10–42), as was folic acid (3.7–6.5 mg/l; n = 1.8–14).

At 3 years of age the neurological exam showed: a stepping walk, marked distal muscle atrophy and weakness of the legs and the hands, mild decrease of proximal muscle strength and absence of all tendon reflexes. There was distal loss of all modalities of sensation. The cranial nerves were intact. These clinical findings and the electromyogram (EMG) remained stable at 1 year follow-up. In spite of normal plasma vitamin levels, the boy was treated with oral vitamin E for 6 months (100 mg/day); however, without variations in the neurological status or in the EMG. Biopsy of the sural nerve showed an axonal neuropathy with a loss of the larger calibre fibres and absence of reparative phenomena. On teased fibre preparation there were no figures of segmental demyelination (Fig. 1). Blood urea, cholesterol, triglycerides, glucose tolerance test, serum lipoprotein, phytanic acid levels, immunoglobulins, urinary porphyrin and lead estimations were normal, as were the vitamins B_6 and B_{12} levels. Furthermore, the search for neurotropic anti-virus antibodies as well as specific and non-specific organ autoantibodies was negative. ECG and EEG were normal. Cerebrospinal fluid examination was not performed.

Both parents are clinically and electrophysiologically normal, and there is no family history of neuromuscular disease.

Discussion

The early symptoms of anorexia with frequent stools, stunted somatic growth, and sideropenic anaemia represent characteristic clinical onset of CD (Auricchio & Troncone, 1993). This 'classic' presentation of the disease, particularly observed in children diagnosed within the first two years of life, is characterized by the prominence of intestinal symptoms. In this case early diagnosis and dietary treatment have allowed a rapid recovery of growth: however it did not change the progression of the sensory-motor polyneuropathy which developed in the meantime. A sural nerve biopsy showed marked fibre loss (particularly of large calibre fibres) and absence of evidence for regeneration, such as clustered, small myelinated fibres.

As far as the aetiology of the PNS involvement, malabsorption of vitamins, such as vitamin E and folic acid, cannot be considered to be the main cause of nerve damage since serum levels of both were normal during the whole course of the disease. Reduced concentration of serum vitamin E has been described in children affected with CD (Muller *et al.*, 1974) and malabsorption of lipids with vitamin E deficiency has been involved in the aetiology of neurologic impairment (Muller *et al.*, 1983). Even if vitamin amounts detected in serum do not fully reflect tissue levels, as may occur in hyperlipidemia (Sokol *et al.*, 1984), this condition can be ruled out since normal blood levels of total lipids were present in this patient. In the only reported paediatric case of CD associated with axonal polyneuropathy which started during a gluten free diet and which was associated with normal blood levels of vitamin E, both clinical and neurophysiological improvement were observed

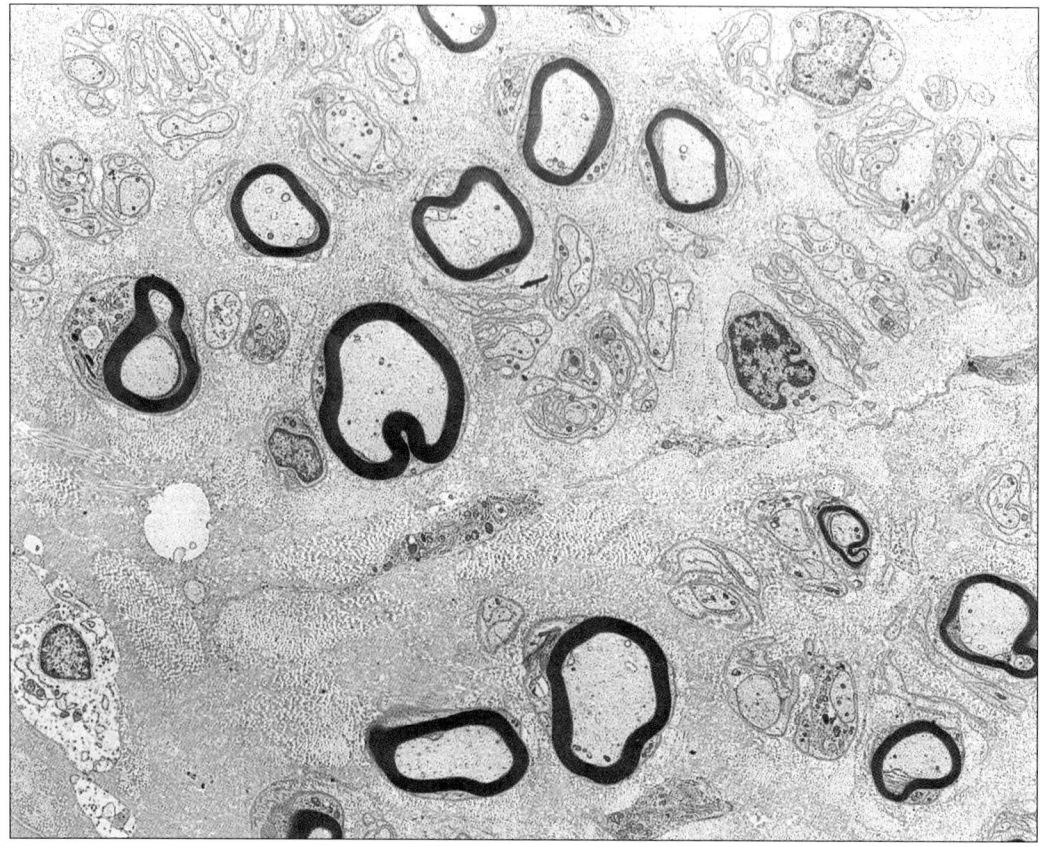

Fig. 1. Sural nerve biopsy: marked reduction of myelinated fibres; increased amount of endoneurial collagen; no evidence of Schwann cell hypertrophy (× 3300).

following vitamin E supplementation (Papadatou *et al.*, 1991). This was not seen in the present case. Chronic vitamin E deficiency is rarely observed and is commonly associated with chronic fat malabsorption, reduced bile salts in the small intestine, or fibrocystic disease. Both physiological and morphological investigations of PNS are consistent with a distal axonopathy (Landrieu *et al.*, 1985; Sokol *et al.*, 1983).

Reports of human PNS involvement following chronic acid folic deficiency are quite rare (Botez *et al.*, 1978, Fehling *et al.*, 1974; Manzoor & Runcie, 1976; Viader *et al.*, 1995). Both clinical and physiological recovery, however, occur following diet supplementation.

As previously mentioned, in some CD patients progression of the neurological complications is not halted by vitamin supplementation, nor does it respond to a gluten-free diet, suggesting that direct toxicity of gliadin is not implicated (Hermaszewski *et al.*, 1991). Moreover, in some cases the neuropathological lesions do not resemble the established pattern of any known deficiency disease, and therefore the depletion of a still unrecognized essential nutrient due to malabsorption remains a possibility (Kinney *et al.*, 1982). Both clinical and pathological features of the present case recall the early onset of hereditary motor and sensory neuropathy (HMSN) of the neuronal type, as described by Ouvrier *et al.* (1981). It is a genetically determined disorder, probably related to altered maturation of both peripheral motor and sensory neurons, leading to chronic atrophy and degeneration of nerve fibres (Gabreels-Festen *et al.*, 1991). The disorder, which starts in early infancy, is transmitted as an autosomic recessive trait, and sporadic cases have also been described. Nothing is known about the molecular genetics of the disease, and therefore any relationship with genetic determinants of CD is purely speculative.

The reported case describes a child affected with CD who developed a progressive axonal poly-neuropathy which did not respond to a gluten-free diet, nor to vitamin supplementation. There was no evidence of malabsorption, nor of blood factor deficiency, such as avitaaminosis, which might cause the nerve damage. The pathological features of the nerve biopsy were consistent with peripheral axonopathy, but the lesion pattern is not like the previously reported one in CD. There-fore, either two different diseases (HMSN and CD) were affecting this child, or the polyneuropathy is the expression of a still unknown pathological effect of CD on peripheral nerve tissue.

References

Auricchio, S. & Troncone, R. (1993): Coeliac disease. In: *Management of digestive and liver disorders in infants and children*, eds. J.P. Buts & E.M. Sokal, pp. 271–283. Amsterdam: Elsevier Science.

Banerji, N.K. & Hurwitz, L.J. (1971): Neurological manifestations in adult steatorrea. *J. Neurol. Sci.* **14,** 125–141.

Bernier, J.J., Buge. A., Rambaud, J.C., Rancurel, G., Hauw, J.J., Modigliani, R. & Denvil, D. (1976): Polyneuropathies chroniques non carentielles au cours de la maladie coéliaque de l'adult. *Ann. Med. Int.* **10,** 721–729.

Binder, H.J., Solitare, G.B. & Spiro, H.M. (1970): Neuromuscular disease in patients with steatorrhea. *Gut* **8,** 605–611.

Botez, M.I., Peyronnard, J.M., Bachevalier, J, & Charron, L. (1978): Polyneuropathy and folate deficiency. *Arch. Neurol.* **35,** 581–584.

Brown Carnegie, E. (1908): *Sprue and its treatment.* Pitman, London.

Catassi, C., Rätsch, I.M., Fabiani, E., Rossini, M., Bordicchia, F., Candela, F., Coppa, G.V. & Giorgi, P.L. (1994): Coeliac disease in the year 2000: exploring the iceberg. *Lancet* **343,** 200–203.

Chapman, R.W.G., Laidlow, J.M., Colin-Jones, D., Eade, O.E. & Smith, C.L. (1978): Increased evidence of epilepsy in coeliac disease. *BMJ* **ii,** 250–251.

Collin, P. & Mäki, M. (1994): Associated disorders in coeliac disease: clinical aspects. *Scand. J. Gastroenterol.* **29,** 769–775.

Collin, P., Pirttilä, T., Nurmikko, T., Somer, H., Erilä, T. & Keyriläinen, O. (1991): Coeliac disease, brain atrophy and dementia. *Neurology* **41,** 372–375.

Connolly, C.E., Kennedy, M., Stevens, F.M. & Mc Carty, C.F. (1994): Brown bowel syndrome occurring in coeliac disease in the West of Ireland. *Scand. J. Gastroenterol.* **29,** 91–94.

Cooke, W.T. (1976): Neurologic manifestations of malabsorption. In: *Handbook of clinical neurology*, vol 28, eds. P.J. Vinken & G.W. Bruyn, pp. 225–241. Amsterdam: North-Holland

Cooke, W.T. & Holmes, G.K.T. (1984): Neurological and psychiatric complications. In: *Coeliac disease,* eds. W.T. Cooke & G.K.T. Holmes, pp. 197–213. Edinburgh: Churchill Livingstone.

Cooke, W.T., Johnson, A.G. & Woolf, A.L. (1966): Vital staining and electron microscopy of the intramuscular endings in the neuropathy of adult coeliac disease. *Brain* **89,** 663–682.

Cooke, W.T. & Smith, W.T. (1966): Neurological disorders associated with adult coeliac disease. *Brain* **89,** 683–722.

Fehling, C., Jagerstad, M., Lindstrand, K. & Elmquist D. (1974): Folate deficiency and neurological disease. *Arch. Neurol.* **30,** 263–265.

Finelli, P.F., Mc Entee, W.J., Ambler, M. & Kostenbaum, D. (1980): Adult celiac disease presenting as cerebellar syndrome. *Neurology* **30,** 245–249.

Gabreëls-Festen, A.A.W.M., Joosten, E.M.G., Gabreëls, F.J.M., Jennekens, F.G.I., Gooskens, R.H.J.M. & Stegeman, D.F. (1991): Hereditary motor and sensory neuropathy of neuronal type with onset in early childhood. *Brain* **114,** 1855–1870.

Gobbi, G., Bouquet, F., Greco, L., Lambertini, A., Tassinari, C.A., Ventura, A. & Zaniboni, M.G. (1992): Coeliac disease, epilepsy, and cerebral calcifications. *Lancet* **i,** 439–443.

Greco, L., Maki, M., Di Donato, F., Visakorpi, J.K. (1992): Epidemiology of coeliac disease in Europe and the Mediterranean area. A summary report on the multicentre study by the European Society of Paediatric Gastroenterology and Nutrition. In: *Common food intolerances 1: epidemiology of coeliac disease*, vol 2, eds. S. Auricchio & J.K. Visakorpi, pp. 25–44. Basel: Karger.

Hallert, C. & Derefeldt, T. (1982): Psychic disturbances in adult coeliac disease. I Clinical observations. *Scand. J. Gastroenterol.* **17,** 17–19.

Hallert, C. & Aström, J. (1982): Psychic disturbances in adult coeliac disease. II Psychological findings. *Scand. J. Gastroenterol.* **17,** 21–24.

Hermaszewski, R.A., Rigby, S. & Dalgleish, A.G. (1991): Coeliac disease presenting with cerebellar degeneration. *Postgrad. Med. J.* **67,** 1023–1024.

Kaplan, J.G., Pack, D., Horoupian, D., DeSouza, T., Brin, M. & Schaumburg, H. (1988): Distal axonopathy associated with chronic gluten enteropathy: a treatable disorder. *Neurology* **38,** 642–645.

Kinney, H.C., Burger, P.C., Hurwitz, B.J., Hijmans, J.C. & Grant, J.P. (1982): Degeneration of the central nervous system associated with celiac disease. *J. Neurol. Sci.* **53,** 9–22.

Kristoferitsch, W. & Pointner, H. (1987): Progressive cerebellar syndrome in adult coeliac disease. *J. Neurol.* **234,** 116–118.

Landrieu, P., Selva, J., Alvarez, F., Ropert, A. & Metral, S. (1985): Peripheral nerve involvement in children with chronic cholestasis and vitamin E deficiency: a clinical, electrophysiological and morphological study. *Neuropediatrics* **16,** 194–201.

Manzoor, M. & Runcie, J. (1976): Folate responsive neuropathy: report of ten cases. *BMJ* **i,** 1176–1178.

Marsh, M.N. (1992): Gluten, major histocompatibility complex, and the small intestine. A molecular and immunobiologic approach to the spectrum of gluten sensitivity ('celiac sprue'). *Gastroenterology* **102,** 330–354.

Mauro, A., Orsi, L., Mortara, P., Costa, P. & Schiffer, D. (1991): Cerebellar syndrome in adult celiac disease with vitamin E deficiency. *Acta Neurol. Scand.* **84,** 167–170.

Morris, J.S., Adjukiewicz, A.B. & Read, A.E. (1970): Neurological disorders and adult coeliac disease. *Gut* **11,** 549–554.

Mulder, C.J.J. & Tytgat, G.N.J. (1987): Coeliac disease and related disorders. *Ned. J. Med.* **31,** 286–299.

Muller, D.P.R., Harries, J.T. & Lloyd, J.K. (1974): The relative importance of the factors involved in the absorption of vitamin E in children. *Gut* **15,** 966–971.

Muller, D.P.R., Lloyd, J.K. & Wolff, O.H. (1983): Vitamin E and neurological function. *Lancet* **i,** 225–228.

Ouvrier, R.A., Mc Leod, J.G., Morgan, G.J., Wise, G.A. & Conchin, T.E. (1981): Hereditary motor and sensory neuropathy of neuronal type with onset in early childhood. *J. Neurol. Sci.* **51,** 181–197.

Pallis, C.R. & Lewis, P.D. (1974): Neurological complications of coeliac disease and tropical sprue. In *The Neurology of Gastrointestinal Disease*, eds. J. Walton, pp. 138–156. Philadelphia: W.B. Saunders.

Papadatou, B., Di Capua, M., Gambarara, M., Castellucci, G., Lucidi, V., Ferretti, V., Ferretti, F., Colombo, A.M., Bella, S. & Castro, M. (1991): Nervous system involvement in paediatric coeliac patients. In: *Coeliac disease*, eds. M.L. Mearin & C.J.J. Mulder, pp. 199. Dordrecht: Kluwer Academic Publishers.

Sokol, R.J., Bove, K.E., Heubi, J.E. & Iannaccone, S.T. (1983): Vitamin E deficiency during chronic childhood cholestasis: presence of sural nerve lesion prior to 2 1/2 years of age. *J. Pediatr.* **103,** 197–204.

Sokol, R.J., Heubi, J.E., Iannaccone, S.T., Bove, K.E. & Balistreri, W.F. (1984): Vitamin E deficiency with normal serum vitamin E concentrations in children with chronic cholestasis. *N. Engl. J. Med.* **310,** 1209–1212.

Ventura, A., Bouquet, F., Sartorelli, C., Barbi, E., Torre, G. & Tommasini, G. (1991): Coeliac disease, folic acid deficiency and epilepsy with cerebral calcifications. *Acta Paediatr. Scand.* **80,** 559–562.

Viader, F., Chapon, F., Doro, T., Rivrain, Y. & Lechevalier, B. (1995): Maladie coeliaque de l'adulte révélée par une neuropathie sensitivo-motrice. *Press. Med.* **24,** 222–224.

Visakorpi J.K. (1992): Silent coeliac disease: the risk groups to be screened. In *Common food intolerance 1: epidemiology of coeliac disease*, Vol. 2, eds. S. Auricchio & J.K. Visakorpi, pp. 84–91. Basel: Dyn Nutr Res, Karger.

Ward, M.E., Murphy, J.T. & Greenberg, G.R. (1985): Celiac disease and spinocerebellar degeneration with normal vitamin E status. *Neurology* **35,** 1199–1201.

Epilepsy and other neurological disorders in coeliac disease, edited by G. Gobbi *et al.*
© 1997 John Libbey & Company Ltd, pp. 301–303.

Chapter 41

Muscular disorders in coeliac disease

Antonella Pini, Claudio Zanacca*, Giacomo Banchini*, Gianna Bertani and Giuseppe Gobbi

*Child Neurology and Psychiatry Service and *Paediatric Department, Arcispedale S. Maria Nuova, Viale Risorgimento 80, Reggio Emilia, Italy*

Introduction

Signs and symptoms of muscular involvement such as muscle wasting and hypotonia are frequently observed in the acute phase of classical coeliac disease (CD). However, although 'loss of muscular power and delayed milestones' has been reported (Walker-Smith, 1975), weakness does not necessarily develop even if marked hypotonia occurs (Dubowitz, 1995). As far as the causes are concerned, these symptoms may be a consequence of malabsorption if malnutrition with protein-calorie deficiency and nutritional myopathy develops (Renault & Quesada,1993; Dubowitz, 1995); moreover, it has been recently demonstrated that total serum carnitine, which is necessary for normal muscle function, is significantly reduced in patients with active CD (Ceccarelli *et al.*, 1992; Lerner *et al.*, 1993).

In chronic malabsorption of silent CD forms, presenting symptoms may be fatiguability, limb pain or muscle cramps, hypotonia and proximal weakness due to muscular involvement secondary to hypovitaminosis D, hypocalcaemia and osteomalacia or rickets (Hardoff *et al.*, 1980; De Boer & Tytgat, 1992; Rakover *et al.*, 1994; Dubowitz, 1995). As for the role of vitamin E, deficiency can occur in CD and its involvement in some neurological disorders has already been demonstrated (Satya-Murti *et al.*, 1986; Trabert, 1992; Mauro *et al.*, 1991). However, although a myopathy can be experimentally induced by vitamin E deficiency and a human myopathy associated with severely reduced plasma levels of the vitamin (reversible by treatment) has been reported (Tomasi, 1979), there is no clear evidence of a primary myopathy due to selective vitamin E deficiency in CD.

Among disorders associated with CD (Collin & Maki,1994; Collin *et al.*, 1994), autoimmune thyroid disorders or rheumatoid arthritis represent well known causes of myopathy, while the association between polymyositis and CD has not been clearly demonstrated, although it has been reported that CD may exceptionally present with symptoms that include polymyositis (Malnik *et al.*, 1994). Polymyositis and adult CD have been reported (Henriksson *et al.*, 1982).

Although some of the findings reported above are indicative of possible muscular involvement in CD, studies specially aimed at checking muscle integrity in CD are still lacking. Therefore, in a group of 64 patients with CD diagnosed or examined at the Paediatric Gastroenterological Day-Hospital of the S. Maria Nuova Hospital in Reggio Emilia between 1991–1994, 36 unselected patients underwent a muscle evaluation protocol.

Material and method

The age-range at the time of study was 18 months–26 years (mean age 9.4 years). Diagnostic criteria for CD were those of ESPGAN 1970–89. The patients were regularly followed by clinical observation and routine biochemical assays of gliadin, endomysium and reticulin antibodies were carried out. Twenty-three patients were examined; the parents of 13 patients were interviewed by phone. Additional information was obtained from medical reports and clinical notes. Details on age of onset, type of CD and latency between age of onset and age at diagnosis are summarized in Table 1. The time range between age at diagnosis (which was coincidental with gluten-free diet introduction) and age at the time of study was 1–20 years for CD with classical onset. All patients but two with atypical CD onset were investigated after 2–11 years after diagnosis; two patients were investigated at the time of diagnosis (after 3 years of untreated CD) and 3 months after diagnosis (after 11 months of untreated CD) respectively. The following data were collected for each patient: presence of relevant weakness before gluten-free diet introduction, motor skills, quality of dietary regime, presence of clinical-laboratory signs of active CD and of symptoms suggesting myopathy (such as weakness, exercise intolerance or cramps) at the time of study. Assessment of muscle power was graded according to a standardized scale and/or functional evaluation (depending on the patient's age), presence of contractures, muscular atrophy, myotonic and myastenic signs. Muscle ultrasound examination (quadriceps and deltoid muscles) was also performed.

To rule out the possibility of mitochondrial disease, needle muscle biopsy was performed in two patients, not included in the previous group, affected by the syndrome of CD, cerebral calcifications and gluten free diet resistant epilepsy.

Table 1.

Age onset of CD	Classical CD	Atypical/subclinical CD
Before 18 months	18 patients (latency: 1 month–3 years)	9 patients (latency: 2 months–11 years)
2–7 years	5 patients (latency: 1 year–17 years)	4 patients (latency: 6 months–8 years)

Results and conclusions

Muscular assessment was carried out in CD patients affected by childhood onset CD, most of whom were investigated at least one year after the diagnosis and the introduction of a gluten free diet. Although no patient was examined during the active phase of classical CD, retrospective information indicated that in no case was there severe prolonged malabsorption with marked nutritional deficit. All patients were on a gluten free diet at time of study and in no case was there clinical or laboratory evidence of active CD.

In this group of patients weakness and delayed motor skills were not reported before diagnosis and gluten free diet introduction, irrespective of the of age onset, type of CD and latency between age of onset and age at diagnosis. No symptoms of muscular involvement were present. Direct evaluation of muscle power and function and muscle ultrasound examination in 23 patients did not show any abnormality. In summary, muscular involvement was not found in 36 patients, with mean age of 9.4 years and childhood onset CD, who were maintained on a gluten-free diet and showed no clinical and laboratory evidence of active disease. Muscle biopsy showed a normal histological, histoenzymatic and histochemical picture at light microscopy in the two patients with CD, cerebral calcifications and epilepsy. In conclusion, as CD is characterized by immunologically mediated intestinal damage induced by dietary gluten intake in susceptible individuals, there could be many reasons for muscular involvement in the course of the disease: secondary myopathy may develop if severe nutritional protein-calorie intake deficiency, hypovitaminosis D, hypocalcaemia, osteomalacia, rickets or carnitine deficiency are present. Although muscle hypotonia and wasting remain typical findings in the acute phase of classical CD, early diagnosis and gluten-free diet introduction now usually prevent the development of severe prolonged malnutrition and, consequently, of true nutritional myopathy with weakness. As regards associated disorders, myopathy may occur in the presence of thyroid disorders or rheumatoid arthritis, while the association between CD and polymyositis is still to be investigated. Finally, direct experience suggests that muscular involvement does not seem to occur in individuals with childhood onset CD maintaining a gluten-free diet and without clinical or laboratory evidence of active disease, in the absence of associated disorders.

References

Ceccarelli, M., Cortigiani, L., Assanta, N., Nutini, P. & Ughi, C. (1992): Concentrazioni plasmatiche di L-carnitina in bambini celiaci. *Minerva Pediatr.* **44**, 401–405.

Collin, P. & Maki, M. (1994): Associated disorders in coeliac disease: clinical aspects. *Scand. J. Gastroenterol.* **29**, 769–775.

Collin, P., Reunala, T., Pukkala, E., Laippala, P., Keyrilainen, O., Pasternack, A. (1994): Coeliac disease-associated disorders and survival. *Gut* **35**, 1215–1218.

De Boer, W.A. & Tytgat, G.N. (1992): A patient with osteomalacia as single presenting symptom of gluten sensitive enteropathy. *J. Int. Med.* **232**, 81–85.

Dubowitz, V. (1995): Nutritional myopathies. In: *Muscle disorders in childhood,* 2nd edu, pp. 320–322. London: W.B. Saunders

Hardoff, D., Sharf, B. & Berger, A. (1980): Myopathy as a presentation of coeliac disease. *Dev. Med. Child Neurol.* **22**, 781–783.

Henriksson, K.G., Hallert, C., Norrby, K. & Walan, A. (1982): Polymiositis and adult coeliac disease. *Acta Neurol. Scand.* **65**, 301–319.

Lerner, A., Gruener, N. & Iancu, T.C. (1993): Serum carnitine concentrations in coeliac disease. *Gut* **34**, 933–935.

Malnick, S.D.H., Lurie, Y., Bass, D.D. & Geltner, D. (1994): Screening for coeliac disease. *Lancet* **343**, 675.

Mauro, A., Orsi, L., Mortara, P., Costa, P., Schiffer, D. (1991): Cerebellar syndrome in adult celiac disease with vitamin E deficiency. *Acta Neurol. Scand.* **84**, 167–170.

Rakover, Y., Hager, H., Nussinson, E. & Luboshitzky, R. (1994): Celiac Disease as a cause of transient hypocalcemia and hypovitaminosis D in a 13 year-old girl. *J. Pediatr. Endocrinol.* **7**, 1 53–55.

Renault, F. & Quesada, R. (1993): Muscle complications of malnutrition in children: a clinical and electromyographic study. *Neurophysiol. Clin.* **23**, 371–380.

Satya-Murti, S., Howard, L., Krohel, G. & Wolf, B. (1986): The spectrum of neurological disorders from vitamin E deficiency. *Neurology* **36**, 917–921.

Tomasi, L.G. (1979): Reversibility of human myopathy caused by vitamin E deficiency. *Neurology* **29**, 1182–1186.

Trabert, W. (1992): Celiac disease and vitamin E deficiency. *Neurology* **42**, 1641.

Walker-Smith, J. (1975): Coeliac disease. In: *Diseases of the small intestine in childhood*. London: Pitman Publishing Ltd, pp 51–88.

Addendum Section

Epilepsy and other neurological disorders in coeliac disease, edited by G. Gobbi *et al.*
© 1997 John Libbey & Company Ltd, pp. 307–369.

1: Screening for gluten intolerance

Klaus Pittschieler and Brigitte Ladinser

Department of Paediatrics, Ospedale Regionale, via L. Böhler 5, I 39100 Bolzano/Bolzen, Italy

In South Tyrol, an alpine region in Northern Italy, one child out of 950 is clinically affected by coeliac disease (Pittschieler *et al.*, 1988). These data are based on patients diagnosed both by clinical symptoms and biopsy. We decided to investigate the epidemiology of coeliac disease in this region by screening a large number of healthy adults.

Sera from 4615 blood donors were firstly analysed for IgA and IgG antigliadin antibodies by ELISA. Positive sera were further evaluated by a modified methodology of the immunofluorescent assay of the endomysial antibody: a new substrate, human umbilical cord instead of the distal part of monkey oesophagus, gave a specificity and sensitivity of 100 per cent and the cost of endomysial antibody testing was greatly reduced (Ladinser *et al.*, 1994).

Out of 140 subjects positive for antigliadin antibodies (IgA, IgG or IgA, and IgG), 33, including the nine positive for endomysial antibody, gave their consent for intestinal biopsy. However, only those nine patients positive for the modified endomysial antibody test showed mucosal abnormalities, i.e. total (six cases) and partial villous atrophy (two cases) or minimal villous changes. All subjects showing positive tests for both endomysial and antigliadin antibodies had, independently from the histological appearance of their mucosa, a pathological ratio of γ/δ to α/β T-cell receptors in the intraepithelial lymphocytes of the intestinal mucosa. However, those subjects tested as positive for antigliadin but negative for endomysial antibodies, showed a normal receptor ratio.

In conclusion, we found positive predictive values for coeliac disease of only 8.1 per cent for TgG antigliadin antibody, of 53 per cent for IgA, of 75 per cent for combined IgA and IgG , and of 100 per cent for endomysial antibody. The umbilical cord assay, although probably similar in cost, is slightly more labour intensive than the antigliadin antibodies test. The umbilical cord endomysial antibody assay is much more sensitive and specific than the traditional AGA-test, making it the first choice as a screening method. Furthermore, mucosas from AGA positive but endomysial antibody negative subjects show no features of overt or latent coeliac disease.

Finally, according to the results of this screening, the prevalence of coeliac disease in the two population groups is not significantly different: 216/100 000 in the German speaking group and 163/100 000 in the Italian one. This prevalence is higher than expected from our previous investigations, but close to that found in similar screenings in Europe (Catassi *et al.*, 1994).

Coeliac disease should therefore no longer be considered as a rare disorder.

2: Dental enamel defects in coeliac disease children and their relatives: the significance of HLA typing

P. Mariani, M.C. Mazzilli[*], G. Margutti[**] , L. Calvani, F. Virgilii, F. Petronzelli[*], L. Ferrante and M. Bonamico

Istituto Clinica Pediatrica, [*]Dipartimento di Medicina Sperimentale e [**]Cl. Odontoiatrica, Università 'La Sapienza', Roma, Italy

Introduction

In coeliac disease (CD) oral lesions can be observed, particularly recurrent aftous stomatitis and dental enamel defects. On the other hand enamel hypoplasia has been described in other conditions with hypocalcaemia (rickets, hypoparathyroidism, neonatal tetany and severe malnutrition (Nikiforuk & Fraser, 1981). Finnish authors (Aine *et al.*, 1990) have given particular attention to the enamel status in CD and have described permanent tooth enamel defects in a high percentage of patients. Moreover the same lesions have

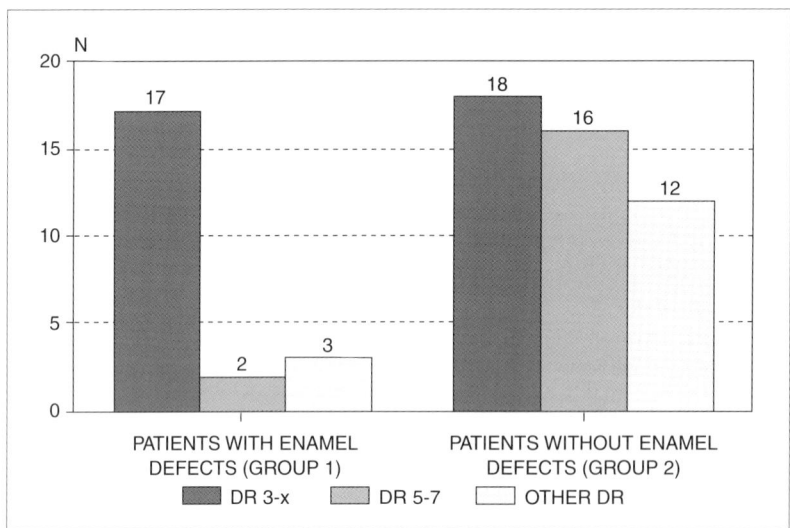

Fig. 1. HLA DR antigens and enamel defects in children with coeliac disease.

been observed in half of CD relatives and, in some of them, CD was subsequently diagnosed. Dental enamel defects are distributed symmetrically in all four sections of dentition, occurring at the same time as the enamel maturation process, and can be classified in four grades: the first one characterized by a defect in colour and the others by slight, evident or severe structural defects (Aine *et al.*, 1990). Conversely the Commission on Oral Health Research and Epidemiology distinguish developmental enamel lesions into *demarcated opacity* and *diffuse opacity*, which involve an alteration in the translucency of the enamel, and *hypoplasia*, a reduced localised thickness of enamel surface (Commission on Oral Health, Research and Epidemiology, 1992).

Aim of this study was to evaluate the prevalence of enamel defects in a group of Italian CD children and their relatives. In children, a possible correlation between enamel lesions, serum calcium levels and HLA DR antigens was also investigated.

Materials and methods

Developmental enamel defects have been researched in 87 coeliacs (29 males and 58 females, mean age 11 years and 9 months ± 4 years and 6 months) diagnosed according to ESPGAN criteria, and in 161 relatives (120 parents and 41 siblings) of 90 coeliac children. As normal controls 189 apparently healthy children, age-matched with CD children, were enrolled in the study.

Dental examination was performed by a dentist; the teeth were cleaned, washed, dried and observed in a good artificial light. Colour, type and site of defects were recorded. In 80 children, at the first biopsy, calcium serum levels were evaluated. 68 children and 77 relatives were HLA class II typed using PCR-based DNA typing.

Relatives were evaluated by an anamnestic record for gastrointestinal disorders, by AGA IgA (131 cases), AGA IgG (129 cases) and EMA (100 cases) determination. According to clinical data, intestinal biopsy was performed in six parents and 14 siblings. Student *t*-test, Fisher's exact test, regression analysis and logistic regression analysis were used to analyse the results.

Results

In 11/87 (12.6 per cent) of CD children we found demarcated opacities or hypoplasia systematically distributed (Group 1A), whereas in 13 (14.9 per cent) enamel lesions distributed symmetrically and chronologically, but involving only the maxilla, were observed (Group 1B). The occurrence of the different enamel defects in Groups 1A and 1B was: five and nine children with demarcated opacities, one and none with diffuse opacities and five and four with hypoplasia. In the remaining 92 cases (Group 2) no dental lesions were detected. No differences in the male/female ratio and in the mean age (Student *t*-test) between children with or without lesions was observed. Nevertheless regression analysis showed a correlation between age at diagnosis and number of teeth with enamel defects. Hypocalcaemia was found in 8/23 (34.8 per cent) patients in Group 1 and in 14/57 (24.6 per cent) in Group 2 (Fisher's test: n.s.). Mean serum calcium did not show differences (Student t test) between Group 1 (9.4 ± 1.1 mg/dl) and Group 2 patients (9.3 ± 0.9 mg/dl).

Thirty-five out of 68 HLA-typed children were DR3,x (51.5 per cent), 18 were DR5,7 (26.5 per cent), 15 (22.0 per cent) were DR4 or other DR positive. The figure shows the distribution of genotypes in Group 1 and 2 children. Relative risk of enamel lesions for genotype DR3,x and DR 5.7 was 5.28 and 0.17 respectively. No differences in the DR antigens in Groups 1A and 1B children were found (Mariani *et al.,* 1994). Logistic regression analysis was performed with enamel status as dependent variable and age at diagnosis, serum calcium, number of affected teeth, type of enamel defect and DR antigens as independent variables. The only variable that enters the model is HLA DR antigens.

Dental lesions, found in 28/189 (14.8 per cent) controls (in 24 demarcated opacities and in 4 hypoplasia) were significantly less frequent than in CD patients (Fisher's exact test: $P < 0.005$). Enamel lesions have been observed in 29 relatives (18 per cent) of CD children, 22 parents (18.3 per cent) and in seven siblings (17.1 per cent). Demarcated opacities, diffuse opacities and hypoplasia were observed in 14 (48.3 per cent), three (10.3 per cent) and 12 (41.4 per cent) cases respectively.

None of the 16 relatives with enamel lesions was HLA-DR5,7, while among 61 subjects without lesions 12 were DR5,7 ($P < 0.05$). In 9/16 HLA DR3,x dental defects have been observed, while 26/61 relatives without lesions were DR3,x (P = n.s.).

Among 20 biopsied relatives CD has been diagnosed in two parents and 12 siblings; enamel lesions have been observed in one parent (HLA not typed) and in three siblings (two HLA DR3,x and one HLA DR4,9).

Discussion

Our observations indicate that little more than a quarter of CD children present peculiar enamel defects. This percentage is much lower than in Finnish children (96 per cent Aine *et al,*. 1990), and is comparable with other Italian studies (Prati *et al.,* 1987; Balli *et al.,* 1988). Results are higher (3.8 per cent) than in a Swiss series (Shmerling *et al.,* 1980). Moreover in respect of Finnish data, in our series enamel lesions, when present, involve a lower number of teeth and were less pronounced, often involving only the maxilla. Since no differences were found between patients of Groups 1A and 1B in respect of the different variables investigated, we suggest that non-systematic enamel defects represent a milder form of systematic lesion. Also in respect of controls in our children, enamel lesions were less frequent (14.8 per cent) than in the Finnish children (31.4 per cent). The different prevalence observed in the various populations could be due partially to genetic factors, as is indicated by the significant prevalence of DR3 antigen in our CD patients with enamel defects. This is in agreement with Maki *et al.,* 1991, who observed such lesions in 15 CD patients, 14 HLA DR3 positive. Our data suggest that HLA factors causing CD risk and dental lesions are not identical: whereas CD appears to be primarily associated with the DQ (α1*0501,β1*0201) heterodimer, present both in DR3 and DR5,7 patients (Mazzilli *et al.,* 1991), enamel defects in CD patients seem to be associated to a greater extent with DR antigens. However, since enamel defects were observed only in a certain number of DR3 patients, other factors are to be considered in the pathogenesis of dental lesions in CD. Another possible explanation for the presence of enamel defects in CD is that enamel hypoplasia is caused by hypocalcaemia due to malabsorption, in agreement with the unifying hypothesis on the aetiology of enamel hypoplasia in various pathological conditions (Nikiforuk & Fraser, 1981). Nevertheless different calcium levels among children with or without dental lesions were not found. Finally, enamel defects could be related to immunological factors. In fact, it is well known that CD is associated with HLA-DR specificities, as well as with a number of alterations in the T-and B-cell activities, thus suggesting that a defect in the immunoregulation may be the basis of this disease (Davidson & Bridges, 1987). Enamel defects have been observed in a lower percentage of relatives of CD children than in CD patients, with similar percentages in parents and siblings. Only 4/14 CD relatives showed enamel lesions, while Maki (1991) observed these defects in all CD relatives.

Results of relatives' HLA typing confirm that genotype DR5,7 seems to protect against the occurrence of dental changes, while the presence of HLA DR3 antigen, different from CD children, does not increase the risk of dental lesions.

3: Epilepsy and coeliac disease: the role of hypofolataemia

V. Galli, A. Guerra, S. Leoni, M.F. Roversi, F. Balli, P. Bertolani, P., Melli and C. Faccini

Paediatric Department, Modena University, 41100 Modena, Italy

Folate deficiency, due to malabsorption, has been described as a pathogenetic factor of neurological impairment in CD. Neurological alterations (ataxia, athetosis, peripheral neuropathy, mental retardation, seizures and cerebral calcifications) have been found in both congenital folate metabolism anomalies and acquired folate deficiency (iatrogenic, malabsorpitive, antiepileptic induced, etc.) (Garwicz & Mortensson, 1976; Gobbi *et al.*, 1992; Lanzkowky *et al.*, 1969; Norris & Pratt, 1971). The hypofolataemia pathogenetic pathway in neurological impairment may show up as an alteration of lecithin metabolism that leads to endothelial inflammation with cerebral calcium deposits (Della Cella *et al.*, 1991). The selective vulnerability of the occipital lobe may be related to the high vascularization and synaptogenesis during the first year of life.

At the Modena University Paediatric Department we follow 300 patients suffering from CD: 210 of them were diagnosed early (70 per cent) and 90 diagnosed late (> 4 years of age). Fifteen patients were selected with the aim of studying the relationship between CD, cerebral calcifications and folic acid deficiency. We identified two groups.

Group 1

Three subjects (1 per cent of the total) affected by CD and epilepsy, are described below.

Case 1

P.D., a 6-year-old girl, was referred to our department because of occipital partial seizures (transient blindness, staring, eye deviation to the left sometimes followed by headache). Developmental milestones were reached at appropriate age. Neurological examination and haematological findings were normal. The EEG showed continuous high-voltage spike waves and slow waves bilaterally in the occipital regions. On computed tomography scanning (CT), bilateral occipital sinuous cortical-subcortical calcifications were observed with no surrounding parenchymal abnormalities. Previously diagnosed as atypical Sturge–Weber disease, at the age of 10 the patient manifested failure to thrive, severe hypochromic anaemia, persistence of seizures despite antiepileptic treatment, and progressive mental impairment. Laboratory tests for CD were performed and found positive. Jejunal biopsy showed villous atrophy. GFD was started with no clinical effect. Serum folate levels were persistently low in spite of a long period of GFD.

Case 2

M.A., a 5-year-old male, hospitalized for generalized epilepsy with several types of seizures including atypical absences, generalized tonic seizures during sleep, drop attacks and impairment of psychomotor development. The EEG showed abnormal background with continuous spike waves discharges at 1.5 c/s. The CT scan was normal. In subsequent years, the patient manifested a Lennox–Gastaut syndrome with intractable epilepsy (multiple daily seizures) and severe mental impairment. At the age of 14 years the subject was at the lower end of the distribution for both weight and height and showed absence of pubertal development and persistent hypochromic anaemia in spite of iron therapy. Tests for antigliadin and antiendomysium antibodies, performed at this age, were positive and jejunal biopsy showed villous atrophy. CT scan was still normal (no cerebral calcifications) while the serum folic acid level was persistently low even after 1 year of GFD.

Case 3

P.E., a girl, was first admitted to our Department at the age of 1 year for classical symptoms of CD. The diagnosis was confirmed by blood test results and jejunal biopsy. At the age of 11 years, on GFD, she manifested generalized seizures (absences) and the EEG showed 3 c/s spike wave discharges. We started antiepileptic therapy until the age of 14 years. The CT scan was consistently normal as well as the neurological development. The serum folic acid level was always normal.

Table 1. Twelve late-diagnosed coeliac disease patients

No. Case	Name	Sex	CD symptomatology	Age of CD diagnosis	Neurological symptomatology	EEG pattern	Cerebral CT	Folataemia before GFD (2–17 ng/ml)	Folataemia after GFD (2–17 ng/ml)
1	B.G.	F	typical	5 years	absent	normal	negative	1.82	2.57
2	S.C.	F	hypochromic anaemia	4 years and 4 months	absent	normal	negative	1.12	5.43
3	M.V.	F	low weight	6 years	absent	normal	negative	0.93	1.47*
4	P.S.	F	low weight and low height	4 years and 3 months	absent	normal	negative	0.98	0.98*
5	D.G.	F	low weight and low height after the age of 9 years	11 years and 3 months	absent	normal	negative	0.95	1.23*
6	M.C.	F	typical	4 years and 2 months	absent	normal	negative	0.97	0.93*
7	R.M.	M	herpetiform dermatitis from the age of 5 years	15 years and 10 months	absent	normal	negative	1.85	2.76
8	B.E.	F	low weight and low height from the age of 9 years	13 years and 3 months	absent	normal	negative	0.78	0.82*
9	B.K.	F	herpetiform dermatitis	16 years and 5 months	absent	normal	negative	0.96	1.03*
10	P.E.	F	frequent vomiting, hypochromic anaemia	18 years and 9 months	absent	normal	negative	1.46	3.85
11	C.G.	F	typical	25 years	absent	normal	negative	1.72	4.03
12	D.L.	M	low weight, herpetiform dermititis	37 years	absent	normal	negative	1.83	4.84

GFD, Gluten-free diet; CD, coeliac disease; *persistent hypofolataemia.

Group 2

Group 2 included 12 subjects, 10 girls and two boys, whose diagnosis was identified after a long illness. Their age at the time of diagnosis ranged from 4 years and 2 months to 37 years, with an average of 13 years and 3 months ± 9 and 9. They had, consequently, a deficient nutrient intake and more extensive malabsorption (Table 1). In nine out of 12 cases (75 per cent) the CD onset was atypical, showing extraintestinal symptoms such as growth failure, iron deficiency with anaemia, herpetiform dermatitis. Only three patients (25 per cent) started with gastroenterological symptoms. Together with the histological diagnosis we carried out EEG, CT and serum folic acid level determination. All patients showed hypofolatemia (mean 1.28 ± 0.42 ng/ml, minimum 0.78 ng/ml, maximum 1.85 ng/ml; n.v.: 2–17 ng/ml), EEG patterns and CT were normal. 1–2 years after the beginning of GFD we repeated the serum folic acid level determination. For six out of 12 subjects the value was persistently low (mean value 1.07 ± 0.23 ng/ml, minimum 0.82 ng/ml, maximum 1.47 ng/ml) in spite of strict GFD and clinical improvement or normalization; the mean value of serum folic acid level in the 12 cases on GFD was 2.49 ± 1.67 ng/ml (minimum 0.82 ng/ml, maximum 5.43 ng/ml).

To sum up all the 12 late diagnosed coeliac patients showed hypofolataemia but did not manifest epilepsy and/or cerebral calcifications while one out of the three cases with neurological involvement (Group 1) did not have hypofolataemia. It is apparent that little is known of the true role of hypofolataemia in the neurological involvement in CD. It is likely that several factors, environmental and genetic, affect the neurological damage due to folate deficiency.

4: The triad of epilepsy, coeliac disease and cerebral calcifications: in search of the missing item

Patrizia Pinto*, Cristina Agostinis** and Carlo Alberto Defanti*

*1st Department of Neurology, Regional Epilepsy Center; ** Department of Neuroradiology, Ospedali Riuniti, Largo Barozzi 1, 24100 Bergamo, Italy

Introduction

In the last few years several cases of association of CD, epilepsy and cerebral calcifications have been reported in (Sammaritano et al., 1988; Molteni et al., 1988; Ventura et al., 1991; Zaniboni et al., 1991; Ambrosetto et al., 1992; Gobbi et al., 1992; Fois et al., 1993; Magaudda et al., 1993; Piattella et al., 1993; Tiacci et al., 1993). This particular pattern of calcifications is documented on CT scan in the posterior regions of cerebral hemispheres at cortico-subcortical level. They are generally bilateral but asymmetrical and were previously considered part of an atypical Sturge–Weber syndrome (Garvitz et al., 1976; Ambrosetto et al., 1983; Gobbi et al., 1988). The pathogenetic mechanism of these lesions is still under investigation. Similar findings have been reported after administration of methotrexate and skull irradiation (Garvitz et al., 1976). Some authors have postulated a role of folate deficiency due to the antifolic effect of methotrexate or due to the malabsorption in CD (Garvitz et al., 1976; Sammaritano et al., 1988; Molteni et al., 1988; Ventura et al., 1991), while others (Magaudda et al., 1993) have supported the hypothesis that a similar HLA pattern could induce susceptibility both for CD and cerebral calcifications.

In order to provide additional data concerning this interesting syndrome we have evaluated neuroradiological, gastroenterological and immunogenetic aspects in seven patients with seizures and at least one other element of the triad.

Patients

We observed a group of seven patients (four males, three females, mean age 18.5 years, range 10–28) affected by CD and seizures.

In a first subgroup we included four epileptic patients (three females, mean age 18.5 years, range 10–28 years) with a previous diagnosis of CD. The mean age of diagnosis of CD was 9.5 years (range 1–25 years). All patients were following a restricted gluten-free diet since the time of diagnosis. In this group the mean age of onset of epilepsy was 10.2 years (range 1–23 years). In two cases the seizures were tonic–clonic during sleep, in one case the seizures were partial motor and in the last case they were polymorphic (visual, versive and tonic-clonic). All patients had complete control of seizures with antiepileptic drugs and in one case the treatment had been discontinued. These patients had a neuroradiological evaluation which included CT scan and MRI.

The second subgroup included three males with mean age 18.6 years (range 16–21 years) suffering from seizures. In these cases a previous CT scan performed at mean age of 11.6 years (range 2–19 years) had shown bilateral hemispheric calcifications, located in the occipital regions in two cases and in the parieto-occipital regions in the third case. No patient had a family history of epilepsy. None had port-wine facial naevus nor history of meningoencephalitis, radio- or chemotherapy, vascular accidents and congenital infections. At the time of observation no malabsorption symptoms were mentioned by any patients. In one patient only, the history revealed previous transient symptoms and signs of malabsorption during the first two years of life. The mean age of onset of seizures was 11.6 years (2–19 years). All patients presented tonic–clonic seizures: patient 7 (Table1) had an isolated seizure during wakefulness at the age of 18: in the other two cases the generalized seizures were associated with partial complex and versive seizures respectively.

In this group we evaluated the presence of IgA and IgG antigliadin antibodies (AGA) and of antiendomysial antibodies (AEA), the serum level of vitamin B_{12} and folates, parathyroid hormone, calcitonin, calcium and phosphates. Small bowel biopsy was performed in all three cases. Fundus oculi was also examined.

All patients underwent EEG, Wechsler Scale evaluation, and HLA typing.

Table 1. Main clinical and radiological features

Patients	Sex	Age	Seizures onset (years)	Type of seizures	Diagnosis of CD (years)	Calcifications	HLA
1	F	19	15	t- c*	1	absent	DR3,DR7
2	F	17	2	t-c*, versive, visual	4	bioccipital	not available
3	F	28	23	t-c*	25	absent	DR11,(5)DR7
4	M	10	1	partial motor	8	absent	DR3,DR7
5	M	21	14	partial complex,t- c*	21	parieto-occipital	DR11(5)DR7
6	M	16	2	t-c*, versive	16	bioccipital	DR3,DR7
7	M	19	19	isolated t-c*	19	bioccipital	DR11(5)DR7

*Tonic–clonic.

Results

In the first subgroup the imaging studies revealed bioccipital calcifications in only one case. In the other patients CT scan and MR examination after contrast medium administration were normal.

The interictal EEG during wakefulness showed epileptiform activity in all cases (sharp waves of high voltage mixed with theta activity) on the occipital regions of both hemispheres in two cases and on the temporal region of one hemisphere in the other two.

In the second subgroup the AGA titer was increased in two cases, the AEA level was elevated in two cases; small bowel biopsy revealed total villous atrophy in all. Folate deficiency was discovered in two cases. All other serum investigations fell within normal limits.

The interictal EEG during wakefulness showed epileptiform activity limited to occipital regions in the cases with isolated seizure: in the other two cases it was recorded from the temporo-occipital regions of one hemisphere.

Mental development was normal in all patients. Fundus oculi examination showed normal findings except for one case who had a unilateral post-traumatic lesion.

HLA typing was performed in 6 patients; the results are reported in Table 1.

Discussion

An increased prevalence of epilepsy among patients suffering from CD has been reported since the early 1970s (Laidlow *et al.*, 1977).

More recently attention focused on the association of CD, brain calcifications and epilepsy (Sammaritano *et al.*, 1988; Molteni *et al.*, 1988; Ventura *et al.*, 1991; Zaniboni *et al.*, 1991; Ambrosetto *et al.*, 1992; Gobbi *et al.*, 1992; Magaudda *et al.*, 1993; Fois *et al.*, 1993; Piattella *et al.*, 1993). In these reports we noticed the frequent diagnosis of clinically silent coeliac disease in epileptic patients with brain calcifications. In most cases the calcifications were cortico- subcortical, gyriform or nodular, occipito or parieto-occipital, often bilateral, rarely with frontal extension. The basal nuclei were spared. Cerebral atrophy, reported in Sturge–Weber syndrome, was absent.

In our study we found silent coeliac disease in all the three patients of the second group, presenting brain calcifications. In this regard we point out the case of a 37 year old woman without history of seizures, in whom a silent CD was diagnosed after a CT scan, performed because of recurrent headache, had demonstrated the typical bioccipital calcifications.

Not all the patients affected by CD and epilepsy present these characteristic CT findings (Ambrosetto *et al.*, 1992): in the first subgroup of our patients, rigorously following a gluten-free diet, the search of cerebral calcifications was positive in one case only.

On the basis of these data and according to the observations of Bardella *et al.* (1994), we could suppose that prolonged malabsorption plays an essential role in the pathogenesis of these calcifications. In particular, some authors (Garvitz *et al.*, 1976; Sammaritano *et al.*, 1988; Molteni *et al.*, 1988; Ventura *et al.*, 1991) have drawn special attention to folate deficiency: in our observations two of the three patients with asymptomatic CD presented hypofolatemia.

All the six patients examined for HLA showed the presence the histocompatibility antigens HLA-DR7. Three of them were DR3 positive and the others were DR5 positive. The 37 year old woman with calcifications and CD, without history of seizures, was DR3 and DR7 positive.

DR3 and DR7 are strongly associated with the susceptibility to CD (De Marchi *et al.*, 1983), while HLA-DR5 is reported to be related to epilepsy (Minev *et al.*, 1987).

In our small group of patients no relation was found between calcifications and specific HLA-DR antigens.

As far as the evolution of epilepsy is concerned in patients with cerebral calcifications, some authors have reported unresponsiveness to antiepileptic drugs evolving to epileptic encephalopathy (Gobbi *et al.*, 1988; Magaudda *et al.*, 1993): our patients showed an excellent control of seizures, independent of the presence or absence of calcifications, except for one case of the second subgroup, who had typical CT findings.

Our impression is that the peculiar pattern of cerebral calcifications must be considered highly evocative for a concurrent CD (symptomatic or not) independent of the presence of seizures. Moreover, the relationship between CD and calcifications is probably closer than the one existing between calcifications and epilepsy.

In patients with CD and epilepsy, the presence of EEG anomalies predominating over posterior regions as well as the high frequency of occipital seizures suggest the possibility that in an early phase a functional alteration is present in these regions; later on, under the influence of unknown factors – nutritional, genetic, immunological, degenerative – in some patients this alteration becomes morphologic, eventually producing the triad of epilepsy, coeliac disease and cerebral calcifications.

Acknowledgements

The authors wish to thank doctors M. Bontempelli and P. Bellavita from the Immunohematologic Laboratory and doctors E. Pellizzari and F. Negrini from the Department of Gastroenterology of OORR, Bergamo, for their kind cooperation.

5: Infantile coeliac disease associated with epilepsy and endocranial calcifications: report of six cases

Bruno Cirillo, Gianmario Della Rotonda, Raffaella Mormile and Salvatore Buono[*]

Divisione di Medicina Pediatrica, Primario Berni Canani Mario, Unita' Operativa di Gastroenterologia;
[*]Reparto di Neurochirurgia, Servizio di Neurofisiologia, Azienda Ospedalieva di Rilievo Nazionale Santobono,
Napoli, Italy

Introduction

Several reports have described the association between epileptic disorders and endocranial calcifications in patients with coeliac disease (CD) (Piatella *et al.*, 1993; Bardella *et al.*, 1994; Gobbi *et al.*, 1992).

From January 1993 to December 1994, we screened a paediatric population of 109 subjects in the age range 8 months to 15 years, sex ratio M > F, for CD by jejunal biopsy. They were selected by history suggestive of CD and positive antiendomysial (AEA) and/or antigliadin (AGA) IgA and IgG antibodies. Examination of biopsy specimens demonstrated a total or a partial villous atrophy with crypt hyperplasia and intraepithelial plasma–cell infiltrate in 91 patients. In our experience, AEA and AGA IgA display better sensitivity and specificity in the diagnosis of CD than AGA IgG. Negative biopsies were found in the patients with positive AGA IgG only. The patients with CD often presented atypical signs such as short stature, poor weight gain without intestinal symptoms, and recurrent anaemia with low serum levels of iron. Six patients in the age range 2 years to 14 years, sex ratio M = F had seizures: in all but one, epilepsy preceded the diagnosis of CD. We report on these six cases with epilepsy, occipital calcifications and CD.

Case reports

Case 1

An 11 year old male was referred to our department for small stature. He was affected by a generalized partial epilepsy with complex symptomatology. The onset of epilepsy had occurred at the age of 2 years in the form of convulsive seizures. From the age of 3 years, his growth had been impaired. Seizures were unsatisfactorily controlled despite various anti-epileptic drug combinations: phenobarbital (PB), (CBZ), valproic acid (VPA) and Sabril. We diagnosed CD by laboratory tests and jejunal biopsy. CT scan of the skull showed bilateral occipital calcifications. A gluten-free diet was started but rendered no benefit. Seizures worsened with increasing frequency and progressive mental deficiency. Last CT scan of the skull was identical to the previous one. Follow-up has been discontinued.

Case 2

A 2 year old female was referred to our department for 'failure to thrive (5th percentile)' without intestinal symptoms. She had partial seizures with complex symptomatology and secondary generalization. Laboratory tests and jejunal biopsy confirmed the diagnosis of CD. CT scan of the skull demonstrated bilateral occipital calcifications. She was treated with PB therapy and a gluten-free diet. Neurological disorder improved with resultant disappearance of seizures. After 18 months PB was ceased without any relapse of seizures.

Case 3

An 8 year old male was referred to our department because of chronic diarrhoea and weight loss. We diagnosed CD by laboratory tests and jejunal biopsy. A gluten-free diet was started but not maintained. At the age of 3 year seizures suddenly began. He was admitted to our department again and suffered a generalized clonic seizure. We confirmed CD. CT scan of the skull showed unilateral occipital calcifications. The seizures are being successfully controlled with PB and a restricted gluten-free diet.

Case 4

An 8 year old male was referred to our department for short stature. He had simple partial motor seizures.

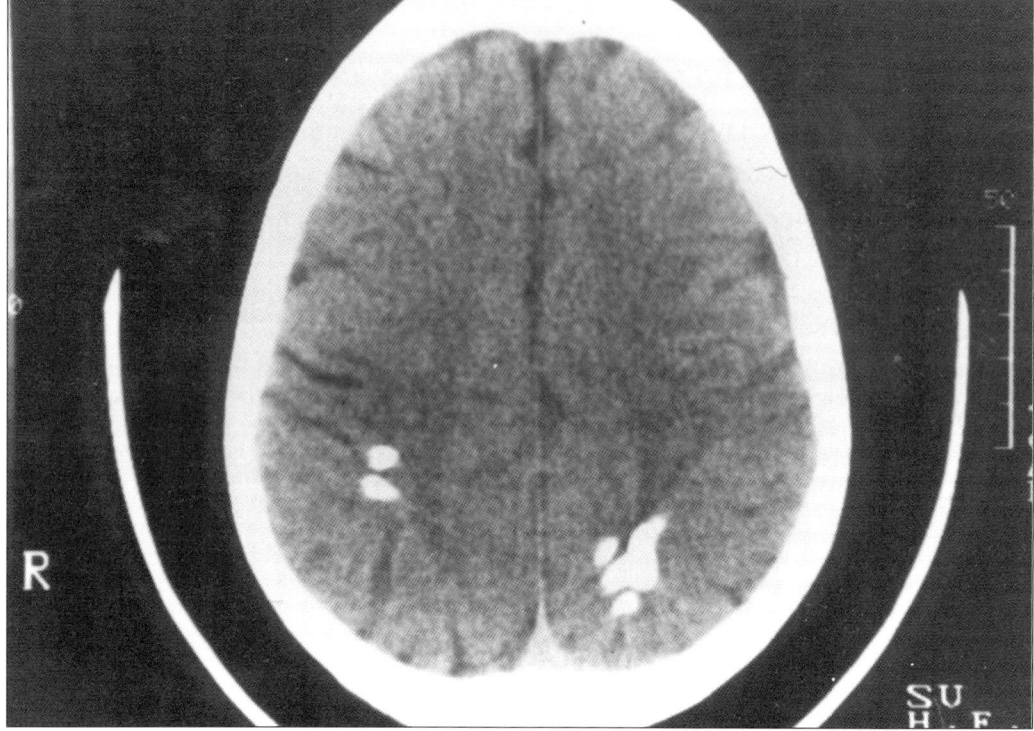

Fig. 1. Case 1, occipital calcifications in an 11-year-old child with coeliac disease.

Laboratory tests and jejunal biopsy confirmed CD. CT scan of the skull showed bilateral occipital calcifications. He is treated only with a gluten-free diet, without any recurrence of seizures.

Case 5

A 3 year old female was referred to our department for poor weight gain (5th percentile) and anaemia with low serum iron levels despite iron therapy. She had generalized clonic seizures. CD was confirmed by laboratory tests and jejunal biopsy. CT scan of the skull demonstrated bilateral occipital calcifications. Although she is currently receiving anti-epileptic therapy (PB) and a gluten-free diet, two brief seizures have recurred.

Table 1.

Features of the six cases observed

* No parental consanguinity
* No family history of epilepsy or neurological diseases
* No family history of coeliac disease
* Epilepsy with unilateral or bilateral occipital calcifications in all
* No epilepsy with occipital symptoms only
* Only one case of a severe drug-resistant epileptic encephalopathy
* Two cases of generalized epilepsy with clonic seizures
* Only one case of partial epilepsy with simple motor symptomatology
* Two cases of partial epilepsy with complex symptomatology and secondary generalization

Case 6

A 12 year old female was referred to our department for short stature and iron deficiency anaemia. She had a partial epilepsy with complex symptomatology. Laboratory tests and jejunal biopsy confirmed CD. CT scan of

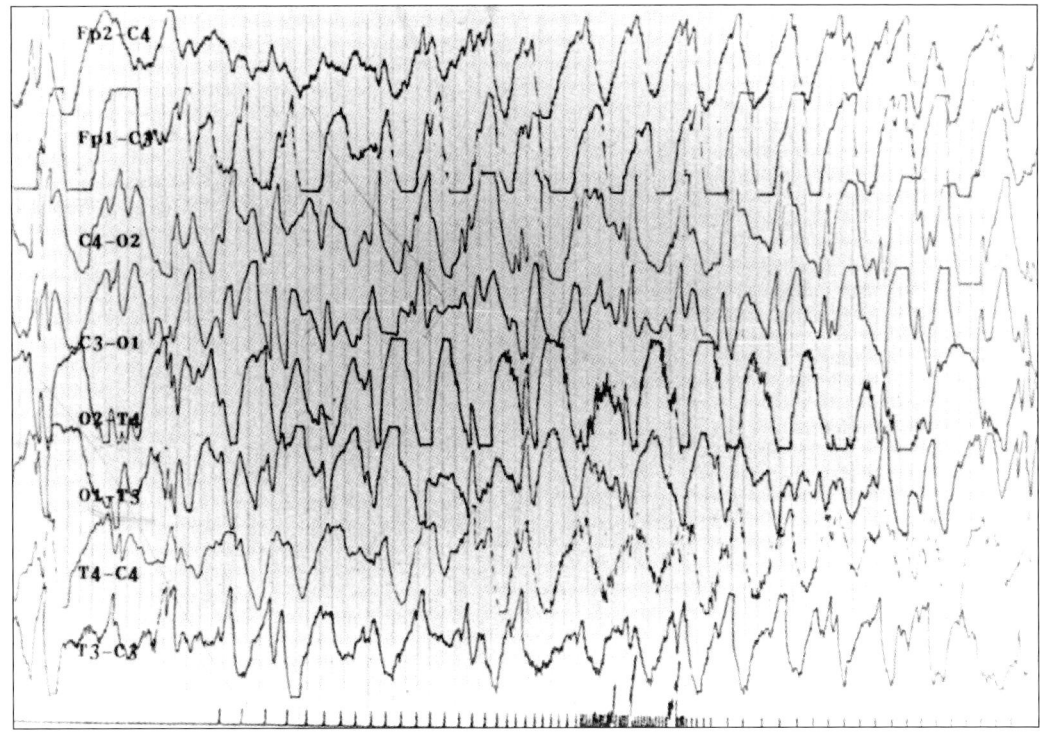

Fig. 2. Case 1, EEG showing diffuse paroxysmal alterations.

the skull showed bilateral occipital calcifications. She is currently on a gluten-free diet and anti-epileptic therapy and (PB) with improvement of neurological symptoms without any relapse of seizures.

Discussion

Numerous reports of severe epilepsy and occipital calcifications have resulted in coining of the acronym EBOC (Tiacci *et al.*, 1993). This combination was considered as a variant of the Sturge–Weber syndrome (SWS) without cutaneous abnormalities (Battistella *et al.*, 1986; Bye *et al.*, 1989; Taly *et al.*, 1987; Tateno *et al.*, 1985). In EBOC the anatomohistologic findings show patchy pial angiomatosis of lesser extent than in SWS, neither leptomeningeal angiomatosis nor signs of phakomatosis (Longo *et al.*, 1992). In addition, EBOC and SWS are different clinically by age of onset, type, course, severity of epilepsy and associated cognitive deficits (Tiacci *et al.*, 1993). So EBOC is still considered as an encephalopathy due to an unidentified mechanism. The existence of a specific syndrome including intracranial calcifications as well as CD and partial seizures was first proposed by Sammaritano and colleagues in 1988 (Sammaritano *et al.*, 1988). Recently there was a veritable explosion of interest in this condition. The largest series of patients are Italian: Gobbi and colleagues from the Bologna School (Gobbi *et al.*, 1988), Magaudda and the group from Verona (Magaudda *et al.*, 1990) and Gobbi and The Italian Working Group on CD and epilepsy (Gobbi *et al.*, 1992; Bye *et al.*, 1993). In the largest study, patients with epilepsy and calcifications were screened for CD by small bowel biopsy and 77 per cent of 31 had characteristic villous atrophy (Gobbi, 1988). Conversely 42 per cent of 12 patients with CD and epilepsy had calcifications on computed tomographic screening (Dickey, 1994). In our study 6.6 per cent of the 91 patients with CD showed the combination of epilepsy and intracranial calcifications. The relationship between epilepsy with cerebral calcifications and CD is still unknown. Some authors stressed the role of the folic acid deficiency in determining the brain lesions (Piatella *et al.*, 1993; Bye *et al.*, 1993; Molteni *et al.*, 1988; Ventura *et al.*, 1991). Folic acid deficiency is often documented in CD (Sammaritano *et al.*, 1988). It can produce neurological disorders with cerebral calcifications, mental retardation, and EEG abnormalities (Arakawa, 1970; Lanzowsky, 1970). Intracranial calcifications have been described in an infant with congenital folate malabsorption (Corbeel *et al.*, 1985). The connection between folic acid deficiency and intracranial calcifications has also been demonstrated in patients treated with methotrexate and central nervous system irradiation or with anti-convulsivant drugs (Molteni *et al.*, 1988; Garwicz & Mortensson, 1976). Even though authors suggest that cerebral calcifications may be caused by folic acid deficiency by means of cerebral vasculitis, their pathogenesis is still not thoroughly understood (Molteni *et al.*, 1988). In the six cases observed, folic acid deficiency was detected in all the three children tested. However seven patients of 91 with CD showed folic acid deficiency without endocranial calcifications and/or convulsive disorders.

The cerebral calcifications are usually located in the occipital region, as in our cases (Tortorella *et al.*, 1993); they can be unilateral or bilateral. We were unable to find any correlation between unilateral or bilateral localization of calcifications and the type of epilepsy. The prognosis of epilepsy seems unrelated either to bilateral localization of the calcifications or to the type of epileptic encephalopathy. An early diagnosis of CD with the start of a gluten–free diet and a possible antiepileptic therapy led to improvement of neurological symptoms and a clear decrease in seizures.

Conclusion

We suggest neurological and neuroradiological investigations in all patients with CD and seizures as well as gastroenterologic examinations in all the patients with convulsive disorders and clear or atypical manifestations compatible with a diagnosis of CD.

6: Report of a case of CEC with onset of epilepsy after one year of gluten-free diet

M. Vignolo, A. Naselli, R. Biancheri[*], P. Garzia and E. Veneselli[*]

Istituto di Puericultura e Medicina Neonatale 'L. Gaslini', Università di Genova;
[*]Divisione e Cattedra di Neuropsichiatria Infantile, Istituto G. Gaslini, Università di Genova, Italy

A patient with late-diagnosed coeliac disease who developed epilepsy after one year on gluten-free diet is reported. A.S., born at term, birthweight 2400 g, presented in the first years of life recurrent episodes of vomiting and diarrhoea, poor growth and height gain and slight psychomotor retardation. She was first admitted at 10.3 years of age for short stature, poor nutritional status, mild anaemia and abdominal distension.

On that occasion coeliac disease was diagnosed (AGA 192.6 AU, jejunal biopsy: subtotal villous atrophy, third degree). Gluten-free diet was started with significant clinical improvement and catch-up of growth (Table 1). After 1 year, she presented partial seizures with secondary generalization. A waking and sleep EEG showed normal background activity but bilateral slow spike and slow waves complexes in parieto-occipital regions, more evident on the right side. These abnormalities were activated by hyperpnoea and sleep, mainly during the first and second stages. Neurological examination showed signs of minimal brain damage; I.Q. was 73 (WISC R scale). Folic acid value was 3.3 ng/ml (n.v. 3–17) and AGA 14.5 AU. Therapy with carbamazepine (20 mg/kg/day) and supplementation with folinic acid were started, with temporary control of seizures. Subsequently, the patient presented atypical absences and an episode of amaurosis, followed by a generalized seizure. At 12 years a tonic–clonic generalized seizure recurred, and therapy with sodium valproate (about 30 mg/kg/day) was started. No more generalized seizures have occurred, although occasional atypical absences and short episodes of amaurosis still do, mainly during the premenstrual period. At last EEG follow up, background activity showed a moderate degree of posterior slow rhythms and diffuse irregular slow-wave discharges, enhanced by eye closure.

A follow-up CT scan remained unchanged; MRI with gadolinium administration did not show any relevant morphological and signal alterations.

It is interesting to observe that this patient, with late diagnosis of coeliac disease, developed epilepsy one year after starting a gluten-free diet without folic acid supplementation, coincidental with a 'dramatic' increase in statural growth (12.7 cm/year), due to the catch-up growth associated with the adolescent growth spurt (Fig. 1). Despite other reports of epilepsy and cerebral calcifications (Gobbi *et al.* 1992, Magaudda *et al.*, 1993, Ventura *et al.* 1991) being associated with untreated coeliac disease, in the present case it is debatable whether this considerable growth spurt was a relevant pathogenetic factor in the development of the epilepsy, in some way linked to an increased need for folic acid.

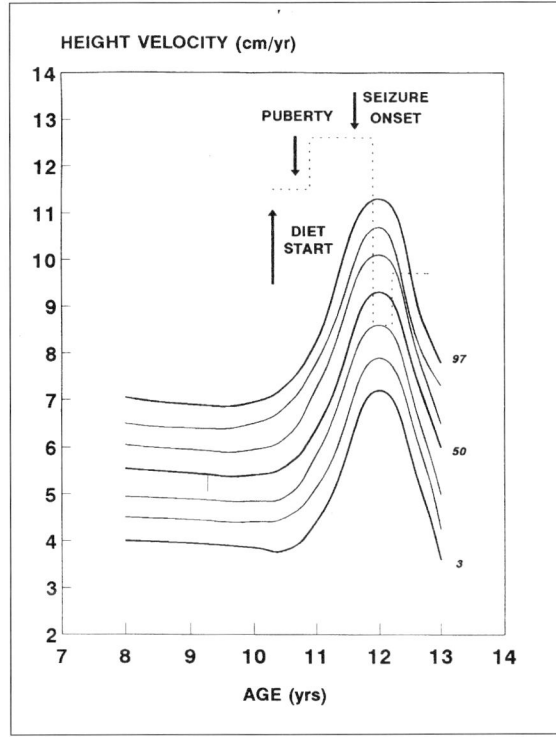

Fig. 1. Height growth velocity plotted on the Tanner et al. height velocity scale.

Table 1. Physical variables on admission and after gluten-free diet

	Age (years)	Height (cm)	Height (SDS[*])	Weight (kg)	Skeletal age (years)**	Breast development stage[***]
On admission Feb. 1990	10.3	115.3	−3.8	20.3	8.5	1
Sept. 1990	10.9	122.2	−3.0	24.6	8.8	1
Seizure onset Feb. 1991						
Sept. 1991	11.9	134.8	−2.3	30.4	10.5	2–3
Jan. 1992	12.2	137.4	−2.4	38.7		3–4
Sept. 1992	12.8	143.2	−2.1	41.1	11.5	4

[*]SDS, standard deviation score, ** Greulich & Pyle method for skeletal age assessment.
[***] According to the method of Tanner *et al.*

7: Neurological and neuroradiological follow-up of a case with CEC

E. Veneselli, R. Biancheri, L. De Santis[*] and M.P. Fondelli[**]

Divisione e Cattedra di Neuropsichiatria Infantile, Università di Genova[*] Servizio di Pronto Soccorso, Accettazione e Osservazione, [**]Servizio di Neuroradiologia, Istituto G. Gaslini, Genova, Italy.

Case report

A 10 year old girl, suffering from recurrent eczema in infancy and asthmatic bronchitis in childhood. A first episode of amaurosis, fixed gaze and clonic seizing in the left arm, followed by unconsciousness for 12 h, occurred at 4 years and 7 months of age. Phenobarbital was started. Post-ictal EEG showed slow waves in the right parieto-occipital regions.

CT scan (Fig. 1a) and T2-weighted MRI (Fig. 1b) revealed isolated hyperdense areas and hyperintense images, respectively, in the right cortico-subcortical temporo-parieto-occipital and left temporo-parietal regions; MRI showed no changes. Cerebral angiography was normal.

During the following year the patient presented three similar but less prolonged episodes. A clear increase in the size and number of temporo-parieto-occipital calcifications and the appearance of a small one in the right frontal region were evident on CT scan (Fig. 1d); MRI (Fig. 1e) showed areas of mild enhancement after gadolinium administration on the left (Fig. 1e). Laboratory investigations, including anti-endomysium antibodies, were normal, except for increased serum AGA and low folic acidemia. The HLA haplotype was B8, DR3, DQw2, typical of coeliac disease. Jejunal biopsy showed total villous atrophy. No further episodes occurred while on a gluten-free diet supplemented with folinic acid and vitamin B_{12}, except for a brief febrile generalized seizure, after three months. The neurological examination and IQ on WISC-R were normal. The awake and sleep EEGs showed posterior slow and sharp waves. The last CT scan at 7 years was unchanged, and at 9 years, MRI showed linear hyperintense areas in the bilateral temporo-parieto-occipital regions, unmodified after gadolinium administration.

Discussion

In our case, repeated neuroradiologic evaluations showed an evolution of lesions rarely reported in the literature (Gobbi *et al.*, 1992; Longo *et al.*, 1995). Magaudda *et al.*, (1993) reported progressive extension of calcifications on CT scan in 2/20 cases: in these cases, the first CT examination was normal, while occipital calcifications were shown on subsequent CT images. MRI, documented only in a few studies, has revealed: normal findings (Magaudda *et al.*, 1993); areas of void signal corresponding to calcifications (Piattella *et al.*, 1993); areas of increased signal on T2-weighted sequences, transiently in one case (Piattella *et al.*, 1993) and progressively in another case (Fois *et al.*, 1993); areas of high-intensity signals in the white matter on T1-weighted sequences in another case (Bye *et al.*, 1993). Neuropathological studies (Bye *et al.*, 1993) showed signs of cortical vascular abnormality with patch pial angiomatosis, fibrosed veins and large jagged microcalcifications, as observed in Sturge–Weber syndrome.

In our patient, the sequence of neuroradiological images on CT scan shows progression of the lesions in about one year and subsequent stabilisation. The mild hyperintense signal observed only on the first T2-weighted MRI, and not on subsequent examinatons, was probably due to localized oedema.

Linear bilateral temporo-parieto-occipital hyperintensity on T1-weighted MRI appeared unilaterally close to the first calcified area, but less extensive compared to the calcifications visible on CT scan; in particular mild enhancement after gadolinium administration was evident but disappeared subsequently.

The different types of lesion localization and signals observed in this study suggest progressive mineralizing microangiopathy with selective involvement of the boundary zone between gray and white matter, more evident in temporo-parieto-occipital regions.

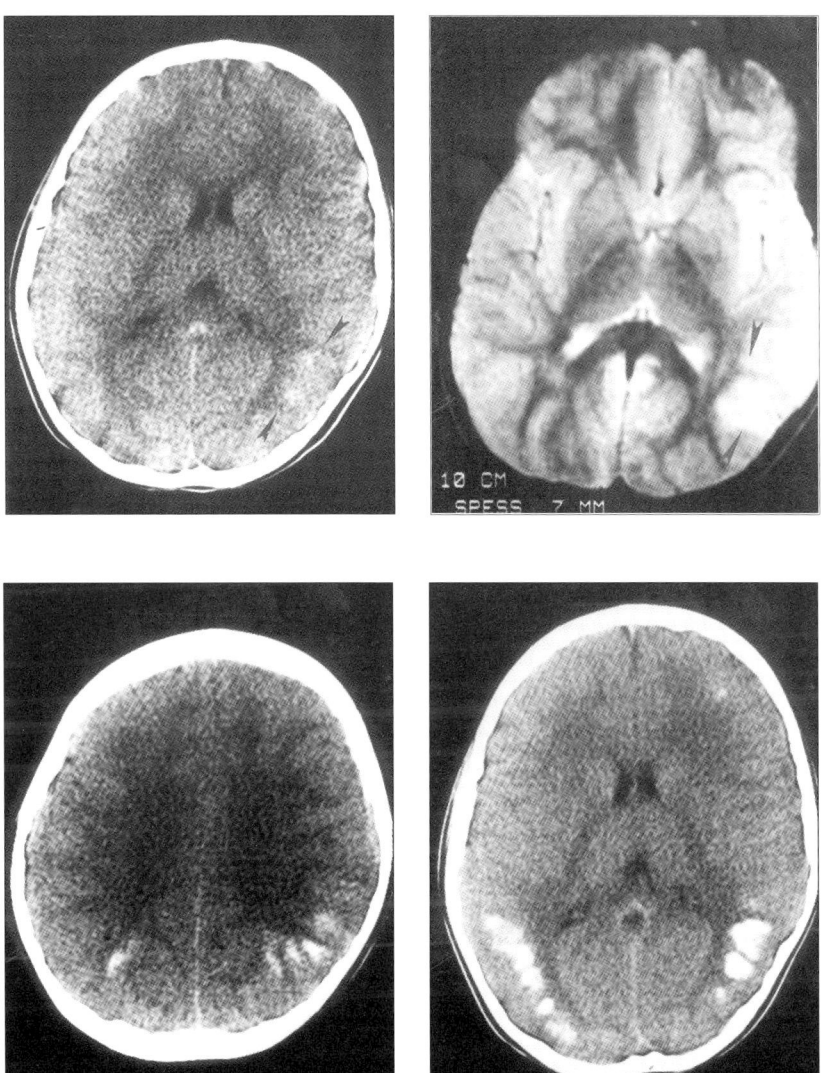

*Fig. 1.(a) CT (4 years 7 months): isolated hyperdense areas in the right
cortico-subcortical temporo-occipital region; (b) T2-weighted MRI
(4 years 7 months): mild hyperintense areas in the same area;
(c) CT (4 years 9 months): multiple calcified areas in parietal regions;
(d) CT (5 years 6 months): bilateral temporo-occipital and right frontal
calcifications.*

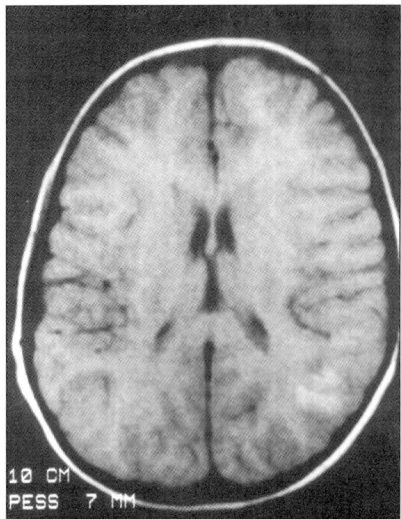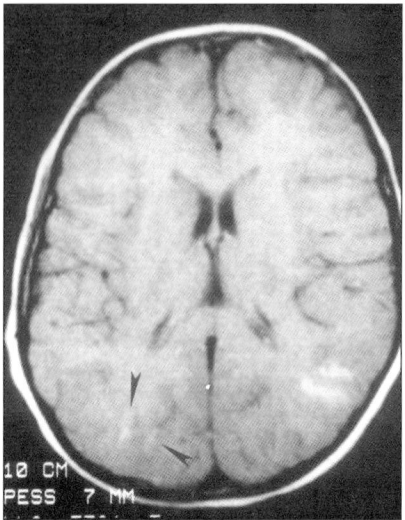

*Fig. 1. (e) T1- weighted MRI (5 years 6 months): hyperintense area in
the right parieto-temporal region; (f) mild enchancement after
gadolinium administration on the left.*

8: Epilepsy and coeliac disease in a case with cerebral calcifications at follow-up

**Ottaviano Martinelli[*], Alessandra Tiberti[*], Daniela Valseriati[*] and
Giuseppe Gobbi[**]**

[*]*Divisione di Neuropsichiatria Infantile, Spedali Civili, Ussl 41, Brescia, Italy;*
[**]*Servizio di Neuropsichiatria Infantile, Ussl 9, Reggio Emilia, Italy*

Introduction

During the last few years a syndrome with coeliac disease (CD), posterior cerebral calcifications and epilepsy has been identified (Gobbi *et al.*, 1992), possibly including cases previously classified as atypical forms of Sturge–Weber syndrome (SWS) (Ambrosetto *et al.*, 1983). The relationship between CD, epilepsy and cerebral calcifications is still unclear.

We report a case with a ten year follow-up period, in which evolution of epilepsy, brain calcifications and EEG recordings were useful in increasing our understanding of this syndrome.

Case report

A boy, born after normal delivery and uneventful gestation, was hospitalized at 26 months for generalized seizures without fever, lasting 30 min. Four further partial seizures occurred, once a month, originating in the occipital regions. Symptoms at onset included vomiting (on two occasions) followed by right ocular and head deviation, and right clonic and generalized seizures. The EEG recordings performed during wakefulness showed sharp wave discharges localized to both occipital regions, disappearing on eye opening. Post-ictal EEG showed slowing of the background activity in the left posterior head region. Brain CT scan (Fig. 1) and

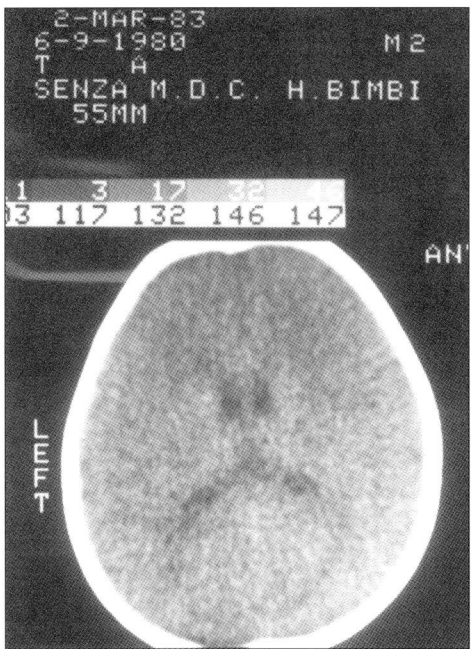

*Fig. 1. Brain CT scan shows normal finding in
occipital regions.*

neurological evaluation were normal. Complete seizure control was obtained with phenobarbital (75 mg/daily), which was withdrawn and no seizures occurred for seven years.

In addition, during the first year of life, the patient had recurrent diarrhoea episodes, which became infrequent. Seven years later, CD was diagnosed using specific tests: antigliadin antibodies (AGA-IgA = 10; n.v. until 7; AGA-IgG = 36; n.v. until 15); one-hour xylose afterload blood level tests (15 mg per cent ; n.v. > 25 mg per cent) and jejunal biopsy (subtotal villous atrophy). At this time the patient began a gluten-free diet (GFD).

Three months later he presented an isolated, nocturnal, generalized seizure followed by brief (< 5 min) visual seizures with hallucinations (coloured steps, moving wheels, turning and smiling men) and ocular deviation towards the left. These seizures increased to daily frequency over two years, when he was re-evaluated. The neurological examination was normal. A new CT scan (Fig. 2) showed bilateral occipital cortico-subcortical calcifications; MRI was normal. The EEG during wakefulness showed spike-and-wave discharges in both temporo-occipital regions, disappearing on eye opening; during sleep, diffuse mainly posterior fast polyspike bursts occurred. The Wechsler Intelligence Scale for Children (WISC-R) showed a significant difference between verbal (VIQ = 130) and performances (PIQ = 61) scores with a global IQ of 112. Further neuropsychological tests revealed a decrease in visuo-spatial and memory functions. Laboratory tests (haematology, serum parathyroid hormone, calcitonin level, FT 3, FT 4, FSH and antigliadin antibodies) were normal. Blood antibodies to Torch, measles virus, parotitis virus and Epstein-Barr virus were normal. Folic acid level was 1.9 (n.v. > 1.9). HLA phenotypes data (DR3 DQw2) were consistent with a diagnosis of CD.

Carbamazepine was administred (20 mg/kg/daily) and, since then, complete control of seizures and improvement of the EEG recordings during wakefulness and sleep has been obtained (with a decrease in paroxysms of more than 75 per cent). Because of CD, the patient has followed a regular GFD.

Discussion

This case report is a further description of the CD, epilepsy and cerebral calcifications syndrome and could provide some important data concerning the correlation between epilepsy and CD.

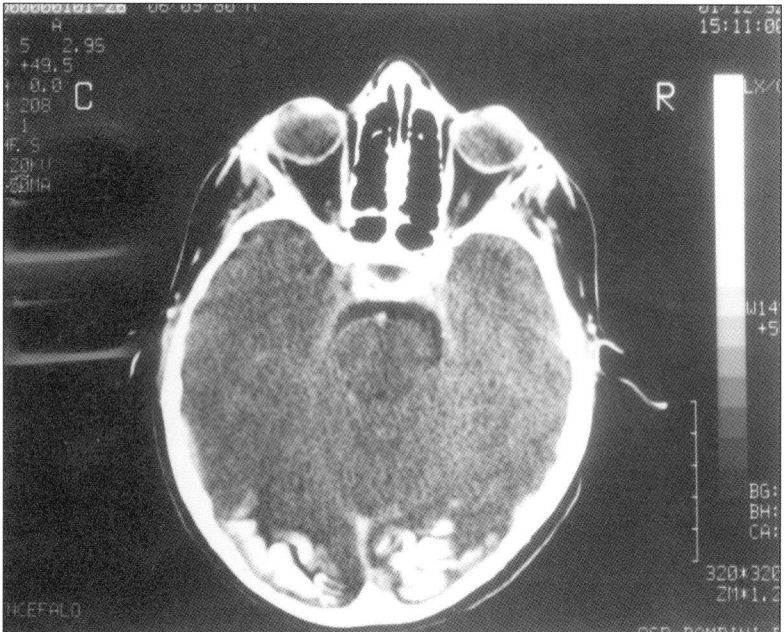

Fig. 2. Brain CT scan shows bilateral occipital cortico-subcortical calcifications.

The origin of the occipital calcifications is still questionable. They could depend on chronic folic acid deficiency due to untreated CD (Ventura *et al.*, 1991). Since CD may be associated with different immune disorders, Gobbi *et al.* (1992) hypothesized that cerebral calcifications could depend on chronic autoimmune or immune-complex-related endothelial inflammation. In this patient with untreated CD, the brain calcifications were not present during the early phases of the disease and appeared during a later phase. Although the CT-scan cuts and angulation are not exactly the same in the first and second illustrations, they unquestionably provide two very close sections of the parietal occipital region, demonstrating that the calcifications appeared only during the later phase. Therefore, we suppose that occipital calcifications appeared as a consequence of long-lasting untreated CD. Since folic acid levels were low but within the normal range, different causes have to be investigated in search of the origin of cerebral calcifications.

In the CD, epilepsy and cerebral calcifications syndrome the seizures, although clinically heterogeneous, are usually focal, originating from the occipital lobe. The evolution of epilepsy can be benign or pharmaco-resistant or sometimes characterized by an early and apparently benign initial phase followed by epileptic encephalopathy, after a seizure-free interval (Gobbi *et al.*, 1988).

Our case confirms the puzzling clinical outcome of occipital epilepsy in a case of CD. In this patient the initial seizures with vomiting and the good control as well as the previous normal CT-scan findings could have suggested an idiopathic occipital epilepsy, such as described by Panayiotopoulos in 1989. On the other hand, the late seizure onset, the late abnormal CT-scan and the EEG sleep findings suggested the diagnosis of a lesional occipital epilepsy. One might hypothesize that this patient had two epilepsies: an idiopathic occipital epilepsy when he was younger, and then a lesional occipital epilepsy due to an untreated CD. On the other hand, the evolution of the epilepsy up to now might suggest an apparently benign initial phase followed by an epileptic encephalopathy, after a seizure-free interval.

Finally, in our patient the cerebral dysfunction resulted not only in epilepsy, but also in impairment of visuo-spatial and memory functions. This type of dysfunction, which has never been explored in previous studies, is consistent which the site of the brain damage.

Conclusion

This report demonstrates that, in the case of epilepsy and CD, bilateral occipital cortico-subcortical cerebral calcifications can appear at a relatively late stage during the evolution of the disease, probably as a consequence of an untreated CD. To our knowledge, only Aldao *et al.* described a similar case in 1992.

In agreement with Ambrosetto *et al.* (1992), this case suggests that all patients with occipital lobe epilepsy should be assessed for CD even in the absence of cerebral calcifications, which could develop at a later stage.

9: Coeliac disease, epilepsy and cerebral calcifications. Report of a typical case with long-term follow-up

P. Tanganelli, L. Malfatto, C. Beluschi[*], S. Babbini[*], G. Giambartolomei[*] and
G. Regesta

Divisione di Neurologia, Centro per l'Epilessia, Ospedale San Martino, Viale Benedetto XV 10, 16132 Genova;
[*]Divisione di Pediatria, Ospedale Civile, Chiavari Genova, Italy

Case Report

The patient (M.A.) was a 25-year-old male, with no family history of epilepsy. He had his first seizure, a simple partial motor versive attack with secondary generalization, at the age of 4 years. Repeated EEGs during wakefulness showed normal background activity and rhythmic (2–3 Hz), high amplitude, spike-and-wave discharges, localized in both occipital regions, mainly occurring when the eyes were closed.

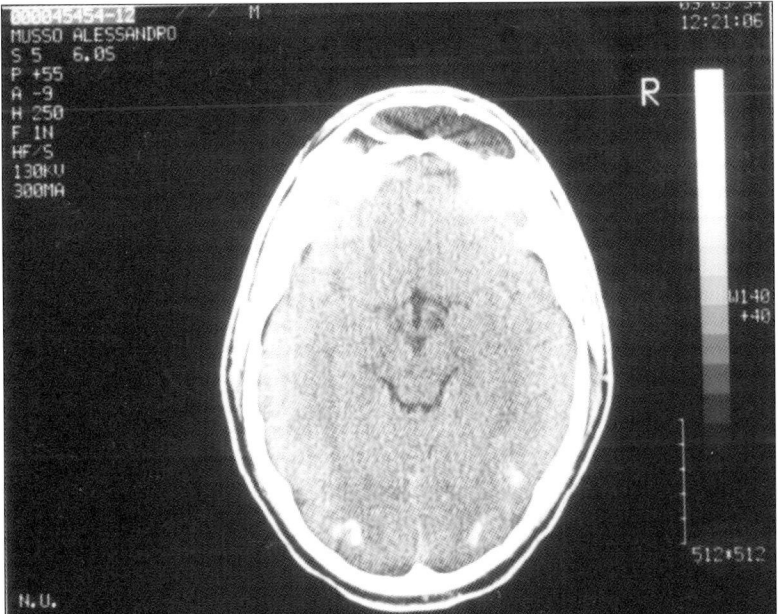

Fig. 1. CT of the patient showing bilateral, cortico-subcortical, parieto-occipital calcifications.

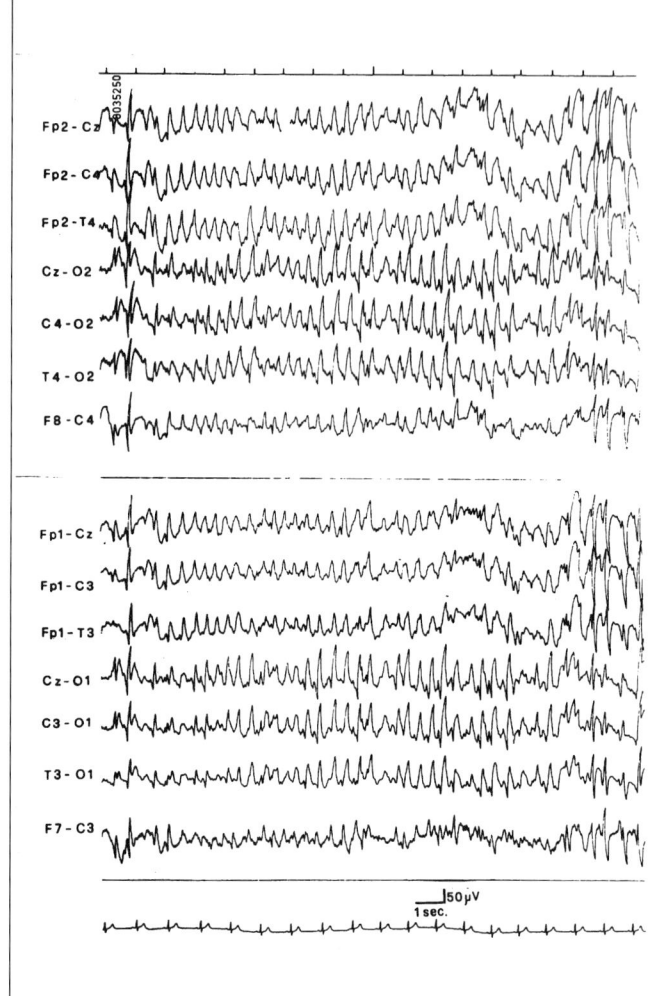

Fig. 2. Diffuse, rhythmic spike-and-wave discharges with prominence in occipital regions.

The neurological examination and growth were normal. Due to the presence of bulky fatty faeces the patient underwent a full gastrointestinal evaluation. Xylose loading test was below the normal range and jejunal biopsy showed atrophy of the villi. The boy was prescribed a coeliac diet and phenobarbital therapy (30 mg/d), after which no attacks occurred during a three-year follow-up. When he was given a regular diet, they occurred again. They were characterized by a sensation of discomfort and nausea, followed by turning of the head to the left and generalized tonic–clonic attacks.

CT scans, performed when he was eight, and repeated when he was fifteen, showed bilateral, cortico-subcortical, parieto-occipital calcifications (Fig. 1).

Neurological status and intellectual level remained normal. No sign of phakomatosis was detectable and the EEG recordings were unchanged. A second jejunal biopsy confirmed the subtotal atrophy of the villi.

From 9 to 14 years the attacks were frequent and persistent despite the use of various combinations of anti-epileptic drugs. The patient, however, was sometimes noncompliant with his diet.

At the age of 15, frequent (more than one per day) atypical absences, often with atonic component, and less frequent complex partial (oro-gestual) and simple partial visual seizures appeared.

During these years the EEGs showed a progressive slowing of background activity while bioccipital and

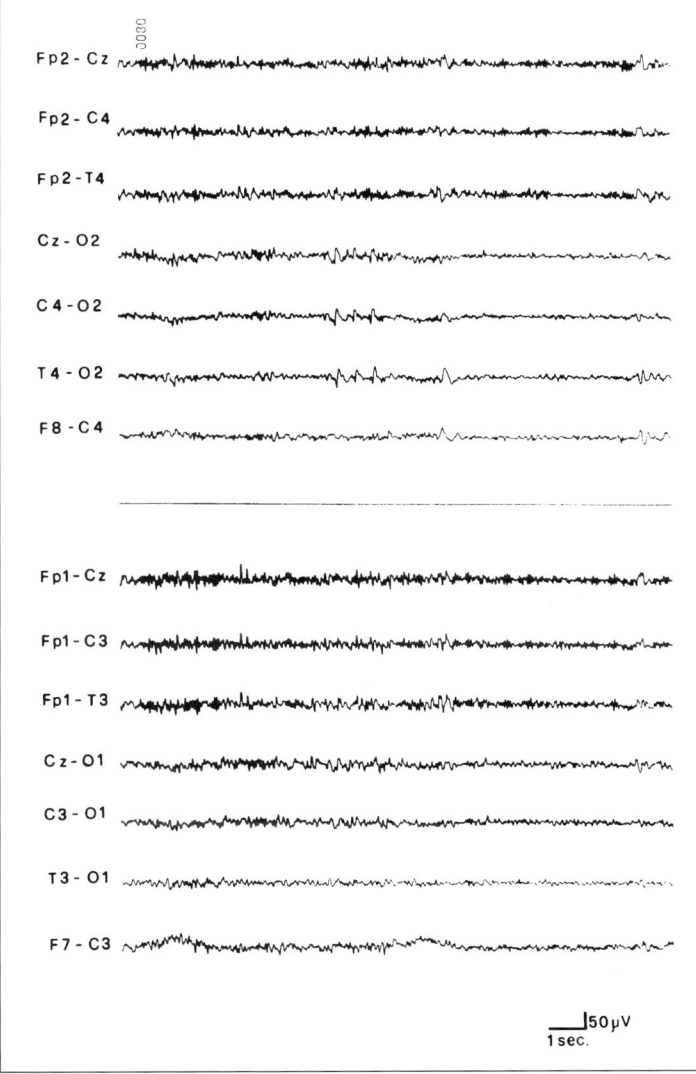

Fig. 3. Dramatic amelioration of the EEG tracing with reduction of the abnormalities and reappearance of background activity.

temporo-occipital discharges became more frequent, often involving anterior regions. However, the reactivity of the spike-and-wave discharges on eye opening persisted.

Sleep organization was disturbed owing to the increase of abnormalities. The different non-REM phases were hardly recognizable.

Fast polyspike bursts and discharges of spikes and polyspike-slow wave complexes of varying duration (up to some minutes), diffuse but always with greater prominence in both occipital regions, were observed. There was no clinical accompaniment. During REM sleep, which was well represented, the discharges tended to disappear.

Despite various therapeutic attempts (including vigabatrin and lamotrigine) and rigorous diet regimen, seizure frequency persisted unchanged for several years. Cranio-facial trauma was frequently reported.

Folic acid levels, which were below the normal range (< 2 ng), returned to normal following a well-conducted dietary regimen.

The presence of high titres of antigliadin antibodies (AGA-IgA and AGA-IgG) resulted on ELISA test. HLA typing showed the presence of class II antigen DQw2 phenotype.

Blood levels of parathyroid hormone and calcitonin were normal.

A Wechsler Intelligence Scale for Adults, performed when he was 24, gave an IQ of 80. A deterioration quotient of 27 per cent was demonstrated. Analysis of score profiles revealed an evident fall in the digit-memory and digit-symbol association items, while logical abilities were well preserved.

A further CT scan did not reveal any alteration in the size or extent of calcifications. No pathological changes were evident on MRI, even after gadolinium administration.

During repeated EEGs, the spikes and spike-and-wave discharges appeared to be almost continuous and generalized, making it difficult to recognize background activity (Fig. 2). The reactivity on eye opening was much less evident. These abnormalities persisted during REM sleep.

At the age of 25 the introduction of felbamate (2400 mg/d), as are adjunctive drug to the therapy with phenobarbital and carbamazepine, led to a dramatic reduction in seizure frequency with a concomitant substantial improvement of the EEG (Fig. 3).

In the course of the following 6 months the patient remained seizure free. The withdrawal of felbamate on request of the patient, having been informed by us about its possible potentially fatal haematological complications, and the substitution of lamotrigine was immediately followed by the reappearance of pre-existing clinical and EEG findings.

After a 3-month interval the patient decided to return to felbamate and was again seizure-free for 4 months.

We conclude that felbamate should be considered as a valid therapeutic option in this type of patient.

Acknowledgement

The authors are grateful to Mr. Bruno De Bernardi, Tech. Neurophysiol., for his assistance.

10: Prevalence of coeliac disease in subjects affected by drug-resistant epilepsy

G. Incorpora, M. Cocuzza, R. Bianchini, N. Rotolo, M. Spina and G. Bottaro

Clinica Pediatria, Universita di Catania, V.le A. Doria 6, 95125 Catania, Italy

Introduction

Forms of epilepsy which are not controlled by a congruous and rational therapy are defined as intractable or drug-resistant (Aicardi, 1992). Many of these forms have a hidden organic cause which is not easily identifiable.

It is now well known that there is a neurological syndrome associated with coeliac disease which is characterized by drug-resistant epilepsy and endocranial calcifications, particularly in the occipital region (Gobbi *et al.*, 1992). This syndrome is prevalent in adolescent patients who have not been diagnosed early or who have not followed the diet. It is also known that other forms of epilepsy are associated with this disease (Fois *et al.*, 1994).

Taking the patients with drug-resistant epilepsy as the starting point of this study, the presence of nondiagnosed coeliac disease was evaluated.

Patients and methods

The study included 20 patients aged between 4 and 21 years (mean age 11.2), affected by different forms of epilepsy with seizures that were not controlled by the administration of at least three of the foremost drugs appropriate to the epilepsy. The seizures presented by the patients were: eight cases generalized tonic–clonic, five myoclonic, four complex partial and three generalized epilepsy with absence-seizures.

The patients' AGA (antigliadin antibody) and EMA (antiendomysium antibody) values were assayed and, in the case of an increased value, an intestinal mucous biopsy was performed.

The AGA and EMA values were altered in three of the 20 patients (15 per cent), and the intestinal biopsy of all three patients showed atrophy of the villi.

Patient No. 1 at 14 years of age, had a negative clinical record except for the presence of occasional episodes of diarrhoea, with somatic development appropriate for the age. The first episode of convulsive generalized tonic–clonic seizures occurred at 8 years. Despite anti-convulsant treatment, the patient continued to present convulsions which were not controlled by the association of several drugs, and began to manifest a deterioration in intellectual function. Today the patient still presents occasional convulsions, although a reduction in the number of seizures and an improvement in intellectual function was noted coincident with the initiation of the diet. CAT examination did not show calcification.

Patient No. 2 was aged 9 years with moderate to severe MR and a severe epilepsy with complex partial and myoclonic seizures. At 9 months, following an endocarditis, the patient had a stroke resulting in severe hemiparesis. From 4 years of age, the patient began to present severe convulsive episodes occurring several times a day. CAT examination showed an extensive porencephalic cavity in the left fronto-temporal region. Subsequent to AGA assay and intestinal biopsy, dietary treatment was started although latterly the patient did not follow the diet regularly. The convulsive seizures initially showed slight improvement, but persist with increased severity at the present time.

Patient No. 3, the oldest of the three was 20 years old in 1995. The clinical record shows only occasional episodes of diarrhoea which occurred from early infancy until 4 years. The patient's history of epilepsy is complex. At 9 years, brief partial oculogyric seizures began. The seizures were repeated many times a day and were resistant to the various drugs administered. The patient attended several medical centres. At 12 years, CAT examination showed a small calcification in the right occipital region.

Two years later the calcification was surgically removed. The convulsive seizures persisted, increasing in intensity and frequency. Because of the patient's drug-resistance, AGA assay and intestine biopsy were performed and coeliac disease was diagnosed at 16 years. Curiously, before the begining of the dietary treatment, there was a spontaneous reduction in the seizures which are still well controlled. Further CAT examinations performed after the removal of the calcification were normal.

Conclusion

Three cases of coeliac disease in 20 patients affected by drug-resistant epilepsy is a relatively high proportion (15 per cent).

Patient No. 1 shows this association but does not present intracerebal calcification. The patient has a below average I.Q. and benefited from the dietary treatment, particularly at the beginning, although the seizures persist. Patient No.2 presents neurological symptomatology which can be related to the stroke at 9 months, and the coeliac disease is presumably a concomitant pathology.

Patient No. 3, instead, represents the most characteristic case of the association convulsions-coeliac disease-calcification and is striking for the gravity of the seizure pattern which led to numerous visits to neurologic and epileptic centres.

Two points appear particularly relevant in this patient's complex history; the excision of the calcification did not lead to improvement in the clinical picture and new calcifications did not form over time.

Two of these three patients benefited from the dietary treatment, although, strangely, patient No. 3 began to show an improvement shortly before beginning the diet. The lack of success with the diet in patient No. 2 probably depends on the fact that in this case the epilepsy is secondary to the porencephalic cyst and the coeliac disease is simply an associated pathology.

Much remains to be clarified in this tangle of pathologies and it would seem evident that AGA evaluation is an essential step in the diagnosis of drug-resistant epilepsy in Italy today.

11: Bioccipital calcifications and coeliac disease with late-onset

Miguel Baquero, Juan J. Vílchez, Francisco J. Domínguez and Manuel García-Fernández

Servicio de Neurología, Hospital Universitari La Fe, Av. Campanar 21, 46009 Valencia, Spain

Introduction

The striking association of epilepsy, bioccipital calcifications (BOC) and coeliac disease (CD) mostly defined after the work of Gobbi *et al.* (1992a, b) is not always uniform in the presentation of its three components. The severity of epilepsy varies from the asymptomatic cases described by Maggauda *et al.* (1993, 1994) to uncontrolable seizures and mental impairment; sometimes a benign disease may become unexpectedly severe later (Gobbi *et al.*, 1988). BOC can also be atypically located in any cerebral lobe, and they may either remain static or grow and multiply (De Marco & Lorenzin, 1990; Fois *et al.*, 1993). CD itself can be either overt or silent. However, age at onset in every reported case has consistently been during the first two decades of life.

We report two patients with CD and BOC in adulthood. These cases also present some peculiar clinical and neuroimaging features.

Case 1

This patient, a 45 year old man, was a light smoker who worked as a carpenter. In the last three years, he suffered from several episodes of alternating brachical monoparesis that completely resolved after a period of a few hours to ten days. Examination during the episodes showed a slight paresis that mainly affected fine movements of upper limb; reflexes, as well as sensation, coordination and other functions, were preserved. Cranial CT showed symmetric BOC and moderate-to-severe brain atrophy. MRI further disclosed T2-weighted hyperintense images, widespread in parietooccipital white matter, affecting mostly arcuate fibres ers and sparing the periventricular white matter. Cervical and cranial angiography was normal. All these features were unchanged on repeated examinations over three years. The diagnosis of CD was known after the last episode because the patient had been presenting gastrointestinal symptoms consisting mainly as attacks of intense abdominal pain. Peroral jejunal biopsy and antigliadin antibodies were confirmatory. Since the patient was submitted to a gluten-free diet two years ago, he has been quite asymptomatic.

Case 2

This female patient aged 53 years suffered from a 20-year history of a biopsy-proven coeliac disease, manifested as a pronounced malabsortion syndrome; she was not adherent to the gluten-free diet. Progressive action myoclonus appeared at the beginning of 1994; she complained of clumsy gait, involuntary jerky movements, and three generalized tonic–clonic seizures preceded by spreading myoclonus. Mental status was preserved. Vibratory sensation was diminished in legs but reflexes, strength and other sensations were normal. Gait was ataxic. Action greatly increased the myoclonic jerks. On laboratory examination, iron deficiency anaemia was often detected; low serum folates and vitamin E levels, and hypocalcaemia were occasionally found in addition. Cranial CT showed typical symmetrical BOC. MRI was normal. Several EEGs showed continuous spikes and polispikes not related to jerking. ENG-EMG studies are unremarkable. She was placed on a variety of drugs and nutritional supplements. Laboratory deficits were corrected, but the course was progressive and disabling. A combination of clonazepam, carbamazepine and piracetam was her most effective therapy. Valproate and other antiepileptic drugs have not proved useful. Nowadays myoclonus is seldom present at rest, but becomes continuous and generalized after drug withdrawal. During activity, arm and hand function is rather preserved, but gait is severely disturbed by leg and truncal myoclonus.

Discussion

CD is believed to be a permanent condition that appears at any age after the introduction of cereals into the diet. Most cases seem to be silent (Catassi *et al.*, 1994). Because of the natural remission that occurs during adolescence, a bimodal distribution of incidence has been observed, with an early peak in infancy and a later peak in the last decades of life. Clinical features of CD are specially variable in these adult cases. Some of these features are true for the BOC-CD association: adult cases of BOC-CD do exist and their clinical appearance is variable. CD-linked BOC pathogenesis is not known. As in CD, a special genetic background seems essential, since most cases come from Italy or Argentina. Some findings suggest that gluten intake can play a key role: gluten-free diet (GFD) can improve epilepsy; a better outcome correlates with lower age at the start of the GFD (Gobbi et al., 1992a); and good adherence to the GFD would preclude BOC development (Bardella et al., 1994). If persistent gluten intake is an important factor in the BOC-CD association, more late onset cases are likely to be detected amongst CD patients that remain undiagnosed, like our case 1, or without good adherence to the GFD, like our case 2.

Apart from the age at onset, case 1 shows two remarkable features. First, the intriguing brachical monoparesis as initial symptom. It is difficult to find an explanation for the origin of this recurrent, reversible, pure motor deficit. Neuroimaging does not support the initial suspicion of ischaemic attacks; postictal paresis of an unnoticed seizure or transient deficit from subcortical demyelination can hardly be involved. On the other hand, the significance of the white matter abnormality is also an enigma. White matter abnormalities can be part of the syndrome, because they have been found in some cases of BOC-CD (Bye et al., 1989; Fois et al., 1993; Sammaritano et al., 1985; Tiacci et al., 1993), but other cases do not show them. CD patients without BOC and affected by other obscure neurologic disorders have white matter damage too (Cooke & Smith, 1966; Kepes et al., 1975; Kinney et al., 1982).

Case 2 presented progressive action myoclonus, rare tonic–clonic generalized seizures and ataxia. This complex association of symptoms fits very well the diagnostic criteria for progressive myoclonic ataxia (Berkovic et al., 1994; Marsden et al., 1989), a rare disorder sharing features of progressive myoclonic epilepsies and of progressive ataxias. The association of myoclonic ataxia and CD was first reported by Lu et al. (1986) in patients without BOC. Other causes of progressive myoclonic ataxia have not been fully ruled out in this case, but CD is an accepted cause and, moreover, BOC were present.

These two patients came from eastern Spain. The clinical pattern of the other reported Spanish cases is more typical (Baigès et al., 1994; Hernández et al., 1994; Montón et al., 1992; Pinilla et al., 1995). Thus, a special geographic variability is not likely.

In summary, BOC appears as the hallmark of CD in the brain, like villous atrophy in the jejunal mucosa. Our CD patients showing BOC, indicate that this unusual pattern on a CT scan must suggest the diagnosis of CD, despite the clinical presentation and the age of the patient.

12: Coeliac disease, headache and epilepsy: report of seven cases

E. Tozzi, T. Gentile, R. Angelini, M.V. Meucci, F. Pace, L. Tobia, A. Marrelli[*],
P. Aloisi[*], F. Papola[**], C. Cervelli[**], F. de Matteis

Clinica Pediatrica, Università' L'Aquila; [*]Servizio di Neurofisiopatologia, USL L'Aquila; [**]Centro regionale di Immunoematologia e Tipizzazione Tissutale, L'Aquila, Italy

Introduction

Among neurological disorders associated with coeliac disease (CD) (Fois et al., 1992; Gobbi et al., 1988; Gobbi et al., 1992; Magaudda et al., 1993; Visacorpi, 1992) we focussed on headache (H). Particularly we proposed to verify if the H presented by coeliac children group is secondary to the malabsorption syndrome and/or is a primary pathology coexisting with CD.

Material and methods

A group of 40 children affected by CD, 7 (six females, one male) aged from 10 months to 14 years, were admitted to this study. All subjects were suffering from H and one from epilepsy (E) as well. Seven children with CD without neurological disorders and seven children with H without CD represented the control group. For each subject we evaluated EEG reports, visual evoked potentials abstained by the checkerboard pattern reversal method (pVEP), CT scan, MR films, serum magnesium level and HLA class I and II alleles studied by Terasaki's method (Hors, 1990). Diagnosis of CD was made according to ESPGAN criteria (1990) (Maki,

1990), for H according to IHS criteria (1988) (I.H.S., 1988), and for E according to ILAE criteria (Commission on Classification and Terminology of the International League against Epilepsy, 1989).

Table 1. Age of diagnosis of coeliac disease (CD) and onset of migraine (M) and/or epilepsy (E)

Patients	Diagnosis of CD (years)	Migraine with aura	Onset (years)	Migraine without aura	Onset (years)	Epilepsy	Onset (years)
1	9.02	*	7				
2	12.02			*	11		
3	11.06			*	16		
4	7.06	*	9				
5	8.10			*	7.06		
6	8	*	10			*	12
7	6	*	6				

Table 2. Percentage values of familiarity with migraine and epilepsy in the parents of three children groups

	Father					Mother				
	CD	TH	MA	MWA	E	CD	TH	MA	MWA	E
Coeliac and migraine patients	0	14%	17%			17%	28%	17%	55%	33%
Migraine patients	0	0	0	0	0	0		17%	33%	
Coeliac patients	0	14%				0		17%		

CD, Coeliac disease; TH, tension headache; MA, migraine with aura; MWA, migraine without aura; E, epilepsy.

Table 3. HLA typing in 2 patients and their parents

HLA alleles	Case 1: Migraine with aura		Mother: Migraine with aura + coeliac disease	
A	1	3	1	3
B	7	22	7	22
C	W1		W1	
DR	2	3	2	3
DQ	W1	W"	W1	22

HLA alleles	Case 6: Migraine with aura + epilepsy		Father	Father	Mother	Mother
A	11	30	24	30	11	28
B	40	41	13	40	35	41
c	W2	W3	W3		W2	W4
DR	4		1	4	4	11
DQ	W3		W1	W3	W3	

Results and discussion

Three children were affected by migraine with aura (MA) and three children by migraine without aura (MWA), one by MA and occipital epilepsy. Among the controls, 17.5 per cent of the cohort of coeliacs were affected by migraine (M) and 2.5 per cent by E: these values are higher than in the general populations. No patient

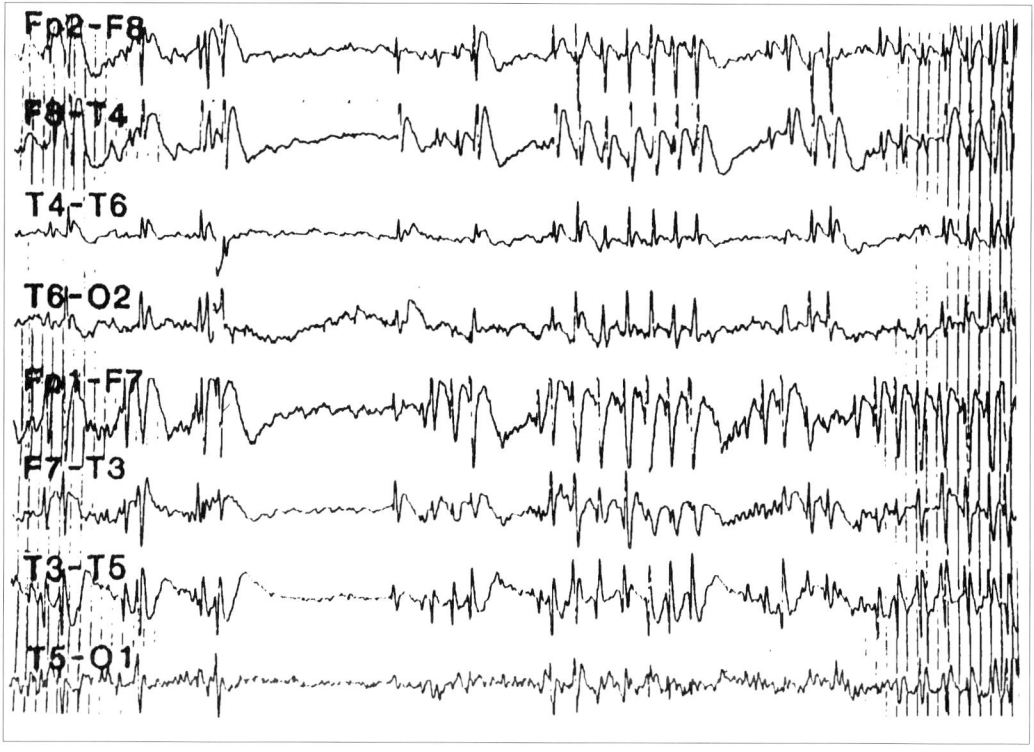

Fig. 1. Case 6: spike and waves discharges with closed eyes.

presented cerebral calcifications. Four coeliac patients showed neurological symptoms after diagnosis of CD and when they were just on a gluten-free diet. In Table 1 we show the age of diagnosis of CD and of onset of M.

Greater familiarity with M and E has been found in the coeliac migrainous children's group (Table 2), compared to the group of parents of migraineurs or of those with coeliac disease. The interictal EEG records of four patients showed slow waves as often seen in migraine, one patient presented atypical slow waves and one patient showed spike and waves discharges when the eyes were closed (Fig. 1). The pVEP showed smaller amplitude of P100 in the coeliac migraineurs (3.39 ± 0.84 µV) compared to the M group (7.84 ± 3.79 µV) and to healthy children of the same age (5.15 ± 0.69 µV). Serum magnesium values in coeliac migraineurs (1.50 ± 0.30 mg per cent) and migraineurs without coeliac disease (1.52 ± 0.30 mg per cent) were significantly lower ($P < 0.01$) compared to coeliac children (1.63 ± 0.15 mg per cent) and healthy children (2.08 ± 0.58 mg per cent). The patients with occipital epilepsy showed progressive severity with high frequency of atypical absences or visual seizures and progressive mental impairment. In the coeliac and migrainous groups the HLA typing was different compared to the coeliac group without H. In fact the alleles very different between two groups were: A1 (50 per cent ⇒ 33 per cent), A2 (65 per cent ⇒ 33 per cent), B7 (33 per cent ⇒ 100 per cent), DQW1 (50 per cent ⇒ 100 per cent), DR6 (0 per cent ⇒ 33 per cent), B14, 17, 18 (0 per cent ⇒ 35 per cent), DR4 (50 per cent ⇒ 35 per cent) (Tsuji *et al.*, 1992). In Table 3 we summarize the HLA alleles of the patients and their parents. The cases examined were few, but we underline two cases: nos. 1 and 6 of Table 1. In case 1, mother and daughter show the same pathology (CD and MA) and the same HLA typing. Furthermore the patient with occipital epilepsy has the DR4 allele as a homozygous condition because this allele is present in both parents. The H of coeliac children examined seems to be the primary pathology associated with CD. High prevalence of M in these coeliac patients is proven, but the causal relationship between the two pathologies still needs to be verified (Battistella *et al.*, 1987; Hernanz & Polanco, 1991; Martelletti *et al.*, 1984; Minev *et al.*, 1987). This association could be causal and genetically determined, as these two patients show in the HLA typing (Martelletti *et al.*, 1984; Minev *et al.*, 1987; Tsuji *et al.*, 1992).

13: Migraine in the bilateral occipital calcification epilepsy–coeliac disease syndrome

L. Perniola, T. Margari, M.G. De Iaco, M. Buttiglione, B. Figliolia, A. Polito, A. De Giacomo and I. Simone*

*Child Neuropsychiatric Service, *Neurological clinic, University of Bari, Italy*

Our experience with epilepsy-occipital calcifications-coeliac syndrome is limited to two cases but we think that their clinical presentation may be of interest.

Case 1

C.G., was born after normal pregnancy, without pre-perinatal risk factors. There was no consanguinity of parents, no family history of epilepsy, headache or myopia. Growth and psychomotor development were normal. In the first year of life visual difficulty was noticed and an important myopia was diagnosed two years later. He had normal learning ability.

At the age of 8 the first complex partial seizure appeared and three more episodes were described in the following month.

Physical and neurological examinations were normal. The neuropsychological evaluation with WISC-R showed a verbal IQ = 84, a performance IQ = 81 and a full scale IQ = 81. The ophthalmologic evaluation revealed severe myopia; a myopic chorioretinosis of the posterior pole was found. VEPs showed an altered morphology of P100 with prolonged latency and slight reduction of amplitude. Routine laboratory tests, folic acid and vitamin B_{12} levels, rubella, toxoplasma, cytomegalovirus and herpes simplex antibodies, thyroid function tests, parathyroid hormone, xylose absorption test, AGA and EMA-test were all normal. Serological HLA typing was as follows: A10, A29, B13, B35, Cw4, Cw-, DR5(11), DR7, DQ2, DQ3. Chest radiography and EKG were normal. Transcranial doppler sonography showed a reduced vascular index in the posterior circulation. Brain CT scan disclosed bilateral occipital coarse parenchymal calcifications; enhancement did not modify the pattern. Cranial MR1 was normal.

A waking EEG record showed intense paroxysmal activity sharp elements, spikes, spikes and polyspikes wave complexes in occipito-temporo-parietal regions without hemispheric predominance, at times with anterior spread. These discharges suppressed by eye opening and activated after about 10–15 seconds by eye closing. Photic stimulation with eyes open and eyes closed did not modify the pattern.

Sleep EEG showed normal sleep organization: the paroxysmal activity was less intense but more diffuse and generalized compared to waking, above all in NREM sleep, in the REM phase this activity was reduced. Carbamazepine therapy was started.

The boy remained in good health until October 1990 when he had a complex partial seizure during sleep and, shortly after awakening, complained of a right frontal pulsating headache associated with general discomfort, pallor and weakness for the whole day. He then had other headache episodes weekly, without premonitory symptoms, frequently associated with general discomfort, pallor, palpebral oedema and sometimes vomiting, photo- and phonophobia. These symptoms lasted some hours, and ended with sleep.

In this period the boy showed attention deficit at school, less interests, learning difficulties in arithmetical skills and slight dysgraphia. For the persistence of headache Nimodipine therapy was started in May 1991, and continued for about two months. The response to therapy was good, and the boy was free of headache for 7 months.

After this period headache episodes with the same features reappeared: firstly they occurred every two weeks, then they became more frequent, occurring daily so that the boy again had difficulties in concentration, in learning and in playing. For this reason he spent most of the day in bed. Other therapies were attempted:

dihydroergotamine metasulphonate, cafergot, L-5-hydroxytryptophan, pizotiphene, all with inadequate response. A reduction of headache attacks was obtained with the use of sumatriptan.

The headache persisted and several months later he was readmitted to our department. Awake and sleep EEG recordings and brain CT scan were unchanged; MR angiography was normal.

He then presented rare epileptic episodes with polymorphic features: right versive head movements; right sided clonic movements followed by loss of muscle tone, impairment of consciousness with right versive eye and head movements; epigastric aura and palpebral clonic movements, without clear loss of consciousness.

Carbamazepine dosage was increased; afterwards vigabatrin therapy was added with only initial and brief benefit; then phenobarbital therapy was introduced.

The patient then presented different episodes characterized by gradual and progressive visual reduction for 30–60 min with adequate contact with the environment and without other signs except headache. Vision returned slowly. During another hospitalization, a jejunal biopsy was carried out and showed villous atrophy, coeliac disease was diagnosed and a gluten-free diet was started.

In the last two years the clinical picture was characterized by aggravation of epileptic seizures with polymorphic features: psychomotor arrest, sudden generalized tonic contraction followed by periods of confusion lasting up to few minutes with or without falling; versive eye, head and arm movements more on the right side with or without generalization, paroxysmal nystagmus for a few minutes associated with visual difficulty. These episodes, that occurred several times a day, and seemed to be provoked by meals, urination, entering in to a dark room, eating ice cream and during active games.

The attacks were frequent and persistent in spite of the use of various combinations of antiepileptic drugs: clobazam, oxcarbazepine, felbamate, lamotrigine and hydrocortisone.

Long-lasting headache often followed the generalized seizures. A brain CT scan after a sudden fall, did not show an increase in size of the calcifications

The gluten-free diet was continued.

Lately the boy became less active: in particularly when the epileptic seizures were long and numerous, and his school performance declined.

The last EEG showed diffuse slowing of the background activity with poor physiological activity, high amplitude spikes, spike-waves and slow spikes-wave discharges, mostly on occipital regions, with, at times, generalized spread; this pattern was not modified by hyperventilation or photic stimulation. Furthermore, they decreased when the eyes were open. During wakefulness a seizure was recorded with an EEG-clinical pattern of a tonic seizure, characterized on the EEG by abrupt onset of diffuse bilateral high amplitude slow waves followed by depression of the background activity and then by a recruiting rhythm lasting 8 s.

Case 2

D.G. was the son of non-consanguinous parents without family history of headache of epilepsy. He was born after a normal pregnancy and delivery and had a normal psychomotor development.

At the age of 5½, after awakening, he had an intense headache followed by an epileptic seizure (loss of consciousness, right versive head and eye movement) that lasted several minutes. Valproate therapy was initiated.

Brain CT scan showed bilateral parieto-occipital cortico-subcortical calcifications. Cranial MRI was normal.

After one month he complained of gastroenteric disturbance and was admitted to the Paediatric Clinic of Bari, where a jejunal biopsy was performed. Coeliac disease was diagnosed, and a gluten-free diet started.

After cessation of valproate, two episodes of visual reduction, intense headache, and vertigo appeared. They lasted about 2 h and ended with transient loss of consciousness. Valproate therapy was restarted.

The boy was seen at the age of 6 and the following examinations were performed: routine laboratory tests, rubella, toxoplasma, cytomegalovirus and herpes simplex antibodies. The ophthalmological evaluation revealed hypermetropic astigmatism. Several waking and sleep EEG recordings showed mild slowing of background activity on posterior regions, more on the left.

A subsequent MRI showed no change, and MR angiography was normal.

During hospitalization he had episodes of sparkling scotoma and pulsating headache lasting for one hour. One of these attacks was described as follows: visual disturbances (coloured circles for about 20 min and then visual reduction for another two hours) followed by violent frontal headache for about two hours with persistence of darkened vision. During the attack no loss or impairment of consciousness was present and EEG recording was unchanged.

During the ensuing two months headaches, occuring three times a week, and a complex partial seizure, were described.

A year later he began to complain again of headache episodes occurring a daily; some reduction of attacks was obtained with the use of nimodipine. These attacks caused difficulties in concentration, in learning ability and in playing. Sumatriptan therapy could not be tried due to the young age.

In May 1995 rare brief headache episodes followed by unresponsiveness and motionless staring appeared. EEG showed brief bilateral and synchronous atypical polyspike-wave discharges during sleep. A cranial NMR showed slight bilateral occipital cortical atrophy. Valproate dosage was increased. The boy attended first grade and did well.

Recently in both cases a combined study of proton magnetic resonance imaging (MRI) and Spectroscopy (MRS) was performed with a 1.5 Tesla Siemens Magnetom. The imaging protocol included SE sequences (TR 2200/TE 12–80 ms, TR 600/TE 20 ms), axial, coronal and sagittal planes of 5 mm thickness and a 0.5 mm interslice gap, obtained by 256×192 matrices. Proton spectra were acquired on a $2.5 \times 2 \times 2$ cm volume of interest localized in occipital regions of both hemispheres, using a spin echo sequence (TR 150O, TE 135 msec). No changes in N-acetylaspartate (NAA)/creatine (Cr), NAA/choline (Cho), Cho/Cr ratios were found in comparison to values of healthy subjects. Lactate signal was detected in the left hemisphere of both patients. These MRS data suggest that the increase of lactate metabolism could depend on impairment of oxygen supply associated with possible anaerobic glycolysis by infiltrating inflammatory cells in this ischaemic brain region. In contrast, normal values of NAA indicate preserved neuronal function.

Discussion

Migraine feature a characterize the clinical story of our two patients. This type of headache in this syndrome has also been described by other authors: Martini *et al.*, 1985; Ciarmatori *et al.*, 1987; Masson *et al.*, 1988; Battistella *et al.*, 1988; Giroud *et al.*, 1990; Veneselli *et al.*, 1991; Galletti *et al.*, 1991. A high incidence of headache, nausea and vomiting associated with occipital seizures in children has been described (Camfield *et al.*, 1978; Panayiotopoulos *et al.*. 1980; Terzano *et al.*, 1980; Newton & Aicardi, 1983; De Romanis *et al.*, 1988).

In our two patients, in the early phase of the illness, the headaches were constant in time and severity, so that family life and scholastic activities suffered, while epileptic seizures were sporadic. The early severity of headache symptomatology has not been described in previous reports.

We also wish to emphasise that both our patients presented episodes of long-lasting amaurosis associated with headache, without loss of consciousness. These features do not seem to be epileptic seizures in which the amaurotic episodes are transient and associated with loss of consciousness, (Salanova *et al.*, 1992; Williamson *et al.*, 1992) and are difficult to diagnose. They might be explained as vertebro-basilar migraine or, on the contrary on the basis of an ischaemic vascular mechanism taking place in the territory of the posterior cerebral artery. Increase of lactate metabolism as detected by MRS in our patients seems to confirm the presence of an ischaemic vascular mechanism.

Recently pathological findings of cortical vascular abnormality with patchy pial angiomatosis, fibrosed veins and microcalcifications were reported by Bye *et al.* (1993) and by Plazzi *et al.* (1994). The oligoemia affecting the territories of distribution of the calcarine artery and consequently a regional hypoxic phenomenon might facilitate the occurrence of epileptic seizures.

14: Neurological disorders in Spanish children with coeliac disease

Antonio Martínez Bermejo, Isabel Polanco[*], Valentín López Martín and Ignacio Pascual Castroviejo

Servicio de Neurologiay Gastroenterologia[*] Hospital Infantil La Paz, Universidad Autónoma, Paseo de la Castellana 261, 28046 Madrid, Spain

Introduction

An increased prevalence of epilepsy and other neurological disorders in patients with coeliac disease (CD) has been reported since the observations of Daynes (1956), Cooke & Smith (1966), Morris *et al.* (1970) and Chapman *et al.* (1978). Furthermore, CD associated with epilepsy and intracranial calcifications has been described in recent years in Italian and Argentinian people (Sammaritano *et al.*, 1988; Molteni *et al.*, 1988; Gobbi *et al.*, 1992; Arroyo *et al.*, 1992). The incidence of bilateral occipital calcifications (BOC) and epilepsy in CD is not yet well defined in Spanish patients. The present investigation was designed to estimate the frequency with which neurological abnormalities occur in Spanish patients with CD.

Patients and methods

Among the 730 patients with CD (ESPGAN criteria) followed at our hospital, 36 were randomly selected (20 girls and 16 boys), aged 8–24 years (mean 13.8), to undergo cerebral computed tomography (CT) scanning, EEG, detailed neurological history and complete clinical examination. All patients had EEG recordings in wakefulness according to the 10–20 International System of electrode placement. The age at diagnosis CD was between 8 months and 8 years (mean 2.3 years). In addition three cases with cryptogenic cerebral calcifications (two of them unilateral occipital), in which clinical and laboratory tests failed to establish the cause of the calcifications, underwent intestinal biopsy. All patients or their parents were asked for informed consent beforehand; 36 patients who underwent CT for headache were considered as a control group.

Results

No cases of BOC were found in our CD patients or in the control group. The intestinal biopsy in the three cases with cryptogenic cerebral calcifications was normal. In the 36 CD patients group, nine (25 per cent) were found to suffer from seizures: one Lennox-Gastaut syndrome, three febrile convulsions (8.3 per cent), one partial complex seizures (at 5 years) and four cases (11.1 per cent) had experienced transient epileptic attacks (generalized tonic or tonic-clonic) with loss of consciousness of unknown aetiology, beginning at 5 months, 3, 10 and 13 years. Except in the patient with Lennox-Gastaut syndrome, the seizures were well controlled.

We also observed a delay in beginning to walk (mean 15 months). There were no disorders of language development and learning. Eight cases (22.2 per cent) presented occasional tension headache and four (11.1 per cent) had migraine.

Discussion

We observed a high incidence of seizures and febrile convulsions in our patients with CD compared with the incidence of these diseases in Spanish children. A high incidence of epilepsy among patients with CD was also observed (Morris *et al.*, 1970; Chapman *et al.*, 1978). At the moment the reason for this is not well understood.

We also observed a high incidence of tension headache and migraine in our series (11.1 per cent), higher than the prevalence of headache observed in other studies (Deubner, 1982). We observed a delay in beginning to walk in our patients with CD (mean 15 months) compared with normal Spanish children (mean 12.5 months) (Fernandez-Alvarez, 1989) which may be explained by the diarrhoea, malnutrition and malabsorption problems.

Table 1. Reported cases of Spanish patients with coeliac disease (CD), epilepsy and cerebral calcifcations

Authors		Sex	Age (y)	Age at onset of epilepsy (y)	Seizure pattern	Cerebral calcifi- cations	Age at diagnosis of CD (y)	Origin in Spain	Comments
Montòn et al. (1992)									
	Case 1	M	12	2	Generalized (2y) Visual (8y)	BO	12	Canary Islands	I.Q. Borderline. Bad control of seizures. HLA A1 A26 B17
Baquero et al. (1994)									
	Case 2	M	41	37	Visual seizures, focal motor	BO	39	Valencia	(*) I.Q. normal
	Case 3	F	53	52	Generalized, multi- focal myoclonic	BO	32	Valencia	Myoclonic ataxia associated with low level of Vit. E.
Baiges et al. (1994)									
	Case 4	M	13	4	Partial with secon- dary generalization	BPO	8	Catalonia	(*) Recurrent seizures at 12 y (visual, adversive, partial complex) with bad control.
Hernàndez et al. (1994)									
	Case 5	F	18	9	Focal motor, adversives	BO	18	Canary Islands	I.Q. 53. HLA DR3
Pinilla et al. (1995)									
	Case 6	F	18	11	Generalized	PO right	14	La Rioja	(*)

F, female; M, male; (y), years; BO, bilateral occipital; BPO, bilateral parieto-occipital; PO, parieto-occipital; I.Q., intelec-tual quotient; (*), good control of seizures with gluten-free diet.

We did not observe bilateral occipital calcifications (BOC) in our study. The association of cerebral calcifica-tions and epilepsy with CD is very rare in Spanish medical reports. To our knowledge only six cases of Spanish origin have been described (Table 1). The reason is unknown. Spain is a country with a high incidence of CD. Moreover the HLA phenotype in Spanish patients with CD is similar to that of Italian patients (Tighe et al., 1992) and the food habits are similar in both countries.

The relatively high incidence in Italian and Argentinian people could be related to unknown environmental agents and/or genetic factors. A lot of Argentinian people have ancestors of Italian origin. Probably this association could represent a new and genetically determined syndrome.

15: Epilepsy and neurological findings in adult coeliac patients

N. Rebaudengo, P. Pignatta, E. Bo, W. Liboni, C. Sategna Guidetti*, M. Bruno and S. Grosso[*]

Dipartmento di Neuroscienze, Osp. Gradenigo, Torino; *Cattedra di gastroenterologia, Università di Torino, Italy

Introduction

The purpose of our study was to evaluate the association of coeliac disease (CD) with neurological disorders, mainly with epilepsy (Bouhnik *et al.*, 1991; Kinney *et al.*, 1982). We analysed 30 patients (mean age 38.7 ± 17.3) by extensive neuroimaging and neurophysiological investigation to determine the presence of any pathological alteration (Table 1).

Table 1.

30 patients with coeliac disease mean age: 38.7 ± 17.3 (range 19–77 years)	
19 females	11 males
Neurophysiological and neuroimaging investigation	
EEG	30 patients
CT	30 patients
MRI	4 patients

Table 2.

Patients	Age (years)	Gastroent. sympt.	2nd Investigation
10	20–30	6 since 1 year old	4 since 3–4 years
11	30–45	6 since 10 year old	5 since 6 months
5	45–60	variable since 10 years	1 since 2 years
4	60–80	variable	2 since 2 years

Results

Considering the onset of malabsorption symptoms and the period before diet, our population was heterogeneous (Table 2). The youngest patients were generally diagnosed in childhood (one year old); on the contrary, older ones were discovered to have coeliac disease later, 10 or more years after the onset of gastroenterological symptoms. In our study few neurological disorders were found. The most frequent psychological symptom was dysthimia in 23 per cent of patients. The clinical examination did not reveal any neurological deficit except for a reduction of achilles tendon reflexes in 13 per cent of patients. The other neurological disorders had a prevalence similar to that in the general population (migraine with and without aura in two young patients, mnesic disorders in four patients older than 60 years) and the difference was not statistically significant We discovered a sporadic arachnoid cyst in a young woman and another one had Basedow disease. Slight cerebellar abnormalities were only diagnosed in one patient. We did not find any clinical history of epileptic seizures (Hanly *et al.*, 1982; Ventura *et al.*, 1991). The EEG pattern was completely normal in 21. In five patients we detected specific slight bilateral electric abnormalities, such as a theta pattern in the anterolateral part of the scalp. We recorded one short episode of generalized sharp waves in a female who never suffered from seizures, but who had migraine with aura, Basedow disease, and dysthimia.

Table 3.

Brain atrophy			
Mild	6 patients	diffuse cortical cerebral atrophy	Mean age: 41.5± 16
Moderate	6 patients	diffuse cortical cerebral atrophy	Mean age: 55 ± 8
Severe		in 2 cases mainly in the posterior regions (52, 54 years)	Mean age: 51 ± 13
		in 1 case left fronto parietal (43)	
		in 1 case in the occipital lobes (50)	
Microcalcifcations	5 patients		
	Basal ganglia		
	Caudate nucleus		
	Lentiform nucleus		
	Occipital cortex		
Cerebellar atrophy			
Slight	6 patients		(57 ± 9)
Moderate	3 patients		(63 ± 12)

We studied CNS degeneration by extensive neuroradiological examination (CT in all patients and MRI in 4 of them). CT investigation revealed a slight degree of cerebral cortical atrophy in six patients (two of them were older than 60 years), suffering from slight amnesic deficits. The other four patients were younger (20 to 40 years old), without any focal neurological symptom. These two male patients suffered respectively from anxiety and migraine; besides, one female had an arachnoid cyst. CT showed a severe degree of atrophy in six patients (Table 3). It was a diffuse cortical atrophy, in three of them mainly in the posterior parietal-occipital region. These patients were asymptomatic and only three of them were suffering from mnesic disturbances. Atrophy in the cerebellar cortex was present in two asymptomatic patients (60 and 70 years old). In seven patients we detected a slight cerebellar atrophy in addition.

All of them were asymptomatic, except for one with a slight left deviation on walking. Our data show slight atrophy in the youngest patients involving both cerebral and cerebellar hemispheres.

Table 4. Vascular disease

Ischaemic lesions	Patients	(Mean age: 55.7 ± 14)
Small	5 patients	
	Bilateral basal ganglia	(52)
	Left fronto parietal	(64)
	Right MCA territory	(64)
	Bilateral frontal lobes	(23)
	Left basal ganglia	(55)
More extensive Hypodensity	3 patients	
	Left Parietotemporooccipital and diffuse vascular disease	(60)
	Left frontoparietal	(64)
	Left temporoparietal lobes	(66)
ICA wall calcifications	2 patients	(43, 65)

Degeneration of the vascular system was also found in our study (Table 4). We detected diffuse vascular disturbances in a 60 year old male. He was asymptomatic, except for slight mnesic deficit. CT examination revealed a hypodense area in the cortical-subcortical parietal-occipital regions and more definite hypodense lesions in the brain stem. One month after this examination, he had a short-lasting episode of diplopia.

Table 5.

Psychiatric symptoms (dysthimia)	10 patients
Diminution of achilles tendon reflexes	6
Migraine	2
Cerebellar symtoms	1
Memory disturbances	4 (more than 60 years old)

Vascular abnormalities, with lacunar lesions, also involved the basal ganglia of a 55 year old man, and the centrum semi-ovale of a 60 year old male. Ischaemic abnormality of the frontal-parietal cortex was evident in three asymptomatic patients: a woman (64 years old), and two males (64 and 65 years old).

We did not find any large calcification pattern in the brain (Gobbi *et al.*, 1992). CT examination revealed microcalcification of the basal ganglia in four patients and a small calcification in the occipital cortex in one patient (54 years old) who never suffered from seizures.

Discussion

We studied a population of coeliac patients with a long history of disease from childhood to presenium. From their clinical history and neurological – neurophysiological and neuroradiological examinations we can deduce the following:

(A) The most frequent psychiatric and neurological symptoms are reported in Table 5. The pathologies frequently associated with coeliac disease are shown in Tables 3 and 4.

(B) The CT / MR finding, are similar in a population of 45 cases of the same age studied for ENT pathologies (otitis, sinusitis) or for minor cranial trauma without any neurologic focal lesions. The only different finding is the atrophy, more frequently involving cerebellar hemispheres, even in young patients of the coeliac population.
Calcifications. We discovered occipital cortical microcalcifications in a patient aged 54 with specific gastro enterologic symptoms for 6 years, without clinical history of seizures. In four patients there were small calcifications in the basal ganglia. In the control group CT examination revealed calcification in five patients out of 45, only in the basal ganglia.
CT/MR vascular alterations. Both cortical and cortical-subcortical lesions were evident, not related to the clinical symptoms.

(C) The EEG patterns were not typical for epileptic seizures.

Our experience suggests the oresence of a vascular condition that could be relelated to an immune vasculitis.

In future studies we plan to clinically follow up and reveal any neuroradiologic finding in young coeliac patients, to investigate cortical atrophy and asymptomatic vascular disturbances, and to prevent ischaemica symptoms.

16: Neurological findings in adults with unknown coeliac disease

G.L. de Angelis, M.E. Street, M. Corna, E. Romanini, C. Capone[*], I. Dodi and C. Faienza[*]

Division of Gastroenterology, Department of Paediatrics, Parma, Italy; [*]Division of Neuropsychiatry, Department of Paediatrics, Parma, Italy

Introduction

Coeliac disease (CD) is a permanent intolerance to the gluten contained in flour made from wheat, barley and oats. The condition is ill-defined and often does not present with the typical growth deficiency in childhood as was thought during the first years following its discovery (Auricchio *et al.*, 1988). This disease may be clinically and/or biologically latent for a long period of time and is extremely heterogeneous (Corazza *et al.*, 1994; Visakorpi & Maki, 1994; Catassi *et al.*, 1994).

In recent years screening with AGA and AEA has helped make the diagnosis of coeliac disease, but new forms of the disease, definitely 'atypical', have emerged and have increased the polymorphic clinical picture (Ferguson *et al.*, 1992; Burgin-Wolff *et al.*, 1991; Volta *et al.*, 1983). At present it is often difficult to distinguish symptoms from complications.

Therefore clinical intuition is still fundamental for the diagnosis which can be made only by the study of intestinal biopsies.

Patients and investigations

Patient no. 1

A 33-year-old male was admitted to a department of neurology for a sudden acute episode of loss of consciousness and generalized tonic-clonic seizures which lasted a few minutes and were followed by post-ictal confusion of about one hour.

Blood samples showed mainly an alteration of the calcium (Ca) phosphate (P) metabolism.

A cerebral CT scan was carried out and showed bilateral gross calcifications of the basal nuclei and of the occipital region bilaterally, with normal ventricles (Fig. 1). This gave rise to the suspicion of Fahr's syndrome.

The medical history revealed chronic diarrhoea during his first year of life, which had led to a decline of his general condition. Anti-gluten antibodies (AGA-IgA) and anti-endomisium antibodies (AEA) were measured and were both positive (AGA IgA: 119 AU; AEA: ++++; normal AGA IgA: < 24 AU and AEA: neg).

Endoscopy carried out in our department showed subtotal villous atrophy. The diagnosis of coeliac disease was confirmed by histopathology, and the patient was put on a gluten-free diet.

The principal laboratory findings at diagnosis were: Ca: 5.4 mg/dl (nl: 8.3–10.5 mg/dl); folic acid: 1.2 ng/ml (nl: 2–16 ng/dl); mean cellular volume of erythrocytes (MCV): 96 μm^3 (nl: 80–95 μm^3); parathormone: 9.3 pg/mL (nl: 9–55 pg/mL).

Bone mineral density was normal. Ophthalmologic examination showed bilateral juvenile cataracts (the patient had never been on glucocorticoids).

The general condition of the patient improved markedly, and after 6 months on the gluten-free diet he stopped the anti-convulant treatment he had been given during his admission. A repeat biopsy 10 months after diagnosis, showed a perfectly normal mucosa.

One year later a second CT scan was performed. This showed periventricular amorphous calcifications and calcifications of the basal nuclei; the bilateral occipital calcifications were not confirmed (Figs. 1–2). The reason for this was the immediate use of contrast during the first examination which created false images.

The patient has been well for more than a year and a half since that time.

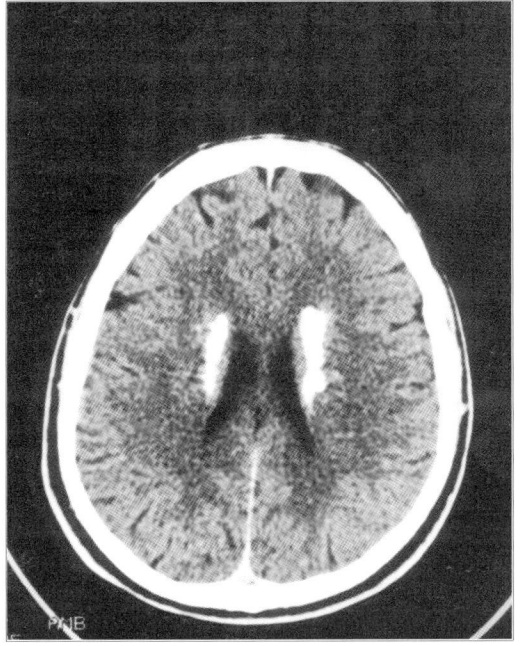

Fig. 1. Amorphous periventricular calcifications.

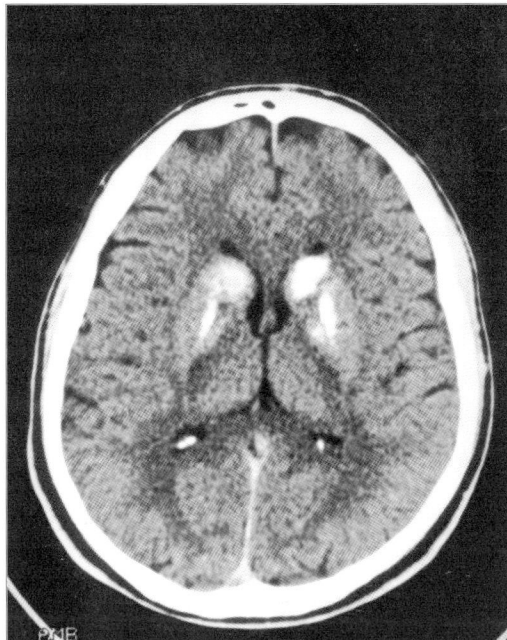

Fig. 2. Calcifications of the basal ganglia.

Patient no. 2

A 59 year-old man presented with a four-year history of chronic diarrhoea associated with anorexia, loss of weight (about 8 kg) and a depressive syndrome which was being treated with tricyclic antidepressant drugs (imipramine, 50 mg/day).

The depressive symptoms had been interpreted as being a reaction to stressing environmental factors (his retirement); the 'gastro-enterological troubles' had been considered as secondary symptoms due to the emotional condition of the patient. Laboratory assays showed a slight macrocythaemic anaemia (Hb: 11.8 g/dL; MCV: 93 μm^3).

The patient was dyspeptic and we carried out an endoscopy. Several duodenal biopsies were taken and on histological examination showed sub-total villous atrophy of the mucosa compatible with active coeliac disease. At the same time blood was drawn for AGA IgA which was positive (150 AU).

Ca-P metabolism and bone mineral density were normal. Concomitant autoimmune diseases were excluded and the patient was put on a gluten-free diet.

A month after beginning the diet the patient stopped his antidepressant treatment, and after a year had regained the weight lost and was in good health. One year later a second duodenal biopsy was performed. The intestinal mucosa, AGA IgA and AEA were normal.

Discussion

Coeliac disease is a syndrome affecting all the organs of the body with variable clinical evidence. Through complex metabolic alterations the central nervous system suffers too. Great aetiopathogenic importance in the development of cerebral calcifications and epilepsy is now ascribed to low blood levels of folic acid, which was extremely low at diagnosis in patient I (Ventura *et al.*, 1991; Gobbi *et al.*, 1992) and CD is known to be the most common cause of secondary low folic acid.

Bilateral occipital calcifications (BOC) are reported to be the most commonly observed in CD (Magaudda *et al.*, 1993). The periventricular calcifications and calcifications of the basal ganglia described in the first patient are not generally reported and are usually suggestive of Fahr's disease (Billard *et al.*, 1989). However, the normal PTH and jejunal biopsies after one year on a gluten-free diet and the disappearance of all symptoms on this treatment suggest confirmation of the diagnosis of CD.

This disease has a markedly progressive course and this justifies a gluten-free diet which, if accompanied by supplementation with folic acid, can normalize clinical features and electroencephalographic alterations.

Among the disorders of visual function (e.g. permanent defects of the visual field and acuity), cataract, which is bilateral in our first patient, is not usually reported and we do not have an explanation for it.

A depressive syndrome is reported as a consequence of malnutrition and may also occur in childhood as can be seen, for example, in proteic-caloric denutrition (Hernanz & Polanco, 1991). It must be borne in mind that a depressive disorder which presents in adulthood is not necessarily due to a primary neurological disorder.

The second patient had a late presentation of CD, which must have been latent clinically and/or biologically for a long time, while in patient no. 1 it is more difficult to understand if this was an atypical presentation of CD or if the disease had always been there in an oligosymptomatic manner. On the basis of our experience we think it would be more correct to define this as an unrecognized complication of coeliac disease which presented in childhood and was untreated rather than an atypical form 'ab initio'. In patients with neurological findings out of 50 of our series who presented after age 15, the determination of AGA IgA and AEA was extremely useful as a first screening (Burgin-Wolff *et al.*, 1991; Ferguson *et al.* 1992). However when there is clinical evidence of disease it is mandatory to carry out rendoscopic biopsies considering also the lower sensitivity of screening with AGA-AEA in adults (Grodzinsky *et al.*, 1990; Scott *et al.*, 1990).

CD may be difficult to diagnose, and it is to a large extent, heterogeneous. To date CD is probably more often undiagnosed in adults than in children due to the process of sensibilization which has been ongoing already for several years among paediatricians. The combined evaluations by different adult specialists (gynaecologists, neurologists, endocrinologists, etc.), could avoid mistakes in the treatment which is fundamental in order to avoid both metabolic-nutritional and severe complications of untreated CD such as malignancies.

17: Neuropsychological evaluation of posterior areas function in coeliac patients with or without epilepsy

Giovanni De Maria, Maria Luisa Gorno, [*]Stefano Francesco Cappa,
Bruno Guarneri and Luisa Antonini

Neurophysiopathology Service, Spedali Civili, Brescia; [*]Institute of Neurology, University of Brescia, Brescia, Italy

Introduction

The association of epilepsy, cerebral calcifications and coeliac disease is a recently described syndrome characterized by an involvement of posterior regions of the brain (Dickey, 1994).

The purpose of the present study was the assessment of the neuropsychological functions of posterior areas of the brain in patients with coeliac disease with or without epilepsy.

Patients and methods

Two groups of patients were included. The first group comprised five patients with epilepsy and coeliac disease, three with cerebral calcifications and two without cerebral calcifications. The second group included 26 subjects (four male, 22 female, age range 21–64 years) with coeliac disease without epilepsy.

The first group of patients were tested with an extensive neuropsychological battery. The second group were tested with Raven's progressive coloured matrices to assess general non-verbal reasoning, and judgment of line orientation and facial recognition test to assess posterior areas function.

Table 1. Cognitive measures in five patients with coeliac disease and epilepsy

Test	Normal scores	Abnormal scores
Judgment of line orientation	0	5
Facial recognition test	2	3
Rey complex figure copy	2	3
Rey complex figure recall	1	4
Spatial span	2	3
Token test	5	0
Raven's progressive matrices	5	0
Digit span	5	0
Short story recall	5	0
Verbal fluency	5	0
Wisconsin card sorting test	5	0
Attentional test	5	0

Table 2. Cognitive measures in 26 coeliac patients without epilepsy

Test	Normal scores
Raven's progressive matrices	26
Judgment of line orientation	20
Facial recognition test	25

Results and discussion

Table 1 presents the results obtained for the coeliac patients with epilepsy. All had abnormal scores in tests sensitive to posterior areas impairment, independent of the presence of cerebral calcification. In contrast, none of them showed a performance below normal on the other tests. Table 2 shows the results obtained by the patients with coeliac disease without epilepsy. Only one patient had pathological scores on both judgment of line orientation and facial recognition test.

Occipital seizures associated with coeliac disease (with or without cerebral calcification) suggest a link between coeliac disease and occipital lobe dysfunction (Ambrosetto *et al.*, 1993). In our patients with coeliac disease and epilepsy, independent of the occipital calcifications, the pattern of cognitive impairment gives further evidence of involvement of posterior areas of the brain. All these patients have pathological scores in tests sensitive to posterior areas function (judgment of line orientation, facial recognition test, Rey complex figure copy, Rey complex figure recall, spatial span).

The relation between coeliac disease and epilepsy with or without occipital calcification is unclear. While posterior areas dysfunction in patients with coeliac disease and epilepsy could be related to a relative vulnerability of the occipital lobe, only one of the 26 coeliac patients without epilepsy had pathological scores in both the tests clearly associated with impairment of posterior areas. Our observations indicate that the neuropsychological pattern of posterior areas dysfunction observed in patients with coeliac disease and occipital lobe seizures is not present in patients with coeliac disease without epilepsy.

18: Coeliac disease, mental retardation and macrocephaly: two affected sisters

Antonia Parmeggiani[*]**, Gianna Bertani**[**]**, Margherita Santucci**[*]**, Gloria Lolli***, **Maria Gilda Zaniboni**[**]**, Giuseppe Gobbi**[**]**, Antonella Pini**[**] **and Paola Giovanardi Rossi***

[*]*Department of Child Neurology and Psychiatry, Neurological Institute, University of Bologna;* [**]*Department of Child Neurology and Psychiatry, S. Maria Nuova Hospital, Reggio Emilia;* [***]*Department of Child Gastroenterology, Maggiore Hospital 'C.A. Pizzardi', Bologna, Italy*

Introduction

Coeliac patients do not necessarily present malabsorption, and coeliac disease (CD) is often clinically silent (Ferguson *et al.*, 1993; Collin & Maki, 1994). Typical CD is less frequent while atypical cases in childhood with symptoms like iron-deficiency anaemia and short stature are increasingly frequent (40 per cent of diagnosed cases) (Zaniboni *et al.*, 1993).

CD is characterized by several clinical aspects including neurologic and psychiatric symptoms (Cooke, 1976). Interestingly the association between CD, epilepsy and cerebral calcifications has been reported by the Italian Working Group on CD and epilepsy (Gobbi *et al.*,1992). Other reports concern the association between CD and cognitive disturbances (Pavone *et al.*, Chapter 39; this book), schizophrenia and autism (Dohan, 1970; Perisic *et al.*, 1990), depression (Hallert & Derefeldt, 1982; Hallert & Aström, 1982; Hernanz & Polanco, 1991), dementia and brain atrophy (Collin *et al.*, 1991), cerebellar syndrome (Finelli *et al.*, 1980), Down Syndrome (Granditsch, 1990) and Williams syndrome (Pittschieler *et al.*, 1993).

We describe two sisters presenting CD, mental retardation (MR) and macrocephaly and discuss this unreported clinical association.

Case report

Sa. and Gr. are two sisters aged 17 years 4 months and 12 years 2 months. Family history was positive for MR, epilepsy, and short stature (Fig. 1).

During pregnancy threatened abortion occurred. Both girls were macrocephalic at birth. The elder (Sa.) showed mild motor retardation, the younger (Gr.) some problems with language development. Both showed irritability and difficulties in social functioning.

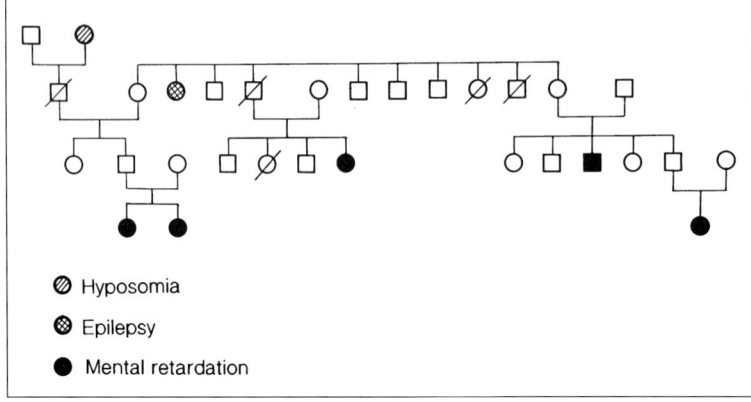

⊘ Hyposomia

⊗ Epilepsy

● Mental retardation

Fig. 1. Family pedigree positive for short stature. epilepsy and mental retardation.

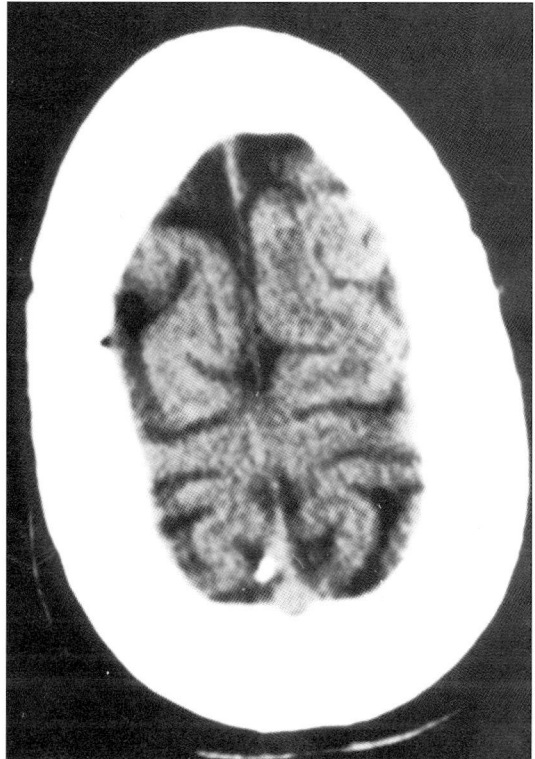

*Fig. 2. Sa. CT scan showing unilateral calcification
and cortical atrophy.*

Sa. at the age of 9 months developed diarrhoea. At that time CD was diagnosed clinically without biopsy and she began a gluten-free diet that was discontinued at the age of 3 years without recurrence of malabsorption symptoms. At the age of 8 years she presented nephrolithiasis.

Gr. had only recurrent vomiting during the first year of life.

At the time of our first examination at the age of 13 years 4 months and 8 years 2 months, respectively they presented macrocrania, normal growth and anaemia with low iron and folic acid levels. Antigliadin and endomysium antibodies, intestinal biopsy and HLA (DR3 - DQw2) were typical for CD and they started with a gluten-free diet.

Neurometabolic, amino-acid screening and karyotypes were negative.

EEG and SPECT were negative. CT scan in the elder (Sa.) showed unilateral right parieto-occipital calcification and cortical atrophy (Fig. 2).

Neuropsychological testing was performed before and during gluten-free diet using the WISC-R, Raven Matrices, Rey test, Children's apperception test, drawing, reading and writing tests, and L. Düss tales.

Both were mildly mentally retarded (IQ 56 and 64) with mild improvement in the younger after gluten-free diet. Neither girl could write or count. Sa. was anxious and Gr. showed phobic neurotic traits.

Discussion

These two cases are interesting because up to now literature reports have not described similar patients. CD has been associated with diseases with MR such as Down syndrome (Grandisch, 1990), Williams syndrome (Pittschieler *et al.*, 1994), or psychiatric disturbances such as schizophrenia, autism (Dohan, 1970; Perisic *et al.*, 1990), depression (Hallert & Derefelt, 1982; Hallert & Aström, 1982; Hernanz & Polanco, 1991) and progressive neurologic pathology (Finelli *et al.*, 1980; Collin *et al.*, 1991).

In our patients we did not find a low plasma level of tryptophan as is seen in patients with depression, behavioural disorder and CD (Hernanz & Polanco, 1991).

Pavone *et al.*; Chapter 39, this book; found in CD patients treated or untreated with a gluten-free diet cognitive disturbances such as impairment in visual discrimination ability and short-term memory.

In our girls, even though they were macrocephalic at birth, Sotos syndrome was excluded; on the other hand macrocephaly may sometimes be associated with MR (Diebler & Dulac, 1990). The association between CD, MR and macrocephaly in our patients might not be simply a coincidence, especially considering the family pedigree where MR and growth deficiency (CD undiagnosed?), were reported. At present, however, it is difficult to explain the aetiopathogenesis of the disorder and other case reports to confirm the existence of this syndrome are necessary.

Acknowledgements

We are grateful to Ms. Silvia Muzzi, Ms. Manuela Zuffi, Mr. Massimo Armaroli and Ms Elena Zoni for technical assistance. We wish to thank Ms. Anne Collins for linguistic revision.

19: Cognitive and psychosocial aspects in 81 coeliac patients and their parents

A. De Pascale, P. Mariani, S. Maello, F. Virgilii, L. Calvani, E. Cipolletta, M. Montuori and M. Bonamico

Paediatric Clinic, Rome University 'La Sapienza', Viale Regina Elena 324, 00161 Rome, Italy

Accdrding to several authors, coeliac disease (CD) patients show peculiar psychological symptoms (Di Cagno & Bonassi, 1977), or frank psychiatric disturbances (Cooke & Holmes, 1984) not directly due to the coeliac enteropathy.

We investigate the cognitive aspects and the emotional and relational styles more often present in coeliac children and their families.

Methods

We studied 81 coeliacs, 47 females and 34 males, aged 1–21 years (mean 8.5 years ± 5.0 years), diagnosed according to ESPGAN (1989), receiving a gluten-free diet for at least six months. Patients were divided into three age groups (at diagnosis): Group 1 – diagnosis before 2 years – 44 children, 21 females and 23 males; Group 2 – diagnosis between 2 and 10 years – 19 children, 14 female and 5 male; Group 3 – diagnosis after 10 years – 18 children, 12 female and 6 male (Table 1).

Subjects and their families were interviewed according to the assessment procedures of a systemic and cognitive approach. Then the subjects' reports and contents were collected in a form including the following items:

Attitude to disease; Adopted solutions; Patient's psychosocial development; Relational family characteristics

Results

Content analysis of data obtained during interviews showed: a well-balanced attitude towards the disease more frequently observed among fathers (71 per cent) and mothers (66 per cent); in almost 25 per cent of subjects there was a denial reaction towards the disease and in 5–6 per cent an inadequate laid-back attitude towards the disturbance. Only 10 per cent adopted completely inadequate strategies to cope with the dietary needs.

Regarding the children's psychosocial development, 72 per cent of fathers, 73 per cent of mothers, and 76 per cent of patients reported a significant level of satisfaction with their school progress and social adjustment.

Regarding the family relations, a prevailing difficulty of parent–child relationship is present in 14 per cent of fathers and 16 per cent of mothers and it is so recognized by both parents and children.

The attitude towards the disease is well-balanced in the group in which the age of diagnosis was between 2 and 10 years. The adopted solutions in most of cases were good in all groups.

The quality of patients' psychosocial development becomes progressively worse from the first to the third group. Table 2 shows that in the second group satisfactory relationships were more frequently encountered (a well-balanced attitude in 69 per cent of fathers, 64 per cent of mothers and 95 per cent of children, versus 59, 59 and 77 per cent in the first group, and 54, 55 and 78 per cent in the third) with only some disturbances in marital and parent–child relationships.

Table 1. 81 Subjects (47 female + 34 male) – CD + gluten-free diet > 6 months

Group 1	Group 2	Group 3
Diagnosis < 2 years	Diagnosis 2–10 years	Diagnosis > 10 years
44 subjects (8 teenagers)	19 subjects (10 teenagers)	18 teenagers
(21 female + 23 male)	(14 female + 5 male)	(12 female + 6 male)

Table 2. Adjustments in the different group's characteristics

Group 1	Group 2	Group 3
Diagnosed < 2 years	Diagnosed 2–10 years	Diagnosed > 10 years
59% F. balanced	69% F. balanced	54% F. balanced
59% M. balanced	64% M. balanced	55% M. balanced
77% C. balanced	95% C. balanced	78% T. balanced

Table 3. Family problems in the different groups

	Total	Total	Adolescents	Adolescents
	N	%	N	%
Group 1	10/44	22.7	4/8	50.0
Group 2	2/19	10.6	2/10	20.0
Group 3	5/18	27.7	5/18	27.7
Total	17/81	20.9	11/36	30.5

Discussion

The best adjustment observed in parents and in subjects diagnosed between the ages of 2 and 10 years seem to be a consequence of the time elapsed between diagnosis and the time of interview. In the second and third groups young children are more easily taught dietary compliance. Observed difficulties in children of the other two groups could be related in the first group to the parents' reaction to the recent diagnosis aand in the third group to the behavioural characteristics of adolescence.

Examining the number and percentage of families with difficulties in paarent–child relationships (Table 3) the data suggest such problems are more often present among adolescents. The presence of a juvenile disease which expresses itself in patterns of conflict towards parents is part of the normal development of psychological growth. One could formulate the hypothesis that in coeliac patients this maturational aspect of disease could take the form of a refusal to be compliant with a gluten-free diet.

The behavioural patterns with which patients and their fanilies deal with the constraints imposed by gluten intolerance and the subsequent psychological development, are linked to the quality of information that parents and coeliac children receive about the disease. This is also linked to the meaning that they attribute to the dietary constraints, to the idea that they are participating in the evolution of the disease itself, and to the subsequent behavioural styles they adopt (Anson *et al.*, 1990; Vella & De Pascale, 1988).

In conclusion, in this coeliac population we did not find psychiatric disturbances, whereas some psychological problems are present especially amond adolescents. Such difficulties could be related more to the parents' age than to the coeliac disease itself. Patients whose diagnosis had been formulated between 2 and 10 years show better dietary compliance annd a more satisfactory level of adjustment.

20: Anxiety and depression in subjects with coeliac disease. A personality 'trait' or a reactive condition?

G. Gasbarrini and G. Addolorato

Institute of Internal Medicine, Universita' Cattolica, Rome, Italy

Introduction

The presence of numerous primary and secondary psychological behavioural pathologies is well known in coeliac disease (Hallert & Aström, 1982). Many studies have been conducted on reactive syndromes which appear to have been caused by the limitations imposed by a gluten-free diet since this must be strictly followed and is very often difficult to apply in everyday life, both in and outside the home. Difficulties are present both in childhood, where subjects undergo the sometimes over-strict control of parents in respecting the gluten-free diet, and in adult life, which is conditioned by the continuous surveillance for unsuspected gluten in desirable foods.

Besides all these 'reactive' conditions, which can lead to a total refusal of the gluten-free diet, personality disturbances or other psychiatric conditions such as schizophrenia or autism may be present in coeliac disease (Dohan, 1970; Dohan, 1969; Perisic *et al.*, 1990; De Santis *et al.*, 1996). For this reason it is important to distinguish in these patients between a reactive anxiety state and an anxious personality trait. The psychometric evaluation of emotional status and personality traits has greatly developed in recent years. Numerous tools are available derived from a model of anxiety clearly formulated in operative terms and easy to use, such as the State and Trait Anxiety Inventory (STAT-TEST).

This test which is based on the difference between 'state' and 'trait' anxiety allows the distinction between existing anxiety and the possibility of anxiety reaction as a personality characteristic. This theory is based on the conceptual distinction between anxiety as a transitory state and anxiety as a relatively stable personality trait. The anxiety state is conceptualized as an emotive state characterized by subjective feelings perceived on a conscious level as apprehension and tension, with an increase in the activity of the autonomous nervous system, which varies with time; anxiety as a trait refers to individuals with a relatively stable continuous disposition towards anxiety and who thus differ from those with anxiety state who react with an increase in the intensity of anxiety to situations perceived as threatening (Spielberg *et al.*, 1970; Sacco *et al.*, 1992).

Aims

The aim of our study was to understand and characterize anxiety levels in both state and trait and also assess the possibility of a including the depressive syndrome in coeliac patients. Ten successive coeliac cases were evaluated and compared with a group of healthy volunteers using a protocol applied by us to numerous other studies of gastrointestinal pathology (Addolorato *et al.*, 1995, 1996).

Patient and methods

Ten patients affected by coeliac disease with a mean age of 30.5 ± 7.8 years, between the ages of 21–40, 6 females (60 per cent) and 4 males (40 per cent), were enrolled in the study (group A). As controls we studied 10 healthy subjects, 6 females (60 per cent) and 4 males (40 per cent), with a mean age of 35 ± 9.6 years, between the age of 20–50 years, selected randomly every time a coeliac patient was admitted to the study (group B). We also studied a group of 10 control subjects affected by inflammatory bowel disease (IBD) chosen consecutively from those under treatment in our centre, 5 females and 5 males, with a mean age of 25 ± 2.6 years, between the ages of 20–30 years (group C).

The following evaluations were carried out in all patients:

    – blood cell count;
    – serum electrolytes (Na, K, Fe, Ca);

– electrophoresis pattern of serum proteins, ESR, transaminases, glycaemia, blood nitrogen, serum and urinary amylase

– abdominal ultrasonography, in particular to exclude biliary pathology and study the thickness of the intestine;

– presence of antigliadin (AGA) and antiendomysium (EMA) antibodies;

– A-xylose absorbtion test;

– endoscopic and biopsy examinations of the small intestine (duodenum, sigmoid and colon), not performed in healthy control;

– skin prick test for foods divided into cereals, fruits, eggs, fish, meat, vegetables, beans, nuts and seeds, milk, olive oil, yeast, garlic and onion.

Most of the coeliac patients (80 per cent) presented with a classical symptomatology of abdominal pain, diarrhoea and meteorism but in two patients (20 per cent) the presentation pattern was monosymptomatic with hypochromic anaemia. In these patients the diagnosis was based on the positivity of AGA and EMA and on the typical atrophy of duodenal mucosal with hypertrophy of the crypts and lymphomonocyte infiltration.

In one case (10 per cent) the skin prick test for foods was positive for shell-fish.

The prevalent abdominal symptomatology of the IBD controls was a moderate diarrhoea with abundant mucous and with variable quantities of blood. Two subjects (20 per cent) presented with a sub-occlusive pattern. The laboratory results in most cases showed iron deficiency anaemia, leucocytosis and an increase in sedimentation rate. The diagnosis was confirmed by the histological biopsy patterns of the ileum and colon. In 8–10 subjects there was thickening of the ileum for lengths between 5 and 10 cm.

All patients were given a questionnaire demanding information on their level of education and economic social status, and containing two different autoevaluation psychometric tests: one for anxiety and the other for depression. Due to their simplicity and affordability, we preferred to use the State and Trait Anxiety Inventory (STAI test), made up of 2 axes ($y1$ for anxiety state and $y2$ for anxiety trait) both consisting of 20 multiple choice items in which a point score superior to 40 is considered to be high (Spielberg *et al.*, 1970), and the IPAT Depression Scale Questionnaire (Krug & Laughlin, 1976), made up of 40 multiple choice items in which a rough point score must be translated into a STEN point score: a STEN point score of 8 or more is considered high. Through these tests the anxiety state and the anxiety trait were evaluated as was the depression and the depressive-anxious syndrome (DAS), when the patients showed a high point score in the $y2$ axis of the STAI-test and in the CDQ test.

Statistical analysis

The Chi-Square test was utilized to compare the percentage of positive test patients and the Student-t test (with mean value and standard error) to study point scores on the tests.

Results

Of the 10 coeliac patients, 6 subjects (60 per cent) (all symptomatic) showed high levels of anxiety state, with a mean value of 54.8 ± 8.2 on the $y1$ axis of the STAI test (mv $y1$); 4 subjects (40 per cent) were shown to have anxiety as a trait (mv $y2$ 50.9 ± 9.7); 6 subjects (60 per cent) ($P > 0.01$) were shown to be positive for depression (mv CDQ 8.1 ± 0.7); DAS was present in 2 subjects (20 per cent) (mv $y2$ 49.9 ± 9.3, CDQ 8.5 ± 0.8) (Tables 1 and 2).

Of the 10 subjects in the healthy control group, 3 (30 per cent) showed high levels of anxiety state (P: n.s.), (mv $y1$ 50.4 ± 6.9); 3 subjects (30 per cent) showed anxiety as a trait (P: n.s.) (mv $y2$ 48.5 ± 7.1); 1 subject (10 per cent) was shown to be positive for depression ($P > 0.01$) (mv CDQ 8.0); DAS was present in 1 subject (10 per cent) (P: n.s.) (mv $y2$ 50.0, CDQ 8.0) (Tables 1 and 2).

Of the 10 patients affected by IBD, 5 subjects (50 per cent) (P: n.s.) showed high levels of anxiety state (mv $y1$ 51.8 ± 9.2); 3 subjects (30 per cent) (P: n.s.) were positive for trait anxiety (mv $y2$ 49.9 ± 9.3); 2 patients were found be depressed (20 per cent) (P: n.s.) (mv CDQ 8.5 ± 0.8); DAS was present in 2 subjects (20 per cent) (P: n.s.) (mv $y2$ 49.9 ± 9.3, CDQ 8.5 ± 0.8) (Tables 1 and 2).

Table 1. Percentage of subjects with coeliac disease (A), healthy (B) and with IBD (C) who were positive on the tests administered and relative statistical significance (P)

Test	A	B	C	P (A vs. B)	P (A vs. C)	P (B vs. C)
Stai Y1	60%	30%	50%	P: n.s.	P: n.s.	P: n.s.
Stai Y2	40%	30%	30%	P: n.s.	P: n.s.	P: n.s.
CDQ	60%	10%	30%	$P > 0.01$	P: n.s.	P: n.s.
SAD	20%	10%	20%	P: n.s.	P: n.s.	P: n.s.

Stai Y1: % of subjects with high anxiety state levels (total score over 40 points); Stai Y2: % of subjects with anxiety trait (total score over 40 points); CDQ: % of subjects with depression (total score over 7 STEN points); SAD: % of subjects with anxiety-depression syndrome (total score with the STAI test, y2 axis, over 40 points, plus total score in the D + CDQ test, over 7 STEN points).

Table 2. Median values (mv) with standard deviation of the point scores achieved by subjects with coeliac disease (A), healthy (B) and with IBD (C) positive to the tests adminsitered and relative statistical significance(P)

Test	A	B	C	P (A vs. B)	P (A vs. C)	P (B vs. C)
Stai Y1	54.8 ± 8.2	50.4 ± 6.9	51.8 ± 9.2	P: n.s.	P: n.s.	P: n.s.
Stai Y2	50.9 ± 9.7	48.5 ± 7.1	49.9 ± 9.3	P: n.s.	P: n.s.	P: n.s.
CDQ	8.1 ± 0.7	8.0 ± 0	8.5 ± 0.8	P: n.s.	P: n.s.	P: n.s.

When comparing the groups the percentage of subjects with high levels of state and trait anxiety did not appear to be significantly different. As regards the level of depression, the percentage of subjects who were shown to be positive with coeliac disease was statistically superior only versus the healthy control group ($P < 0.01$).

Discussion

Although we did not observe a significant statistical difference in the levels of anxiety in the groups studied (probably due to the low number of patients evaluated for each group) 'reactive' type anxiety state was positive in a higher percentage of coeliac subjects and in the patients affected by IBD compared to the healthy control group (respectively 60 per cent and 50 per cent vs. 30 per cent) (Table 1). This could be linked to the symptomatology (abdominal pain, diarrhoea, meteorism in coeliac subjects and diarrhoea with mucous and blood in patients with IBD) present at the time of the clinical and psychometric observation and reported by the patients to cause problems in social relationships. This hypothesis can be supported by the fact that 6 of 8 symptomatic coeliac patients had high point-scores on the yl axis of STAI-test (reactive anxiety), while the total point score of the yl axis of 2 non-symptomatic coeliac patients was very low.

Anxiety trait, on the contrary, was present in a similar percentage in all the groups evaluated and according to our observation, such data indicate that personality anxiety trait, identifiable as a 'tendency towards anxiety', has no effect in coeliac and IBD patients.

As regards depression, the coeliac patients showed a high total point score in the CDQ test in a significantly higher percentage compared to the healthy control group (Table 1), in accordance with Hallert & Aström (1982), and higher, but not significantly, than patients with 1BD. Such data could confirm a possible linkage between brain functions, depression in particular, and malabsorption, a frequent characteristic of coeliac disease and IBD. Malabsorption could interfere with the regulation of mood, bearing in mind that the pathogenesis of depression could be the result of abnormalities in the metabolism of monoamines (serotonin, dopamine and noradrenalin) by the central nervous system (CNS) and that a high number of food factors are involved in this synthesis (Sourkes, 1979).

Based on this assumption, Hallert et al. (1982) found a statistically significant reduction, compared with controls, in serotonin metabolites (in particular of 5-hydroxyindoleacetic acid, homovanillic acid and 4-hydroxy-3-methoxy-phenyl-ethylene-glycol), and in dopamine and serotonin in cerebral spinal fluid in nine out of the 10 coeliac patients studied.

In conclusion, the anxiety and depression found in coeliac patients could be secondary to a reduced neuronal production of monoaminergics substances, a mechanism currently implicated in the pathogenesis of behavioural disturbances, and to the emotional reaction to the symptoms of disease which often determine a reduction in the quality of life of these patients. It would therefore always be advisable to evaluate not only clinical, laboratory and biopsy parameters in these patients but also to carry out a psychometric evaluation to determine the level of anxiety and depression and to distinguish between 'reactive' and 'trait' forms. The correction of such disturbances would improve the quality of life and the patients' compliance to treatment which is particularly important in subjects with coeliac disease in which adherence to a gluten-free diet, though difficult to accept, is the cornerstone of therapy.

Acknowledgements

We are indebted to G. H. Leefield for his assistance in correcting the English text. Supported by grants from the 'Associazione Ricerca in Medicina', Bologna, Italy.

21: Neuropsychiatric complaints in the clinical pattern of coeliac disease

G. Bottaro, M. Spina, N. Rotolo, M. Cocuzza, A. Franzo and R. Bianchini

1st Paediatric Clinic, University of Catania, Policlinico, Viale A. Doria 6, 95125 Catania, Italy

Since the first report of Samuel Gee in 1888 (Gee, 1888), emotional symptoms have been considered common in children with coeliac disease (CD). Gee describes the child as extremely irritable, fretful, capricious or peevish when he separated from mother. Moreover, the coeliac child is often emotionally withdrawn and this may even resemble autism (Walker-Smith, 1991). In addition anorexia is present in about 50 per cent of cases.

Various neuropsychic disturbances including schizophrenia as well as chronic progressive neurological disorders, have been described in association to CD, especially in adults patients (Hallert & Derefeldt, 1982; Collin *et al.*, 1991). Recently, an Italian multicentric study has pointed out that epilepsy (never controlled by drugs) and cerebral calcifications with epilepsy of unexplained origin, seem to be associated with CD (Gobbi *et al.*, 1992; Ventura *et al.*, 1991). These conditions have been found to be strictly dependent on CD because of improvement a complete regression of symptoms after withdrawal of gluten from the diet (Ventura *et al.*, 1991).

In our experience coeliac children under two years of age, often present anorexia, irritability and muscular hypotonia, simulating a peripheral neuropathy (Bottaro *et al.*, 1993), while epileptic attacks and cerebral calcifications are characteristic in older children.

In order to evaluate the incidence of neuropsychiatric complaints in childhood CD we performed a retrospective clinical study on all coeliac subjects diagnosed in our department in the last 10 years.

Patients and methods

The patients were identified between 1985–94 in the Paediatric Clinic at the University of Catania. Diagnosis of CD was based on the results of intestinal biopsy, demostrating villous atrophy (Walker-Smith *et al.*, 1990). In addition, clinical examination, with particular reference to neuropsychiatric and neurological complaints, patient's age at the time of diagnosis, and other relevant data, were reviewed.

Main neuropsychatric complaints taken into consideration were anorexia, bulimia and irritability, while main neurological disorders were epilepsy (controlled by drugs), and cerebral calcifications.

To evaluate the differences in frequency over time, we divided the observations (1985–94) in two five-year periods. On the basis of the year of diagnosis, the patients were divided in two groups: group A included the cases diagnosed in the between 1985–1989, and group B included those diagnosed between 1990–94.

Statistic analysis was attempted using Chi-square and student *t*-test.

Results

Data from 550 subjects suffering from CD (age range 7 months to 17 years, 237 males and 313 female) were collected. Group A was composed of 283 subjects, 130 male and 153 female (F/M 1.2) mean age 2.3 ± 2.7 years, while group B was composed of 267 subjects, 107 male and 160 female (F/M 1.5) mean age 5.6 ± 9.7 years.

Data analysis of mean age at diagnosis showed statistically significant difference by the student t test ($P < 0.001$) among the two groups, while the frequency of distribution showed a mode around the second year of life in both groups. In group A, 221 subjects (78.1 per cent) had the diagnosis under the second year, 28 (9.9 per cent) through the fifth year, 16 (5.6 per cent) through the tenth year and 18 (6.4 per cent) beyond 10 years of age. In group B 159 subjects (59.5 per cent) had the diagnosis under the second year, 33 (12.4 per cent) through the fifth year, 23 (8.6 per cent) through the tenth year, and 52 (19.5 per cent) beyond 10 years of age. Statistical comparison, using the Chi-square test, showed a statistically significant difference ($P < 0.001$) among subjects of the two groups that had a diagnosis under the second year and beyond 10 years of age (Table 1).

Table 1. Age at diagnosis

	Group A	Group B
> 2 years	221 (78.1%)	159 (59.5%)
2–5 years	28 (9.9%)	33 (12.4%)
5–10 years	16 (5.6%)	23 (8.6%)
> 10 years	18 (6.4%)	52 (19.5%)

*$P < 0.001$ using Chi-square test.

Table 2. Frequency of symptomatology in the two groups

	Group A Main	Group A Associated	Group B Main	Group B Associated
Psychic complaints				
Anorexia	19 (6.7%)	74 (26.1%)	9 (3.4%)	33 (12.3%)
Irritability	–	37 (13.1%)	2 (0.7%)	21 (7.9%)
Bulimia	1 (0.4%)	2 (0.8%)	1 (0.4%)	3 (1.1%)
Neurological disorders				
Drug Resistant epilepsy	–	–	1 (0.4%)	–
Cerebral calcifications	–	–	1 (0.4%)	–

As concerns the clinical pattern, that psychic complaints were present as the main symptoms in 20 subjects (7.1 per cent) of group A, and in 12 subjects (4.5 per cent) of group B, showing no statistically significative difference. In group A, 19 subjects (6.7 per cent) presented anorexia, and 1 (0.4 per cent) bulimia, while in group B, 9 subjects (3.4 per cent) had anorexia, 1 (0.4 per cent) bulimia and 2 (0.7 per cent) irritability. The same neuropsychiatric complaints were present as associated symptoms in 113 subjects (40 per cent) of group A, and in 57 subjects (21.3 per cent) of group B, showing a significant statistical difference using the Chi-square test $P < 0.001$. In roup A, 74 subjects (26.1 per cent) presented anorexia, 2 (0.8 per cent) bulimia, and 37 (13.1 per cent) irritability, while in group B, 33 subjects (12.3 per cent) had anorexia, 3 (1.1 per cent) bulimia, and 21 (7.9 per cent) irritability. There was also a significant statistical difference using the Chi-square test ($P < 0.001$) among the subjects of the two groups that presented anorexia (Table 2).

Considering neurological disorders, no subject in group A had symptoms, while in group B two subjects (0.7 per cent) presented epilepsy and one (0.4 per cent) epilepsy and cerebral calcifications.

None of these data showed significant statistical differences (Table 2).

Discussion

Our results clearly demonstrate that behaviour disturbances are more frequent than neurological disorders, expecially when considered as first symptoms or as associated symptoms in the clinical pattern.

Seventy one per cent of the patients of group A and 4.5 per cent of the patients of group B presented behaviour disturbances as main complaints; while 40 per cent of the cases of group A and 21.3 per cent of group B presented behaviour disturbances as associated complaints. Only three patients had neurological disorders. This difference is remarkable if we consider that psychic complaints are not a direct consequence of the intestinal damage and malabsorption, but mainly represent a reaction of the child to its environment, and reflect the distress of the mother to her child's diarrhoea and worsening nutritional status.

Estimating the presence of the behaviour disturbances in the two five-year periods, we notice its tendency to decrease over time, especially when considered as associated symptoms, showing a reduction by nearly half (40 per cent in group A, versus 21.3 per cent in group B). The explanation might be related to the patients age at the time of diagnosis. The subjects of group B were diagnosed in the last years, when laboratory tests (antigliadin antibodies and antiendomysium antibodies) became available and these are more effective than the former diagnostic tests (one-hour-xylose test, evaluation of steatorrhoea). These new tests have shortened the gap between onset of clinical symptoms and time of diagnosis of the disease, allowing also diagnosis older patients who are usually oligosymptomatic or silent. In fact, complaints like anorexia and irritability are characteristic in small children under two years of age, in whom CD was not diagnosed early but only after several months.

The increase in the mean age at diagnosis might be due to the fact that in the last five years we diagnosed two cases of resistant epilepsy and one case of epilepsy with associate cerebral calcifications. These conditions, recognized in the last years, are characteristic of children beyond 10 years of age and of teenagers.

In our cases behaviour disturbances are frequently present as associated symptoms. Although, during the last period, neuropsychiatric complaints markedly decreased most probably due to diagnosis.

On the contrary neurological disorders, are recently diagnosed more often expecially since we now can recognize them more easily and because we are able to identify the disease even in older children and in adults.

22: Coeliac disease in Down's syndrome: EEG, brain CT-scan and HLA findings

P. Failla, A. Ragusa[*], C. Ruberto[*], M.C. Pagano[**], M. Lombardo[**], F. Colabucci and C. Romano

Department of Pediatrics, Oasi Institute (IRCCS), Troina, (EN); [*]Laboratory of Hematology, Oasi Institute (IRCCS), Troina (EN); [**]S.I.T., USL 36, Catania, Italy

Introduction

The association between Down's Syndrome (DS) and coeliac disease (CD) has been confirmed by several authors (Howell *et al.,* 1983; Levo & Drin, 1977; Mc Culloch, 1982; Milunsky & Neurath, 1968; Ruch *et al.,* 1985; Sare *et al.,* 1978). We report our results on a sample of 57 Down's syndrome subjects (sDS), highlighting the incidence of CD, the potential association with serological and molecular class I and II HLA markers, the EEG features, and the brain CT-scan results.

Patients and methods

The sample is made up of 57 Sicilian sDS with Mean Age 14.9 years, 29 males and 28 females; 53 have a classical trisomy 21, and the remaining four have, respectively, a 14–21 translocation, a 21–21 translocation, a 47XY,+21/46XY mosaicism, and a 47XY,+21/47XY,+21 del (14) (pter→q11) mosaicism. All subjects have been submitted, as a screening test for CD, to IgA-AGA and IgG-AGA assay. We use an immunoenzymatic fluorescence assay (Eurospital a-gliatest, Trieste, Italy). Values are expressed as the percentage of fluorescence in comparison with the standard positive serum. Jejunal biopsy (JB) is made through endoscopy, and the histologic diagnosis has been made according to ESPGAN criteria (Walker-Smith *et al.,* 1990). Class I and II serological HLA typing has been carried out in seven sDS affected by CD and randomly in 22 sDS without CD, using a standard two-stage microlymphocytotoxicity assay (Biotest). Class II HLA has been typed by PCR. This analysis has also been carried out in all HLA serologically typed patients and in 20 unrelated healthy subjects. Allele specific oligonucleotide probes have been used to discriminate DQA1*0101 from DQA1*0102. Family studies has been possible in all sDS with CD and in several without CD. EEG has been performed during sleep. Five subjects have had brain CT-scans.

Table 1. Clinical features, biopsy, EEG and CT-scan results in sDS with CD

Patients.	Symptoms	Atrophy	EEG	CT-Scan
1	D	Subtotal	Normal	Focal atrophy of left temporal lobe
2	D,F	Subtotal	Normal	
3	D	Subtotal	Normal	
4	D,A	Subtotal	Normal	Wide sulci of convexity
5	D,F,A	Total	Normal	Normal
6	D,F,A	Total	Normal	Atrophy of temporal lobes
7	D	Total	Normal	Normal

D, diarrhoea; F, failure to thrive; A, anaemia.

Results

The results in 7 sDS with CD are shown in the Table 1. The villous atrophy is total in three subjects and subtotal in four, leading up to a diagnosis of CD in seven DS children, mean age 10.7 years (range 2.7–14.7 years). The incidence of CD in our sample is 12.2 per cent. EEG is normal in all patients. CT-scan results show the following features: one patient has focal atrophy of the left temporal lobe, the second one presents with wide sulci on the convexity, the third one shows mild atrophy of the temporal lobes, the last two are normal. Neither cerebral calcifications nor seizures are shown by our sDS. All seven sDS with CD have been on a gluten-free diet, with rapid disappearance of symptoms. On HLA typing no statistically significant difference was found for each serological HLA class, matching the group of sDS with CD versus those without CD. All patients have inherited at least one DQA1*0101 allele but only one exhibits the heterodimer DQA1*0501/DQB1*0201 which has a predominant role in the susceptibility to CD. Indeed, only the DQA1*0101 allele is significantly associated with the sDS with CD group matched with sDS without CD or the healthy control group.

Discussion

An alteration of the autoimmune system is thought to be the linking point between CD and DS by several authors. A derangement in the immune system, common in DS, could well explain the AGA behaviour in these patients.

Our sample, as has been found by several authors (Castro *et al.,* 1993; Storm, 1990), exhibits a positive but weaker AGA sensitivity and specificity in comparison with the control group (Burgin Wolff *et al.,* 1989; Guandalini *et al.,* 1989). All subjects submitted to JB presented with a variable combination of gastrointestinal symptoms, such as intermittent diarrhoea, failure to thrive and iron deficiency anaemia, and only two showed the typical symptomatology of CD. The high incidence of CD in sDS (12.2 per cent), found by us, has been reported by several authors and, in the light of current knowledge, we are not able to explain the pathogenesis of such an association. EEGs were normal and CT-scans showed nonspecific lesions in only three subjects. We have examined HLA antigens: while the group with DS with CD exhibits a statistically significant increase in the DQA1*0101 allele, associated with different DQB1 alleles, only one subject of this group shows the presence of the peculiar heterodimer presumptively associated with CD. The results shown here prompt us to respect a different pathogenetic basis for CD associated with DS compared with classic CD.

23: Triatiated impramine binding in coeliac disease – a preliminary report

G. Chiaravalloti[*], D. Marazziti[**], A. Insolvibile[*], S. Quinti[*], C. Ughi[*], M. Ceccarelli[*], A. Batistini[**], G.B. Cassano[**]

[*]*Istituto di Clinica Paediatrica, University of Pisa;* [**]*II Cattedra di Clinica Psichiatrica, University of Pisa, Italy*

Introduction

The peculiar behaviour of children with coeliac disease (CD) in its typical form has been investigated by several authors. Prugh & MacMahon in 1951 stated that these patients appeared to be 'passive, often introverted, with an inhibited personality and they showed obsessive-compulsive tendencies' (Asperger, 1961). Haas & Haas (1951) pointed out the high rate of emotional disorders and the fact that these symptoms improved before intestinal symptoms did after treatment with an appropriate diet (Bonamico *et al.,* 1982). Kaser (196i) Asperger (1961) observed that the psychiatric symptoms of coeliac children could be very similar to those of schizophrenic or autistic children, and improved or worsened depending on the diet (Briley *et al.,* 1979; Challacombe & Wheeler, 1987).

We should not forget the atypical forms of CD, among which cases of severe anorexia and depression in pubertal and adolescent age have been described, regressing after a gluten diet free (gFD) (Haas & Haas, 1951). Psychoses and schizophrenia have been described as late complications of CD when non-diagnosed or non-treated during childhood (Kaser, 1961).

The improvement in mood after a few days of (gFD) and its reversibility if the patients went back to a free diet suggested possible involvement of a humoral agent in this process (Marazziti *et al.,* 1988).

Patients and methods

Since serotonin has been implicated in the physiopathology of depression and since alterations of its metabolism have been described in coeliac disease, we thought of possible involvement of this neurotransmitter in the genesis of behavioural disorders in CD. Blood 5-HT is almost completely contained in platelets, which represent a reliable peripheral model of serotinergic presynaptic nervous terminals; they share morphological, biochemical and functional characteristics with 5-HTergic synaptosomes: presence of a limiting membrane, mitochondria, accumulation granules, microtubules and microfilaments, accumulation of 5-HT via passive transport and an active uptake, probably modulated by the binding sites for tritiated imipramine (^{3}H-IMI), similar to the neuronal transport (Marazziti & Cassano, 1992; Meltzer & Lowy, 1987; Peroutka, 1990).

The use of platelets in biological psychiatry as an instrument for studying some of the properties of the 5-tryptaergic system highlighted several alterations relating to depressive pathology: a reduction of the total content and the uptake of 5-HT, and a reduction of the binding sites for ^{3}H-IMI (Prugh & MacMahon, 1951; Quintana, 1992).

In our study we evaluate the kinetic parameters (B_{max} and Kd) of platelet binding of ^{3}H-IMI in 20 patients with CD (16 females and 4 males aged between 8 months and 24 years); our results are compared with those of 20 healthy controls of comparable age.

B_{max} values (maximum capacity of fmol/mg-binding proteins) in coeliac children were 185.5 ± 60.3 (m $\pm$ DS) *vs.* 521.4 ± 132.2 in healthy children; Kd (dissociation constant – nM) values were respectively 1.58 ± 0.31 and 1.53 ± 0.27. Statistical processing of these data showed a highly significant difference between controls and coeliac subjects ($P < 0.0001$) as to B_{max}, while the Kd difference was not significant (P: n.s.). No correlation has been found between B_{max} and Kd in coeliac subjects and in controls.

Discussion

The 5-HTergic system is involved in the regulation of several functions and cerebral activities (Sleiger, 1961). It has an important control function as a modulator and integrator of sensory stimuli: it thus affects several aspects of behaviour, from aggressiveness to food habits (Sleiger, 1961). It performs its many actions by interacting with specific binding sites placed both at a pre- and post-synaptic level: recently, four classes of receptors with different subtypes have been identified (Sneddon, 1973).

Anomalies of serotoninergic function have been correlated with most depressive symptoms: mood, appetite, dysfunction of sleep and circadian rhythms (Sleiger, 1961). The reduction in plasma tryptophan and in the tryptophan ratio observed in celiac patients following a free diet with alterations of behaviour has been ascribed to an alteration of tryptophan metabolism rather than to an anomaly in intestinal absorption (Hallert *et al.*, 1982; Hernanz & Polanco, 1991). This would involve a reduction of cerebral tryptophan with a consequent alteration of cerebral serotonin synthesis. The latter could be involved in the pathogenesis of behavioral disorders observed in celiac children in their florid phase.

Results

Our data suggest that in celiac subjects there is a reduction of the binding sites for ^{3}H-IMI compared to healthy subjects, while affinity for this receptor was normal in both groups. Such a result bears out the assumption that serotoninergic dysfunction is a predisposing or causal factor of depression, as has been shown by postmortem, CSF, platelet, neuroendocrine and pharmacological data in depressed patients (Stahl, 1977).

We can thus assume that the psychic disorders observed in CD could be due to dysfunction in the serotoninergic system.

These parameters will be evaluated after six months of gluten diet free in order to see if clinical improvement will coincide with increase in the number of receptor sites for tritiated imipramine.

24: Endocranial calcifications and epilepsy: familial encephalopathy with progressive evolution. A study of two brothers

A.F. Crisanti, V. Marchiani, M.R. Migliore and E. Franzoni

Centre of Paediatric Neurology, University of Bologna, Via Massarenti II, 40138 Bologna, Italy

Introduction

Endocranial calcifications are almost always a sign of disease in childhood in contrast with the possibly physiological calcifications found in adults, especially in the older age group (Koller, 1979; Murphy, 1979; Puvanendran 1982).

Different aetiologies metabolic, neoplastic, or as a result of perinatal asphyxia must be considered. The CT scan, has made it possible to detect even small intracranial calcifications with greater detail. Most calcifications occur at the level of the basal ganglia where they were first discovered at pathology (Brannan, 1980; Harrington, 1981; Hilton, 1982). Familial cases of intracranial calcifications with associated neurological disorders are rare: Fahr's disease is still not clearly understood (Boller, 1980; Kuroiwa, 1982; Morgante, 1986; Smits, 1983).

We report two brothers with such problems to bring a further contribution to the understanding of this clinical entity.

Case reports

Patient 1

F.B. was born at term with a birthweight of 2850 g and mild perinatal asphyxia. Left hemiclonic seizures made their appearance at 8 weeks of age and were stopped by phenobarbital (PB). Subsequently a right-sided hemiclonic status developed with lethargy and required a hospital admission. At that time no intracranial calcifications were detected by skull X-ray. For the following 10 years he had no more seizures and was not followed. A second episode of status again brought the patient to hospital. Clinical examination revealed mental retardation, dysarthria, right hemiparesis and with behavioural problems. The EEG was characterized by isolated high amplitude spikes over the left posterior central areas. CT scan of the head showed dilated ventricles and numerous large, mainly periventricular, calcifications. A control CT scan, 4 months later, showed exclusion of brain calcifications at the level of the basal ganglia and of the white matter which also appeared hypodense. EEGs constantly exhibited medium-high voltage slow waves over the left anterior and posteriorl cerebial areas: no spikes were detected. Clinical follow-up documented progressive deterioration of neurological and intellectual functions. MRI of the brain performed at 10 years of age, revealed apart from a void signal, a hyperintense signal of cerebral white matter and a moderate dilatation of the subarachnoid spaces of the convexity. Laboratory investigations including search for alterations in calcium metabolism, endocrinological dysfunctions, mitochondrial abnormalities, had always been normal. Somatosensory and brainstem auditory evoked potentials were normal; visual evoked potentials were asymmetrical (higher amplitude on the left).

Patient 2

R.B. was born at term after normal pregnancy and delivery. Birthweight was 3450 g. When he was 7 days old he presented generalized tonic-clonic status epilepticus stopped with PB. CT scan of the head was normal. He had no further seizures until he was 11 years old but progressive motor difficulties with slow speech, learning and behavioural problems became evident from the first years of life. At 11 years of age the child experienced a secondarily generalized partial seizure. The EEG showed an excess of diffuse slow waves. The levels of Ca, P, T3, T4, TSH, PHT and calcitonin were normal. CT scan showed a picture very similar to his brother's with many calcifications in the interhemispheric and periventricular white matter and in the basal ganglia, more evident on the left side. MRI of the brain with gadolinium enhancement also showed hyperintensity of the periventricular and hemispheric white matter with dilation of the right ventricule. The visual evoked potentials showed a symmetric delay of the latency in the cortex. The brainstem auditory potentials showed an abnormal morphology. The somatosensory evoked potentials were normal.

Our study was completed by CT of the brain of both parents, which were normal.

Discussion

The presence of a familial progressive encephalopathy with epilepsy and endocranial calcifications in our two patients, raised the diagnostic possibility of Fahr's disease. We examined the older boy during the neonatal period and then both brothers after an interval of 10 years. It was therefore impossible to follow in detail the clinical evolution in those years and to study the younger brother until the second epileptic status: no calcifications were evident at birth on skull X-rays but many were found 10 years later.

Fahr's disease was first described in 1930 and is characterized by different clinical pictures. Therefore, the diagnosis is often made by exclusion based on the neuroradiological and neuropathological data.

However, the reports in the literature point to symmetrical calcifications mainly of the basal ganglia as an essential feature of the diagnosis. It is reasonable to think that the heterogeneous clinical findings in Fahr's disease represent different underlying conditions (sharing endocranial calcification as a main sign), which will undoubtedly be identified and clarified with the progress of medical knowledge.

25: Coeliac disease and tuberous sclerosis

B. Papadatou, M. Di Capua[*], F. Ferretti, A. Montaldo[*], R. Cerminara, L. Baldassare[*], V. Lucidi and M. Castro

Gastroenterology Division, [*]Neurophysiology Service, Ospedale Bambino Gesù, Piazza S.Onofrio 4, Rome 00165, Italy

Introduction

In some patients coeliac disease (CD) is associated with clinical involvement of the nervous system, expressed variably as encephalopathy, cerebellar syndrome, seizures, epilepsy with occipital calcifications, psychiatric disorders, myelopathy, myopathy and peripheral neuropathy (Cooke & Smith, 1966; Cooke, 1976; Finelli *et al.*, 1980; Kepes *et al.*, 1975; Cordonnier *et al.*, 1983; Collin *et al.*, 1991; Tison *et al.*, 1989; Kaplan *et al.*, 1988; Kinney *et al.*, 1982; Gobbi *et al.*, 1992; Ward *et al.*, 1985; Brücke *et al.*, 1988).

Such disorders are described in adult patients generally within 10 years after the diagnosis of CD is established. We report the case of a child affected by CD and tuberous sclerosis (TS).

Case report

A 2–year-old girl presented with an 18 months history of diarrhoea, vomiting and failure to thrive. Important weight loss was documented in the last three months. From the age of 12 months the child presented sporadic partial complex seizures with head deviation to the right side of brief duration.

Clinical examination revealed impaired growth. Height and weight were below the third percentile; the abdomen was prominent; meteorism was present; neurological examination showed muscle wasting with hypotonia. Results of initial laboratory investigations were: haemoglobin: 11.0 g/100 ml; white cell count $15.00 \times 10^3/\mu1$; blood iron 71 µg/dl; glucose 64 mg/dl, total serum proteins 6.9 g/dl with albumin 4.6 g/dl; Na^+ 137 mEq/l, K^+: 4.7 mEq/l, Cl^-: 110 mEq/l; SGOT: 90 UI/l, SGPT: 73 UI/l γ-glutamyl-transpeptidase: 13 UI/l; prothrombin time: 117 per cent; partial thromboplastin time: 30 s; fibrinogen: 254 mg/dl; serum immunoglobulins: IgA 249 mg/dl; IgG: 646 mg/dl, IgM: 123 mg/dl.

Further investigation demonstrated high levels of IgA antigliadin antibodies and the presence of antiendomysium antibodies in the patient's serum.

The EEG showed slow and epileptiform abnormalities on the left temporal lobe (focal spikes and slow waves). The CT scan (Fig. 1) showed periventricular calcifications and the cerebral MRI (Fig. 2)revealed two high-intensity signal areas in the frontal and in the temporal lobe of the left hemisphere (tubers).

Jejunal mucosa biopsy was performed at endoscopy. Histological examination of the specimens showed total villous atrophy suggesting CD.

A gluten-free diet was started. Within one month gastrointestinal symptoms disappeared. Medical treatment of the epilepsy with carbamazepine was also started.

After 18 months follow-up, the child achieved normal ponderal and statural growth and normal motor and intellectual development. She presents multiple depigmented ash leaf spots on the legs. Her seizures are partially controlled.

Discussion

TS is characterized by the growth of benign tumours and malformation in one or more organs. The disease shows autosomal dominant inheritance with variable expressivity and high penetrance. When the cerebral cortex is involved, it contains characteristic tubers. The symptoms caused by these tubers are partial or

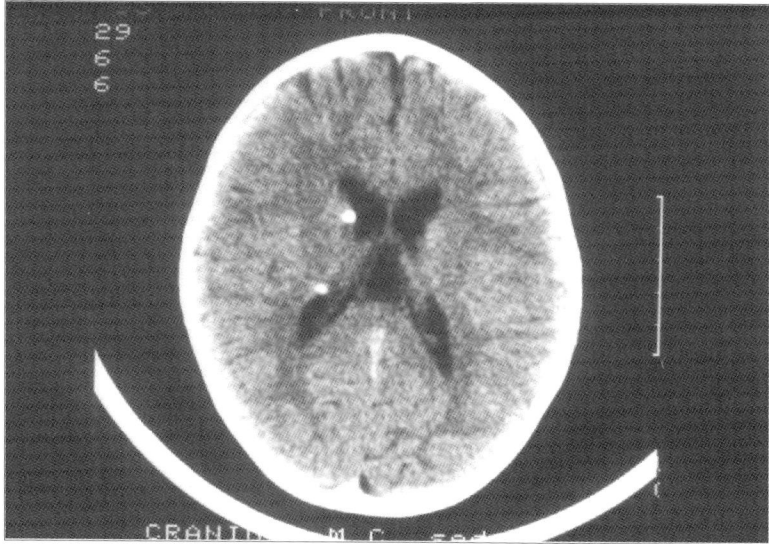

Fig. 1. Cerebral CT scan: periventricular calcifications.

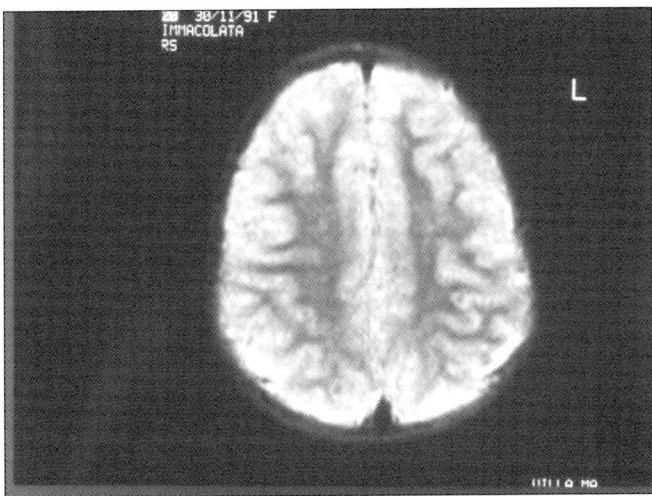

Fig. 2. Cerebral MRI high intensity signal area in the frontal lobe of

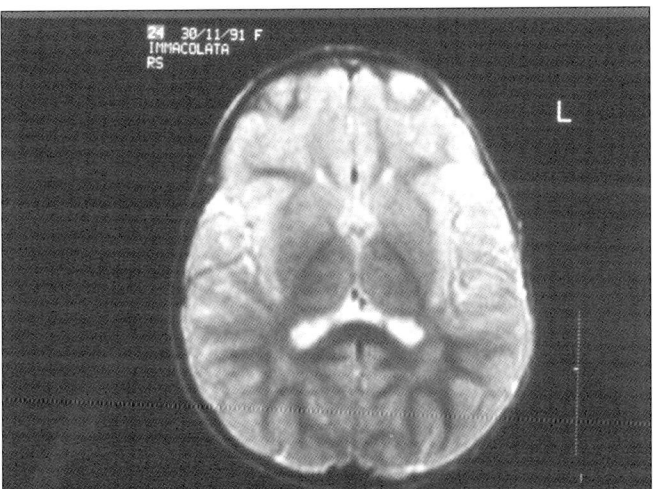

Fig. 3. Cerebral MRI high intensity signal area in the temporal lobe of the left hemisphere.

generalized seizures. The diagnosis of TS in our patient was made because of the presence of partial complex seizures and of tubers in the frontal and temporal lobes of the left hemisphere shown by the MRI.

The diagnosis of CD was based on the presence of gastrointestinal symptoms, the presence in the serum of the specific antigliadin and antiendomysium antibodies and the characteristic flat jejunal mucosa (Bürgin-Wolff *et al.*, 1989; Report of Working Group of European Society of Pediatric Gastroenterology and Nutrition, 1990; Kapuscinska *et al.*, 1987).

The diagnosis of CD in a patient with epilepsy induced us at first to think of the presence of cerebral calcifications as described elsewhere (Gobbi *et al.*, 1992). The neuroimaging helped us formulate the diagnosis.

This is the first report on the coexistence of CD with TS.

The prevalence of CD in Italy is about 1:300 (Catassi *et al.*, 1994) while the TS prevalence is variably assessed from 1:10,000 to 1:100,000 (Wiederholt *et al.*, 1985; Sampson *et al.*, 1989; Nevin & Pearce, 1968) and the coexistence of the two diseases in this child may be fortuitous. Only the description of more cases showing up this association will permit us to consider it to be related.

References

Addolorato, G., Marsigli, L., Caputo, F., Dall'Aglio, Mingrone, G., Capristo, E., Gasbarrini, A. & Gasbarrini, G. (1995): Valutazione dei livelli di ansia e depressione in soggetti con IBD, IBS, allergic e intolleranze alimentari: risultati preliminari. Volume degli atti del IV Congress Nazionale Club del Tenue.

Addolorato, G., Marsigli, L., Stefanini, G.F. & Gasbarrini, G. (1996): Irritable bowel syndrome and food allergy: are they associated via anxiety and depression? *Gastroenterology* (in press).

Aicardi, J. (1992): Epilepsy and other seizure disorders. In: *Diseases of the nervous system in childhood,* p. 91. London: Mac Keith press.

Aine, L., Maki, M., Collin, P. & Keyrilainen, O. (1990): Dental enamel defects in celiac disease. *J. Oral. Pathol.* **19,** 241–245.

Aldao, M. Del Rosario. (1992): Oligosymptomatic coeliac disease and progressive cerebral calcifications with seizures. *Pediat. Neurol.* **8,** 5

Ambrosetto, G, Antonini, L. & Tassinari, A. (1992): Occipital lobe seizures related to clinically asymptomatic coeliac disease in adulthood. *Epilepsia* **33,** (3) 476–481.

Ambrosetto, P., Ambrosetto, G., Michelucci, R. & Bacci, A. (1993): Sturge–Weber syndrome without port-wine facial nevus: report of two patients. *Child's Brain* **10,** 387.

Anson, O., Weizman, Z. & Zeevi, N. (1990): *Pediatrics* **85,** 98–103.

Arakawa, T. (1970): Congenital defects in folate utilization. *Am. J. Med.* **48,** 594.

Arroyo, H.A., Massaro, M., De Rosa, S., Caraballo, R., Di Blasi, M., Taratuto, A. & Fejerman, N. (1992): Epilepsy, posterior calcifications and celiac disease. *Abstracts 6th Intern. Cong. Child Neurol.* Assoc. Buenos Aires, Argentina, 176.

Asperger, C. (1961): Psychopathology of children with celiac disease. *Ann. Pediat.* **197,** 346–351.

Auricchio, S., Greco, L. & Troncone, R. (1988): Gluten-sensitivity in childhood. *Pediatr. Clin. North Am.* **35** 157-187.

Baiges, L., Gine, J.J., Viedma, P., Afani, O. & Merce (1994): Epilepsia, calcificaciones cerebrales y celiaca. *Neurologia* **9,** 485.

Balli, M.P., Balli, M.E., Mengoli, M., Balli, C. & Balli, F. (1988): Studio dell'accrescimento, dell'età schelettica e dentale nella diarrea cronica in età pediatrica. *Ped. Med. Chir.* **10,** 277–282.

Baquero, M., Dominguez, F., Garcia Fernandez, M., Perla & Martinez Lozano, M.D. (1994): Sindrome calcificaciones occipitales-epilepsia-celiaca: dos caves tardios. *Neurologia* **9,** 438.

Bardella, M.T., Molteni, N., Prampolini, L., Giunta, .M., Baldassari, A.R., Morganti, D. & Bianchi, P.A. (1994): Need for follow up in coeliac disease. *Arch. Dis. Child* **70,** 211–213.

Battistella, P.A, Casara, G.L., Condini, A. *et al.* (1987): Calcificazioni cerebrale bi-occipitali e cefalea di tipo emicranico. Atti VII Conv. *Neurologia Infantile,* L'Antologia Ed., Napoli.

Battistella, P.A., Casara, G.L., Carollo, G. *et al.* (1986): Bilateral cerebral calcifications without cutaneous angioma: atypical form of Sturge–Weber Syndrome, *Riv. Ital. Ped.* (IJP) **12,** 417–418.

Battistella, P.A., Laverda, A.M., Drigo, P., Boniver, C., Suppiej, A. & Casara, G.L. (1991): Calcificazioni endocraniche. Iter diagnostico. *Minerva Pediatrica.***43,** 219–221.

Battistella, P.A., Mattesi, P., Casara, G.L., Carollo, C., Condini, A., Allegri, T. & Rigon, F. (1987): Bilateral cerebral occipital calcifications and migraine-like headache. *Cephalalgia* **7,** 125–129.

Berkovic, S.F., Cochius, J., Andermann, E. & Andermann, F. (1993): Progressive myoclonus epilepsies: clinical and genetic aspects. *Epilepsia* **34,** S19–S30.

Billard, C., Dulac, O., Bouloche, J., Echenne, B., Lebon, F., Motte, J., Robain, O. & Santini, J. (1989): Encephalopathy with calcifications of the basal ganglia in children. A reappraisal of Fahr's syndrome with respect to 14 new cases. *Neuropediatrics* **20,** 12–19.

Boller, F., Boller, M. & Gilbert, J. (1983): Familial idiopathic cerebral calcifications. *J. Neurol. Neurosurg. Psych.* **43,** 403–406.

Bonamico, M. *et al.* (1982): Il polimorfismo clinico della malattia celiaca. *Min. Ped.* **34,** 517–521.

Bottaro, G., Failla, P., Rotolo, N., Sanfilippo, G., Azzaro, F., Spina, M. & Patane, R. (1993): Changes in coeliac disease behaviour over the years. *Acta Paediatr.* **82**, 566–568.

Bouhnik, Y. & Rambaud, J.C. (1991): Manifestations systemiques associèes à la maladie coeliaque de l'adulte. *Gastroenterol. Clin. Biol.* **15** 28–33.

Brannan, T.S, Burger, A.A. & Chaudhary, M.Y. (1980): Bilateral basal ganglia calcifications visualised on CT scan. *J. Neurol. Neurosurg. Psych.* **43,** 403–406.

Briley, M.R., Raisman, R. & Langer, S.Z. (1979): Human platelets possess high-affinity sites for 3H-Imipramine. *Eur. J. Pharmac.* **58,** 347–348.

Bruche, T., Kolleger, H., Schmidbauer, M., Muller, C., Podreka, I. & Deecke, L. (1988): Adult coeliac disease and brain stem encephalitis. *J. Neurol. Neurosurg. Psych.* **51**, 456–457.

Burgin Wolff, A., Berger, R., Gaze, H., Huber, H., Lentze, M.J. & Nussle, D. (1989): IgG, IgA and IgE gliadin antibody determinations as screening test for untreated coeliac disease in children, a multicentre study. *Eur. J. Pediatr.* **148,** 496–502.

Burgin-Wolff, A., Gaze, H., Hadziselimovic, F. *et al.* (1991): Antigliadin and antiendomysium antibody determination for coeliac disease. *Arch. Dis. Child* **66,** 941–947.

Bye, A.M., Matheson, J.M. & Mackenzie, R.A. (1989): Epilepsy surgery in Sturge–Weber syndrome. *Aust. Paediatr. J.* **25,** 103–105.

Bye, A.M.E., Andermann, F., Robitaille, Y., Oliver, M., Bohane, T. & Andermann, E. (1993): Cortical vascular abnormalities in the syndrome of celiac disease, epilepsy, bilateral occipital calcifications and folate deficiency. *Ann. Neurol.* **34** (3) 399–403.

Camfield, P.R., Metrakos, K. & Andermann, F. (1978): Basilar migraine, seizures and severe epileptiform EEG abnormalities. *Neurology* **28**, 584–588.

Castro, M., Crinò, A., Papadatou, B., Purpura, M., Giannotti, A., Ferretti, F., Colistro, F., Mottola, L., Digilio, M.C., Lucidi, . & Borrelli, P. (1993): Down's syndrome and celiac disease: the prevalence of high IgA-Antigliadin antibodies and HLA-DR and DQ antigens in Trisomy 21. *J. Pediatr. Gastroenterol. Nutr.* **16,** 265–268.

Catassi, C., Ratsch, I.M., Fabiani, E., Rossini, M., Borrdicchia, F., Candela, F., Coppa, G.V. & Giorgi, P.L. (1994): Coeliac disease in the year 2000: exploring the iceberg. *Lancet* **343,** 200–203.

Challacombe, D.N. & Wheeler, E.E. (1987): Are the changes of mood in children with celiac disease due to abnormal serotonin metabolism? *Nutr. Health* **5,** 145–152

Chapman, R.W.G., Laidlow, J.M., Colin-Jones, D., Eade, . & Smith, C.L (1978): Increased prevalence of epilepsy in coeliac disease. *BMJ* **ii** 250–251.

Ciarmatori, C., Alesi, C., Michelucci, R. *et al.* (1987): Epilessia e calcificazioni occipitali: un caso con crisi visive riflesse e dislessia. *Boll. Lega It. Epil.* **58/59,** 93–97.

Ciccarone, V., Rozzi, N., Balli, F. & Galli, V. (1987): Calcificazioni endocraniche simulanti la malattia di Sturge-Weber in una bambina con malattia celiaca. *Riv. Ital. Ped.* (IJP), **13**, 186.

Collin, P. & Maki, M. (1994): Associated disorders in coeliac disease: clinical aspects. *Scand. J. Gastroenterol.* **29,** 769–765.

Collins, P., Pirtilla, T., Nurmikko, T., Somer, H., Erilla, T. & Keyrilainen, O. (1991): Celiac disease, brain atrophy and dementia. *Neurology* **41,** 372–375.

Commission on Classification and Terminology of the International League Against Epilepsy (1989): Proposal for revised classification of epilepsies and epileptic syndromes. *Epilepsia* **30**, 389–399.

Commission on Oral Health, Research and Epidemiology: review of the developmental defects of enamel index (DDE Index) (1992): *Intern. Dent. J.* **42**, 411–426.

Cooke, W.T. & Holmes, G.K.T. (1984): Coeliac disease. In: *Neurological and psychiatric complications.* eds. W.T. Cook & J.K.T. Holmes, pp. 197–213. Edinburgh: Churchill Livingstone.

Cooke, W.T. & Smith, W.T. (1966): Neurological disorders associated with adult coeliac disease. *Brain* **89,** 683–722.

Cooke, W.T. (1976): Neurologic manifestations of malabsorption. In: *Handbook of clinical neurology*, vol. **28** (Metabolic and deficiency diseases of the nervous system, part II), eds. P.J. Vinken & G.W. Bruyn, pp. 225–241. Amsterdam: North-Holland Publ. Co.

Corazza, G.R., Di Sario, A., Sacco, G., Zoli, G., Treggiari, E.A., Brusco, G. & Gasbarrini, G. (1994): Subclinical coeliac disease: an anthropometric assessment. *J. Intern. Med.* **236** 183–187.

Corbeel, L., Van der Berghe, G. *et al.* (1985): Congenital folate malabsorption. *Eur. J. Pediatr.* **143,** 284–290.

Cordonnier, M., Robin, M., Cornelte, M., Brassine, A. & Pirolte, J. (1983): Neuro-myélo encephalopathie de la maladie coeliaque. *Acta Gastroenterol. Belgica.* **46,** 47–54.

Crosato, F. & Senter, S. (1992): Cerebral occipital calcifications in coeliac disease. *Neuropediatrics* **23**, 214–217.

Davidson, A.G.F. & Bridges, M.A. (1987): Coeliac disease: critical review of aetiology and pathogenesis. *Clin. Chim. Acta* **163**, 1–40.

Daynes, G. (1956): Bread and tears–naughtiness, depression and fits due to wheat sensitivity. *Proc. Roy. Soc. Med.* **49,** 391-394.

De Marchi, M., Carbonara, A., Ansaldi, N., Santini, B., Barbera, C., Borele li I., Rossino, P. & Rendine, S. (1983): HLA-DR3 nd DR7 in coeliac disease: immunogenetic and clinical aspects. *Gut* **24,** 706–712.

De Marco, P. & Lorenzin, G (1990). Growing bilateral occipital calcifications and epilepsy. *Brain Dev.* **12**, 342–344.

De Romanis, F., Feliciani, M. & Cerbo, R. (1988): Migraine and other clinical syndromes in children affected by EEG occipital spike-waves complexes. *Funct. Neurol.* **3**, 187–203.

De Santis, A., Addolorato, G., Romito, A., Caputo, S., Gambassi, G., Taranto, C., Giordano, A., Manna, R. & Gasbarrini, G. (1996): Regression of schizophrenic symptoms and single photon emission computed tomography normalization in a coeliac patient after gluten free diet. *(unpublished).*

Della Cella, G., Beluschi, C. & Cipollina, F. (1991): Calcificazioni endocraniche - convulsioni - celiachia: presentazione di un caso. *Ped. Med. Chir. (Med. Surg. Ped.)* **13**, 427–430.

Deuhner, D.C. (1982): An epidemiologic study of migraine and headache in 10–20 year olds. *Headache* **22**, 268–275.

Di Cagno, L. & Bonassi, E. (1977): *Minerva. Pediatr.* **29,** 2207–2220.

Dickey, W. (1994): Epilepsy, cerebral calcifications, and coeliac disease. *Lancet* **344,** 1585–86.

Diebler, C. & Dulac, O. (1990): *Neurologie et neuroradiologie infantile*, 2nd Edn., p. 443. Paris: Springer-Verlag.

Dohan, F.C. (1969): Is celiac disease a clue to the pathogenesis of schizophrenia? *Ment. Hygiene* **53,** 525–529.

Dohan, F.C. (1970): Celiac disease and schizophrenia. *Lancet* **25**, 897–898.

Ferguson, A., Arranz, E. & O'Mahony, S. (1992): Definitions and diagnostic criteria of latent and potential coeliac disease. In: *Common food intolerances 1: epidemiology of coeliac disease.* Dyn. Nutr. Res., **2,** pp. 119–127. Basel: Karger.

Ferguson, A., Arranz, E. & O'Mahony, S. (1993): Clinical and pathological spectrum of coeliac disease-active, silent, latent, potential. *Gut* **34,** 150–151.

Fernandez-Alvarez, E. (1989): Factores que influyen en el desarrollo de la marcha: el desplazamiento autonomo inicial. *Int. Pediatr.* **4** (suppl.), 19–24.

Finelli, P.F., McEytel, W.J., Ambler, M. & Kostenbaum (1980): Adult celiac disease presenting as a cerebellar syndrome. *Neurology* **30**, 245–249.

Fois, A., Balestri, P., Vascotto, M., Farnetani, A., DiBartolo, R., Di Marco, V. & Vindigni, C. (1993): Progressive cerebral calcifications, epilepsy and celiac disease. *Brain Dev.* **15,** 79–82.

Fois, A., Balestri, P., Vascotto, M., Farnetani, M.A., Di Bartolo, R.M. & Di Marco, V. (1992): Epilepsy, progressive cerebral calcifications and coeliac disease. *Lancet* **340,** 1095.

Fois, A., Easy, T., Vascotto, M., Di Bartolo, R. M. & Di Marco, V. (1994): Celiac disease and epilepsy in pediatric patients. *Child's Nerv. Syst.* **10**, 15–20.

Galletti, F., Cerquiglini, A., Guidetti, V. *et al.* (1991): Occipital spike–waves epilepsies and headache. In: *Juvenile headache*, eds. V. Gallai. & V. Guidetti. *Excerpta Medica Internat. Congr. Series,* 189.

Garwicz, S. & Mortensson, W. (1976): Intracranial calcification mimicking the Sturge-Weber syndrome. A consequence of cerebral folic cid deficiency? *Pediatr. Radiol.* **5,** 5–9.

Gee, S. (1888): On the coeliac affection. *St Bartholomew's Hospital Report* **24**, 17–20.

Giroud, M., Borsotti, J.P., Michiels, R. *et al.* (1990): Epilepsie et calcifications occipitales bilaterales: 3 cast *Rev. Neurol.* **146,** 288–292.

Gobbi, G, Bouquet, F, Greco, L, Lambertini, A, Tassinari, A., Ventura, A. & Zaniboni, M.G. (1992): Coeliac disease, epilepsy and cerebral calcifications. *Lancet* **340,** 439–443.

Gobbi, G, Sorrenti, G, Santucci, M, Giovanardi-Rossi, P, Ambrosetto, P, Michelucci, R. & Tassinari, C.A. (1988): Epilepsy with bilateral occipital calcifications: a benign onset with progressive severity. *Neurology* **38**, 913–920.

Gobbi, G., Ambrosetto, P., Zaniboni, M.G., Lambertini, A., Ambrosioni, G. & Tassinari, C.A. (1992): Celiac disease, posterior cerebral calcifications and epilepsy. *Brain Dev.* **14**, 23–29.

Granditsch, G. (1990): Down's syndrome and celiac disease. *MIJ Pediatr. Gastroenterol. Nutr.* **11**, 279.

Grodzinsky, E., Hed, J., Lieden, G., Sjogren. F. & Strom, M. (1990): Presence of IgA and IgG antigliadin antibodies in healthy adults as measured by micro-ELISA. *Int. Arch. Allergy Appl. Immunol.* **92**, 119–123.

Guandalini, S., Ventura, A., Ansaldi, N., Giunta, A.M., Greco, L., Lazzari, R., Mastella, G. & Rubino, A. (1989): Diagnosis of coeliac disease: time for a change? *Arch. Dis. Child.* **64**, 1320–1325.

Haas, M.P. & Haas S.V. (1951): *Management of celiac disease.* Philadelphia: J.B. Lippincott Company.

Hallert *et al.* (1982): Brain availability of monoamine precursors in adult celiac disease. *Scand. J. Gastroenterol.* **17**, 87–89.

Hallert C. & Derefeldt, T. (1982): Psychic disturbances in adult coeliac disease. I. Clinical observations. *Scand. J. Gastroenterol.* **17**, 17–19.

Hallert, C. & Aström, J. (1982): Psychological disturbances in adult coeliac disease. II Psychological findings. *Scand. J. Gastroenterol.* **17**, 21–24.

Hallert, C. Aström, J. & Sedvall, G. (1982): Psychological disturbances in adult coeliac disease. III Reduced central monoamine metabolism and sign of depression. *Scand. J. Gatroenterol.* **17**, 21–24.

Hanley, H., Stassen, W., Whelton, M. & Callaghan, N. (1982): Epilepsy and coeliac disease. *J. Neurol. Neurosurg. Psych.* **45**, 729–730.

Harrington, M.G., Macpherson, P. & Mcintosh, W.B. (1981): The significance of the incidental finding of basal ganglia calcification on computed tomography. *J. Neurol. Neurosurg. Psych.* **44**, 1168–1170.

Hernandez, M.A., di la Colina, G., Ortigosa, J.M., Togores, J., Flores, J. & Urriza, J. (1994): Epilepsia, calcificaciones bioccipitales y anticuerpos antiendomisio. *Rev. Neurol.* **22**, 727.

Hernanz, A. & Polanco, I. (1991): Plasma precursor amino acids of central nervous system monoamines in children with coeliac disease. *Gut* **32**, (12) 1478l–1481.

Hilton, J. (1982): The significance of the incidental findings of basal ganglia calcification on CT. *J. Neurol. Neurosurg. Psych.* **45**, 942–943.

Hors, J. (1980): Microlymphocytotoxicity (Groupage pour les antigens HLA des locus A,B,C,) In: *Techniques d'étude des antigenès d'histocompatibilité,* Ed INSERM; Paris. 1–7

Howell, S.J., Foster, K.J. & Reckless, J. (1983): Protracted survival in patients with Down's syndrome. *BMJ* **287**, 1429.

I.H.S. (1988): Classification and diagnostic criteria for headache disorders, cranial neuralgias and facial pain. *Cephalalgia* **8** (suppl.); 9–93.

Kaplan, J.G., Pack, D., Horoupian, D., Desoura, T., Brin, M. & Schaumburg, H. (1988): Distal axonopathy associated with chronic gluten enteropathy: a treatable disorder. *Neurology* **38**, 642–645.

Kapuscinska, A., Zalewski, T., Chorzelski, T.P., Suley, J., Beutner, E.H., Kumar, V. & Rossi, T. (1987): Disease specificity and dynamics of changes in IgA class anti-endomysial antibodies in celiac disease. *Ped. Gastroenterol. Nutr.* **6**, 529–534.

Kaser, H. (1961): *Ann. Pediatr.* **197**, 320.

Kazis, A.D. (1985): Contribution on CT scan to the diagnosis of Fahr's syndrome. *Acta Neurol. Scand.* **71**, 206–211.

Kepes, J.J., Chon, S.M. & Price, L.W. (1975): Progressive multifocal leukoencephalopathy with 10-year survival in a patient with nontropical sprue. *Neurology* **25**, 1006–1012.

Kinney, H.C., Burger, P.C., Hurwitz, B.J., Humans, J.C. & Grant, J.P. (1982): Degeneration of the central nervous system associated with celiac disease. *J. Neurol. Sci.* **53**, 9–22.

Koller, W.C., Cochran, J.W. & Klawans, H.L. (1979): Calcification of the basal ganglia: computerized tomography and clinical correlation. *Neurology* **29**, 328–333.

Krug, S.E. & Laughlin, J.E. (1976): Manual for the IPAT expression Scale Questionnaire. Champaign, Illinois, USA.

Kuroiwa, Y. (1982): Computed tomography visualisation of extensive calcinosis in a patient with idiopathic familial basal ganglia calcification. *Arch. Neurol.* **39**, 603.

Ladinser, B., Rossipal, E. & Pittschieler, K. (1994): Endomysium antibodies in coeliac disease: an improved method. *Gut* **35**, 776–778.

Laidlow, J.M., Chapman, R.G., Colin-Jones, D.G., Eade, O. & Smith, C.I. (1977): Increased prevalence of epilepsy in coeliac disease. *Gut* **18**, A 943.

Lanzkowsky, P.H., Erlandson, M.E. & Bezan, A.I. (1969): Isolated defect of folic acid absorption associated with mental retardation and cerebral calcification. *Blood* **34**, 452–465.

Lanzowsky, P. (1970): Congenital malabsorption of folate. *Am. J. Med.* **48**, 580.

Levo, V. & Drin, P. (1977): Down's syndrome and autoimmunity. *Am. J. Med. Sc.* **273**, 95.

Longo, M., Magaudda, A., Blandino, A. & Oddone, M. (1995): Sindrome delle calcificazioni occipitali bilaterali, epilessia e malattia celiaca. In: *Malformazioni cranio-encefaliche: neuroradiologia*, eds. P. Tortori Donati, A. Taccone & M. Longo, cap. 17. Torino: Minerva Medica.

Longo, M.A., Magaudda, A., Dalla Bernardina, B. *et al.* (1992): Sindrome delle calcificazioni occipitali bilaterali, epilessia e malattia celiaca. Diagnosi differenziale con la Sturge–Weber. In: *Neuroradiologia*, ed. G. Scotti, pp. 109–112. Udine: D del Centauro

Lu, C.S., Thompson, P.D., Quinn, N.P., Parkes, J.D. & Marsden, C.D. (1986). Ramsay Hunt syndrome and coeliac disease: a new association? *Mov. Disord.* **1**, 209–219.

Magaudda, A., Colamaria, V., Narbone, M.C., *et al.* (1990): Calcificazioni occipital bilateral senza nevo flammeo. Studio di 8 casi. *Boll. Lega. Ital. Epil.* **70/71**, 251–254.

Magaudda, A., Dalla Bernardina, B., De Marco, P., Sfaello , Z., Longo, M., Colamaria, V., Daniele, O., Tortorella, G., Tata, A., Di Perri, R. & Meduri, M. (1993): Bilateral occipital calcifications, epilepsy and celiac disease: clinical and neuroimaging features of a new syndrome. *J. Neurol. Neurosurg. Psych.* **56**, 885–889.

Magaudda, A., Magazzu, G., Longo, M., Romano, C. & Di Perri, R. (1994): Frequency of occipital calcification and epilepsy in coeliac patients. *Epilepsia* **35**, S12.

Maki, M. (1990): Normal small bowel biopsy followed by coeliac disease. *Arch. Dis. Child* **65**, 1137–1141.

Maki, M., Aine, L., Lipsanen, V. & Koskimies, S. (1991): Dental enamel defects in first-degree relatives of coeliac disease patients. *Lancet* **i**, 763–764.

Marazziti, D. & Cassano, G.B. (1992): Sistema serotoninergico e depressione. *Aggiorn. Medico,* **16**, 509–515.

Marazziti, D. *et al.* (1988): High affinity ^{3}H-Imipramine binding: a possible state-dependent marker for major depression. *Psych. Res.* **23**, 229.

Mariani, P., Mazzilli, M.C., Margutti, G., Lionetti, Triglione, P., Petronzelli, F., Ferrante, E. & Bonamico, M. (1994): Coeliac disease, enamel defects and HLA typing. *Acta Paediatr.* **83**, 1272–1275.

Marsden, C.D., Harding, A.E., Obeso, J.A. & Lu, C.S. (1990): Progressive myoclonic ataxia (the Ramsay Hunt syndrome). *Arch. Neurol.* **47**, 1121–1125.

Martelletti, P., Romiti, A. & Gallo, M.F. (1984): HLA B14 antigen in cluster headache. *Headache* **24**, 152–156.

Martini, C., Bollani, T., Dellanoce, F., *et al.* (1985): Caso di Sturge–Weber con calcificazioni endocraniche bilaterali e senza angioma cutaneo. *Riv. It. Ped.* **11**, 729.

Masson, C. Gallet, J.P., Cheron, F., *et al.* (1988): Epilepsie avec calcifications corticales bilaterales *Rev. Neurol.* **144**, 499–502.

Mazzilli, M.C., Ferrante, P., Mariani, P., *et al.* (1991): A study of Italian pediatric celiac disease patients confirms that the primary HLA association is due to the DQ(α1*0501, β1*0201) heterodimer. *Hum. Immunol.* **33**, 133–139.

Mc Culloch, A.J., Ince, P.C. & Kendall-Taylor, P. (1982): Autoimmune chronic active hepatitis in Down's syndrome. *J. Med. Genet.* **19**, 232.

Meltzer, H.Y. & Lowy, M.T. (1987): The serotonin hypothesis of depression 513–526, ediz. H.V. Meltzer.

Milunsky, A. & Neurath, P.W. (1968): Diabetes mellitus in Down's syndrome. *Arch. Environ. Health* **17**, 372.

Minev, M., Martinova, F. & Belopitova, L. (1987): On the association of the HLA system with epilepsy in children. *Epilepsia* **28**, 74–76.

Molteni, N., Bardella, M.T., Baldassarri, A.R. & Bianchi, P.A. (1988): Celiac disease association with epilepsy and intracranial calcifications: report of two patients. *Am. J. Gastroenterol.* **83**, 992–994.

Monton, F. Perez Senas, M.T., Perez, J., Zurita, A. & Manas, S. (1992): Epilepsia, calcificaciones occipitales y enfermedad celiaca. *Neurologia* **7**, 92.

Morgante, L., Vita, G. & Meduri, M. (1986): Fahr's syndrome: local inflammatory factors in the pathogenesis of calcification. *J. Neurol.* **233,** 19–22.

Morris, J.S., Ajdukiewic, A.B. & Read, A.E. (1970): Neurological disorders and adult coeliac disease. *Gut* **11,** 549–554

Murphy, M. (1979): Clinical correlations of CT-scan detected calcifications of the basal ganglia. *Ann. Neurol.* **6,** 507–511.

Nevin, N.C. & Pearce, W.G. (1968): Diagnostic and genetic aspects of tuberous sclerosis. *Med. Genet.* **5,** 273–280.

Newton, R. & Aicardi, J. (1983): Clinical findings in children with occipital spike-wave complexes suppressed by eye opening. *Neurology* **33,** 1526.

Nikiforuk, G. & Fraser, D. (1981): The etiology of enamel hypoplasia: a unifying concept. *J. Pediatr.* **98,** 888–893.

Norris, J.W. & Pratt, R.F. (1971): A controlled study of folic acid in epilepsy. *Neurology* **21,** 659–664.

Panayiotopoulos, C.P. (1980): Basilar migraine? seizures and severe epileptic EEG abnormalities. *Neurology* **30,** 1122–25.

Panayiotopoulos, C.P. (1989): Benign nocturnal childhood occipital epilepsy: a new syndrome with nocturnal seizures, tonic deviation of the eyes, and vomiting. *J. Child Neurol.* **4,** 43–48.

Pavone, L., Mazzone, D., Incorpora, G., Drago, F. & Bottaro, G. Cognitive disturbances in children with coeliac disease (Chapter 39; this book).

Perisic, V.N., Lopicic, Z. & Kokai, G. (1990): Celiac disease and schizophrenia: Family occurrence. *J. Ped. Gastroenterol. Nutr.* **11,** 279.

Peroutka, S.J. (1990): Receptor families for 5-hydroxytryptamine. *J. Cardiovasc. Pharmacol.* **16,** (suppl.3), 8

Piattella, L., Zamponi, N., Carinali, C., Porfiri, L. & Tavoni, M.A. (1993): Endocranial calcifications, infantile celiac disease, and epilepsy. *Child's Nerv. System* **19,** 172–175.

Pinilla Moraza, J., Gil Pujades, A., Labarga Echeverria, P. & Astiazaran Echeverria, F. (1995): Epilepsia, calcificaciones cerebrales y enfermedad celiaca. Un nuevo caso. *Neurologia* **10,** 214–215.

Pittschieler, K., Morini, G. & Crepaz, R. (1993): Williams syndrome and coeliac disease. *Acta Paediatr.* **82,** IV.

Pittschieler, K., Reissigl, H. & Mengarda, G. (1988): Celiac disease in two different population groups in South Tyrol. *J. Pediatr. Gastroenterol. Nutr.* **7,** 400–02.

Plazzi, G., Tinuper, P., Provini, F., *et al.* (1984): Epilepsy, occipital calcifications and coeliac disease: anatomopathologic findings and response to a gluten-free diet. *Epilepsia* **35,** supp. 7, 81.

Prati, C., Santopadre, A. & Baroni, C. (1987): Ritardata eruzione, ipoplasia dello smalto e carie in corso di malattia celiaca dell'infanzia. *Minerva Stomatol.* **36,** 749–752.

Prugh, D.G. & MacMahon, B. (1951): A preliminary report on the role of emotional factors in idiopathic celiac disease. *Psychosom. Med.* **13,** 220–241,

Puvanendran, K., Low, C.H. & Boey, H.K. (1982): Basal ganglia calcification on computed tomographic scan *Acta Neurol. Scand.* **66,** 309–315.

Quintana, J. (1992): Platelet serotonin and plasma tryptophan decreases in endogenous depression. Clinical, therapheutic and biological correlations. *J. Affect. Dis.* **24,** 55–62.

Revised criteria for diagnosis of coeliac disease: report of Working Group of the European Society of Paediatric Gastroenterology and Nutrition. (1990) *Arch. Dis. Child* : **65,** 909–911.

Ruch, W., Shurmann, K., Gordon, P., Burgin-Wolf, A. & Girard, J. (1985): Coexistence of coeliac disease, Graves disease and diabetes mellitus type 1 in a patient with Down's syndrome. *Eur. J. Pediatr.* **144,** 89.

Sacco, M., Serio, G., Ghezzi, T., Vaglio, P. & Fanelli, M. (1992): Ansia ed ospedalizzazione. Studio epidemiologico su 496 pazienti ricoverati nel policlinico di Bari. Psichiatria e medicina, **3,** 7.

Salanova, V., Andermann, F., Olivier, A., *et al.* 1992): Occipital lobe epilepsy: electroclinical manifestations electrocorticography, cortical stimulation and outcome in 42 patients treated between 1930–91. *Brain* **115,** 1655–1680.

Sammaritano, M., Andermann, F., Melanson, D., *et al.* 1988): The syndrome of intractable epilepsy bilateral occipital calcifications and folic acid deficiency. *Neurology* **38,** 239.

Sammaritano, M., Andermann, F., Melanson, D., Guberman, Tinuper, P. & Gastaut, H. (1985): The syndrome of epilepsy and bilateral occipital cortical calcifications. *Epilepsia* **26,** 532.

Sampson, J.R., Scahill, S.J., Stephenson, J.B.P., *et al.* (1989): Genetic aspects of tuberous sclerosis in the West of Scotland. *Med. Genet.* **26,** 28–31.

Sare, Z., Ruvalcaba, R.H.A. & Kelly, V.C. (1978): Prevalence of thyroid disorder in Down's syndrome. *Clin. Genet.* **14**, 54.

Scott, H., Fauso, O., Ek, J., Valnes, K., Blystad, L. & Brandtzaeg, P. (1990): Measurements of serum IgA and IgG activities of dietary antigens. A prospective study of the diagnostic usefulness in adult coeliac disease. *Scand. J. Gastroenterol.* **25**, 287–292.

Shmerling, D.H., Sacher, M., Widmer, B. & Ben Zur, E.D. (1980): Incidence of dental caries in coeliac children. *Arch. Dis. Child* **55**, 80–81.

Simmat, G., Lelong, B. & Morin, M. (1984): Aspects cliniques et tomodensitometriques peculiers de la maladie de Sturge–Weber. Calcifications occipitales bilaterales sans angiome facial. *J. Radiol.* **65**, (4) 279–283.

Sleiger, M.H. (1961): Clinical and metabolic studies on non-tropical sprue. *N. Engl. J. Med.* **265**, 49–56.

Sneddon, J.M. (1973): Blood platelets as a model for monoamine-containing neurons. In*: Progress in neurobiol*, eds. G.A. Kerkurt & J.W. Phillis, pp 151–198. Oxford: Pergamon Press.

Spielberg, C.D., Gorsuch, R.L. & Lushene R.E. (1970): *Manual for the State-Trait Anxiety Inventory*. Ed. Palo Alto, California: Consulting Psychologist Press.

Stahl, S. (1977): The human platelet. A diagnostic and research tool for the study of biogenic amines in psychiatric and neurologic disorders. *Arch. Gen. Psychiatr.* **34**, 509–516.

Storm, W. (1990): Prevalence and diagnostic significance of gliadin antibodies in children with Down syndrome. *Eur. J. Pediatr.* **149**, 833–834.

Taly, A.B., Nagaraja, D., Dos, S., *et al.* (1987): Sturge–Weber Dimitry disease without facial nevus. *Neurology* **37**, 1063–1064.

Tateno, A., Matsui, A., Sakuragawa, N., *et al.* (1985): Two siblings with multiple intra-cranial haemangiomatosis with calcifications, *J. Neurol.* **232**, 112–114.

Terzano, M.G., Manzoni, G.C., Maione, R., *et al.* (1990): Epilessia benigna con parossismi occipitali ed emicrania: problema delle crisi intercalate. Atti IX Congresso It. S.I.N.P.I. San Marino, p.827.

Tiacci, C., D'Alessandro, P., Cantisani, T.A., Piccirilli, M., Signorini, E., Pelli, M.A., Cavalletti, M.L., Castellucci, G., Palmeri, S., Battisti, C. & Federico, A. (1993): Epilepsy with bilateral occipital calcifications: Sturge–Weber variant or a different encephalopathy? *Epilepsia* **34**, 528–539.

Tighe, M.R., Hall, M.A., Barbado, M., Cardi, E., Welsh, K.I. & Ciclitira, P.J. (1992): HLA class II alleles associated with celiac disease susceptibility in a Southern European population. *Tiss. Antigens* **40**, 90–97.

Tison, F., Arne, P. & Henry, P. (1989): Myoclonus and adult coeliac disease. *Neurology* **236**, 307–308.

Tortorella, G., Magaudda A., *et al.* (1993): Familial unilateral and bilateral occipital calcifications and epilepsy. *Neuropediatrics* **24**, 341–342.

Tsuji, K., Aizawa, M. & Sasazuki, T. (1992): In: *HLA 1991*, 11th International histocompatibility workshop and conference held in Yokohama, Japan, 6–13 Nov., 1991. Oxford University Press.

Vella, G. & De Pascale, A. Il bambino e i suoi sistemi. Rome: Kappa.

Veneselli, E., Baglietto, M.G., Oddone, M., *et al.* (1991): Migraine and epilepsy with bilateral occipital calcifications. In: *Juvenile headache*, eds. V. Gallai & V. Guidetti. *Excerpta Medica Internat. Congr. Series,* 197.

Ventura, A., Bouquet, F., Sartorelli, C., Barbi, E., Torre, G. & Tommasini, G. (1991): Case report: Coeliac disease, folic acid deficiency and epilepsy with cerebral calcifications. *Acta paediatr. Scand.* **80**, 559–562.

Visacorpi, J.K. (1992): Silent coeliac disease: the risk groups to be screened for common food tollerance. In: *Epidemiology of coeliac disease,* eds. S. Auricchio & J.K. Visacorpi, pp. 84–92. Dyn. Nutr. Res. Basel: Kargel.

Visakorpi, J.K. & Maki, M. (1994): Changing clinical features of coeliac disease. *Acta Pediatr. Suppl.* **83**, 10–13.

Volta, U., Lenzi, M., Cassani, F., Lazzari, R., Bianchi, F.B. & Pisi, E. (1983): Gliadin antibodies in coeliac disease. *Lancet* **i**, 1285.

Walker-Smith, J.A. (1991): Celiac disease. In: *Pediatric gastrointestinal disease,* eds. A.W. Walker, P.R. Durie, J.R. Hamilton, J.A. Walker-Smith & J.B. Watkins pp. 700–718. Philadelphia: B.C. Decker Inc.

Walker-Smith, J.A,, Guandalini, S., Schmitz, J., Shmerling, D.H. & Visakorpi, J.K. (1990): Revised criteria for diagnosis of coeliac disease. Report of working Group of European Society of Paediatric Gastroenterology and Nutrition. *Arch. Dis. Child* **65**, 909–911.

Ward, M.E., Murphy, J.T. & Greenberg, G.R. (1985): Coeliac disease and spinocerebellar degeneration with normal vitamin E status. *Neurology* **35**, 1199–1201.

Wiederholt, W.C., Gomez, M.R. & Kurland, L.T. (1985): Incidence and prevalence of tuberous sclerosis in Rochester, Minnesota: 1950 through 1960. *Neurology* **35**, 600–603.

Williamson, P.D., Thadani, V.M. & Darcey, T.M. *et al.* (1992): Occipital lobe epilepsy: clinical characteristics, seizure spread patterns and results of surgery. *Ann. Neurol.* **31,** 3–13.

Zaniboni, M.G., Ambrosetto, P., Lambertini, A., Parmeggiani, Santucci, M., Gobbi, G. & Tassinari, C.A. (1991): Epilessia, calcificazioni endocraniche, malattia celiaca. *Minerva. Pediatr.* **43**, 215–218.

Zaniboni, M.G., Lambertini, A. & Brusa, S. (1993): La malattia celiaca: ieri, oggi, domani. *Medico e bambino* **1,** 26–31.

Subject Index

Author Index